GERIATRIC NEUROPSYCHOLOGY

GERIATRIC NEUROPSYCHOLOGY

Assessment and Intervention

edited by
DEBORAH K. ATTIX
KATHLEEN A. WELSH-BOHMER

THE GUILFORD PRESS
New York   London

© 2006 The Guilford Press
A Division of Guilford Publications, Inc.
72 Spring Street, New York, NY 10012
www.guilford.com

Printed in the United States of America

This book is printed on acid-free paper.

Last digit is print number: 9   8   7   6   5   4   3   2   1

Library of Congress Cataloging-in-Publication Data

Geriatric neuropsychology : assessment and intervention / edited by
    Deborah K. Attix, Kathleen A. Welsh-Bohmer.
      p. cm.
    Includes bibliographical references and index.
    ISBN 1-59385-226-6 (cloth)
    1. Geriatric neuropsychiatry. 2. Cognition disorders in old age
—Diagnosis. 3. Neuropsychological tests.   I. Attix, Deborah K.
II. Welsh-Bohmer, Kathleen A.
    [DNLM: 1. Mental Disorders—diagnosis—Aged. 2. Mental Disorders
—therapy—Aged. 3. Behavioral Symptoms—Aged. 4. Neuropsychological Tests—Aged.   WT 150 G36855 2005]
    RC451.4.A5G4665   2006
    618.97′68—dc22

                                    2005017534

For Eva, Ted, Noah, and Maximus
—D. K. A.

For Patrick, Elise, and Nathan
—K. A. W.-B.

About the Editors

Deborah K. Attix, PhD, completed her postdoctoral fellowship in Clinical Neuropsychology at the Cleveland Clinic Foundation. She joined the Department of Psychiatry and Behavioral Sciences (Division of Medical Psychology) and Department of Medicine (Division of Neurology) at Duke in 1995 and is now an Assistant Clinical Professor there. Dr. Attix worked with the Joseph and Kathleen Bryan Alzheimer's Disease Research Center and subsequently organized and became the Medical Director of the Clinical Neuropsychology Service at Duke University Medical Center. Her clinical work focuses on geriatric neuropsychological assessment and intervention. Dr. Attix is best known for her intervention work involving cognitive training and compensation and for psychotherapeutic techniques targeting memory, function, and mood in dementia.

Kathleen A. Welsh-Bohmer, PhD, is a Professor within the Department of Psychiatry and Behavioral Sciences (Division of Medical Psychology) at Duke University Medical Center and holds a joint appointment in the Department of Medicine (Division of Neurology). Dr. Welsh-Bohmer was recruited by Duke University Medical Center in 1987 to join the newly formed Joseph and Kathleen Bryan Alzheimer's Disease Research Center, and she currently is the Director of that center. Dr. Welsh-Bohmer is best known for her work in the clinical detection of early-stage Alzheimer's disease (AD) and related dementias and the relationship of these diseases to genetic and environmental factors. She has been a leader in many multicenter collaborative studies of AD and currently leads the nationally known Cache County Memory Study, a population-based epidemiological investigation of mild cognitive impairment and AD. Dr. Welsh-Bohmer's clinical work focuses on neuropsychological assessment in neurodegenerative disorders, including AD and related dementias.

Contributors

Amarilis Acevedo, PhD, Department of Psychiatry and Behavioral Sciences, Miller School of Medicine, University of Miami, Miami Beach, Florida

Deborah K. Attix, PhD, Department of Psychiatry and Behavioral Sciences, (Medical Psychology) and Medicine (Neurology), Duke University Medical Center, Durham, North Carolina

Ann Louise Barrick, PhD, Psychology Department, John Umstead Hospital, Butner, North Carolina, and Department of Psychology, University of North Carolina–Chapel Hill, Chapel Hill, North Carolina

Mark W. Bondi, PhD, Psychology Service, VA San Diego Health Care System, and Department of Psychiatry, University of California–San Diego, San Diego, California

Michelle S. Bourgeois, PhD, Regional Rehabilitation Center, College of Communication, Florida State University, Tallahassee, Florida

Robyn M. Busch, PhD, Department of Psychiatry and Psychology, Cleveland Clinic Foundation, Cleveland, Ohio

Cameron J. Camp, PhD, Myers Research Institute, Beachwood, Ohio

M. Allison Cato, PhD, VA RR&D Brain Rehabilitation Research Center, Malcolm Randall Veterans Affairs Medical Center, and Department of Clinical and Health Psychology, University of Florida, Gainesville, Florida

Gordon J. Chelune, PhD, The Mellen Center, Cleveland Clinic Foundation, Cleveland, Ohio

Cory K. Chen, MA, Department of Psychology, University of North Carolina–Chapel Hill, Chapel Hill, North Carolina

Linda Clare, PhD, School of Psychology, University of Wales, Bangor, Wales

Bruce A. Crosson, PhD, Department of Clinical and Health Psychology, University of Florida, Gainesville, Florida

Joanne Green, PhD, Wesley Woods Health Center, Department of Neurology, Emory University, Atlanta, Georgia

Kathleen Hayden, PhD, Joseph and Kathleen Bryan Alzheimer's Disease Research

Center, Division of Neurology, Department of Medicine, Duke University Medical Center, Durham, North Carolina

Katina R. Hebert, MS, Department of Psychology, University of Alabama, Tuscaloosa, Alabama

Wes S. Houston, PhD, Department of Neurology, University of Iowa, Iowa City, Iowa

Nancy Johnson, PhD, Cognitive Neurology and Alzheimer's Disease Center, Feinberg School of Medicine, Northwestern University, Chicago, Illinois

David Loewenstein, PhD, Department of Psychiatry and Behavioral Sciences, Miller School of Medicine, University of Miami, Miami Beach, Florida

Rebecca G. Logsdon, PhD, Northwest Aging Research Group, School of Nursing, University of Washington, Seattle, Washington

Jennifer J. Manly, PhD, G. H. Sergievsky Center and Taub Institute for Research on Alzheimer's Disease and the Aging Brain, Department of Neurology, Columbia University Medical Center, New York, New York

Daniel Marson, PhD, Department of Neurology and Alzheimer's Disease Research Center, University of Alabama–Birmingham, Birmingham, Alabama

Susan M. McCurry, PhD, Psychosocial and Community Health, University of Washington, Seattle, Washington

Guy G. Potter, PhD, Department of Psychiatry and Behavioral Sciences, Duke University Medical Center, Durham, North Carolina

Beth K. Rush, PhD, Department of Psychiatry and Psychology, Mayo Clinic and Foundation, Jacksonville, Florida

Mary Sano, PhD, Department of Psychiatry, Mount Sinai School of Medicine, New York, New York, and Bronx VA Medical Center, Bronx, New York

Glenn Smith, PhD, Department of Psychiatry and Psychology, Mayo Clinic and Foundation, Rochester, Minnesota

Yana Suchy, PhD, Department of Psychology, University of Utah, Salt Lake City, Utah

Linda Teri, PhD, Psychosocial and Community Health, University of Washington, Seattle, Washington

Cynthia K. Thompson, PhD, Communication Sciences and Disorders and Neurology, Northwestern University, Chicago, Illinois

Lauren H. Warren, MA, Department of Psychology, University of North Carolina–Chapel Hill

Kathleen A. Welsh-Bohmer, PhD, Department of Psychiatry, Joseph and Kathleen Bryan Alzheimer's Disease Research Center, Division of Neurology, Duke University Medical Center, Durham, North Carolina

Preface

In the pages that follow, readers will find the essentials of geriatric neuropsychological assessment and intervention. The first half of the volume focuses on assessment; presentation of an assessment model is followed by chapters outlining common age-related conditions and the special considerations critical to the neuropsychological evaluation process. The second half of the volume focuses on intervention; presentation of an intervention model is followed by approaches to cognitive training and compensation as well as psychotherapeutic techniques.

Our intent in this book is to provide a uniquely different text for the field of geriatric neuropsychology, one that integrates not only assessment methods and issues of differential diagnosis but also emphasizes intervention and management approaches available to neuropsychologists. Our contributors detail the current state of knowledge regarding the neuropsychological, medical, pathological, and genetic aspects of the most common geriatric conditions. They also offer the latest intervention approaches involving the use of nonpharmacological treatments with geriatric patients who have cognitive dysfunction that is not expected to resolve. These interventions utilize modified techniques and therapeutic approaches designed to maximize use of residual capacities, enhance compensatory functioning, and increase adjustment. These leaders in the field of geriatric dementia present models for assessment and intervention, and also provide a thorough review of geriatric central nervous system disorders, cognitive training, psychotherapy, and considerations specific to this population.

In providing a synthesized approach to assessment and intervention, our intention is to provide neuropsychologists with a practical reference source with which they are able to (1) recognize common dementias in their diverse clinical manifestations, (2) identify the diagnostic issues central to each, and (3) become familiar with how assessment extends beyond diagnostics to facilitate treatment planning. Likewise, we detail the use of assessment data and neurobehavioral principles to maximize the likelihood of treatment gains, and our contributors provide in-depth coverage of specific treatment approaches. This text draws together practice techniques, theory, and evidence-based outcome data to provide a conceptual framework for professionals involved in geriatric neuropsychological assessment and intervention. We thank our contributors, who have helped us to present and integrate these important aspects of practice.

DEBORAH K. ATTIX
KATHLEEN A. WELSH-BOHMER

Acknowledgments

I would like to thank all the authors and editors involved with the creation of this book; your careful work allowed the volume to exceed its original vision and I am grateful. I also want to acknowledge my family, friends, mentors, colleagues, and patients. I especially want to thank Ted, who captures me with all of who he is, and my mother, who gave me the world. I also want to acknowledge the powerful examples I have had in my Uncle Laci and late Feri Bacsi, who always cheered me on, and the late Mel Stroupe, whose lessons became a part of the fabric of who I am. Thanks also to Sally, who walks with me and reads my whispers, and to Gordon Chelune, who taught me neuropsychology with inspiration, cheer, and a horrible red pen. Thanks to "The Guys" and all the patients who have given me the privilege of joining them on their journeys. Thanks also to Warren Strittmatter, Ron Beauvais, and Joel Morgenlander—my cavalry—who gave me the balance that brings me such joy. And most of all, thanks to my little one Noah, who will always be my moon, stars, and life—your laugh sets me free—and to my new Maximus, my cherished, thoughtful moose. We, too, will dance in the sunlight.

—D. K. A.

It is a privilege to be associated with this volume of collected works from so many notable and respected scholars in the field. I wish to thank Deborah Attix for the tremendous opportunity she has given me to serve as a coeditor on this work. I would like to acknowledge my loving family, Patrick, Elise, and Nathan, who show me daily the joy of life reflected through their creative, youthful, and energetic lenses. I also wish to thank my parents for their example in living and aging with love, grace, and wisdom. A special note goes to my siblings, Karen, Greg, and Eric, and to the entire extended Welsh-Bohmer family, who together give my life so much meaning and dimension. Finally, I thank my many students, colleagues, patients, and their families, with whom I have had the pleasure to work over the years. You constantly remind me of the importance of human discovery and why we do what we do in clinical neuropsychology.

—K. A. W.-B.

Contents

PART I

GERIATRIC NEUROPSYCHOLOGICAL ASSESSMENT

The first part of the book is divided into two sections designed to introduce the reader to geriatric neuropsychological assessment and special considerations in clinical interpretation. A conceptual model of the standard neuropsychological evaluation in geriatrics initiates Section A. The chapters that follow the assessment model review common geriatric conditions ranging from normal aging to dementia. Each of the chapters in this section outlines our current understanding of various clinical syndromes or diseases by describing their most typical neuropsychological presentation and underscoring the related neuropathology, histopathology, and genetic etiology (when known). Section B delineates topics of particular importance in the assessment of the geriatric population, including normative and multicultural considerations, functional capacity and competency, and the use of feedback.

Section A

Assessment of Common Geriatric Conditions

Section A presents an assessment model and reviews geriatric conditions ranging from normal aging to dementia.

Chapter 1 introduces the broad issues of neuropsychological assessment in elderly groups: goals of the evaluation, commonly employed instruments, factors influencing test performance, interpretation of findings, and the importance of supportive medical data. Rather than present the assessment model as any definitive method of evaluation, we offer it as an evolving dynamic model that is meant to be introductory and orienting for the reader. This chapter sets the stage for the chapters that follow, in which more detailed discussion is given to specific diagnostic conditions, their etiology, and clinical management.

Chapter 2 takes us into the realm of neurocognitive impairment that exceeds normal aging with a consideration of mild cognitive disorders, commonly referred to as mild cognitive impairment (MCI), and conditions that presage Alzheimer's disease and other dementias. This chapter reviews the historical evolution of the definition of MCI and key classification issues that affect our clinical and research conceptualizations of this condition.

Chapter 3 details the typical presentation of the three most commonly encountered neurodegenerative conditions of aging that are invariably progressive: Alzheimer's disease, frontotemporal dementia, Parkinson's disease dementia, and diffuse Lewy body dementia. A thorough consideration of these fundamental clinical conditions provides a firm basis for recognizing the less commonly encountered progressive conditions.

Chapter 4 presents an analysis of geriatric conditions that are more variable in their longitudinal course, with either slow progression or stability. The emphasis again is on the most common illnesses affecting elders in this category: Parkinson's disease, vascular cognitive impairment and dementia, alcoholic dementia, and traumatic brain injury.

In Chapter 5 we consider conditions that have been regarded as either partially or totally reversible with adequate, timely treatment. Specifically reviewed are the conditions associated with normal-pressure hydrocephalus, hypothyroidism, vitamin B_{12} deficiency, thiamine deficiency, sleep breathing disorders, and late-life depression. This latter topic introduces the notion of *pseudodementia* and *the dementia of depression*, which is of

3

particular importance to elderly patient groups. We have stated elsewhere that evaluation of mood is indispensable to any comprehensive evaluation, and that any evaluation that does not carefully consider this dimension runs a high risk of inaccuracy. It is well understood that depression alone can result in diminished cognition. In addition, it must also be considered as a comorbid condition to other central nervous system disorders, potentially—and in all probability—altering the overall constellation of findings. It is well known that the prevalence of depression decreases across the lifespan among normal community dwellers, although some believe that the prevalence of mild subclinical emotional distress is notable among elders. It is extraordinarily important not to underestimate the prevalence of dysthymia and major depression in samples of memory-disordered elders, in whom prevalences rise sharply.

In offering a volume focused on both assessment and intervention, we intend to emphasize the fact that specific factors related to cognitive compromise are *treatable*. Depression and other sources of emotional unrest are perhaps the most common appropriate target of intervention. Improvement leading to adaptive, successful coping and adjustment in the context of neurological change can have a perceptible, meaningful impact on quality of life. In addition to the importance of considering mood for accurate diagnosis, it is this potential for improvement in quality of life through identification and treatment of a treatable factor that we would like to underscore.

Of course, an entire volume could be devoted to this topic, as well as almost any other condition or disease reviewed in Section A. The reader is encouraged to consider this when reviewing the common geriatric conditions, syndromes, and diseases that are presented. We also appreciate the fact that we offer views based upon our current state of knowledge—which is but a snapshot in a continuously evolving field of research and practice. We look forward to the enhanced discernment in each area that will come with time.

An Integrated Model for Geriatric Neuropsychological Assessment

GUY G. POTTER
DEBORAH K. ATTIX

Declining memory and cognitive losses are common with age (Blanchard-Fields & Hess, 1996; Craik & Salthouse, 1992). Because similar changes often present as the early signs of progressive cognitive disorders such as Alzheimer's disease (AD), distinguishing the relatively benign changes of normal aging from the more adverse changes associated with progressive cognitive disorders is a critical issue in the neuropsychological assessment of older adults. Fortunately, the field of neuropsychology has made great strides in distinguishing "normal" and "abnormal" processes of cognitive aging and in characterizing the numerous disease processes that can impair the cognitive functioning of older adults. For instance, the prevailing diagnostic consensus for mild cognitive impairment (MCI) includes characterization based on neuropsychological performance (Winblad et al., 2004), whereas the diagnosis of AD has long recognized the role of neuropsychological measures in objectively assessing cognitive function (McKhann et al., 1984). The neuropsychologist's ability to detect and diagnose age-related cognitive disorders depends not only on a knowledge of psychometrics and brain–behavior relationships that is the bedrock of neuropsychological training, but also on an ability to integrate data from other disciplines concerning the health and function of older adults, including epidemiology, cognitive neuroscience, and geriatric medicine.

The purpose of this chapter is to present a model of geriatric neuropsychological assessment that encompasses the range of information that may be involved in the detection and diagnosis of age-related cognitive disorders. We present a framework for interpreting neuropsychological findings in relation to our current knowledge of the presentation and course of these disorders. We begin by considering the prevailing uses of neuropsychological assessment for older adults, followed by consideration of variables relevant to the geriatric evaluation. The remainder of the chapter focuses on neuropsychological interpretation, including consideration of factors related to an older individual's presentation and performance, the role of a core neuropsychological knowledge base, and the use of attendant data.

APPLICATIONS OF GERIATRIC NEUROPSYCHOLOGICAL ASSESSMENT

There are three major applications of neuropsychological testing in the clinical assessment of older adults: diagnostics, estimation of functional status, and intervention planning.

Neuropsychological Assessment and Clinical Diagnosis

The most common application of geriatric neuropsychological assessment continues to be differential diagnosis of cognitive disorders of aging. Consequently, this focus tends to play the major role in the planning of most neuropsychological evaluations. Frequently, neuropsychological assessment is requested in cases of suspected early dementia, where the patient's or family's report of cognitive loss may be ambiguous or undetected in a clinician's interview. Because a neuropsychological evaluation provides characterization of deficits based on objective data, it potentially avoids many sources of error inherent in subjective observational methods (Davison, 1974; Lezak, Howieson, & Loring, 2004). The neuropsychological evaluation can characterize the presence and severity of cognitive compromise independent of structural imaging and other correlates of neuropathology, and also provide domain-based profiles of impairment that can assist in the inclusion or exclusion of diagnoses that appear viable based on other aspects of the clinical presentation. Because of its clinical utility, the neuropsychological examination is now recognized as playing a central role in the medical evaluation of Alzheimer's disease and other cognitive disorders of aging (Cummings et al., 1996).

Neuropsychology and Estimation of Functional Status and Competency

Although diagnosis remains the primary referral issue for most geriatric neuropsychological evaluations, neuropsychologists are frequently called upon to address how cognitive impairments might affect a patient's ability to function in his or her daily life. Because most neuropsychological tests were developed to detect and differentiate brain dysfunctions, rather than to provide ecological validity, prediction of functional outcomes cannot typically be answered on the basis of test data alone. Until fairly recently there have been few data on the predictive relationship between functional outcomes and neuropsychological test performance, but an emerging body of research suggests that neuropsychological test performance does predict function in activities of daily living, such as medication management and bill paying (Cahn-Weiner, Boyle, & Malloy, 2002; Diehl, Willis, & Schaie, 1995). Related outcomes such as health care utilization and need for institutional care appear to be related to neuropsychological performance as well (Rockwood, Stolee, & McDowell, 1996; Willis & Marsiske, 1991). Questions about fitness to operate a motor vehicle are frequently raised in geriatric referrals, and it does appear that driving ability is adversely affected by neuropsychological deficits (Lesikar, Gallo, Rebok, & Keyl, 2002) and dementia severity (Dubinsky, Stein, & Lyons, 2000).

Despite these informative findings, unresolved questions remain about (1) the degree of shared variance between neuropsychological tests and functional outcomes, (2) the neurocognitive domains that are most predictive of functional ability, and (3) how these associations generalize across different diagnostic populations (Farias, Harrell, Neumann, & Houtz, 2003; McCue, Rogers, & Goldstein, 1990; Richardson, Nadler, & Malloy, 1995). McCue and colleagues (1990) have argued that neuropsychological tests have greater utility in predicting performance for complex functional tasks than for simple activities. Other researchers have found support for this assertion (Farias et al., 2003), but also note that the strength of association for neuropsychological measures in general may be greater for performance-based functional assessment than for informant report of function. These researchers also note that a considerable amount of variance in functional performance is not explained by neuropsychological performance. On the whole, current research suggests that neuropsychological assessment and functional assessment measure related but non-overlapping domains, indicating that neuropsychological data are complementary to assessments of functional performance, rather than substitutes for them.

In some instances cognitive impairment becomes a legal as well as a clinical issue, particularly when it applies to an individual's competency to make medical and financial decisions. In such cases a neuropsychologist may be called upon to provide information relevant to a legal determination of competency. Competency, in this context, is a legal term whose meaning is not under the purview of the clinician; however, the determination of whether or not a person is deemed to be legally competent can be influenced by a neuropsychologist's characterization of how an individual's observed neurocognitive performance may affect specific decision-making capacities. Although there is some support for the use of neuropsychological tests in helping to characterize an individual's decision-making capacity, there is no consensus about which specific cognitive constructs or test scores best predict competency (e.g., Marson, Cody, Ingram, & Harrell, 1995; Stanley, Stanley, Guido, & Garvin, 1988; Tymchuk, Ouslander, Rahbar, & Fitten, 1988). One consistent finding across studies is that although dementia patients may be like non-cognitively impaired older adults in their ability to make reasonable choices, they differ from their cohorts in their ability to provide a rationale for their decision and to appreciate the consequence of one decision versus another (Marson, Ingram, Cody, & Harrell, 1995). Although a diagnosis such as dementia can be informative in characterizing decision-making capacity, characterization based on diagnosis alone provides limited information about specific questions of capacity; an individual's functioning may be intact in an area such as financial decision making but impaired in a different area such as medical decision making (Scogin & Perry, 1986). Neuropsychological testing holds promise as an objective counterpart to clinical impressions of decision-making capacity. Nevertheless, it should be viewed as one facet of information in a comprehensive assessment. For further discussion of this issue, see Marson and Hebert (Chapter 7, this volume).

Neuropsychological Assessment and Intervention Planning

In addition to functions of diagnosis and prognosis, clinical neuropsychologists have become increasingly involved in intervention and treatment planning. Neuropsychological evaluations often serve as a baseline reference of cognitive performance from which changes in an individual's performance may be tracked over time. It is desirable to track cognitive changes in order to assess the efficacy of an intervention, whether it is pharmacotherapy or psychotherapy. To track therapeutic progress, serial assessment of neuropsychological function may be advised. Psychotherapeutic interventions may include traditional approaches to treatment, such as behavioral therapy (Teri, Logsdon,

Uomoto, & McCurry, 1997), or more focused cognitive rehabilitation methods (Prigatano, 1997). Most individuals with MCI can benefit from such interventions, and information from their neuropsychological evaluations may suggest strategies to capitalize on cognitive strengths and to accommodate weaknesses. Information from assessment may also indicate whether mnemonic aids such as calendars, diaries, or alarms can be utilized effectively. An in-depth discussion of how neuropsychological data are utilized for intervention planning appears in Attix (Chapter 10, this volume).

EXAMINATION FACTORS

Whether the purpose of neuropsychological evaluation with older adults is diagnosis, functional estimation, intervention planning or (most likely) all three, several testing factors need to be considered when working with this population. Much as cognitive function can decline with age, decline in physical functions can present confounding variables to test administration and interpretation. Clinicians often explore potential testing confounds at the beginning of a visit, which allows them to modify their approach as needed. If neuropsychological data are collected by psychometricians, they should be trained to identify potential confounds and to interact with the supervising neuropsychologist about how to make appropriate modifications to testing (e.g., use of voice amplification device to accommodate hearing impairment). In some cases, the clinician may face the prospect of omitting a measure if the confound cannot be accommodated, such as the problem of administering tests of visual memory to someone who is profoundly visually impaired. In other cases, procedures can be modified so that the individual can complete a test, albeit in a nonstandardized fashion. Such "testing of limits" can provide valuable diagnostic information even when the validity of normative interpretation is questionable. Consider the case of an individual who cannot draw visual memory figures due to paresis or severe tremor in his or her drawing hand. If that individual studies the figures visually for an equivalent length of time and later performs flawlessly on forced-choice recognition of those figures, the clinician at least has qualitative information about the individual's ability to store visual information in memory. When testing of limits does occur, clinicians must consider how any modifications to standard protocol may affect their interpretation of norms based on standardized administration. With that caveat in mind, the following section addresses several potential confounds that can occur in geriatric neuropsychological assessment.

Vision

Vision problems are overrepresented among adults ages 65 and over, in that this group makes up approximately 13% of the U.S. population but accounts for roughly 30% of the visually impaired (Desai, Pratt, Lentzer, & Robinson, 2001). Vision is an important issue to geriatrics as a whole because visual impairment is related to decreased functional independence among older adults. For instance, impairments in visual acuity and contrast sensitivity are significant predictors of functional impairments in such skills/actions as reading, telephone dialing, and descending and ascending stairs (West et al., 2002). One study of cognitive outcomes reported significant improvement on a dementia screening measure following cataract surgery, even when items related specifically to visual function were excluded (Tamura et al., 2004).

As it relates to neuropsychological assessment, poor vision can be a confound to test validity and interpretation. It may require specific test selection and modification of procedures. Among blind patients, for instance, an informal evaluation of naming ability can be obtained by having an individual name common objects that are placed in his or her hand (given that there is no additional deficit in tactile discrimination). Tactile stimuli can also be substituted in some memory testing; for instance, the Fuld Object Memory Evaluation (Fuld, 1977) utilizes touch in the identification of objects to be remembered. A more common problem than outright blindness is impaired vision due to problems such as macular degeneration or diabetic retinopathy. In many cases, the print and visual stimuli on neuropsychological tests are too small and complex to be perceived adequately by individuals with poor vision. Some tests, such as the Wide Range Achievement Test–3 (WRAT-3; Wilkinson, 1993), provide versions of their materials in larger type. In other cases, visual stimuli may be enlarged in a photocopier or placed under magnification. When evaluating older patients, a pocket eye chart is often useful to help identify individuals who may have difficulty perceiving print and other visual stimuli.

Hearing

Hearing loss is another common problem among older adults. One estimate from the Centers for Disease Control and Prevention is that 37% of all hearing problems occur in individuals over the age of 65 (Desai et al., 2001). Moreover, hearing loss may be harder to detect than visual problems because older adults are found to be less likely to get hearing evaluations and to wear hearing aids than they are to get consultation and correction for poor vision. As is the case with poor vision, hearing deficits are associated with increased cognitive and functional difficulties. One study that investigated hearing loss among nondemented individuals versus those with AD found it to be associated with increased cognitive impairment among both groups, including a dose-dependent relationship among those with AD (Uhlmann, Larson, Rees, Koepsell, & Duckert, 1989). Moreover, concurrent visual and hearing deficits may be associated with greater cognitive and functional impairment than each impairment alone (Lin et al., 2004). In the context of a neuropsychological evaluation, examiners can address the potential confound of minor hearing loss by speaking clearly, making eye contact, and positioning themselves to face the ear with the best hearing. Hearing aids are typically helpful, as are systems that amplify sound via headphone. In cases of severe hearing deficits, test instructions may have to be presented to the examinee in written form. Administration of verbal memory tests is particularly challenging in the context of hearing impairment, and it is useful to note that the word-list learning items from the CERAD battery (Consortium to Establish a Registry for Alzheimer's Disease; Morris et al., 1989) appear in printed form, which can be read by the patient to minimize the risk of information loss due to poor hearing.

Motor Function

Like vision and hearing deficits, impairments of upper extremity motor function are common among older adults but vary considerably in type and severity. Stroke is one condition that is more prevalent with age and which commonly produces dyscoordination, paresis, or even paralysis of an extremity. Arthritis and peripheral neuropathy are conditions with greater prevalence among older adults that can compromise speed and dexterity. Motor impairment can make it difficult to administer the many neuropsychological tests that rely on writing or drawing. Visual study, as mentioned previously, is a useful "test of limits" for drawing-dependent visual memory tasks when there is a subsequent visual recognition trial that can be used to assess recall. There are a few tests of psychomotor processing that provide limited normative values for oral administration, including the Symbol Digit Modalities Test (Smith, 1982) and the Trail Making Test (Ricker & Axelrod, 1994).

Fatigue

Another factor to consider when assessing older adults is the reasonable length of the test battery. Lengthy testing may produce fatigue effects that adversely affect performance among older adults and individuals with cognitive disorders in general (Lezak et al., 2004). Consequently, clinicians may need to modify testing into a shorter, more focused, and less taxing session than is used with a younger population. Testing might also be structured so that assessment of a specific neurocognitive domain does not occur all at the same time, so as to minimize the differential effects of fatigue on functions assessed later in the examination. The final consideration for limiting the length of an assessment for older adults is evidence that suggests that most elders perform significantly better on effortful cognitive tasks in the morning than they do in the afternoon (Hasher, Chung, May, & Foong, 2002; May, Hasher, & Stoltzfus, 1993); hence, a test battery that can be completed in the course of a morning has the advantage of assessing older adults at their optimum time of day while also minimizing test fatigue.

Literacy

The rate of illiteracy among adults ages 65 and over has been estimated at 44%, with increasing rates as a function of age (Kirsch, Jungeblut, Jenkins, & Kolstad, 1993). Literacy should be considered an important domain in geriatric neuropsychological assessment because higher literacy appears protective of memory decline (Manly, Touradji, Tang, & Stern, 2003), whereas lower literacy is a risk factor for negative outcomes such as hospitalization and poor disease management (Baker, Parker, Williams, & Clark, 1998; Williams, Baker, Parker, & Nurss, 1998). It is well known that many neuropsychological measures have strong education effects. Research by Manly and colleagues has highlighted the negative bias that low-literacy level can have on test interpretation (Manly et al., 1999; Manly, Jacobs, Touradji, Small, & Stern, 2002). Our clinical experience suggests that the prevalence of low literacy levels is greater among the populations of inpatient hospital wards and state psychiatric hospitals that serve the underprivileged than among the typical outpatient population of tertiary care clinics. It can be difficult to identify low literacy in an individual who is embarrassed or otherwise reluctant to acknowledge this fact; for instance, an individual may refuse to take tests rather than reveal his or her inability to read the stimuli. Low literacy is also problematic in that many neuropsychological tests and test items are based on reading or providing written responses and thus are fundamentally compromised by an individual's low literacy level. The clinician needs to keep these factors in mind when deciding which tests will be the most valid indicators of cognitive function for a patient with low reading ability. The Reading subtest of the WRAT-3 (Wilkinson, 1993) may be useful for estimating the grade reading level of examinees.

Rapport and Motivation

Rapport and motivation are important variables that can influence neuropsychological assessment performance, and certain aspects of these variables are particularly relevant to a geriatric population. The neuropsychological evaluation may be an older adult's first contact with a professional psychologist, and it may be viewed with trepidation if the outcome of the assessment is perceived as potentially contributing to an unwanted diagnosis of cognitive impairment and possible major life changes. Moreover, some examinees may arrive at their appointment reluctantly, at the urging of family members, rather than of their own accord. For such individuals, additional attention may be needed to educate them about the causes of cognitive impairment and the possibility of both positive and negative outcomes of an evaluation. Reassuring reluctant patients that participation in testing is voluntary while also explaining ways in which testing provides valuable information for their care can help them find ways to feel personally invested in the process. The clinician may also need to "normalize" the testing experience for patients by informing them that although they may find some tests to be difficult, this does not necessarily mean that they have dementia; rather, easy and difficult items are part of the normal testing experience. Taking the time to address patient concerns at the beginning of the evaluation can place the process in an informative and potentially less threatening context, which may optimize motivation while reducing test anxiety and other forms of emotional distress that could adversely affect test performance. Any distress or signs of poor motivation that do emerge should be addressed promptly with appropriate reassurances, or if necessary, temporary or terminal discontinuation of testing. Continued assessment of an agitated or unmotivated patient is likely to compromise test validity and interpretation.

ASSESSMENT STRATEGIES

The clinician's approach to selecting tests to administer in a neuropsychological evaluation is typically guided by (1) the referral question, and (2) the utility of a test to answer the referral question for an individual patient (i.e., the availability of appropriate normative data). Although a referral question often dictates attention to a particular cognitive domain, such as extensive language assessment for an individual with suspected primary progressive aphasia, test batteries are typically selected with comprehensiveness in mind. Most clinicians would agree that a comprehensive neuropsychological evaluation should include assessment in the domains of (1) orientation, (2) attention, (3) executive functions, (4) memory, (5) expressive and receptive language, (6) visuospatial functions, (7) motor skills, (8) emotional status and personality, (9) estimated premorbid function, and (10) functional status.

Although the proliferation of new neuropsychological measures over the past decade has made it easier for the clinician to select test instruments that are tailored to specific populations and referral questions, shortcomings still remain in the assessment of older adults. For instance, there are still few measures that effectively accommodate impairments in vision, hearing, and motor functions. However, the most salient issue is the need for tests with norms that correct for multiple demographic variables of age, education, ethnicity, and gender. The application of normative standards in test interpretation is based on the assumption that the individual who is being evaluated is similar in most respects to the population that comprised the normative sample. That assumption is invalid, however, when an individual's characteristics are not a good fit with the normative population, which has historically occurred when an individual has a low level of education, is a member of a minority ethnic group, or is older. Regarding education, for instance, Pittman and colleagues found that neuropsychological tests can overdiagnose dementia among individuals with low levels of formal schooling (Pittman et al., 1992). Fortunately, the recent generation of neuropsychological instruments has been developed with greater attention to validation on large, demographically representative samples. For instance, the normative sample for the Wechsler Adult Intelligence Scale—3rd Edition (WAIS-III, Wechsler, 1997a) and Wechsler Memory Scale—3rd Edition (WMS-III, Wechsler, 1997b) was collected to broadly reflect the demographic representation of the U.S. population. These tests also have a scoring supplement that corrects for specific demographic factors.

In addition, work by Heaton and colleagues (Heaton, Miller, Taylor, & Grant, 2004) has resulted in a compilation of demographically corrected norms for neuropsychological measures that provide norms for specific demographic subpopulations; these corrected norms include combinations for age, education, African American versus European American ethnicity, and sex. While the field of clinical neuropsychology continues to make progress in the development of demographically representative norms, it is important to note that even when norms are carefully collected to represent the general population, the application of these norms to geographic and ethnic subpopulations can still be misleading (Spreen & Strauss, 1998), particularly if members of that subpopulation do not have English as their native language. Ultimately, it is incumbent on clinicians to be well informed about the normative properties of the tests they use to assess older adults. An informative discussion of criteria for evaluating normative properties appears in Mitrushina, Boone, and D'Elia's (1999) thorough collection and review of neuropsychological test norms.

Another aspect of assessment that affects test selection is the overall approach to test battery construction; that is, fixed versus flexible assessment batteries. Bearing in mind that the nomenclature itself may be misleading, the "fixed battery" approach to neuropsychological assessment is to administer the same collection of tests in the same order to every patient, perhaps best exemplified by the Halstead–Reitan Neuropsychological Battery (HRB). A "flexible battery," in contrast, is composed of neuropsychological measures tailored to each individual's specific referral question. One way to summarize the two approaches is that the former collects the data before generating interpretive hypotheses, whereas the latter often collects data guided by hypotheses. Whereas a fixed battery approach, specifically the HRB, has a strong tradition in forensics and the assessment of focal neurological conditions, there are disadvantages to this approach for geriatric assessment; the time required to administer a large fixed battery is fatiguing to many older adults, and many tests may not necessarily be suitable to the functional levels of demented patients. In practice, many clinicians typically administer a certain core collection of tests to all patients, while also selecting additional tests to address specific referral issues. This approach retains one advantage that is often attributed to the fixed battery approach, which is that consistent administration of tests across different diagnostic groups builds a sense of how different illness groups may perform on a particular test. In addition, it also maintains the flexibility to add to these tests as circumstances dictate. Thus, a core of well selected, age-sensitive measures in a geriatric neuropsychological assessment battery can improve diagnostic specificity without compromising the clinician's flexibility.

One caveat to consider in test selection is that cognitive function among older adults is heterogeneous; administering tests that are too hard or too easy for patients' functional levels can lead to both false negative and false positive errors in diagnosing impairment. One example is the word-list learning task in the CERAD battery, which was developed to assess AD and to be tolerable for individuals with mid- to late-stage impairments. When administered to high-functioning individuals with mild or non-AD impairments, however, this 10-item word list may produce a ceiling effect (see Welsh-Bohmer & Mohs, 1997). On the other hand, tests that generate floor effects due to a high level of difficulty can be demoralizing, which may lead to diminished effort.

Some clinicians administer screening tests as either a core or starting point for their assessments. These measures typically sample a few items from several cognitive domains and range in administration time from 5 to 45 minutes. An example that is on the brief end of the screening spectrum is the long- and oft-used Mini-Mental State Examination (MMSE; Folstein, Folstein, & Fanjiang, 2001). The MMSE is pervasive in clinical research studies involving cognition and is widely used by physicians to screen for cognitive impairment. One drawback to using the MMSE as a global screen for cognitive impairment is its poor sensitivity to right-hemisphere dysfunction and subtle cerebral dysfunctions (Naugle & Kawczak, 1989). Another drawback is adherence to the common convention that an MMSE score below 25 is indicative of dementia. In fact, there are significant effects of age, education, and lifetime principal occupation on the MMSE (Anthony, LeResche, Niaz, Von Korff, & Folstein, 1982; Frisoni, Rozzini, Bianchetti, & Trabucchi, 1993; Launer, Dinkgreve, Jonker, Hooijer, & Lindeboom, 1993), which can result in overdiagnosis of impairment in older and lower-educated individuals and underdiagnosis of impairment among individuals who are younger, more highly educated, and more mildly impaired. Although many neuropsychologists include the MMSE in research batteries because of its brevity and status as a lingua franca for cognitive status, its utility as a stand-alone measure of cognitive function is limited.

Several other screening batteries are more extensive in length and consequently demonstrate higher levels of sensitivity and specificity for age-related cognitive impairments. The Cognistat (formerly Neurobehavioral Cognitive Screening Examination; Kiernan, Mueller, & Langston, 2001) and the Repeatable Battery for the Assessment of Neuropsychological Status (RBANS; Randolph, 1998) are examples of screening batteries used in general neuropsychological assessment that have been validated as stand-alone assessments in demented populations. Each of these batteries yields information about the presence and severity of cognitive deficits by sampling cognitive processes that tend to change in the context of neurological dysfunction. The drawback to screening batteries is that they can fail to detect subtle cognitive deficits or may lack the necessary comprehensiveness to inform differential diagnosis. One way to address the latter drawback is to administer additional tests in the domains that are positive for impairment on the screening measure, thus making the instrument the "core" of a larger flexible assessment. A screening approach may also be used effectively in an inpatient setting where time constraints preclude the administration of a comprehensive battery for all referrals, and where test specificity may be a lesser priority. Although there is potential utility in measures that broadly screen for cognitive dysfunction, appreciation of their limitations is an important part of test selection and interpretation.

INTERPRETATION OF NEUROPSYCHOLOGICAL DATA

The interpretive process essentially defines the neuropsychological evaluation; it is the process by which a standardized laboratory procedure becomes clinically relevant and meaningful. Test interpretation is an inferential process that begins with the use of standardized normative information and extends consideration to information about onset and course of illness, neurobehavioral signs and symptoms, medical history, family history, and other data that provide an important context for the test scores themselves. It is this essential integration of test data with clinical knowledge that sets the neuropsychologist apart from a psychometrician or computer algorithm.

The following section details key aspects of integrated neuropsychological interpretation. We consider how individual presentation and history provide context for neuropsychological interpretation, and how clinical knowledge of neuropathological processes can provide an organizational framework for relating individual profiles to broader diagnostic entities. Although these aspects are recognized elements of most neuropsychological evaluations, we consider them as they pertain to the assessment of geriatric cognitive disorders.

Core Neuropsychological Knowledge Base

Functional Neuroanatomy

A comprehensive understanding of brain–behavior relationships is an intellectual cornerstone in the specialty practice of clinical neuropsychology. Familiarity with the neurobehavioral manifestations of changes to central nervous system structures, pathways, and systems allows for an informed generation of hypotheses regarding the etiology of a patient's presenting condition. Also important is an understanding of how neuroanatomy is related to specific neurological and psychiatric disorders. From this starting point, the neuropsychologist can proceed to test interpretive hypotheses based on the relationship between patient data and established clinical knowledge.

Diagnostic Criteria

Many geriatric cognitive disorders can be defined by diagnostic criteria that have been developed to formally characterize the relationship between patient presentation and established profiles of neurocognitive change. For instance, numerous diagnostic guidelines have been developed to aid the diagnosis and differential diagnosis of dementia. One of the most prevalent sets of diagnostic criteria for dementia was developed for the fourth edition of the *Diagnostic and Statistical Manual of Mental Disorders* (DSM-IV; American Psychiatric Association, 1994). These criteria require memory impairment in addition to at least one of the following cognitive disorders: (1) aphasia, (2) apraxia, (3) agnosia, or (4) executive dysfunction. These cognitive impairments must also (1) be associated with impairments in social or occupational function, (2) reflect a decline from premorbid performance, and (3) not be better explained by other conditions, including delirium and psychiatric disorder. Additional criteria in the DSM-IV differentiate AD from vascular and other dementias. Other diagnostic criteria have been developed in clinical research to diagnose AD (National Institute of Neurological and Communicative Disorders and Stroke–Alzheimer's Disease Related Disorders Association [NINCDS-ADRDA]; McKhann et al., 1984) and vascular dementia (National Institute of Neurological Disorders and Stroke and Association Internationale pour la Recherche et l'Enseignement en Neurosciences [NINDS-AIREN]; Roman et al., 1993). The chapters that follow in Part I, Section A, of this book outline many formalized diagnostic criteria, including those for MCI, which is non-normal cognitive performance that does not produce the level of impairment consistent with dementia (Winblad et al., 2004). In the absence of formalized or widely accepted criteria, clinicians often look to key studies to guide their conceptualization of typical presentations of disorders linked to specific etiologies.

Although diagnostic criteria are useful to guide clinical diagnosis, it is important to bear in mind that their nature is to capture the typical profile of a condition. There is, however, considerable interindividual heterogeneity in the aging process, in risk factors for neuropsychological dysfunction, and in presentation of the cognitive disorders themselves. It is thus important to recognize that some presentations of a cognitive disorder may be atypical or influenced by comorbid conditions and, as such, may not precisely fit a specific nosology. Therefore, divergence from typical diagnostic criteria does not necessarily rule out specific interpretive hypotheses; rather, they should be considered in light of each patient's specific presentation, including knowledge of the base rates and age distributions of typical and atypical presentations of the etiologies under consideration.

Neurobehavioral Presentations

Although neuropsychological testing is the primary source of interpretive information for the neuropsychologist, knowledge of behavioral manifestations in specific cognitive disorders is complementary to the interpretation process. Many geriatric cognitive disorders have characteristic behavioral presentations, with the dementia syndrome of depression as a common example. Frontal lobe dementias are often notable for disinhibited behavior that typically accompanies the disorder (Liu et al., 2004). Depressed affect often accompanies Parkinson's disease (Leentjens, 2004), whereas dementia with Lewy bodies often produces visual hallucinations early in the course of the illness (Rampello et al., 2004).

Although some manifestations of abnormal behavior can be observed in the course of an evaluation, deficits in patient insight or unwillingness to report behavioral symptoms often makes collateral reports an important source of these data. Instruments that help quantify the presence and severity of neuropsychiatric problems in geriatric populations include the Geriatric Depression Scale (GDS; Yesavage et al., 1983), the Neuropsychiatric Inventory (NPI; Cummings, 1997), and the Clinical Assessment Scales for the Elderly (CASE; Reynolds, 2001). Beyond the diagnostic utility of the behavioral presentation, it is important to consider the role of behavior in treatment prognosis, given that behavioral disruption in dementia increases the likelihood of institutionalization and decreases quality of life for both patients and caregivers (Finkel, Costa e Silva, Cohen, Miller, & Sartorius, 1996).

Characteristic and Pathognomonic Signs

Another important aspect of a geriatric neuropsychologist's core knowledge should be the ability to recognize presentations that are highly specific to a particular disorder. For instance, the neuropsychological assessment of a patient following stroke may reveal a constellation of dysgraphia, dyscalculia, right–left disorientation, and finger agnosia, which represent the characteristic signs of Gerstmann's syndrome (Benton, 1992). In a patient who presents with Parkinsonian features, it may be useful to assess for the impairment in downward gaze that characteristically appears in the early course of progressive supranuclear palsy (Golbe, 2001). When neuropsychological findings of confusion, disorientation, and memory impairment are accompanied by observation of an apractic gait and a reported history of urinary incontinence, a diagnosis of normal-pressure hydrocephalus is a strong diagnostic possibility (Lezak et al., 2004). These examples illustrate the importance of evaluating neuropsychological test results in the context of other aspects of the assessment process, such as behavioral observations and medical history. This theme of integrative interpretation continues throughout the discussion that follows.

Patient Presentation and Performance

Integrative neuropsychological interpretation proceeds as the clinician applies his or her base of clinical knowledge to the patient's specific presentation. In addition to data from neuropsychological testing, patient presentation and history are valuable to the interpretive process. Other chapters in this text are devoted to the neuropsychological profiles of specific cognitive disorders, and we refer the reader to these for more detailed information. Here we address the more general interpretive aspects of patient presentation, which include estimation of premorbid function, behavioral observations, and characterization of normal versus abnormal performance. Following these considerations we consider aspects of clinical and medical history that are key to the interpretive process. Finally, we discuss neuroimaging and genetic data that are supplemental to the neuropsychological interpretive process.

Patient Data

Estimating Premorbid Function. One of the key criteria for diagnosing a cognitive disorder is whether an individual's observed performances differ from expected performances based on evidence or estimates from prior healthy function. Without a valid estimate of premorbid function, interpretation based on normative standards alone may still underdiagnose impairment among individuals with high premorbid ability or overdiagnose individuals with low premorbid function. Unfortunately, few older individuals have neuropsychological test results or formal estimates of intellect from earlier in their life, so premorbid abilities must be estimated based on (1) educational and academic achievements, (2) demographic factors (Barona, Reynolds, & Chastain, 1984), (3) tests of verbal intellect or reading that are typically resistant to early cognitive decline (e.g., Shipley Institute of Living Scale, Shipley, 1946; North American Adult Reading Test, Blair & Spreen, 1989; WRAT-3, Wilkinson, 1993), or (4) combined demographic–performance estimates (e.g., Oklahoma Premorbid Intelligence Estimate–3 [OPIE-3], Schoenberg, Scott, Duff, & Adams, 2002). Each of these methods has utility in estimating premorbid neurocognitive performance, but all require caution in their application to older adults. Educational level or occupational background may not reliably predict intelligence in this age cohort, because economic, geographic, and cultural barriers limited the educational and occupational opportunities of many individuals. Further, education level does not influence performance in all cognitive domains equally (Heaton, Ryan, Grant, &

Matthews, 1995). In addition, caution must be exercised when using estimates based on performance in such areas as reading, because these estimates may not be stable in conditions such as stroke or traumatic injury (e.g., Johnstone & Wilhelm, 1996). Thus the clinician needs to be appropriately judicious in the use of these approaches in cases when these estimates may be prone to over- or underestimation of premorbid function.

Behavioral Observations. One source of nontest data that is nonetheless critical to neuropsychological interpretation is that of behavioral observations. Observations of behavior during testing and other patient contact provide important contextual information for interpreting test performances. For instance, consistent evidence of word-finding deficits and circumlocution during conversation may alert the clinician to the possibility of primary progressive aphasia, whereas perseverative responses and echolalia might raise consideration of frontal-lobe dementia. There are also many diagnostic behaviors that contribute to poor test performance that would go unnoticed in the examination of test scores alone. For instance, poorer performances that appear influenced by inattentive and impulsive behavior might suggest frontal-lobe involvement, whereas poorer performances due to inattention and slowed cognitive processing might suggest a subcortical etiology. Observation of behaviors such as these during the course of testing can help the clinician make determinations regarding test validity. Behavioral observation is also an important way to assess emotional presentation and thought processes. Depressed affect, for instance, is important to assess via observation because self-report of mood is not always veridical. The presence of insight into cognitive deficits is a key behavioral observation, for example, because depressed individuals typically overreport their cognitive difficulties, whereas individuals with AD or frontal-lobe dementia tend to underreport (Breitner & Welsh, 1995).

Characterizing Normal versus Abnormal Performance. Perhaps the most critical element of neuropsychological interpretation are the data themselves. The objective, standardized information generated from a comprehensive neuropsychological evaluation is the primary source of data in establishing the presence or absence of deficits, the degree of compromise, the specific neurocognitive domains affected, and the overall constellation of test results—all of which allow for inferences regarding neuroanatomical correlates and diagnosis. An analysis of deviations from expected performances typically involves both normative comparisons and consideration of the overall pattern of test findings. The principal purpose of normative data is to compare an individual's performance to what is expected of his or her peer group (see Busch & Chelune, Chapter 6, this volume). Given that many older adults experience slowing and other mild cognitive changes as they age, it is particularly important in geriatric assessment to distinguish normal age-related decline from abnormal performances indicative of a cognitive disorder. Thus a brief review of the neuropsychology of normal aging is provided for this purpose.

Normal aging of the nervous system is the most common explanation for relatively mild changes in cognitive functioning occurring after the fifth decade (Albert & Heaton, 1988). The profile of change with normal aging is often characterized as a loss of "fluid" abilities that are associated with problem solving and novel task performance (Horn, 1982). "Crystallized" abilities, by contrast, are those skills that have been well learned over time and tend to be less susceptible to age effects. It is important to recognize, however, that there is a great deal of interindividual variability in the rate and profile of change among normally functioning older adults. Research suggests that some individuals may carry more of a cognitive reserve against age-related decline than others (Stern, 2002), which may be related to number factors such as genetic inheritance, intellectual engagement, and health status. Establishing normal and abnormal performances within a given evaluation rests upon normative comparisons, but also considers the overall constellation of test findings. In this manner, suspected changes in patient function are considered in the context of relevant individual factors, such as estimated premorbid ability and key developments in clinical history. Nonetheless, even with adherence to these practices, there can be considerable ambiguity in a cross-sectional assessment of neuropsychological status. In these instances, longitudinal follow-up is often essential to document whether there is a progression of deficits that typifies dementia or a pattern of stability or improvement that may suggest normal aging.

Historical Data: Clinical Presentation and Medical History

Clinical Presentation. Understanding the history of a patient's presenting symptoms is important to the neuropsychological assessment process because it is a key source of information about the onset, course, and presentation of deficits. This information allows the neuropsychologist to compare the patient's presentation to those that typify specific cognitive disorders. Important aspects of the clinical presentation include type of onset along with the rate and course of neurocognitive and behavioral changes.

Onset. The etiologies of many geriatric cognitive impairments can often be segregated by whether the onset of symptoms was gradual or sudden. As a general rule, the impairments that characterize AD and associated progressive dementias tend to develop over the course of months and years, and may even have a preclinical period extending decades prior to diagnosis (Hulette et al., 1998; Snowdon et al., 1996). In the case of vascular dementia, progression is often characterized as "stepwise," in that overall progressive decline is interspersed with periods of stable function, gradually reflecting the cumulative effects of acute episodes of cerebrovascular insults (Roman et al., 1993). In contrast to gradual or stepwise onset, sudden changes in cognitive function are often linked to acute events, such as cerebrovascular accidents, metabolic dysregulations, or psychiatric disturbances. In some cases, the etiology of an acute change can be corroborated by clinical signs or laboratory results.

Rate and Course. Although it is important to establish a patient's symptom onset, it is equally important to understand the rate and manner in which subsequent changes in function have occurred. Neurocognitive performance can decline slowly or rapidly, remain stable, or even demonstrate improvement. For instance, although most dementias present a progression from mild to severe impairment that can be measured in years, a patient who progresses from mild to severe dementia in the course of months may be suspected of having an uncommon, rapidly progressive illness such as Creutzfeldt–Jakob disease (Brown, Cathala, Castaigne, & Gajdusek, 1986). As mentioned previously, cognitive impairments that present suddenly and remain stable often suggest the occurrence of cerebrovascular occlusion or hemorrhage. The "dementia of depression" syndrome is a common etiology of acute cognitive decline among older adults, which potentially can resolve as depressive symptomatology remits (Alexopoulos, Meyers, Young, Mattis, & Kukuma, 1993; McNeil, 1999). Metabolic dysregulation and medication effects often contribute to cognitive impairment in older adults, but can resolve in response to medical intervention. Attention to progressive, reversible, and stable presentations of neurocognitive impairment may aid the neuropsychologist with intervention planning as well as with differential diagnosis.

Relative Decline In addition to considering the general rate and course of cognitive impairment, neuropsychological interpretation is also aided by consideration of how specific neurocognitive domains decline relative to each other. The classic presentation of AD, for instance, is characterized by an early disproportionate decline in memory abilities, whereas frontal-lobe dementias are characterized by an early disproportionate decline in executive functions. True to their names, progressive movement disorders such as Parkinson's disease present with early motor abnormalities (Tröster, 1998), whereas early impairment in speech production in the context of general neurocognitive preservation is the hallmark of primary progressive aphasia (Mesulam, 2001). Non-neuropsychological but associated features such as extrapyramidal symptoms (EPS) can also have diagnostic and prognostic utility when they are prominent factors in the disease course. For instance, individuals who present with early EPS are more likely to have neuropathological signs of Parkinson's disease and Lewy body disease, and their clinical course is associated with greater cognitive decline and behavioral disturbances (Green, 2001).

Informant Reports. Ideally, the neuropsychologist's primary tool for evaluating the direction and rate of neurocognitive changes involves longitudinal neuropsychological comparisons; however, longitudinal test data are not present nearly as often as the clinician would like. In the absence of previous testing, the clinician can attempt to estimate direction and rate of progression from patient and family report by comparing the magnitude of cognitive deficits observed in current testing relative to the reported course of cognitive compromise.

Medical History

Information regarding past or current medical conditions and medications is important to neuropsychological interpretation because these factors can cause cognitive impairment in their own right as well as influence the presentation of an underlying dementing process. Medical history is particularly important because many medical illnesses become more prevalent with age, and increased medical burden is associated with decreased cognitive function. Primary hypothyroidism, for instance, is more common with age and can result in neurocognitive decline that is potentially reversible with treatment (Dugbartey, 1998). Postoperative cognitive dysfunction is also common among older adults (Lewis, Maruff, & Silbert, 2004). Overmedication is a cause of neurocognitive impairment that is more prevalent among older adults (Moore & O'Keefe, 1999); thus it is important to obtain a list of current medications as part of the medical history. Prior medical history can also be a significant aid to neuropsychological interpretation. For instance, brain trauma in early life can change the organization of the brain in atypical ways (Bates et al., 1997; Cioni, Montanaro, Tosetti, Canapicchi, & Ghelarducci, 2001), and head trauma in early adulthood may be a risk factor for later dementia (Plassman et al., 2000). Finally, family medical history is salient to diagnostic interpretation because many late-life cognitive disorders have familial influences (Plassman & Breitner, 1996).

Attendant Data

The previous section discussed the integration of patient presentation with essential clinical knowledge of disease characteristics as a method for interpreting neuropsychological data. The following section briefly highlights additional data that are not deemed essential to the interpretation process, but which are certainly important to refining or supporting the interpretation of neuropsychological data.

Neuroimaging

The neuroimaging of brain structures and functions has produced some revolutionary advances in the study of brain–behavior relationships and can be very useful in neuropsychological diagnosis when used appropriately. Imaging can be used to confirm areas of neuropathology that would be expected in a given disorder, such as evidence of brain lesions in suspected vascular dementia. In conditions such as stroke, imaging data can also support hypotheses about lesion localization derived from neuropsychological testing. Imaging also has emerging prognostic capability; for instance, regional brain metabolism on positron emission tomography (PET) imaging was found to predict later development of a neurodegenerative disorder (Silverman et al., 2001). Structural imaging such as computed tomography (CT) and magnetic resonance imaging (MRI) provide useful information about the location and volume of lesions in specific areas of the brain, but do not provide information related to brain function per se. Although functional imaging techniques such as PET, functional magnetic resonance imaging (fMRI), and electroencaphalography (EEG) are useful in identifying relationships between brain functions and structure, there is still an incomplete understanding of how these relationships relate to many specific neurological conditions, to the severity of cognitive impairment, and to neuropsychological strengths and weaknesses of a specific individual. Studies relating imaging findings to treatment intervention are currently limited as well.

Genetics

One of the most promising developments in medicine is the use of genes and other biomarkers to diagnose and treat medical conditions. Information from genetic investigations has proven useful in the diagnosis of AD (Welsh-Bohmer, Gearing, Saunders, Roses, & Mirra, 1997) and some familial frontotemporal dementias (e.g., Yamaoka et al., 1996). Apolipoprotein E (apoE), in particular, has been studied for its relationship to AD and cognitive decline (Saunders, Hulette, Welsh-Bohmer, et al., 1996; Small, Mazziotta, Collins, et al., 1995; Welsh-Bohmer, et al., 1997). As promising as these developments may be, it is important to note that understanding of the diagnostic and treatment implications of such information is complex. For instance, one study found that the inclusion of apoE genotyping to the information available for diagnosing AD increased the specificity of diagnosis from 55 to 84%, but decreased the sensitivity of the diagnosis from 93 to 61% (Mayeux et al., 1998). Unlike the deterministic genotyping for Huntington's disease and rare familial forms of AD, apoE and other biomarkers will likely provide only probabilistic information about disease susceptibility—which raises ethical issues about disclosing the results of this testing. Because the diagnostic utility of biomarker information is not yet well validated and there is potential psychological harm in disclosure of this information, its use is not currently recommended outside of specialized research centers operating within protocols that include genetic counseling (Hedera, 2001).

CONCLUSIONS

The previous section on neuropsychological interpretation reviewed key factors that should be synthesized with test data to arrive at diagnostic and functional impressions that are beneficial to both the patient and other treatment professionals involved in his or her care. Whereas some of these factors are addressed in the neuropsychological assessment itself, other factors require the clinician to remain abreast of findings regarding the etiology and diagnosis of cognitive disorders that occur among older adults, and to apply this knowledge to the patient's profile with the same intellectual rigor that is applied to psychometric data.

As the proportion of elderly in the United States and other developed Western nations continues to increase, the practice of geriatric neuropsychology becomes increasingly integral to the care of older adults. The utility and relevance of neuropsychological assessment are enhanced by attention to the characteristics and needs of this population. Because there is a high degree of heterogeneity in the aging process, the specificity of neuropsychological assessments can be improved by consideration of all relevant sources of information. It is important for clinicians to remain abreast of developments in related areas such as cognitive neuroscience and neuroepidemiology, which can provide valuable information concerning the detection and treatment of age-related cognitive disorders. Evaluations are enriched when they occur in conjunction with other sources of information, such as historical information, functional change measures, and behavioral observations. Although the ultimate goal of eliminating dementing conditions altogether remains immensely challenging, research across disciplines has made considerable progress in earlier and more reliable detection of AD and other dementias. Treating these conditions before symptoms become overt offers the greatest likelihood of preventing or minimizing decline. One goal for the field of geriatric neuropsychology should be to assure that our expertise in intervention and management of cognitive disorders keeps pace with our expertise in detection and diagnosis.

REFERENCES

Albert, M., & Heaton, R. (1988). Intelligence testing. In M. S. Albert & M. B. Moss (Eds.), *Geriatric neuropsychology* (pp. 13–32). New York: Guilford Press.

Alexopoulos, G. S., Meyers, B. S., Young, R. C., Mattis, S., & Kakuma, T. (1993). The course of geriatric depression with "reversible dementia": A controlled study. *American Journal of Psychiatry*, *150*, 1693–1699.

American Psychiatric Association. (1994). *Diagnostic and statistical manual of mental disorders* (4th ed.). Washington, DC: Author.

Anthony, J., LeResche, L., Niaz, U., Von Korff, M., & Folstein, M. (1982). Limits of the Mini-Mental State as a screening test for dementia and delirium among hospital patients. *Psychological Medicine*, *12*, 397–408.

Baker, D. W., Parker, R. M., Williams, M. V., & Clark, W. S. (1998). Health literacy and the risk of hospital admission. *Journal of General Internal Medicine*, *13*, 791–798.

Barona, A., Reynolds, C., & Chastain, R. (1984). A demographically based index of premorbid intelligence for the WAIS-R. *Journal of Consulting and Clinical Psychology, 52,* 885–887.

Bates, E., Thal, D., Trauner, D., Fenson, J., Aram, D., Eisele, J., et al. (1997). From first words to grammar in children with focal brain injury. *Developmental Neuropsychology, 13,* 275–344.

Benton, A. L. (1992). Gerstmann's syndrome. *Archives of Neurology, 49,* 445–447.

Blair, J., & Spreen, O. (1989). Predicting premorbid IQ: A revision of the National Adult Reading Test. *Clinical Neuropsychologist, 3,* 129–136.

Blanchard-Fields, F., & Hess, T. M. (Eds.). (1996). *Perspectives on cognitive change in adulthood and aging.* New York: McGraw Hill.

Breitner, J. C. S., & Welsh, K. A. (1995). Diagnosis and management of memory loss and cognitive disorders among elderly persons. *Psychiatric Services, 46,* 29–35.

Brown, P., Cathala, F., Castaigne P., & Gajdusek, D. (1986). Creutzfeldt–Jakob disease: Clinical analysis of a consecutive series of 230 neuropathologically verified cases. *Annals of Neurology, 20,* 597–602.

Cahn-Weiner, D. A., Boyle, P. A., & Malloy, P. F. (2002). Tests of executive function predict instrumental activities of daily living in community-dwelling older individuals. *Applied Neuropsychology, 9,* 187–191.

Cioni, G., Montanaro, D., Tosetti, M., Canapicchi, R., & Ghelarducci, B. (2001). Reorganisation of the sensorimotor cortex after early focal brain lesion: a functional MRI study in monozygotic twins. *Neuroreport, 12,* 1335–1340.

Craik, F., & Salthouse, T. A. (Eds.). (1992). *The handbook of aging and cognition.* Hillsdale, NJ: Erlbaum.

Cummings, J. L. (1997). The Neuropsychiatric Inventory: assessing psychopathology in dementia patients. *Neurology, 48,* S10–S16.

Cummings, J. L., and the Technology and Therapeutics Assessment Subcommittee. (1996). Assessment: Neuropsychological testing of adults: Considerations for neurologists. Report of the Therapeutics and Technology Assessment Subcommittee of the American Academy of Neurology. *Neurology, 47,* 592–599.

Davison, L. (1974). Introduction. In R. Reitan & L. Davison (Eds.), *Clinical neuropsychology: Current status and applications* (pp. 1–18). Washington, DC: VH Winston & Sons.

Desai, M., Pratt, L. A., Lentzer, H., & Robinson, K. N. (2001). *Trends in vision and hearing among older Americans.* Hyattsville, MD: National Center for Health Statistics.

Diehl, M., Willis, S., & Schaie, K. (1995). Everyday problem solving in older adults: Observational assessment and cognitive correlates. *Psychology and Aging, 10,* 478–491.

Dubinsky, R. M., Stein, A. C., & Lyons, K. (2000). Practice parameter: Risk of driving and Alzheimer's disease (an evidence-based review). *Neurology, 54,* 2205–2211.

Dugbartey, A. T. (1998). Neurocognitive aspects of hypothyroidism. *Archives of Internal Medicine, 158,* 1413–1418.

Farias, S. T., Harrell, E., Neuman, C., & Houtz, A. (2003). The relationship between neuropsychological performance and daily functioning in individuals with Alzheimer's disease: Ecological validity of neuropsychological tests. *Archives of Clinical Neuropsychology, 18,* 635–672.

Finkel, S. I., Costa e Silva, J., Cohen, G., Miller, S., & Sartorius, N. (1996). Behavioral and psychological signs and symptoms of dementia: A consensus statement on current knowledge and implications for research and treatment. *International Psychogeriatrics, 8,* 497–500.

Folstein, M. F., Folstein, S. E., & Fanjiang, G. (2001). *Mini-Mental State Examination: Clinical guide and user's guide.* Lutz, FL: Psychological Assessment Resources.

Frisoni, F., Rozzini, R., Bianchetti, A., & Trabucchi, M. (1993). Principal lifetime occupation and MMSE score in elderly persons. *Journal of Gerontology: Social Sciences, 48,* 310–314.

Fuld, P. (1977). *Fuld Object-Memory Evaluation—Instruction Manual.* Wood Dale, IL: Stoelting.

Golbe, L. I. (2001). Progressive supranuclear palsy. *Current Treatment Options in Neurology, 3,* 473–477.

Green, R. C. (2001). *Diagnosis and management of Alzheimer's disease and other dementias.* Caddo, OK: Professional Communications.

Hasher, L., Chung, C., May, C. P., & Foong, N. (2002). Age, time of testing, and proactive interference. *Canadian Journal of Psychology, 56,* 200–207.

Heaton, R. K., Miller, S. W., Talor, M. J., & Grant, I. (2004). *Revised comprehensive norms for an expanded Halstead–Reitan Battery: Demographically adjusted neuropsychological norms for African-American and Caucasian adults.* Lutz, FL: Psychological Assessment Resources.

Heaton, R. K., Ryan, L., Grant, I., & Matthews, C. G. (1995). Demographic influences on neuropsychological test performance: Differences in neuropsychological test performance associated with age, education, and sex. In I. Grant & K. M. Adams (Eds.), *Neuropsychological assessment of neuropsychiatric disorders* (pp. 141–163). New York: Oxford University Press.

Hedera, P. (2001). Ethical principles and pitfalls of genetic testing for dementia. *Journal of Geriatric Psychiatry and Neurology, 14,* 213–221

Horn, J. (1982). The theory of fluid and crystallized intelligence in relation to concepts of cognitive psychology and aging in adulthood. In F. Craik & S. Trehub (Eds.), *Aging and cognitive processes* (pp. 237–278). New York: Plenum Press.

Hulette, C. M., Welsh-Bohmer, K. A., Murray, M. G., Saunders, A. M., Mash, D. C., & McIntyre, L. M. (1998). Neuropathological and neuropsychological changes in "normal" aging: Evidence for preclinical Alzheimer's disease. *Journal of Neuropathology and Experimental Neurology, 57,* 1168–1174.

Johnstone, B., & Wilhelm, K. (1996). The longitudinal stability of the WRAT-R Reading subtest: Is it an appropriate estimate of premorbid intelligence? *Journal of the International Neuropsychological Society, 2,* 282–285.

Kiernan, R. J., Mueller, J., & Langston, J. W. (2001). *Cognistat professional manual.* Odessa, FL: Psychological Assessment Resources.

Kirsch, I. S., Jungeblut, A., Jenkins, L., & Kolstad, A. (1993). *Adult literacy in America: A first look at the findings of the National Adult Literacy Survey.* Washington, DC: National Center for Education Statistics.

Launer, L. J., Dinkgreve, M. A., Jonker, C., Hooijer, C., & Lindeboom, J. (1993). Are age and education independent correlates of the Mini-Mental State Exam performance of community-dwelling elderly? *Journal of Gerontology: Psychological Sciences, 48,* P271–P277.

Leentjens, A. F. (2004). Depression in Parkinson's disease: Conceptual issues and clinical challenges. *Journal of Geriatric Psychiatry and Neurology, 17,* 120–126.

Lesikar, S. E., Gallo, J. J., Rebok, G. W., & Keyl, P. M. (2002). Prospective study of brief neuropsychological measures to assess crash risk in older primary care patients. *Journal of the American Board of Family Practice, 15,* 11–19.

Lewis, M., Maruff, P., & Silbert, B. (2004). Statistical and conceptual issues in defining post-operative cognitive dysfunction. *Neuroscience and Biobehavioral Reviews, 28,* 433–440.

Lezak, M. D., Howieson, D. B., & Loring, D. W. (2004). *Neuropsychological assessment* (4th ed.). New York: Oxford University Press.

Lin, M. Y., Gutierrez, P. R., Stone, K. L., Yaffe, K., Ensrud, K. E., Fink, H. A., et al. (2004). Vision impairment and combined vision and hearing impairment predict cognitive and functional decline in older women. *Journal of the American Geriatrics Society, 52,* 1996–2002.

Liu, W., Miller, B. L., Kramer, J. H., Rankin, K., Wyss-Coray, C., Gearhart, R., et al. (2004). Behavioral disorders in the frontal and temporal variants of frontotemporal dementia. *Neurology, 62,* 742–748.

Manly, J. J., Jacobs, D. M., Sano, M., Bell, K., Merchant, C. A., Small, S. A., et al. (1999). Effect of literacy on neuropsychological test performance in non-demented, education-matched elders. *Journal of the International Neuropsychological Society, 5,* 191–202.

Manly, J. J., Jacobs, D. M., Touradji, P., Small, S. A., & Stern, Y. (2002). Reading level attenuates differences in neuropsychological test performances between African-American and white elders. *Journal of the International Neuropsychological Society, 8,* 341–348.

Manly, J. J., Touradji, P., Tang, M. X., & Stern, Y. (2003). Literacy and memory decline among ethnically diverse elders. *Journal of Clinical and Experimental Neuropsychology, 25*, 680–690.

Marson, D., Cody, H., Ingram, K., & Harrell, L. (1995). Neuropsychologic predictors of competency in Alzheimer's disease using a rational reasons legal standard. *Archives of Neurology, 52*, 955–959.

Marson, D., Ingram, K., Cody, H., & Harrell, L. (1995). Assessing the competency of patients with Alzheimer's disease under different legal standards. *Archives of Neurology, 52*, 949–954.

May, C. P., Hasher, L., & Stoltzfus, E. R. (1993). Optimal time of day and the magnitude of age differences in memory. *Psychological Science, 4*, 326–330.

Mayeux, R., Saunders, A. M., Shea, S., Mirra, S., Evans, D., Roses, A. D., et al., for the Alzheimer's Disease Centers Consortium on Apolipoprotein E and Alzheimer's Disease. (1998). Utility of the apolipoprotein E genotype in the diagnosis of Alzheimer's disease. *New England Journal of Medicine, 338*, 506–511.

McCue, M., Rogers, J., & Goldstein, G. (1990). Relationships between neuropsychological and functional assessment in elderly neuropsychiatric patients. *Rehabilitation Psychology, 35*, 91–99.

McKhann, G., Drachman, D., Folstein, M., Katzman, R., Price, D., & Stadlan, E. (1984). Clinical diagnosis of Alzheimer's disease: Report of the NINCDS–ADRA work group under the auspices of Department of Health and Human Services Task Force on Alzheimer's disease. *Neurology, 34*, 939–944.

Mesulam, M. M. (2001). Primary progressive aphasia. *Annals of Neurology, 49*, 425–432.

Mitrushina, M. N., Boone, K. B., & D'Elia, L. F. (1999). *Handbook of normative data for neuropsychological assessment.* New York: Oxford University Press.

Moore, A. R., & O'Keefe, S. T. (1999). Drug-induced cognitive impairment in the elderly. *Drugs and Aging, 15*, 15–28.

Morris, J., Heyman, A., Mohs, R., Hughes, P., Van Belle, G., Fillenbaum, G., et al. (1989). The Consortium to Establish a Registry of Alzheimer's Disease (CERAD): I. Clinical and neuropsychological assessment of Alzheimer's disease. *Neurology, 39*, 1159–1165.

Naugle, R., & Kawczak, K. (1989). Limitations of the Mini-Mental State Examination. *Cleveland Clinic Journal of Medicine, 56*, 277–281.

Pittman, J., Andrews, H., Tatemichi, T., Link, B., Struening, E., Stern, Y., et al. (1992). Diagnosis of dementia in a heterogenous population. *Neurology, 49*, 461–467.

Plassman, B. L., & Breitner, J. (1996). Recent advances in the genetics of Alzheimer's disease and vascular dementia with an emphasis on gene–environment interactions. *Journal of the American Geriatrics Society, 44*, 1242–1250.

Plassman, B. L., Havlik, R. J., Steffens, D. C., Helms, M. J., Newman, T. N., Drosdick, D., et al. (2000). Documented head injury in early adulthood and risk of Alzheimer's disease and other dementias. *Neurology, 55*, 1158–1166.

Prigatano, G. P. (1997). Learning from our successes and failures: Reflections and comments on "Cognitive rehabilitation: How it is and how it might be." *Journal of the International Neuropsychological Society, 3*, 497–499.

Rampello, L., Cerasa, S., Alvano, A., Butta, V., Raffaele, R., Vecchio, I., et al. (2004). Dementia with Lewy bodies: A review. *Archives of Gerontology and Geriatrics, 39*, 1–14.

Randolph, C. (1998). *Repeatable Battery for the Assessment of Neuropsychological Status manual.* San Antonio, TX: Psychological Corporation.

Reynolds, C. R. (2001). *Clinical Assessment Scales for the Elderly: Professional Manual for the CASE and CASE-SF.* Odessa, FL: Psychological Assessment Resources.

Richardson, E., Nadler, J., & Malloy, P. (1995). Neuropsychologic prediction of performance measures of daily living skills in geriatric patients. *Neuropsychology, 9*, 565–572.

Ricker, J. H., & Axelrod, B. N. (1994). Analysis of an Oral Paradigm for the Trail Making Test. *Assessment, 1*, 47–51.

Rockwood, K., Stolee, P., & McDowell, I. (1996). Factors associated with institutionalization of older people in Canada: Testing a multi-factorial definition of frailty. *Journal of the American Geriatrics Society, 44,* 578–582.

Roman, G. C., Tatemichi, T. K., Erkinjuntti, T., Cummings, J. L., Masdeu, J. C., Garcia, J. H., et al. (1993). Vascular dementia: Diagnostic criteria for research studies. Report of the NINDS–AIREN International Workshop. *Neurology, 43,* 250–260.

Saunders, A., Hulette, C., Welsh-Bohmer, K., Schmechel, D., Crain, G., Burke, J., et al. (1996). Specificity, sensitivity, and predictive value of apolipoprotein E genotyping for sporadic Alzheimer's disease. *Lancet, 348,* 90–93.

Scogin, F., & Perry, J. (1986). Guardianship proceedings with older adults: The role of functional assessment and gerontologists. *Law and Psychology Review, 10,* 123–128.

Schoenberg, M. R., Scott, J.G., Duff, K., & Adams, R. L. (2002). Estimation of WAIS-III intelligence from combine performance and demographic variables: Development of the OPIE-3. *Clinical Neuropsychologist, 16,* 426–438.

Shipley, W. (1946). *Institute of Living Scale.* Los Angeles: Western Psychological Services.

Silverman, D. H., Small, G. W., Chang, C. Y., Lu, C. S., Kung De Aburto, M. A., Chen, W., et al. (2001). Positron emission tomography in evaluation of dementia: Regional brain metabolism and long-term outcome. *Journal of the American Medical Association, 286,* 2120–2127.

Small, G., Mazziotta, J., Collins, M., Baxter, L., Phelps, M., Mandelkern, M., et al. (1995). Apolipoprotein E type 4 allele and cerebral glucose metabolism in relatives at risk for familial Alzheimer disease. *Journal of the American Medical Association, 273,* 942–947.

Smith, A. (1982). *Symbol–Digit Modalities Test.* Los Angeles: Western Psychological Services.

Snowdon, D. A., Kemper, S. J., Mortimer, J. A., Greiner, L. H., Wekstein, D. R., & Markesbery, W. R. (1996). Linguistic ability in early life and cognitive function and Alzheimer's disease in late life: Findings from the Nun Study. *Journal of the American Medical Association, 275,* 528–532.

Spreen, O., & Strauss, E. (1998). *A compendium of neuropsychological tests.* New York: Oxford University Press.

Stanley, B., Stanley, M., Guido, J., & Garvin, L. (1988). The functional competency of elderly at risk. *Gerontologist, 28,* 53–58.

Stern, Y. (2002). What is cognitive reserve? Theory and research application of the reserve concept. *Journal of the International Neuropsychological Society, 8,* 448–460.

Tamura, H., Tsukamoto, H., Mukai, S., Kato, T., Minamoto, A., Ohno, Y., Yamashita, H., & Mishima, H. K. (2004). Improvement in cognitive impairment after cataract surgery in elderly patients. *Journal of Cataract and Refractive Surgery, 30,* 598–602.

Teri, L., Logsdon, R., Uomoto, J., & McCurry, S. (1997). Behavioral treatment of depression in dementia patients: A controlled clinical trial. *Journal of Gerontology: Psychological Sciences, 52B:* P159–P166.

Tröster, A. (1998). Assessment of movement and demyelinating disorders. In P. J. Snyder & P. D. Nussman (Eds.), *Clinical neuropsychology: A pocket handbook for assessment.* Washington, DC: American Psychological Association.

Tymchuk, A., Ouslander, J., Rahbar, B., & Fitten, L. (1988). Medical decision-making among elderly people in long term care. *Gerontologist, 28,* 59–63.

Uhlmann, R. F., Larson, E. B., Rees, T. S., Koepsell, T. D., & Duckert, L. G. (1989). Relationship of hearing impairment to dementia and cognitive dysfunction in older adults. *Journal of the American Medical Association, 261,* 1916–1919.

Wechsler, D. (1997a). *Wechsler Adult Intelligence Scales—Third Edition.* San Antonio, TX: The Psychological Corporation.

Wechsler, D. (1997b). *Wechsler Memory Scale—Third Edition.* San Antonio, TX: Psychological Corporation.

Welsh-Bohmer, K. A., Gearing, M., Saunders, A. M., Roses, A. D., & Mirra, S. M. (1997). Apolipoprotein E genotypes in a neuropathological series from the Consortium to Establish a Registry for Alzheimer's Disease (CERAD). *Annals of Neurology, 42,* 319–325.

Welsh-Bohmer, K. A., & Mohs, R. C. (1997). Neuropsychological assessment of Alzheimer's disease. *Neurology, 49*, S11–S13.

West, S. K., Rubin, G. S., Broman, A. T., Munoz, B., Bandeen-Roche, K., Turano, K., et al. (2002). How does visual impairment affect performance on tasks of everyday life? *Archives of Ophthalmology, 120*, 774–780.

Wilkinson, G. S. (1993). *Wide Range Achievement Test 3—Administration Manual*. Wilmington, DE: Jastak Associates.

Williams, M. V., Baker, D. W., Parker, R. M., & Nurss, J. R. (1998). Relationship of functional health literacy to patients' knowledge of their chronic disease: A study of patients with hypertension and diabetes. *Archives of Internal Medicine, 158*, 166–172.

Willis, S., & Marsiske, M. (1991). Life span perspective on practical intelligence. In D. Tupper & K. Cicerone (Eds.), *The neuropsychology of everyday life: Issues in development and rehabilitation* (pp. 183–198). Boston: Kluwer.

Winblad, B., Palmer, K., Kivipelto, M., Jelic, V., Fratiglioni, L., Wahlund, L. O., et al. (2004). Mild cognitive impairment—beyond controversies, towards a consensus: Report of the International Working Group on Mild Cognitive Impairment. *Journal of Internal Medicine, 256*, 240–246.

Yamaoka, L., Welsh-Bohmer, K. A., Hulette, C. M., Gaskell, P. C., Murray, M., Rimmler, J. L., et al. (1996). Linkage of frontotemporal dementia to chromosome 17: Clinical and neuropathological characterization of phenotype. *American Journal of Human Genetics, 59*, 1306–1312.

Yesavage, J., Brinks, T., Rose, T., Lum, O., Huang, O., Adley, V., et al. (1983). Development and validation of a geriatric depression screening scale: A preliminary report. *Journal of Psychiatric Research, 17*, 37–49.

2

Normal Aging and
Mild Cognitive Impairment

GLENN SMITH
BETH K. RUSH

Dating back to the writings of V. A. Kral (1958, 1962) and perhaps before, two forms of cognitive change have been associated with aging. One form is proposed to involve typical, *benign*, and perhaps "developmental" changes in cognition associated with nonspecific histopathological brain changes. The second is a *malignant*, atypical form that may reflect specific brain histopathology. An extensive nomenclature has arisen out of attempts to diagnose each form of cognitive aging. A number of these diagnoses are depicted in Figure 2.1. This chapter discusses these two forms of cognitive aging. There is a vast literature that seeks to describe the fundamental processes of cognitive aging. We do not attempt to survey this entire literature in one chapter. We do, however, discuss the implications of cognitive aging for geriatric neuropsychological assessment. We then proceed to discuss mild cognitive impairment and related concepts that have arisen out of attempts to find prodromes for dementia. Finally, we discuss mild cognitive impairment as one of several "risk factors" for dementia.

WHAT IS COGNITIVE AGING?

Studies of cognitive aging typically involve either cross-sectional (interindividual comparison) or longitudinal (intraindividual comparison) design. Most cross-sectional studies of cognitive aging compare the performance of older adults to the performance of younger adults at a single point in time. This approach is favored for its practicality and its ability to appreciate obvious dimensions of difference between age groups on a given cognitive task. However, a major disadvantage to this approach is that between-group comparisons do not take into account cohort effects (e.g., differential access to quality education) or selective attrition (the tendency for lower scoring members of a cohort to drop out of

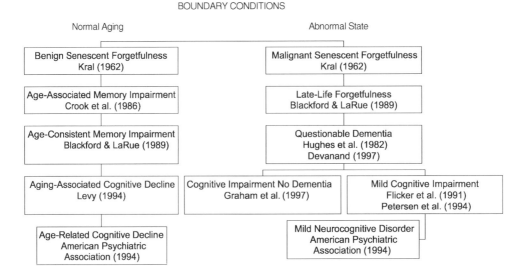

FIGURE 2.1. Proposed terms for benign and malignant cognitive aging.

studies more rapidly). Therefore, cross-sectional studies can provide evidence of cognitive differences between older and younger adult cohorts but may provide misleading information about patterns of functioning over time or rates of decline within individuals.

In contrast, longitudinal studies of cognitive aging are labor intensive with regard to execution and time. Studies that can model single individuals' cognitive change over decades are few. Longitudinal studies compare levels of performance across serial evaluations within individuals and therefore provide information about patterns of performance over time. These studies yield a great deal of information about cognitive change over time. Longitudinal studies advance our understanding of benign cognitive aging by allowing us to examine individual differences in rates of cognitive change. Such investigations lead to a greater understanding of the role that both biological (e.g., genes, metabolism, physical health) and environmental (e.g., lifestyle, demography) factors play in determining the level of cognitive functioning across the lifespan.

Most researchers agree that cognitive change is a nearly inevitable part of advancing age (e.g., Schaie, 1994). A few "optimally" aging people may avoid cognitive decline as they age (Powell & Whitla, 1994). For most, however, childhood development that involves increasing efficiency and abstraction ability, peaks in the middle of our second decade, followed by a slow loss of cognitive efficiency that may accelerate during the fifth decade. A hallmark of cognitive aging is a reduction in mental processing speed (Salthouse, 1996) and an associated reduction in the amount of information that can be processed at a single point in time. Multiple studies have demonstrated that limitations in mental processing speed consequently result in age-related changes in performance across many cognitive domains (e.g., Fisher, Duffy, & Katskiopoulos, 2000; Meyerson, Adams, Hale, & Jenkins, 2003; Meyerson, Jenkins, Hale, & Sliwinski, 2000; Salthouse, 1996). Indeed, changes in processing speed influence attention, language, memory, and executive functions (e.g., Finkel & Pederson, 2000; Hertzog & Bleckley, 2001; Keys & White, 2000; Parkin & Java, 2000; Sliwinski & Buschke, 1997, 1999; Zimprich, 2002). For example, studies of "normal" memory change reveal that, compared to younger adults, healthy older adults are less efficient at encoding to-be-learned information and therefore have greater difficulty recalling information following a delay period (e.g., Brebion, Smith, & Ehrlich, 1997; Frieske & Park, 1999; Light, 1996; Park et al., 1996; Sliwinski & Buschke, 1997). In this case, limitations in the extent of early processing limit the yield of later processing. Indeed, changes in general cognitive speed with advancing age impact performance across cognitive domains.

The cognitive changes that accompany advancing age result from several neurophysiological changes. The most recent research in this area suggests that benign aging involves minor deposition of beta-amyloid peptide and neurofibrillary tangles, as well as a loss of synapses, neurons, neurochemical input, and neuronal networks (Fillit et al., 2002). Additionally, normal aging can result in mild cerebral atrophy, slight ventricular enlargement, and mild hippocampal atrophy. However, actual gliosis or cell death is now thought to be less common in benign aging than it is in malignant aging processes such as dementia (West, Coleman, Flood, & Tronosco, 1994). Senescence-related neurophysiological changes appear to reduce the efficiency and net productivity of the neural system without dramatically altering its structural integrity. This characterization of benign aging sharply contrasts with the more dramatic structural neurological compromise typically associated with malignant aging processes. Interestingly, the same quality and magnitude of contrast are evident when the neurocognitive profiles of benign versus malignant aging are compared.

In the differential diagnosis of benign versus malignant cognitive change, serial assessment (e.g., a longitudinal approach) might be seen as ideal. This approach allows for the appreciation of performance across time, establishing evidence either in favor of or against "excess" cognitive decline over time. However, serial assessment, especially over the time frame it takes for clinical manifestation of malignant aging to develop, is a luxury. This type of data is rare in clinical situations. Most clinicians must rely on data from a single neuropsychological evaluation in order to contribute to an individual's diagnosis. These clinicians must thus consider several factors that could imitate or mask a malignant decline in cognitive functioning. These factors include the age, education, ethnicity, health status, and motivation of the patient.

In summary, benign or "healthy" cognitive aging results in cognitive change. It is evidence of deviation from benign changes that leads to the diagnostic consideration of a malignant aging process. Decreased cognitive processing speed is the hallmark of cognitive aging, impacting the efficiency of cognitive functioning across multiple domains. Age-related changes in processing speed likely result from senescence-related neurophysiological changes that compromise the efficiency and net yield of the neurocognitive system. Although serial assessments over time may aid in appreciating an individual's pattern of cognitive functioning over time, such assessments are not routinely available in clinical practice. The clinician must thus consider a variety of demographic factors to determine if a person might be deviating from expected, typical, or benign cognitive change. This need for normative referents creates a need for appropriate normative data. For a detailed discussion, see Busch and Chelune (Chapter 6, this volume).

NORMATIVE STUDIES OF AGING

The benign cognitive changes of aging can mask the presence of malignant cognitive change. Specifically, normal age-related changes in performance on neuropsychological tests reduce the specificity of these tests for pathological conditions. Test specificity is very important clinically because tests with high specificity are used to rule in the presence of a condition (Sackett, Straus, Richardson, Rosenberg, & Haynes, 2000). Normative data based on age help to improve the specificity of neuropsychological tests (Smith, Ivnik, & Lucas, in press). Historically, the utility of neuropsychological tests in detecting malignant aging processes such as Alzheimer's disease (AD) has been limited by a lack of age-appropriate normative data. This point was made clear as early as 1984, when the National Institute of Neurological and Communicative Disorders and Stroke (NINCDS) met and combined with the Alzheimer's Disease Related Disorders Association (ADRDA) to establish standard diagnostic criteria for AD (McKhann et al., 1984). The incidence of AD is highest over age 75 (Kokmen, Chandra, & Schoenberg, 1988), yet in 1984, 75 was the upper age limit of the standardization samples for most neuropsychological tests. Thus the NINCDS-ADRDA criticism was quite reasonable and valid. Since then, however, a number of investigators has helped to provide norms for older persons on a wide variety of neuropsychological measures (cf. Mitrushina, Boone, & D'Elia, 1999).

Our own studies, named the Mayo Older Americans Normative Studies (MOANS; Ivnik et al., 1992) and the Mayo Older African Americans Normative Studies (MOAANS; Busch & Chelune, Chapter 6, this volume) are discussed in Chapter 6. Collectively we refer to these studies as the MO(A)ANS. These normative works have provided age and education norms for comparing clinical populations to normal populations for persons up to 95 years of age for a variety of tests (see Table 2.1 for test listing, test author, and MOA(A)NS publications). Many of our normative analyses have focused on the Mayo Cognitive Factor Scores (MCFS) (Smith, Ivnik, Malec, Petersen, et al., 1992, 1994; Smith, Ivnik, Malek, & Tangalos, 1993), which are confirmatory-factor-analysis-derived indices based on coadministration of the Wechsler Adult Intelligence Test—Revised (WAIS-R), Wechsler Memory Scale—Revised (WMS-R; Wechsler, 1987), and Auditory Verbal Learning Test (AVLT; Rey, 1964).

The MOANS and MOAANS studies are longitudinal; in the course of repeat testing at quasi-annual intervals we have found that MCES stabilities are comparable to long-term stabilities of traditional Wechsler indices for comparable cognitive domains (Ivnik, Smith, Malec, Petersen, & Tangalos, 1995). Our cross-sectional and longitudinal data document that some cognitive domains are less stable and more susceptible to age-related change (see Figure 2.2).

However, we also find it important to highlight the limitations of this group data for making clinical inferences about individuals. For example, stability coefficients arising from group data tell us little about how much change over time in an individual's score is normal versus abnormal. This information is indicated by the more clinically relevant data on frequencies of difference scores for factors over time. Table 2.2 shows percentile scores for intrafactor change scores from the MOANS cohort. This is the minimum degree of change that most clinicians would require to be present at a 1-year interval to be sure that the change is beyond normative bounds. Relatively small changes in Verbal Comprehension, on the order of 10 points or greater, are statistically rare in normal populations over the interval of 3–5 years. However, it requires changes of 25 standard score points for us to suggest that a drop in Retention score is statistically abnormal (Ivnik et al., 1995).

Of course, longitudinal data from which to consider the meaning of magnitudes of change is a luxury in neuropsychological assessment. Often neuropsychologists must in-

TABLE 2.1. Tests with MOA(A)NS Norms

Test	Author (year)	MOA(A)NS norms papers
Wechsler Adult Intelligence Scale—Revised (WAIS-R)	Wechsler (1981)	Ivnik et al. (1992); Lucas et al. (2005a); Pedraza et al. (2005)
Wechsler Memory Scale— Revised (WMS-R)	Wechsler (1987)	Ivnik et al. (1992); Lucas et al. (2005b); Smith et al. (1997)
Auditory Verbal Learning Test (AVLT)	Rey (1964)	Ivnik et al. (1992); Harris et al. (2002); Ferman et al. (2005)
Visual Spatial Learning Test	Malec et al. (1992)	Malec et al. (1992)
Boston Naming Test	Kaplan, Goodglass, & Weintraub (1978)	Ivnik et al. (1996); Testa et al. (2004)
Controlled Oral Word Association Test	Benton, Hamsher, Varney, & Spreen (1983)	Ivnik et al. (1996)
Stroop Neuropsychological Screening Test	Golden (1978)	Ivnik et al. (1996)
Trail Making Test	Spreen & Strauss (1991)	Ivnik et al. (1996)
Judgement of Line Orientation Test	Benton et al. (1983)	Ivnik et al. (1996)
Multilingual Aphasia Examination Token Test	Benton & Hamsher (1978)	Ivnik et al. (1996)
Wide Range Achievement Test	Jastak & Wilkinson (1984)	Ivnik et al. (1996)
(U.S. modification) Nelson Adult Reading Test	Grober & Sliwinski (1991)	Smith, Bohac, Ivnik, & Malec (1997)
Dementia Rating Scale	Mattis (1988)	Lucas et al. (1998a); Rilling et al. (2005)
Category Fluency Test		Lucas et al. (1998b); Cerhan et al. (2002)
Free and Cued Selective Reminding Test	Grober & Buschke (1987)	Ivnik et al. (1997)

terpret the cognitive data from assessment at a single point in time. In this context neuropsychologists often assume that cognitive skills are highly intercorrelated and roughly comparable. Thus discrepancies among cognitive skills at a given point in time are assumed to be an indicator of decline in those areas that are out of line with other cognitive functions (Lezak, 1995). In a second set of analyses reported by Ivnik et al. (1995), intraindividual, interfactor variability across different MCFS cognitive domains was examined. Table 2.3 depicts the frequency of cross-sectional interfactor discrepancy scores in the MOANS population. Note that even with Verbal Comprehension to Perceptual Organizational comparisons, relatively small discrepancies in scores are necessary before the discrepancy falls outside normal limits. In comparisons of Learning and Reten-

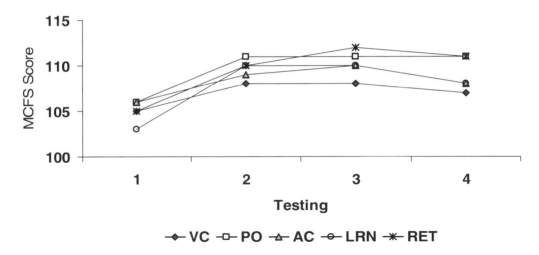

FIGURE 2.2. Mean Mayo Cognitive Factor scores on repeat testing at approximately annual intervals.

tion to verbal comprehension, splits of 25 points or greater are necessary before clinicians can reasonably assume that this variation is outside normal limits. These data extend to the MCFS scores, with cautions previously presented in the literature (Matarazzo & Prifitera, 1989; Ryan & Paolo, 1992) about interpreting discrepancies between cognitive performances as indicative of some underlying neurological insult. Moderate levels of discrepancy may simply represent normal individual differences in cognitive strengths and weaknesses. It is important to develop test norms not only for performance at a single time but also for discrepancies between coadministered measures and for performance change over clinically relevant intervals.

Through these studies of typically aging individuals, we have been able to better understand normative patterns of performance on cognitive tests. Establishing these patterns also elucidates patterns of abnormal performance. These studies have thus helped to clarify the boundary zone between benign and malignant cognitive changes (see Figure 2.1). We now turn to a fuller explication of several of these concepts.

TABLE 2.2. Percentage of Normal People with MCFS Test–Retest "Change Scores" of Different Magnitudes

MCFS	Test–retest change scores[a]					
	≥5	≥10	≥15	≥20	≥25	≥30
VC	30	7	2	< 1	—	—
PO	57	27	9	2	< 1	—
AC	53	28	6	3	1	< 1
LRN	64	35	13	6	2	1
RET	65	43	23	9	5	3

Note. MCFS, Mayo Cognitive Factor Scales; VC, Verbal Comprehension; PO, Perceptual Organization; AC, Attention/ Concentration; LRN, Learning; RET, Retention. From Ivnik, Smith, Malec, Petersen, and Tangalos (1995). Copyright 1995 by the American Psychological Association. Reprinted by permission.

[a] Change scores are the absolute values of Test 1–Test 2 difference scores.

TABLE 2.3. Percentage of Normal Older Persons with MCFS Difference Scores of Varying Magnitudes

MCFS difference score dyad	Magnitude of the difference score					
	≥5	≥10	≥15	≥20	≥25	≥30
VC–PO	64	37	20	9	4	1
VC–AC	66	40	20	11	5	2
VC–LRN	70	45	28	18	10	6
VC–RET	70	49	32	18	9	3
PO–AC	71	53	25	14	6	3
PO–LRN	70	46	29	17	9	4
PO–RET	69	46	27	16	8	4
AC–RET	73	48	31	20	12	6
AC–LRN	75	53	33	20	10	4
LRN–RET	69	41	25	14	5	2

Note. MCFS, Mayo Cognitive Factor Scales; VC, Verbal Comprehension; PO, Perceptual Organization; AC, Attention/Concentration; LRN, Learning; RET, Retention. From Ivnik, Smith, Malec, Petersen, and Tangalos (1995). Copyright 1995 by the American Psychological Association. Reprinted by permission.

BENIGN COGNITIVE CHANGE

Age-Associated Memory Impairment

In 1986 a National Institute of Mental Health work group proposed the diagnosis of age-associated memory impairment (AAMI; Crook et al., 1986). This diagnosis was intended to identify age-related changes in memory performance. As originally proposed, the concept of AAMI was predicated on the comparison of older persons to young adult norms on a variety of memory tests (Crook et al., 1986).

We criticized the method of establishing AAMI diagnoses because it did not recognize that traditional memory measures in clinical neuropsychology have tremendous heterogeneity in terms of their sensitivity to age effects (Smith et al., 1991). We suggested that it would require greater specificity in which aspects of memory were assessed in order for the concept to be applied reliably. Studies using the concept and definition of AAMI continue. Many of these studies originate in Europe, and many represent clinical trials aimed at mitigating age-related cognitive changes (cf. van Dongen, van Rossum, Kessels, Sielhorst, & Knipschild, 2003). Ultimately, instead of becoming more rigorously defined in DSM-IV, the AAMI concept evolved into a much more loosely defined concept of age-related cognitive decline (ARCD; American Psychiatric Association, 1994).

Age-Related Cognitive Decline

The definition of ARCD is not linked to psychometric test performance but is specifically tied to an intervention approach that focuses on memory that is normal in relation to age. Individuals diagnosed with ARCD are sometimes described colloquially as "worried well." In other words, it applies best to the clinical situation in which an older person is worried about his or her memory function, but there is no objective evidence of memory impairment. In recent practice the term is sometimes used interchangeably with normal aging (cf. Caccappolo van Vlict et al., 2003).

MALIGNANT COGNITIVE CHANGE

There is now an extensive literature on early detection of Alzheimer's-type dementia using neuropsychological instruments (Becker, Boller, Saxton, & McGonigle-Gibson, 1987; Berg, 1992; Masur, Sliwinski, Lipton, Blau, & Crystal, 1994; Morris et al., 1991; Petersen, Smith, Ivnik, Kokmen, & Tangalos, 1994; Robinson-Whelen & Storandt, 1992; Storandt & Hill, 1989; Welsh, Butters, Hughes, Mohs, & Heyman, 1991). Most of these studies however, have utilized a case–control methodology comparing normal controls to persons who have previously established clinical diagnoses of dementia, albeit early in the course of the disease. Moving beyond these studies, the question arises of just how "early" can dementia be detected. For example, can the evolution of dementia be predicted in persons assessed while still considered to be clinically not demented?

Dementia researchers and clinicians have improved their ability to diagnose and study "at risk" or malignant boundary conditions (see Figure 2.1). Again a variety of terms and criteria have been promoted. Figure 2.3 presents the combined results of MEDLINE and PsycINFO searches on isolated memory impairment, questionable dementia, cognitive impairment not demented, AAMI, and mild cognitive impairment (MCI) for the period 1985–2003. Clearly the concept of MCI (Petersen et al., 2001) has gained wide acceptance. MCI receives the greatest attention here.

Late-Life Forgetfulness

Historically, late-life forgetfulness (LLF) as suggested by Blackford and LaRue (1989) as modification to AAMI, was probably the forebear of MCI. LLF was defined as having borderline to impaired memory function relative to age-matched peers but the absence of dementia.

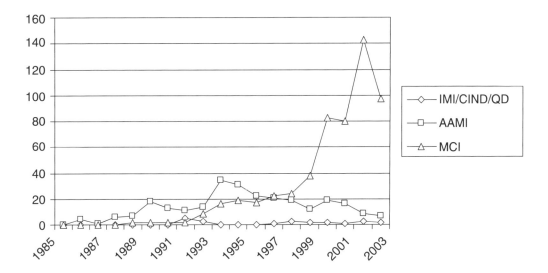

FIGURE 2.3. Frequency of studies of various boundary conditions as listed on MEDLINE and PsycINFO.

Questionable Dementia/Possible Dementia Prodrome

Prior to the evolution of the MCI concept, it was very difficult to label the growing numbers of elderly patients presenting to outpatient clinics when complaints included cognitive impairment, but formal diagnostic criteria for dementia were not met. For this reason, many groups began using a diagnostic category referred to as questionable dementia (QD), with which patients were classified if they obtained a Clinical Dementia Rating (CDR; Morris, 1993) score of 0.5. Longitudinal follow-ups of these patients yielded mixed outcomes; some researchers found good prognosis in QD groups (Reisberg, Ferris, Franssen, Kluger, & Borenstein, 1986; Youngjohn & Crook, 1993) whereas others showed full conversion from QD to Alzheimer's dementia (Hughes, Berg, Danziger, Cohen, & Martin, 1982; Rubin et al., 1993; Storandt & Hill, 1989). The heterogeneity of diagnostic outcomes emerging from the QD classification established the feasibility of clinical research programs aimed at defining specific clinical (and more specifically, cognitive) markers for improving diagnostic accuracy in AD and dementia.

Welsh-Bohmer and colleagues (Welsh-Bohmer, Hulette, Schmechel, Burke, & Saunders, 2001) and others have proposed that preclinical AD is characterized by a continuum of cognitive changes that is paralleled in course by a continuum of histopathological change representative of disease. Neuropsychological studies from the Consortium to Establish a Registry for Alzheimer's Disease (CERAD) and other groups have identified very specific cognitive markers for Alzheimer's-type dementia prodromes. Unsurprisingly, recent memory measures (particularly those requiring delayed free recall) appear to be most sensitive in identifying possible dementia prodromes (Welsh et al., 1991; Welsh, Butters, Hughes, Mohs, & Heyman, 1992). Most recently, Welsh-Bohmer and colleagues (2001) proposed that testing recent memory over multiple brief delays provides the greatest sensitivity in detecting possible AD prodromes.

Aging-Associated Cognitive Decline

The International Psychogeriatric Association and the World Health Organization criticized AAMI as a concept because it presumes that early malignant cognitive aging surfaces exclusively within the learning and memory domain, and not in other cognitive domains (Ritchie & Touchon, 2000). As an alternative to AAMI, the term "aging-associated cognitive decline" (AACD) was introduced (Levy, 1994) and defined by (1) performance on a standardized cognitive test that is at least one standard deviation below age-adjusted norms in at least one of any of the following cognitive domains: learning and memory, attention and cognitive speed, language, and visuoconstructional abilities; (2) exclusion of any medical, psychiatric, or neurological disorder that could cause cognitive impairment; and (3) normal activities of daily living and exclusion of dementia according to DSM-IV criteria. AACD differs from AAMI because it is defined by age-adjusted normative data, allows for cognitive impairment in cognitive domains other than memory, and allows for mild cognitive impairment in multiple cognitive domains. Recent work by Pantel, Kratz, Essig, and Schroder (2003) demonstrated that parahippocampal volumes in patients meeting AACD criteria were intermediate between cognitively intact elderly individuals and individuals meeting criteria for AD. As such, AACD criteria appear to be a feasible approach for establishing diagnostic criteria for preclinical or potentially prodromal Alzheimer's dementia.

Cognitive Impairment No Dementia

The Canadian Study of Health and Aging (CSHA) has utilized multicenter studies to characterize the epidemiology of cognitive impairment among Canadians ages 65 and older (Graham et al., 1997). A diagnostic concept known as "cognitive impairment no dementia" (CIND) has emerged in these population studies to describe individuals with demonstrated cognitive impairment (using a modified Mini-Mental State Examination cutoff score) but no clinical evidence of dementia. The CIND classification is a heterogeneous diagnostic category that is nonspecific with regard to etiology of cognitive impairment. CIND applies to individuals with delirium, chronic alcohol and drug use, depression, psychiatric illness, and mental retardation, although the most popular diagnostic subcategory of CIND relates to circumscribed memory impairment. The prevalence of CIND among the Canadian elderly is about twice that of all dementias combined (Graham et al., 1997). A recent longitudinal study revealed that despite etiological subcategories of CIND, individuals with CIND have higher rates of conversion to dementia, admission to facility care, and mortality than individuals without cognitive impairment (Tuokko et al., 2003). MCI has been recognized as a subcategory of CIND (Fisk, Merry, & Rockwood, 2003), but it remains unclear whether all etiological subcategories of CIND represent malignant cognitive change (i.e., prodromal stages of dementia).

Mild Cognitive Impairment

Flicker, Ferris, and Reisberg (1991) used the term mild cognitive impairment for a group scoring 3 on the Reisberg Global Deterioration Scale (Reisberg, Ferris, de Leon, & Crook, 1982). The score is based on clinician assessment/judgment and ranges from 1 (no impairment) to 7 (a vegetative state due to dementia). A score of 2 on this scale represents a subjective cognitive concern but no objective evidence of cognitive impairment. A score of 3 reflects the earliest clear deficits identified only upon intensive interview conducted by a trained clinician (Reisberg et al., 1982). These deficits are evident in the person who gets lost in unfamiliar environments, performances poorly at work, shows name-finding problems, loses objects of value, etc.

We (Petersen et al., 1995) adopted the term mild cognitive impairment (MCI) for studies of a boundary condition. At the level of the individual who will develop dementia, MCI was conceptualized as epoch in the longitudinal course of the disease, wherein cognition is no longer normal relative to age expectations, but also wherein daily function is not sufficiently disrupted to warrant the diagnosis of dementia. Figure 2.4 depicts this epoch. The initial clinical definition of MCI was proposed to include (1) the presence of a memory complaint, (2) the performance of normal activities of daily living, (3) evidence of normal global cognitive function, and (4) evidence of abnormal memory function compared to the age and education norms described in the first section of this chapter. A CDR (Morris, 1993) of 0.5 is used to corroborate the criteria. The ability to identify this group has been enhanced substantially by the MOANS studies.

With regard to groups of people, MCI constitutes that level of cognitive function wherein low-functioning normals and high-functioning dementia patients cannot be reliably distinguished. Figure 2.5 depicts this overlap. This figure is a bit misleading because it seems to suggest three different groups along the continuum of cognitive function. However, our initial concept of MCI was not as a "condition" present in the patient but as a state of uncertainty in the clinician. We conceived of all persons labeled as MCI as

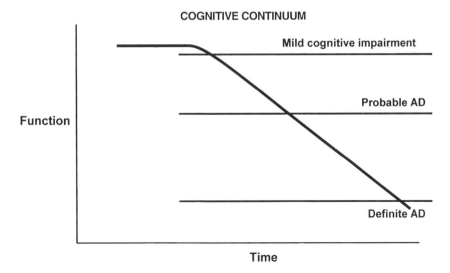

FIGURE 2.4. Theoretical trajectory for an individual progressing to Alzheimer's disease. From Petersen (2000). Copyright 2000 by Elseiver. Reproduced by permission.

belonging in either a normal population, not destined to develop dementia, or from a population that is developing dementia. Because we could not know from which group that individual arose, we turned to the MCI label to reflect our uncertainty. As it turns out, that state of uncertainty can be thought of as constituting a risk factor for the patient with regard to subsequent development of dementia.

We have found that, on average, persons with MCI have intermediate degrees of hippocampal atrophy impairment compared to controls and patients with AD (Jack et al., 1999), and intermediate changes in regional cerebral metabolic patterns (Kantarci et al., 2000). However, we note that these previously reported data represent mean values

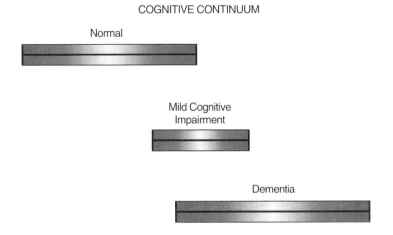

FIGURE 2.5. Mild cognitive impairment at the overlap of distributions of low normal cognitive function versus early dementia. Adapted from Petersen (1995). Copyright 1995 by Lippencott, Williams, & Wilkens. Adapted by permission.

TABLE 2.4. Comparison of Studies of Boundary Conditions

Study	Condition of interest	Annual conversion rate	Sampling method	Sampling frame	Memory tests	Other cognitive domains	Memory complaint
Petersen et al. (1999)	Mild cognitive impairment	12%	Community internal medicine practice	Community	Immediate and delayed recall of unstructured verbal material	Attention, language, visuospatial	Spontaneous
Goldman et al. (2001)	CDR –0.5 a. DAT b. incipient DAT c. Questionable dementia	a. 12% B. 7% C. 4%	Advertisement solicited volunteers	Convenience	None (only immediate structured recall in other research)	None	Spontaneous
Ritchie et al. (2001)	a. "MCI" b. age-associated cognitive decline	a. 6.5% b. 28%	General practitioner network	Population	Immediate and delayed recall of structured verbal material	Attention, language, visuospatial	Solicited
Albert et al. (2001)	Questionable dementia	6%	Advertisement solicited volunteers	Convenience	Immediate and delayed recall of structured and unstructured verbal material	Attention, language, visuospatial, executive function	Not required

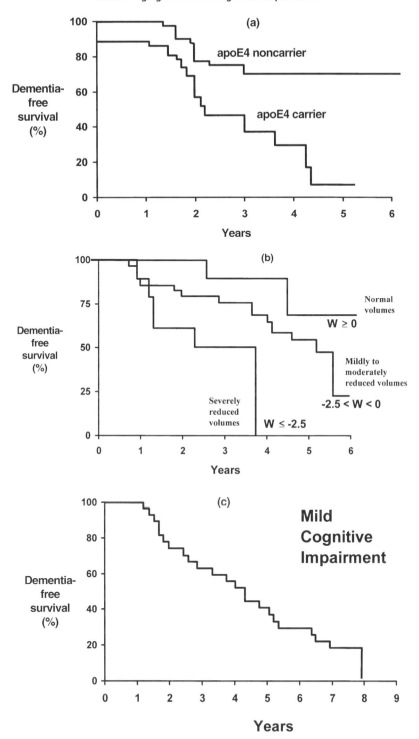

FIGURE 2.6. Survival time from MCI to dementia diagnosis by risk factor (a) by apoE status, (b) by hippocampal volume, and for (c) overall MCI group. Peterson (2001). Copyright 2001 by Wiley. Reproduced by permission.

and could reflect average measurements taken from patients developing dementia with those of normals. We have also found that patients with MCI show similar apolipo-protein E allelic frequencies to patients with AD (Petersen et al., 1995). Finally we have found that these same neuroimaging and genetic variables help predict progression to de-mentia. See Figure 2.6.

In following their group of patients with MCI, Flicker et al. (1991) found a conver-sion rate to the full syndrome of dementia of approximately 72% over 2 years of follow-up. Our conversion rate is about 12% per year over the initial 7 years of follow-up (see Figure 2.6c). An age- and gender-matched group of normal controls had only a 5% rate of developing cognitive impairment in the comparable interval (Petersen et al., 1995). Other researchers have found progression to dementia rates ranging from 6 to 28%. A summary of selected studies is provided in Table 2.4. A review of this literature reveals at least four important dimensions along which studies of boundary conditions must be compared in order to understand their discrepant findings: (1) the population sampled, (2) the nature of memory complaint, (3) the types of memory assessment used, and (4) the number and type of other cognitive domains assessed.

Population Sampled

It is important to distinguish MCI studies that use clinical samples from studies for which MCI "patients" are culled from a population sample or a normal volunteer sample of older adults. Our studies, and those of several others (e.g., Bowen et al., 1997; Tierney et al., 1996), have used clinical samples. The fact that a clinical concern exists for these pa-tients increases the likelihood that they are drawn for the predementia group shown in Figure 2.5.

Other studies of boundary conditions have identified their cohorts by recruiting nor-mal older adults (e.g., Albert, Moss, Tanzi, & Jones, 2001; Ritchie & Touchon, 2000). These samples are composed of individuals who either served as controls in clinical trials or longitudinal aging studies, or were selected as a community sample of older adults in order to describe cognitive function in a group conceived to be representative of older adults from the general U.S. population. MCI "patients" are often culled from these nor-mal samples by using a psychometric cutoff based on their memory performance. Thus, by definition, normal patients scoring at the lowest end of the memory score distributions receive a diagnosis of MCI. Selection in this fashion necessarily increases the likelihood that these MCI patients arise from the normal population rather than from a cognitively impaired population, as depicted in Figure 2.5.

Nature of Memory Complaint

The Mayo criteria for MCI (Petersen et al., 1999) propose that a memory complaint must be present. Differences in the nature of memory complaints across studies are a corollary of differences in recruitment methods. In clinical samples, memory complaints are gener-ally "spontaneous." Complaints arise as a concern from some member of the health care process (e.g., patient, family, provider). Such memory concerns, especially from family or physicians, may have a better correspondence with objectively established cognitive dys-function (cf. Carr, Gray, Baty, & Morris, 2000). In studies that recruit general or normal samples, a memory complaint is typically established by administration of standardized subjective ratings of memory function. Numerous studies have demonstrated that scores on such instruments are more likely to be associated with mood or self-efficacy than with actual cognitive dysfunction (Smith, Petersen, Ivnik, Malec, & Tangalos, 1996; Taylor, Miller, & Tinklenberg, 1992)

Nature of Memory Assessment

Another key difference across studies of boundary conditions involves the manner in which memory is assessed. The term *memory impairment* has been used to describe a wide variety of cognitive impairments that may have different neural substrates. Most studies have focused on episodic memory. However, even within the realm of episodic memory, differences may exist in the extent to which impairments are associated with risk for subsequent decline to dementia. It may be important to distinguish between encoding and retrieval phases of memory tasks. Encoding is typically assessed by aspects of immediate recall, whereas retrieval is assessed by delayed recall. The encoding phase of memory is sensitive to aging effects alone, but may be insensitive for detecting incipient dementia relative to indices of delayed recall (Petersen, Smith, Kokmen, Ivnik, & Tangalos, 1992; Petersen et al., 1994). For example, a recent study of nine people who died and were observed to have healthy brains, compared to five people who were nondemented at death but observed to have Alzheimer's disease changes in the brain, revealed no difference in the cognitive profiles between groups. However, all memory test scores in this very small study focused on immediate recall (Goldman et al., 2001). Numerous studies suggest that delayed recall measures appear to be most sensitive for early discrimination of dementia (Bondi et al., 1994; Ivnik et al., 2000; Tierney et al., 1996). Studies that focus on immediate recall (encoding) versus delayed recall (retrieval) in establishing the memory impairment criteria for MCI may engender very different samples.

Number and Type of Cognitive Domains Assessed

The number and type of non-memory-related cognitive domains assessed in studies of MCI are important because MCI criteria typically stipulate "no dementia." Commonly accepted dementia criteria require impairment in at least two cognitive domains. Because MCI patients have memory impairment, rigid statistical applications of dementia criteria exclude from MCI samples any person with scores falling below some cutoff in any non-memory-related domain. As the number of non-memory-related measures assessed in a given individual increases, there is an increasing probability that at least one other cognitive measure will fall below a given cutoff by chance alone. Because all cognitive domains tend to be correlated to at least a moderate degree, excluding nondemented persons with memory impairment from MCI samples because of low scores in other domains increases the probability that the memory scores for those patients are spuriously low. A study by Ritchie, Artero, and Touchon (2001) provides an example of this problem. In this study, seven non-memory-related domains were assessed. Seventy-five percent of persons with a (loosely defined) memory impairment (scores < −1 standard deviation below age norms) also had at least one non-memory-related score fall below this cutoff. Of the remaining 25% of "MCI" patients, only 7% continued to have memory scores below their cutoff at follow-up. By excluding persons with modestly low non-memory-related scores from their sample, these investigators appeared to exclude persons with true memory impairments.

The common finding that MCI patients show poor performance on sensitive measures in other cognitive domains as well as the relatively common presentation of persons with isolated cognitive concerns in non-memory-related domains has led to an evolution in the concept of mild cognitive impairment.

EVOLUTION OF THE MCI CONCEPT

Of course, not all dementia is Alzheimer's disease, so the idea that MCI could include only memory problems was quickly recognized to be a limitation of the concept (Petersen et al., 2001). For example, we know that early in subcortical dementias such as Parkinson's dementia, memory is spared but basic attention and processing speed are compromised. This knowledge led to the recognition of the need to broaden the concept of MCI to include presentations that are not amnestic or not exclusively amnestic in nature. Petersen and colleagues (2001) proposed at least three subtypes of MCI. All forms of MCI include basic criteria of (1) normal general cognitive functioning, (2) normal activities of daily living, and (3) no dementia. The three subtypes are suggested as follow:

1. Amnestic MCI (aMCI)
   - Memory complaint
   - Memory impaired for age
2. Single non-memory-domain MCI (sMCI)
   - Impairment in one of the following cognitive domains:
     - Attention/concentration
     - Executive functioning
     - Language functioning
     - Visuospatial functioning
3. Multiple-domain MCI (mMCI)
   - Two or more impaired domains, often including memory

Although this conceptualization of MCI is relatively new, preliminary studies argue that multiple-domain MCI and single non-memory-domain MCI may be more common than amnestic MCI (Lopez, Kuller, DeKosky, & Becker, 2002). Single and multi-domain MCIs with an amnestic component progress at roughly equal rates to AD (Petersen et al., 2004). Nonamnestic MCI is also a risk factor for AD but may give rise to non-AD dementias, such as Lewy body dementia or frontotemporal dementia more commonly than does amnestic MCI (Boeve, Ferman, Smith, et al., 2004, Ferman et al., 2005; Petersen et al., 2002).

With regard to multiple-domain MCI, an astute observer will ask, "How can a person have scores in the impaired range in two cognitive domains and not have dementia?" Two fundamental principles of neuropsychology are relevant in this regard. First, a low score is not necessarily equal an impairment. A certain percentage of the normal population scores below clinical cutoffs on any measure. If the cutoff is liberally set at –1 standard deviation, as in the Ritchie study cited above, 16% of the general population will fall below the cutoff. In persons with appropriate histories (e.g., low academic attainment, low IQ), it is entirely possible for a score below this cutoff to be deemed clinically normal for those individuals. *Dementia criteria require a decline from a higher level of cognitive function.* The second fundamental issue is that low scores on tests do not necessarily imply "significant impairment in social or occupational functioning" (American

Psychiatric Association, 1994). There are plenty of people who live normal day-to-day lives who would "fail" the Wisconsin Card Sorting Test.

NOT ALL MCI IS EARLY DEMENTIA: A CAUTIONARY NOTE

If all aMCI and most mMCI patients converted to AD, than it might be unnecessary to have a concept of MCI at all. Morris et al. (1991) and others have argued that MCI is simply early AD and that clinicians need to be brave enough to say so. These investigators base this opinion, in part, on their neuropathological study of 10 patients who died with questionable dementia. In all 10 cases there was sufficient neuropathological burden to justify the CERAD (Gearing et al., 1995; Mirra et al., 1991) diagnosis of AD. However, the neuropathological substrate of MCI is not fully known. We (Jicha et al., in press) studied 15 Mayo Alzheimer's Disease Patient Registry cases who died while their clinical classification was still aMCI. The brains were processed using standard neuropathological techniques and classified according to Katchaturian (1985), CERAD (Mirra et al., 1991), and the National Institute on Aging—Reagan (Hyman & Trojanowski, 1997) neuropathological criteria. Eight of these cases did not meet any of the three neuropathological criteria for AD, although their pathology suggested a transitional state of evolving AD. In addition, there was a great deal of concomitant pathology, including argyrophilic grain disease, hippocampal sclerosis, and vascular lesions. One of these 15 subjects had no identifiable neuropathology. These findings would argue that is not appropriate to simply conclude that all MCI, including aMCI, is simply early AD. In addi-

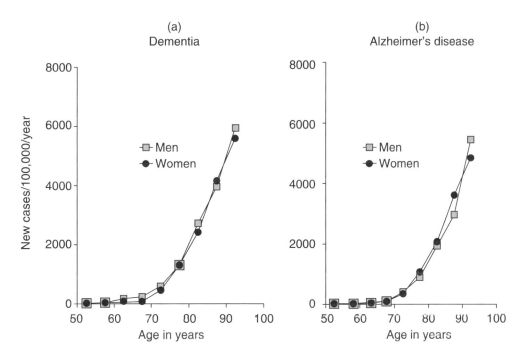

FIGURE 2.7. (a) Incidence of dementia by age group and gender; (b) incidence of Alzheimer's disease by age group and gender. Edland et al. (2002). Copyright 2002 by the American Medical Association. Reproduced by permission.

tion, these neuropathological findings suggest that MCI is not just a state of uncertainty in the clinician, but that the clinical syndrome of MCI may reflect a transitional neuropathological state in many but not all patients. If it is ultimately possible to arrest the development of neuropathology at this point, it would be tantamount to preventing dementia. As such, maintaining the concept of a boundary condition seems valuable.

Incidence of Dementia and Prevalence of MCI

The prevalence (number of cases at a given point in time) of MCI has not been well established. In contrast, the annual incidence (number of new cases in a year) of dementia in the over-65 population is well established at 1–2% (Edland, Rocca, Petersen, Cha, & Kokmen, 2002). This incidence is strongly associated with age (see Figure 2.7). We also believe that about 12% of MCI patients will progress to dementia per year (Figure 2.6c) and that 7–10% of MCI patients will not show a progressive neuropathology at autopsy. If we assume that all dementia patients will pass through the MCI state before displaying dementia, then we can use the percentages above to estimate MCI prevalence. Estimated prevalence of MCI that will progress to dementia would be 1–2% divided by 12% or 8.3–16.6%. Total prevalence would then be 8.3–16.6% divided by (roughly) 90%, which results in an estimated prevalence of 9–18%.

A few studies have investigated the prevalence of MCI and MCI-like conditions (Bennett et al., 2002; Larrieu et al., 2002; Lopez et al., 2002). The prevalence varies widely from 3 to 54% mainly because of the different methods and criteria used. The Cardiovascular Health Study (CHS) evaluated several definitions of MCI in their nondemented cohort (ages 65 years and older) and provided useful prevalence figures (Lopez et al., 2002). The CHS included amnestic and multiple-domain MCIs defined in a very similar fashion to that above. They concluded that the prevalence of MCI among nondemented individuals was 19%, and that it increased with increasing age. These results are strikingly similar to the estimate of MCI prevalence calculated above. In addition, they found a ratio of 2.5:1 for the prevalence of multiple-domain-type MCI (which included memory impairment) compared to amnestic MCI (Lopez et al., 2002). The CHS findings provide preliminary support for the idea that almost all dementia patients pass through the MCI state, and possibly for the idea that MCI cohorts should include a proportion of people that will not develop dementia.

OTHER RISK FACTORS FOR DEMENTIA

As we have noted, certain patterns of cognitive function, described as MCI, may signal the presence of malignant brain changes. These syndromes identify increased risk for a dementia process. Several other risk factors for dementia are known or postulated.

Age

Age is typically thought of as the least equivocal risk factor for dementia. However, at least three studies (Breitner et al., 1999; Ritchie, Kildea, & Robine, 1992; Wernicke & Reischies, 1994) have suggested that the prevalence of dementia and AD increases exponentially up to age 80 or 85 years but then either remains stable or declines. A number of prevalence studies do not support this hypothesis, either for dementia (Hofman et al., 1991) or for AD (Rocca et al., 1991). Moreover, because prevalence reflects the combination of incidence and survival, prevalence can be a misleading statistic in terms of risk (as explained below). We think of "risk" as more associated with the chance of "developing" a disorder (incidence) as opposed to the chance of "having" a disorder (prevalence). Thus information on age and incidence is desirable. Unfortunately, information on incidence of dementia and AD past age 80 years is more limited. Incidence rates from three European studies (Brayne et al., 1995; Fratiglioni et al., 1997; Letenneur, Commenges, Dartigues, & Barberger-Gateau, 1994) and the Framingham study (Bachman et al., 1993) consistently show a continuing increase in the incidence of AD at extreme ages. As shown in Figure 2.7 above, there is a continuous increase in incidence with age (Edland et al., 2002). Data from the Cache County, Utah study showed an increased incidence of dementia and AD until ages 85–90, with a decline in incidence around age 93 for men and age 97 for women (Miech et al., 2002). Finer-grained analyses suggested that an interaction between age and the apolipoprotein E (apoE) genotype further influences AD incidence; homozygous E4 carriers demonstrated accelerated onset of AD compared to non-E4 carriers. Heterozygous E4 carriers also demonstrated accelerated onset of AD compared to non-E4 carriers, although the acceleration effect was more modest than that observed for homozygotes.

Gender

We noted above that prevalence data may be misleading when considering risk factors because prevalence reflects the combination of incidence and survival. Thus a factor (such as gender) will increase prevalence through its impact on survival rather than increasing incidence (i.e., risk). The prevalence of AD appears higher in women than in men (Breteler, Claus, van Duijn, Launer, & Hofman, 1992; Rocca et al., 1991). The Cache County study showed that the prevalence of AD appears higher in women than men, specifically when women are positive for the E4 allele of apoE (Breitner et al., 1999). The Framingham study did not show higher age-specific incidence rates in women; the sex pattern was inconsistent over age (Bachman et al., 1993). As shown in Figure 2.7, Mayo data reveal an inconsistent sex pattern over age and, in general, small differences in incidence between men and women (Edland et al., 2002). On the other hand, Fratiglioni and colleagues (1997) showed a consistently higher incidence of AD in women from Stockholm, Sweden. Data from the Cache County study showed that the incidence of AD after age 90 is higher among women than men, despite the fact that the incidence of AD after age 90 declines for both men and women (Miech et al., 2002).

Head Injury

Numerous population-based studies (Graves et al., 1990; Heyman et al., 1984; Mayeux, Ottman, et al., 1993; Mayeuz et al., 1995; Mortimer, French, Hutton, & Schuman, 1985; Van Duijn et al., 1992) and case-control studies (Fleminger, Oliver, Lovestone, Rabe-Hesketh, & Giora, 2003; Mortimer et al., 1991; Van Duijn et al., 1994) have indicated an association between history of traumatic brain injury (TBI) and risk of Alzheimer's disease or other dementias. Other case–control studies have failed to show an association (Broe et al., 1990; Chandra, Kokmen, Schoenberg, & Beard, 1989; Ferini-Strambi, Smirne, Garancini, Pinto, & Franceschi, 1990; Fratiglinoni, Ahlbom, Viitanen, & Winblad, 1993). Longitudinal studies are also mixed (Katzman et al., 1989; Launer et al., 1999; Schofield et al., 1997; Williams, Annegers, Kokmen, O'Brien, & Kurland, 1991). Several prospective studies of cognitive decline after TBI suggest the possibility of long-term cognitive decline (Corkin, Rosen, Sullivan, & Clegg, 1989; Plassman et al., 2000; Walker & Blumer, 1989).

The findings of several studies suggest that history of TBI may shorten time to onset of AD in persons who were predisposed to develop the condition (Gedye, Beattie, Tuoko, Horton, & Korsarek, 1989; Nemetz et al., 1998; Schofield et al., 1997). Nemetz and colleagues (1998) used the population-based resources of the Rochester Epidemiology Project to examine whether persons with a history of TBI had reduced time to onset of AD among persons at risk of developing AD. Although a similar proportion of persons with TBI as without TBI developed AD, the observed time from TBI to AD was significantly less than the expected time to onset of AD (median = 10 years vs. 18 years). Schofield and colleagues (1997) suggested a time-dependent relationship between TBI and AD. Persons with a history of TBI within the past 30 years were diagnosed with AD at a younger age than those with remote history of TBI (greater than 30 years). The role of head injury as a risk factor for dementia remains unclear.

Genetics

At the time of this writing, there are three genetic mutations that appear to have a causative link to AD. These genes are the APP gene on chromosome 21, the presenilin 1 gene on Chromosome 14, and the presenilin 2 gene on chromosome 1. In addition, a few other genes have been identified that cause related forms of dementia. For example, mutations on chromosome 17 cause a form of frontotemporal dementia (Hutton, 2001; Hutton et al., 1998). These genetic mutations occur in only a small number of families. Thus it is estimated that these genes explain less than 5% of all the AD present in the world today (Bird, 1994). These gene mutations are called *causative* because whenever the genetic mutation is present, and the carrier of the gene lives to the age of risk, he or she invariably develops dementia. Moreover, members of the family who live through the age of risk without developing dementia are not carriers. All of the AD causative gene mutations are associated with early onset (AD occurring before the age of 65). The identification of these genes is significant because it demonstrates that AD can have a genetic etiology. It is possible that a portion of the common late-onset form of AD will have a genetic cause as well.

In addition to genetic mutations that apparently cause AD, at least one genetic variation has been identified that increases AD susceptibility to AD: the apoE gene on chromosome 19 (Strittmatter et al., 1993). This gene has three common forms, labeled E2, E3, and E4. People who possess the E4 genotype are at increased risk for developing AD. However, unlike causative genes, some people with the E4 genotype do live through the age of risk without developing AD. Moreover, over 45% of people with late-onset AD do not carry the E4 genotype. Thus the E4 genotype is neither necessary nor sufficient for development of AD. Still, inheriting one E4 gene increases risk for AD approximately 4 times, and inheriting two E4 genes increases risk on the order of 16 times. Identifying such a significant increased risk for AD may justify intervention E4 carriers before signs of dementia emerge.

Whether the apoE genotype directly influences cognitive function remains a source of debate. Studies have shown that by the time of diagnosis there is a genotype effect on persons with AD such that memory performance is more impaired in E4 carriers (Smith et al., 1998). Several reports have also suggested that in persons who are older than 50 years (i.e., less than two decades from age of risk), E4 carriers perform more poorly on memory and executive function tests. However, these differences may disappear when persons who subsequently develop dementia are removed from the sample (Bondi, Salmon, Galasko, Thomas, & Thal, 1999). Whether or not cognitive differences exist in E4 carriers younger than 50 years of age is equivocal. Reiman et al. (1996) report deficits on reduced cerebral glucose metabolism in the cingulate and prefrontal cortex in E4 homozygotes. Some researchers have postulated that differences may exist in genetic carriers that cannot be detected on crude neuropsychological measures alone. The concept is that persons at risk muster equivalent performance but have to "work harder" to do so (Bookheimer et al., 2000).

CONCLUSIONS

Cognitive aging typically involves a reduction of processing speed or "cognitive efficiency." Longitudinal cognitive aging studies and normative neuropsychological studies with older persons have enhanced our ability to distinguish typical cognitive aging from early signs of neurodegenerative diseases associated with aging.

Boundary concepts remain important to dementia research and clinical practice. One such concept, MCI, appears associated with biomarkers of AD even before patients meet AD criteria. MCI patients are at elevated risk for progressing to dementia. MCI samples are probably comprised of patients with incipient dementia, persons with static neuropathology, *and* normal older persons with poor cognitive function. The relative proportion of each group in an MCI sample will be influenced by the sampling frame (clinical vs. general or normal), the nature of the memory complaint (spontaneous vs. elicited), the type of memory assessment used in selecting patients (e.g., immediate vs. delayed recall) and the number, type, and interpretation of measures of non-memory-related domains. These factors need to be considered when comparing outcomes from studies of boundary conditions.

Using a boundary group conceptualization avoids the problem of knowing for sure whether a person at the boundary between normal and dementia has a disease entity or not. It enables an alternative to attempts to predict which individual normal people will develop dementia. Instead, boundary conditions themselves can be diagnosed. These diagnoses acknowledge the overlapping distributions but still identify risk status. Identifying persons in this way would not preclude their involvement in intervention research. In fact, being able to identify such persons may give impetus to early intervention research. In DSM-IV (American Psychiatric Association, 1994) "mild neurocognitive disorder" (MND) is listed as a diagnosis for future consideration. This concept is congruent with the idea of a boundary area or preclinical status. The DSM criteria for mild neurocognitive disorder are similar but not identical to MCI. Regardless of whether the CIND, MCI, MND, or other labels and criteria ultimately gain widest acceptance, there is likely to be substantial research and clinical benefit to including a boundary condition as a "legitimate" diagnosis in the next DSM.

REFERENCES

Albert, M. S., Moss, M. B., Tanzi, R., & Jones, K. (2001). Preclinical prediction of AD using neuropsychological Tests. *Journal of the International Neuropsychological Society, 7*, 639–639.

American Psychiatric Association. (1994). *Diagnostic and Statistical Manual of Mental Disorders— Fourth Edition*. Washington, DC: Author.

Bachman, D. L., Wolf, P. A., Linn, R. T., Knoefel, J. E., Cobb, J. L., Belanger, A. J., White, L. R., & D'Agostino, R. B. (1993). Incidence of dementia and probable Alzheimer's disease in a general population: The Framingham study. *Neurology, 43*, 515–519.

Becker, J. T., Boller, F., Saxton, J., & McGonigle-Gibson, K. L. (1987). Normal rates of forgetting of verbal and non-verbal material in Alzheimer's disease. *Cortex, 23*, 59–72.

Bennett, D. A., Wilson, R. S., Schneidre, J. A., Evans, D. A., Beckett, L. A., Aggarw, N. T., et al. (2002). Natural history of mild cognitive impairment in older persons. *Neurology, 59*, 198–205.

Benton, A. L., & Hamsher, K. (1978). *Multilingual aphasia examination: Manual.* Iowa City: University of Iowa.

Benton, A. L., Hamsher, K., Varney, N. R., & Spreen, O. (1983). *Contributions to neuropsychological assessment.* New York: Oxford University Press.

Berg, L. (1992). Detection of early (very mild) Alzheimer's disease. In J. E. Morley, R. M. Coe, R. Strong, & G. T. Grossberg (Eds.), *Memory function and aging-related disorders* (pp. 223–236). New York: Springer.

Bird, T. D. (1994). Clinical genetics of familial Alzheimer's disease. In R. D. Terry, R. Katzman, & K. L. Bick (Eds.), *Alzheimers disease* (pp. 65–74). New York: Raven Press.

Blackford, R. C., & LaRue, A. (1989). Criteria for diagnosing age associated memory impairment. *Developmental Neuropsychology, 5*, 295–306.

Boeve, B. F., Ferman, T. J., Smith, G. E., Knopman, D. S., Jicha, G. A., Gela, Y., et al. (2004). Mild cognitive impairment preceding dementia with Lewy bodies. *Neurology* (abstract), *62*, A86S.

Bondi, M., Monsch, A., Galasko, D., Butters, N., Salmon, D., & Delis, D. (1994). Preclinical cognitive markers of dementia of the Alzheimer's type. *Neuropsychology, 8*, 374–384.

Bondi, M. W., Salmon, D. P., Galasko, D., Thomas, R. J., & Thal, L. J. (1999). Neuropsychological function and apolipoprotein E genotype in the preclinical detection of Alzheimer's disease. *Psychology and Aging, 14*, 295–303.

Bookheimer, S. Y., Strojwas, M. H., Cohen, M. S., Saunders, A. M., Pericak-Vance, M. A., Mazziotta, J. C., et al. (2000). Patterns of brain activation in people at risk for Alzheimer's disease. *New England Journal of Medicine, 343*, 450–456.

Bowen, J., Teri, L., Kukall, W., McCormick, W., McCurry, S. M., & Larson, E. B. (1997). Progression to dementia in patients with isolated memory loss. *Lancet, 349*, 763–765.

Brayne, C., Gill, C., Huppert, F. A., Barkley, C., Gehlhaar, E., Girling, D. M., et al. (1995). Incidence of clinically diagnosed subtypes of dementia in an elderly population: Cambridge project for later life. *British Journal of Psychiatry, 167*, 255–262.

Brebion, G., Smith, M. J., & Ehrlich, M. F. (1997). Working memory and aging: Deficit or strategy differences. *Aging, Neuropsychology, and Cognition, 4*, 58–73.

Breiman, L., Friedman, J. H., Olshen, R. A., & Stone, C. J. (1984*). Classification and regression trees.* Pacific Grove, CA: Wadsworth & Brooks.

Breitner, J. C. S., Wyse, B. W., Anthony, J. C., Welsh-Bohmer, K. A., Steffens, D. C., Norton, M. C., et al. (1999). APOE ε4 count predicts age when prevalence of AD increases, then declines: The Cache County Study. *Neurology, 53*, 321–331.

Breteler, M. M., Claus, J. J., van Duijn, C. M., Launer, L. J., & Hofman, A. (1992). Epidemiology of Alzheimer's disease. *Epidemiologic Reviews, 14*, 59–82.

Broe, G. A., Henderson, A. S., Creasey, H., McCusker, E., Korten, Λ. E., Jorm, A. F., et al. (1990). A case-control study of Alzheimer's disease in Australia. *Neurology, 40*, 1698–1707.

Caccappolo-van Vliet, E., Manly, J., Tang, M., Marder, K., Bell, K., & Stern, Y. (2003). The neuropsychological profiles of mild Alzheimer's disease and questionable dementia as related to age-related cognitive decline. *Journal of the International Neuropsychological Society, 9*, 720–732.

Carr, D. B., Gray, S., Baty, J., & Morris, J. C. (2000). The value of informant versus individual's complaints of memory impairment in early dementia. *Neurology, 55*, 1724–1727.

Cerhan, J. H., Ivnik, R. J., Smith, G. E., Tangalos, E. C., Petersen, R. C., & Boeve, B. F. (2002). Diagnostic utility of letter fluency, category fluency, and fluency difference scores in Alzheimer's disease. *Clinical Neuropsychologist, 16,* 35–42.

Chandra, V., Kokmen, E., Schoenberg, B. S., & Beard, C. M. (1989). Head trauma with loss of consciousness as a risk factor for Alzheimer's disease. *Neurology, 39,* 1576–1578.

Colcombe, S. J., Erickson, K. I., Raz, N., Webb, A. G., Cohen, N. J., McAuely, E., et al. (2003). Aerobic fitness reduces brain tissue loss in humans. *Journal of Gerontology Series A—Biological and Medical Sciences, 58,* 176–180.

Colcombe, S. J., & Kramer, A. F. (2003). Fitness effects on the cognitive function of older adults: A meta-analytic study. *Psychological Science, 14,* 125–130.

Corkin, S., Rosen, T. J., Sullivan, E. V., & Clegg, R. A. (1989). Penetrating head injury in young adulthood exacerbates cognitive decline in later years. *The Journal of Neuroscience, 9,* 3876–3883.

Crook, T., Bartus, R. T., Ferris, S. H., Whitehouse, P., Cohen, G. D., & Gershon, S. (1986). Age-associated memory impairment: Proposed diagnostic criteria and measures of clinical change. Report of a National Institute of Mental Health Work Group. *Developmental Neuropsychology, 2,* 261–276.

Devanand, D. P., Folz, M., Gorlyn, M., Moeller, J. R., & Stern, Y. (1997). Questionable dementia: Clinical course and predictors of outcome. *Journal of the American Geriatrics Society, 45,* 321–328.

Edland, S. D., Rocca, W. A., Petersen, R. C., Cha, R. H., & Kokmen, E. (2002). Dementia and Alzheimer's disease incident rates do not vary by sex in Rochester, Minnesota. *Archives of Neurology, 59,* 1589–1593.

Ferini-Strambi, L., Smirne, S., Garancini, P., Pinto, P., & Franceschi, M. (1990). Clinical and epidemiological aspects of Alzheimer's disease with presenile onset: A case control study. *Neuroepidemiology, 9,* 39–49.

Ferman, T. J., Lucas, J. A., Ivnik, R. J., Smith, G. E., Willis, F. B., Petersen, R. C., et al. (2005). Mayo's Older African American Normative Studies: Auditory Verbal Learning Test norms for African American elders. *The Clinical Neuropsychologist, 19,* 214–228.

Ferman, T. J., Smith, G. E., Boeve, B. F., Graff-Radford, N., Lucas, J., Knopman, D., et al. (in press). Neuropsychological differentiation of dementia with Lewy bodies from normal aging and Alzheimer's disease. *The Clinical Neuropsychologist.*

Fillit, H. M., Butler, R. N., O'Connell, A. W., Albert, M. S., Birren, J. E., Cotman, C. W., et al. (2002). Achieving and maintaining cognitive vitality with aging. *Mayo Clinic Proceedings, 77,* 681–696.

Finkel, D., & Pederson, N. L. (2000). Contribution of age, genes, and environment to the relationship between perceptual speed and cognitive ability. *Psychology and Aging, 15,* 56–64.

Fisher, D. L., Duffy, S. A., & Katskiopoulos, K. V. (2000). Cognitive slowing among older adults: What kind and how much? In T. J. Perfect & E. A. Maylor (Eds.), *Models of cognitive aging: Debates in Psychology* (pp. 87–124). New York: Oxford University Press.

Fisk, J. D., Merry, H. R., & Rockwood, K. (2003). Variations in case definition affect prevalence but not outcomes of mild cognitive impairment. *Neurology, 61,* 1179–1184.

Fleminger, S., Oliver, D. L., Lovestone, S., Rabe-Hesketh, S., & Giora, A. (2003). Head injury as a risk factor for Alzheimer's disease: The evidence 10 years on; a partial replication. *Journal of Neurology, Neurosurgery, and Psychiatry, 74,* 857–862.

Flicker, C., Ferris, S. H., & Reisberg, B. (1991). Mild cognitive impairment in the elderly: Predictors of dementia. *Neurology, 41,* 1006–1009.

Fratiglioni, L., Ahlbom, A., Viitanen, M., & Winblad, B. (1993). Risk factors for late-onset Alzheimer's disease: A population-based, case-control study. *Annals of Neurology, 33,* 258–266.

Fratiglioni, L., Viitanen, M., von Strauss, E., Tontodonati, V., Herlitz, A., & Winblad, B. (1997). Very old women at highest risk of dementia and Alzheimer's disease: Incidence data from the Kungsholmen Project, Stockholm. *Neurology, 48,* 132–138.

Frieske, D. A., & Park, D. C. (1999). Memory for news in young and old adults. *Psychology and Aging, 14,* 90–98.

Gearing, M., Mirra, S. S., Hedreen, J. C., Sumi, S. N., Hansen, L. A., & Heyman, A. (1995). The Consortium to Establish a Registry for Alzheimer's Disease (CERAD): Part X. Neuropathology confirmation of the clinical diagnosis of Alzheimer's disease. *Neurology, 45,* 461–466.

Gedye, A., Beattie, B. L., Tuokko, H., Horton, A., & Korsarek, E. (1989). Severe head injury hastens age of onset of Alzheimer's disease. *Journal of the American Geriatrics Society, 37*, 970–973.

Golden, C. J. (1978). *The Stroop Color and Word Test (Manual).* Chicago: Stoelting.

Goldman, W. P., Price, J. L., Storandt, M., Grant, E. A., McKeel, D. W., Jr., Rubin, E. H., et al. (2001). Absence of cognitive impairment or decline in preclinical Alzheimer's disease. *Neurology, 56*, 361–367.

Graham, J. E., Rockwood, K., Beattie, B. L., Eastwood, R., Gauthier, S., Tuokko H., et al. (1997). Prevalence and severity of cognitive impairment with and without dementia in an elderly population. *Lancet, 349*, 1793–1796.

Graves, A. B., White, E., Koepsell, T. D., Reifler, B. V., van Belle, G., Larson, E. B., et al. (1990). The association between head trauma and Alzheimer's disease. *American Journal of Epidemiology, 131*, 491–501.

Grober, E., & Buschke, H. (1987). Genuine memory deficits in dementia. *Developmental Neuropsychology, 3*, 13–36.

Grober, E., & Sliwinski, M. (1991). Development and validation of a model for estimating premorbid verbal intelligence in the elderly. *Journal of Clinical and Experimental Neuropsychology, 13*, 933–949.

Harris, M. E., Ivnik, R. J., & Smith, G. E. (2002). Mayo's Older Americans' Normative Studies: Expanded AVLT recognition trials norms for ages 57–98. *Journal of Clinical and Experimental Psychology, 24*, 214–220.

Hertzog, C., & Bleckley, M. K. (2001). Age differences in the structure of intelligence: Influences of information processing speed. *Intelligence, 29*, 191–217.

Heyman, A., Wilkinson, W. E., Stafford, J. A., Helms, M. J., Sigmon, A. H., & Weinberg, T. (1984). Alzheimer's disease: A study of epidemiological aspects. *Annals of Neurology, 15*, 335–341.

Hofman, A., Rocca, W. A., Brayne, C., Breteler, M. M., Clarke, M., Coopoer, B., et al. (1991). The prevalence of dementia in Europe: A collaborative study of 1980–1990 findings. *International Journal of Epidemiology, 20*, 736–748.

Hughes, C. P., Berg, L., Danziger, W. L., Cohen, L. A., & Martin, R. L. (1982). A new clinical scale for the staging of dementia. *British Journal of Psychiatry, 140*, 566–572.

Hutton, M. (2001). Missense and 5'-splice-site mutations in tau associated with FTDP-17: Multiple pathogenic mechanisms. *Neurology, 56*, S21–S25.

Hutton, M., Lendon, C. L., Rizzu, P., Baker, M., Froelich, S., Houlden, H., et al. (1998). Association of missense and 5'-splice-site mutations in tau with the inherited dementia FTDP-17. *Nature, 18*, 702–705.

Hyman, B. T., & Trojanowski, J. Q. (1997). Consensus recommendations for the postmortem diagnosis of Alzheimer's disease from the National Institute on Aging and the Reagan Institute Working Group on diagnostic criteria for the neuropathological assessment of Alzheimer's disease. *Journal of Neuropathology and Experimental Neurology, 56*, 1095–1097.

Ivnik, R. J., Malec, J. F., Smith, G. E., Tangalos, E. G., Petersen, R. C., Kokmen, E., et al. (1992). Mayo's Older Americans Normative Studies: WAIS-R, WMS-R and AVLT norms for ages 56 through 97. *Clinical Neuropsychologist, 6*(Suppl.), 1–104.

Ivnik, R. J., Malec, J. F., Smith, G. E., Tangalos, E. G., & Crook, T. H. (1996). Neuropsychological Tests' norms above age 55: COWAT, BNT, MAE Token, WRAT-R Reading, AMNART, STROOP, TMT and JLO. *Clinical Neuropsychologist, 10*, 262–278.

Ivnik, R. J., Smith, G. E., Lucas, J. A., Tangalos, E. G., Peterscn, R. C., & Kokmen, E. (1997). Free and cued selective reminding test: MOANS norms. *Journal of Clinical and Experimental Neuropsychology, 19*, 676–691.

Ivnik, R. J., Smith, G. E., Malec, J. F., Petersen, R. C., & Tangalos, E. G. (1995). Long-term stability and inter-correlations of cognitive abilities in older persons. *Psychological Assessment: A Journal of Consulting and Clinical Psychology, 7*, 155–161.

Ivnik, R. J., Smith, G. E., Malek, J. F., Petersen, R. C., & Tangalos, E. G. (1995). Long-term stability and inter-correlations of cognitive abilities in older persons. *Psychological Assessment, 7*, 155–161.

Ivnik, R. J., Smith, G. E., Petersen, R. C., Boeve, B. F., Kokmen, E., & Tangalos, E. (2000). Diagnostic accuracy of four approaches to interpreting neuropsychological test data. *Neuropsychology, 14,* 163–177.

Jack, C. R. , Jr., Petersen, R. C., O'Brien, P. C., & Tangalos, E. G. (1992). MR-based hippocampal volumetry in the diagnosis of Alzheimer's disease. *Neurology, 42,* 183–188.

Jack, C. J., Petersen, R. C., Xu, Y. C., O'Brien, P. C., Smith, G. E., Ivnik, R. J., et al. (1999). Prediction of AD with MRI-based hippocampal volume in mild cognitive impairment. *Neurology, 52,* 1397–1403.

Jastak, S., & Wilkinson, G. S. (1984). *The Wide Range Achievement Test-Revised. Administration manual.* Wilmington, DE: Jastak Associates.

Jicha, G., Petersen, R. C., Parisi, J. E., Dickson, D. W., Johnson, K. A., Knopman, D. S. Boeve, B. F., et al. (in press). Neuropathology of mild cognitive impairment. *Neurology.*

Kantarci, K., Jack, C. R., Jr., Xu, Y. C., Campeau, N. G., O' Brien, P. C., Smith, G. E., et al. (2000). Regional metabolic patterns in mild cognitive impairment and Alzheimer's disease: A ¹H-MRS study. *Neurology, 55,* 210–217.

Kaplan, E. F., Goodglass, H., & Weintraub, S. (1978). *The Boston Naming Test.* Boston: Kaplan & Goodglass.

Katchaturian, Z. S. (1985). Diagnosis of Alzheimer's disease. *Archives of Neurology, 42,* 1097–1105.

Katzman, R., Aronson, M., Fuld, P., Kawas, C., Brown, T., Morgenstern, H., et al. (1989). Development of dementing illnesses in an 80-year-old volunteer cohort. *Annals of Neurology, 25,* 317–324.

Keys, B. A., & White, D. A. (2000). Exploring the relationship between age, executive abilities, and psychomotor speed. *Journal of the International Neuropsychological Society, 6,* 76–82.

Kokmen, E., Chandra, V., & Schoenberg, B. S. (1988). Trends in incidence of dementing illness in Rochester, Minnesota, in three quinquennial periods, 1960–1974. *Neurology, 38,* 975–980.

Kral, V. A. (1958). Neuro-psychiatric observations in an old peoples home: Studies of memory dysfunction in senescence. *Journal of Gerontology, 13,* 169–176.

Kral, V. A. (1962). Senescent forgetfulness: Benign and malignant. *Canadian Medical Association Journal, 86,* 257–260.

Larrieu, S., Letenneur, L., Orgogozo, J. M., Fabrigoule, C., Amieva, H., Le Carret, N., Barberger-Gateau, P., & Dartigues, J. F. (2002). Incidence and outcome of mild cognitive impairment in a population-based prospective cohort. *Neurology, 59,* 1594–1599.

Letenneur, L., Commenges, D., Dartigues, J. F., & Barberger-Gateau, P. (1994). Incidence of dementia and Alzheimer's disease in elderly community residents of South-Western France. *International Journal of Epidemiology, 23,* 1256–1261.

Levy, R. (1994). Aging-associated cognitive decline. *International Psychogeriatrics, 6,* 63–68.

Lezak, M. D. (1995). *Neuropsychological assessment.* New York: Oxford University Press.

Light, L. L. (1996). Memory and aging. In E. L. Bjork & R. A. Bjork (Eds.), *Memory: Handbook of perception and cognition* (2nd ed., pp. 443–490). New York: Academic Press.

Lopez, O. L., Kuller, L. H., DeKosky, S. T., & Becker, J. T. (2002). Prevalence and classification of Mild Cognitive Impairment in a population study. *Neurobiology of Aging, 23,* S138.

Lucas, J. A., Ivnik, R. J., Smith, G. E., Ferman, T. J., Willis, F. B., Petersen, R. C., et al. (2005a). A brief report on WAIS-R normative data collection in Mayo's older African Americans normative studies. *The Clinical Neuropsychologist, 19,* 184–188.

Lucas, J. A., Ivnik, R. J., Smith, G. E., Ferman, T. J., Willis, F. B., Petersen, R. C., et al. (2005b). Mayo's older African American normative studies: WMS-R norms for African American elders. *The Clinical Neuropsychologist, 19,* 189–213.

Lucas, J. A., Ivnik, R. J., Smith, G. E., Bohac, D. L., Tangalos, E. G., Kokmen, E., et al. (1998a). Normative data for the Mattis Dementia Rating Scale. *Journal of Clinical and Experimental Neuropsychology, 20,* 536–547.

Lucas, J. A., Ivnik, R. J., Smith, G. E., Bohac, D. L., Tangalos, E. G., Graff-Radford, N. R., et al. (1998b). Mayo Older Amcrican Studies: Category fluency norms. *Journal of Clinical and Experimental Neuropsychology, 20,* 194–200

Malec, J. F., Ivnik, R. J., Smith, G. E., et al. (1992). Visual Spatial Learning Test (VSLT): Normative data and further validation. *Psychological Assessment, 4*, 433–441.

Masur, D. M., Sliwinski, M., Lipton, R. B., Blau, A. D., & Crystal, H. A. (1994). Neuropsychological prediction of dementia and the absence of dementia in healthy elderly persons. *Neurology, 44*, 1427–1432.

Matarazzo, J. D., & Prifitera, A. (1989). Subtest scatter and premorbid intelligence: Lessons from the WAIS-R standardization sample. *Psychological Assessment: A Journal of Consulting and Clinical Psychology, 1*, 186–191.

Mattis, S. (1988). *Mattis Dementia Rating Scale (MDRS)*. Odessa, Fl: Psychological Assessment Resources.

Mayeux, R., Ottman, R., Maestre, G., Ngai, C., Tang, M. X., Ginsberg, H., et al. (1995). Synergistic effects of traumatic head injury and apolipoprotein-epsilon 4 in patients with Alzheimer's disease. *Neurology, 45*, 555–557.

Mayeux, R., Ottman, R., Tang, M. X., Noboa-Bauza, L., Marder, K., Gurland, B., et al. (1993). Genetic susceptibility and head injury as risk factors for Alzheimer's disease among community-dwelling older persons and their first-degree relatives. *Annals of Neurology, 33*, 494–501.

Mayeux, R., Stern, Y., Ottman, R., Tatemichi, T. K., Tang, M., Maestre, G., et al. (1993). The apolipoprotein E4 allele in patients with Alzheimer's disease. *Annals of Neurology, 34*, 752–754.

McKhann, G., Drachman, D., Folstein, M., Katzman, R., Price, D., & Stadlan, E. M. (1984). Clinical diagnosis of Alzheimer's disease: Report of the NINCDS–ADRDA work group under the auspices of Department of Health and Human Services Task Force on Alzheimer's Disease. *Neurology, 34*, 939–944.

Meyerson, J., Adams, D. R., Hale, S., & Jenkins, L. (2003). Analysis of group differences in processing speed: Brinley plots, Q-Q plots, and other conspiracies. *Psychonomic Bulletin and Review, 10*, 224–237.

Meyerson, J., Jenkins, L., Hale, S., & Sliwinski, M. (2000). Individual and developmental differences in working memory across the life span: Reply. *Psychonomic Bulletin and Review, 7*, 734–740.

Miech, R. A., Breitner, J. C. S., Zandi, P. P., Khachaturian, A. S., Anthony, J. C., & Mayer, L., for the Cache County Study Group. (2002). Incidence of AD may decline in the early 90s for men, later for women: The Cache County Study. *Neurology, 58*, 209–218.

Mirra, S. S., Heyman, A., McKeel, D., Sumi, S. M., Crain, B. J., Brownlee, L. M., et al. (1991). The Consortium to Establish a Registry for Alzheimer's Disease (CERAD): Part II. Standardization of the neuropathologic assessment of Alzheimer's disease. *Neurology, 41*, 479–486.

Mitrushina, M., Boone, K. B., & D'Elia, L. F. (1999). *Handbook of normative data for neuropsychological assessment*. New York: Oxford University Press.

Morris, J. C. (1993). The Clinical Dementia Rating (CDR): Current version and scoring rules. *Neurology, 43*, 2412–2414.

Morris, J. C., McKeel, D. W., Storandt, M., Rubin, E. H., Price, J. L., Grant, E. A., et al. (1991). Very mild Alzheimer's disease: Informant based clinical, psychometric, and pathologic distinction from normal aging. *Neurology, 41*, 469–478.

Mortimer, J. A., French, L. R., Hutton, J. T., & Schuman, L. M. (1985). Head injury as a risk factor for Alzheimer's disease. *Neurology, 35*, 264–267.

Mortimer, J. A., van Duijin, C. M., Chandra, V., Fratiglioni, L., Graves, A. B., Heyman, A., et al. (1991). Head trauma as a risk factor for Alzheimer's disease: A collaborative re-analysis of case-control studies. EURODEM Risk Factors Research Group. *International Journal of Epidemiology, 20*, S28–S35.

Nemetz, P. N., Leibson, C., Naessens, J. M., Beard, M., Kokmen, E., Annegers, J. F., et al. (1998). Traumatic brain injury and time to onset of Alzheimer's disease: A population-based study. *American Journal of Epidemiology, 149*, 32–40.

Pantel, J., Kratz, B., Essig, M., & Schroder, J. (2003). Parahippocampal volume deficits in subjects with aging-associated cognitive decline. *American Journal of Psychiatry, 160*, 379–382.

Park, D. C., Smith, A. D., Lautenschlager, G., Earles, J. L., Frieske, D., Zwahr, M., et al. (1996). Mediators of long-term memory performance across the life span. *Psychology and Aging, 11,* 621–637.

Parkin, A. J., & Java, R. I. (2000). Determinants of age-related memory loss. In T. J. Perfect & E. A. Maylor (Eds.), *Models of cognitive aging: Debates in psychology* (pp. 188–203). New York: Oxford University Press.

Pedraza, O., Lucas, J. A., Smith, G. E., Willis, F. W., Graff-Radford, N. R., Ferman, T. J., et al. (2005). Mayo's older African Americans normative studies: Confirmatory factor analysis of a core battery. *Journal of the International Neuropsychological Society, 11,* 184–191.

Petersen, R. C. (1995). Normal aging, mild cognitive impairment, and early Alzheimer's disease. *The Neurologist, 1,* 326–344.

Petersen, R. C. (2000). Aging, mild cognitive impairment, and Alzheimer's disease. *Neurologic Clinics, 18,* 789–806.

Petersen, R. C. (2001). Mild cognitive impairment: Transition from aging to Alzheimer's disease. In K. Iqbal, S. S. Sisodia, & B. Winblad (Eds.), *Alzheimer's disease: Advances in etiology, pathogenesis, and therapeutics* (pp. 141–151). Chichester, UK: Wiley.

Petersen, R. C., Doody, R., Kurz, A., Mohs, R. C., Morris, J. C., Rabins, P. V., et al. (2001). Current concepts in mild cognitive impairment. *Archives of Neurology, 58,* 1985–1992.

Petersen, R. C., Ivnik, R. J., Boeve, B. F., Knopman, D. S., Smith, G. E., & Tangalos, E. G. (2004). Outcome of clinical subtypes of MCI. *Neurology* (abstract), *62,* A29S.

Petersen, R. C., Smith, G. E., Ivnik, R. J., Kokmen, E., & Tangalos, E. G. (1994). Memory function in very early Alzheimer's disease. *Neurology, 44,* 867–872.

Petersen, R. C., Smith, G. E., Ivnik, R. J., Tangalos, E. G., Schaid, D. I., Thibodeau, S., et al. (1995). Apolipoprotein E status as a predictor of the development of Alzheimer's disease in memory-impaired individuals. *Journal of the American Medical Association, 273,* 1274–1278.

Petersen, R. C., Smith, G. E., Kokmen, E., Ivnik, R. J., & Tangalos, E. (1992). Memory function in normal aging. *Neurology, 42,* 396–401.

Petersen, R. C., Smith, G. E., Waring, S., Ivnik, E. G., & Kokmen, E. (1999). Mild cognitive impairment: Clinical characterization and outcome. *Archives of Neurology, 56,* 303–308.

Plassman, B. L., Havlik, R. J., Steffens, D. C., Helms, M. J., Newman, T. N., Drosdick, D., et al. (2000). Documented head injury in early adulthood and risk of Alzheimer's disease and other dementias. *Neurology, 55,* 1158–1166.

Powell, D. H., & Whirla, D. K. (1994). *Profiles in cognitive aging.* Boston: Harvard University Press.

Reiman, E. M., Caselli, R. J., Yun, L. S., Chen, K., Bandy, D., Minoshima, S., et al. (1996). Preclinical evidence of Alzheimer's disease in persons homozygous for the epsilon 4 allele for apolipoprotein E. *New England Journal of Medicine, 21,* 752–758.

Reisberg, B., Ferris, S. H., de Leon, M. J., & Crook, T. (1982). The Global Deterioration Scale for assessment of primary degenerative dementia. *American Journal of Psychiatry, 139,* 1136–1139.

Reisberg, B., Ferris, S. H., Franssen, E., Kluger, A., & Borenstein, J. (1986). Age-associated memory impairment: The clinical syndrome. *Developmental Neuropsychology, 2,* 401–412.

Rey, A. (1964). *L'examen clinique en psychologie* [The clinical and psychological examination]. Paris: Presses Universitaires de France.

Rilling, L. R., Lucas, J. A., Ivnik, R. J., Smith, G. E., Ferman, T. J., Willis, F. B., et al. (2005). Mayo's older African American normative studies: DRS norms for African American elders. *The Clinical Neuropsychologist, 19,* 229–242.

Ritchie, K., Artero, S., & Touchon, J. (2001). Classification criteria for mild cognitive impairment: A population-based validation study. *Neurology, 56,* 37–42.

Ritchie, K., Kildea, D., & Robine, J. (1992). The relationship between age and the prevalence of senile dementia: A meta-analysis of recent data. *International Journal of Epidemiology, 21,* 763–769.

Ritchie, K., & Touchon, J. (2000). Mild cognitive impairment: Conceptual basis and current nosological status. *Lancet, 15,* 225–228.

Robinson-Whelen, S., & Storandt, M. (1992). Immediate and delayed prose recall among normal and demented adults. *Archives of Neurology, 49,* 32–34.

Rocca, W. A., Hofman, A., Brayne, C., Breteler, M. M., Clarke, M., Copland, J. R., et al. (1991). Frequency and distribution of Alzheimer's disease in Europe: A collaborative study of 1980–1990 prevalence findings. *Annals of Neurology, 30,* 381–390.

Rubin, E. H., Storandt, M., Miller, J. P., Grant, E. A., Kinscherf, D. A., Morris, J. C., et al. (1993). Influence of age on clinical and psychometric assessment of subjects with very mild or mild dementia of the Alzheimer type. *Archives of Neurology, 50,* 380–383.

Ryan, J. J., & Paolo, A. M. (1992). Verbal-performance IQ discrepancies on the WAIS-R: An examination of the old-age standardization sample. *Neuropsychology, 6,* 293–298.

Sackett, D. L., Straus, S. E., Richardson, W. S., Rosenberg, W., & Haynes, R. B. (2000). *Evidence-based medicine: How to practice and teach evidence-based medicine* (2nd ed.). New York: Churchill Livingston.

Salthouse, T. A. (1996). The processing-speed theory of adult age differences in cognition. *Psychological Review, 103,* 403–428.

Schaie, K. W. (1994). The course of adult intellectual development. *American Psychologist, 49,* 304–313.

Schofield, P. W., Tang, M., Marder, K., Bell, K., Dooneief, G., Chun, M., et al. (1997). Alzheimer's disease after remote head injury: An incidence study. *Journal of Neurology, Neurosurgery, and Psychiatry, 62,* 119–124.

Sliwinski, M., & Buschke, H. (1997). Processing speed and memory in aging and dementia. *Journals of Gerontology Series B—Psychological and Social Sciences, 52B,* P308–P318.

Sliwinski, M., & Buschke, H. (1999). Cross-sectional and longitudinal relationships among age, cognition, and processing speed. *Psychology and Aging, 14,* 18–33.

Smith G. E., Bohac, D. L., Ivnik, R. J., & Malec, J. F. (1997). Using word recognition scores to predict premorbid IQ in dementia patients: Longitudinal data. *Journal of the International Neuropsychological Society, 3,* 528–533.

Smith, G. E., Bohac, D. L., Waring, S., Ivnik, R. J., Petersen, R. C., Tangalos, E. G., Kokmen, E., & Thibodeau, S. (1998) Apolipoprotein E genotype influences cognitive "phenotype" in patients with Alzheimer's disease but not in healthy control subjects. *Neurology, 50,* 355–362.

Smith, G. E., Ivnik, R. J., & Lucas, J. A. (in press). Assessment techniques: Tests, test batteries, norms and methodological approaches. In J. Morgan & J. Ricker (Eds.), *Textbook of Clinical Neuropsychology.*

Smith, G. E., Ivnik, R. J., Malec, J. F., Kokmen, E., Tangalos, E., & Petersen, R. C. (1994). Psychometric properties of the Mattis Dementia Rating Scale. *Assessment, 1,* 123–131.

Smith, G. E., Ivnik, R. J., Malec, J. F., Petersen, R. C., Kokmen, E., & Tangalos, E. G. (1994). Mayo cognitive factor scales: Derivation of a short battery and norms for factor scores. *Neuropsychology, 8,* 194–202.

Smith, G. E., Ivnik, R. J., Malec, J. F., Petersen, R. C., Tangalos, E. G., & Kurland, L. T. (1992). Mayo's Older Americans Normative Studies (MOANS): Factor structure of a core battery. *Psychological Assessment: A Journal of Consulting and Clinical Psychology, 4,* 382–390.

Smith, G. E., Ivnik, R. J., Malec, J. F., & Tangalos, E. G. (1993). Factor structure of the MOANS core battery: Replication in a clinical sample. *Psychological Assessment: A Journal of Consulting and Clinical Psychology, 5,* 121–124.

Smith, G. E., Ivnik, R. J., Petersen, R. C., Malec, J. F., Kokmen, E., & Tangalos, E. (1991). Age-associated memory impairment diagnoses: Problems of reliability and concerns for terminology. *Psychology and Aging, 6,* 551–558.

Smith, G. E., Petersen, R. C., Ivnik, R. J., Malec, J. F., & Tangalos, E. G. (1996). Subjective memory complaints, psychological distress, and longitudinal change in objective memory performance. *Psychology and Aging, 11,* 272–279.

Smith G. E., Wong, J. S., Ivnik, R. J., & Malec, J. F. (1997). Mayo's Older American Normative Studies: Separate norms for WMS-R logical memory stories. *Assessment, 4,* 79–86.

Spreen, O., & Strauss, E. (1991). *A compendium of neuropsychological tests: Administration, norms, and commentary.* New York: Oxford University Press.

Storandt, M., & Hill, R. D. (1989). Very mild senile dementia of the Alzheimer Type II: Psychometric test performance. *Archives of Neurology, 46,* 383–386.

Strittmatter, W. J., Saunders, A. M., Schmechel, D., Pericak-Vance, M., Enghild, J., Salvesen, G. S., et al. (1993). Apolipoprotein E: High avidity binding to beta-amyloid and increased frequency of type 4 allele in late-onset familial Alzheimer disease. *Proceedings of the National Academy of Science*, *90*, 1977–1981.

Taylor, J. L., Miller, T. P., & Tinklenberg, J. R. (1992). Correlates of memory decline: A four-year longitudinal study of older adults with memory complaints. *Psychology and Aging*, *7*, 185–193.

Testa J. A., Ivnik R. J., Petersen, R. C., Boeve, B., Knopman, D. S., & Smith, G. E. (2004). Diagnostic utility of Boston Naming Test in MCI and Alzheimer's disease. *Journal of the International Neuropsychogical Society, 10*, 504–512.

Tierney, M. C., Szalai, J. P., Snow, W. G., Fisher, R. H., Nores, A., Nadon, G., et al. (1996). Prediction of probable Alzheimer's disease in memory-impaired patients: A prospective longitudinal study. *Neurology*, *46*, 661–665.

Tuokko H., Frerichs, R., Graham, J., Rockwood, K., Kristjansson, B., Fisk, J., et al. (2003). Five-year follow-up of cognitive impairment with no dementia. *Archives of Neurology*, *60*, 577–582.

van Dongen, M., van Rossum, E., Kessels, A., Sielhorst, H., & Knipschild, P. (2003). Ginkgo for elderly people with dementia and age-associated memory impairment: A randomized clinical trial. *Journal of Clinical Epidemiology, 56*, 367–376.

Van Duijn, C. M., Clayton, D. G., Chandra, V., Fratiglioni, L., Graves, A. B., Heyman, A., et al. (1994). Interaction between genetic and environmental risk factors for Alzheimer's disease: A re-analysis of case-control studies. EURODEM Risk Factors Research Group. *Genetic Epidemiology, 11*, 539–551.

Van Duijn, C. M., Tanja, T. A., Haaxma, R., Schulte, W., Saan, R. J., Lameris, A. J., et al. (1992). Head trauma and the risk of Alzheimer's disease. *American Journal of Epidemiology, 135*, 775–782.

Walker, A. E., & Blumer D. (1989). The fate of World War II veterans with post-traumatic seizures. *Archives of Neurology, 46*, 23–26.

Wechsler, D. A. (1981). *Wechsler Adult Intelligence Scale—Revised*. New York: Psychological Corporation.

Wechsler, D. A. (1987). *Wechsler Memory Scale—Revised*. New York: Psychological Corporation.

Welsh, K. A., Butters, N., Hughes, J., Mohs, R., & Heyman, A. (1991). Detection of abnormal memory decline in mild cases of Alzheimer's disease using CERAD neuropsychological measures. *Archives of Neurology, 48*, 278–281.

Welsh, K. A., Butters, N., Hughes, J., Mohs, R., & Heyman, A. (1992). Detection and staging of dementia in Alzheimer's disease: Use of neuropsychological measures developed for the Consortium to Establish a Registry for Alzheimer's Disease (CERAD). *Archives of Neurology, 49*, 448–452.

Welsh-Bohmer, K. A., Hulette, C., Schmechel, D., Burke, J., & Saunders, A. (2001). Neuropsychological detection of preclinical Alzheimer's disease: Results of a neuropathological series of "normal" controls. In K. Iqbal, S. S. Sisodia, & B. Winblad (Eds.), *Alzheimer's disease: Advances in etiology, pathogenesis, and therapeutics* (pp. 111–122). New York: Wiley.

West, M. J., Coleman, P. D., Flood, D. G., & Tronosco, J. C. (1994). Differences in the pattern of hippocampal neuronal loss in normal ageing and Alzheimer's disease. *Lancet, 344*, 769–772.

Williams, D. B., Annegers, J. F., Kokmen, E., O'Brien, P., & Kurland, L. T. (1991). Brain injury and neurologic sequelae: A cohort study of dementia, parkinsonism, and amyotrophic lateral sclerosis. *Neurology, 41*, 1554–1557.

Youngjohn, J. R., & Crook, T. H., III. (1993). Stability of everyday memory in age-associated memory impairment: A longitudinal study. *Neuropsychology, 7*, 406–416.

Zimprich, D. (2002). Cross-sectionally and longitudinally balanced effects of processing speed on intellectual abilities. *Experimental Aging Research, 28*, 231–251.

Neurodegenerative Dementias

KATHLEEN A. WELSH-BOHMER
LAUREN H. WARREN

Alzheimer's disease (AD), Parkinson's disease dementia (PD-D), Lewy body dementia (LBD), and frontotemporal dementia (FTD) account for nearly 70% of the cases of dementia occurring in late life (Breitner et al., 1999). These conditions are often contrasted to one another and conceptualized as unique clinical entities. And yet, with the advances in neuroepidemiology and genetics, it is becoming clear that these conditions may share a number of common features and underlying etiological mechanisms (Mayeux, 2003). All of the conditions are neurodegenerative in nature, with onset of symptoms occurring typically in mid- to late life. There are strong genetic underpinnings at least to some forms of each of the disorders. AD, PD-D, LBD spectrum disorders, and FTD each has an apparent inherited version as well as a more common sporadic form of disease. Finally, new advances in clinical genetics suggest that at least some of the basic biological mechanisms governing disease onset and perhaps other features of symptom expression are shared across the disorders (Li et al., 2002, 2003).

The goal of this chapter is to present a detailed overview of the clinical presentation of these seemingly disparate neurodegenerative disorders. Central to the consideration is AD, an illness that, alone or in combination with other neurological disorders, accounts for nearly 50–75% of all late-life dementias. Other common neurodegenerative conditions leading to dementia in late life are also discussed. The chapter is not inclusive of all dementing disorders, but rather focuses attention on the major neurodegenerative conditions of aging that can be clinically mistaken for AD. Specifically we contrast two disorders whose clinical features overlap with AD: frontotemporal dementia and the PD spectrum of dementing disorders (PD-D and LBD). Within each section that follows we discuss the prevalence of the condition, the typical clinical features, the associated neuropsychological profile, and, when appropriate, the role of emerging biomarkers and surrogate markers in diagnosing and tracking the disorder in question.

ALZHEIMER'S DISEASE

AD is the most common cause for late-life dementia, currently affecting 4.5 million Americans (Hebert, Scherr, Bienias, Bennett, & Evans, 2003) and accounting for nearly 50% of the prevalent cases of dementia in nearly all epidemiological and case-based series (Breitner et al., 1999). Vascular dementia (VaD), discussed by Cato and Crosson (Chapter 4, this volume), is the second most common cause of dementia, but in isolation likely only accounts for approximately 12–20% of the late-life dementias (Bowler, 2002; Lobo et al., 2000; Rockwood et al., 2000). More commonly, VaD co-occurs with AD (Graves et al., 1996; Knopman, Parisi, et al., 2003). Consequently, when these mixed dementia etiologies (AD and VaD) are considered in calculating AD prevalence, the rates of AD dementia occurrence approach nearly 75%. There is some variation in these relative prevalence figures across countries, with AD being more prominent overall than VaD in North American countries and Europe, and VaD tending to be more common in Asian countries (Fratiglioni, De Ronchi, & Aguero-Torres, 1999), suggesting differences either in environmental exposures or genetic factors that may account for differences in dementia rates. It is possible that these relative distributions simply reflect methodological differences in case ascertainment. However, more recent studies suggest that they are real and that dietary and other environmental factors related to culture may be responsible, because the rates vary by geographic location, with Asian Americans showing similar rates to European Americans in the United States but different rates in mainland Japan (Graves et al., 1996).

AD and related dementias of late life present enormous public health challenges. With current survival trends and in the absence of preventive treatments, it is anticipated that the disease will affect over 8 million individuals in the U.S. by midcentury (Brookmeyer, 1998) and likely will exceed 13.2 million (Hebert et al., 2003). As such, the United States faces a public health crisis of phenomenal proportions, with current personal and societal expenditures related to long-term care of dementia patients generally quoted at $80–100 billion annually (DeKosky & Orgogozo, 2001; Fillit & Hill, 2002). However, some recent figures based on the state of California alone suggest that the $100 billion price tag for dementia care may be a gross underestimate (Fox, Kohatsu, Max, & Arnsberger, 2001). Consequently, there is both a scientific and a public policy priority to quickly develop effective treatments and preventive strategies for AD and related disorders. In this context, a challenge for clinicians is the ability to reliably recognize the disease early in its expression to facilitate effective treatment implementation at a point in the illness when it is likely to be most effective.

Illness Characterization

AD dementia has been well studied since its initial description nearly a century ago (Alzheimer, Stelzmann, Schnitzlein, & Murtagh, 1907/1995) and is now well understood both in terms of its clinical presentation and symptom heterogeneity. Typically the disease emerges in later years, after the age of 50, although in rare instances (under 2% of the cases) it can present at earlier ages. Generally, causal factors for the earlier-than-expected onset can be identified, such as a strong genetic predisposition for the illness, including the rare autosomal dominant familial forms of the illness, or the confluence of risk factors leading to brain compromise (e.g., serious head trauma, Down syndrome). Throughout the illness the disease is characterized by prominent memory impairment for recent events (Welsh, Butters, Hughes, Mohs, & Hayman, 1991). This impairment is evident even in the earliest symptomatic stages, including the prodromal stage of AD and in cases of mild cognitive impairment (MCI; Petersen et al., 1999), a risk condition for AD (Bowen et al., 1997; Flicker, Ferris, & Reisberg, 1991; Morris et al., 2001; Ritchie et al., 2001). Ultimately, as the illness progresses there is a slow erosion of general cognition (Welsh, Butters, Hughes, Mohs, & Hayman, 1992), resulting in increasing functional dependence and eventually death (Tschanz et al., 2004).

The memory impairment of AD is not a singular problem, but it is highly characteristic and distinguishable from other neurocognitive disorders of later life (Cummings & Benson, 1992; Geldmacher & Whitehouse, 1997). The hallmark feature of forgetfulness in everyday life is typically attributable to a disturbance in the consolidation of new information into episodic memory stores (Hart, Kwentus, Taylor, & Harkins, 1987; Hart et al., 1988). The neurocognitive problem parallels the underlying pathobiology in the mediotemporal lobe (Braak & Braak, 1991), where input pathways from the entorhinal cortex and hippocampus are fundamentally disturbed over the course of AD, leading to a functional isolation of the structure from association areas in the neocortices (Hyman, Van Hoesen, Damasio, & Barnes, 1984). As a consequence of this problem, rapid forgetting deficits are observed on formal testing, such as on list-learning procedures and similar tasks (Salmon et al., 2002; Welsh et al., 1991). Unlike normal aging (Nebes & Madden, 1988) and in other neurocognitive disorders, such as VaD, performance of patients with AD on memory tests benefits little by reminder cues (Looi & Sachdev, 1999; Matsuda, Sito, & Sugishita, 1998; Tierney et al., 2001). Semantic memory, including past knowledge of the world and events acquired over many experiences in life, tends to remain more patent until much later in the illness. However, subtle problems can be detected in semantic knowledge at the middle stages of disease, for example, on tasks involving knowledge of detailed information that was once known (Chertkow & Bub, 1990; Hodges, Patterson, Qcbury, & Funnell, 1992). Working memory, a process of holding and manipulating information in more transient short-term memory stores, is also affected early in the illness (Becker, 1988), whereas immediate registration of information and basic stimulus encoding tends to remain well preserved until late stages (Hart et al., 1988).

Episodic memory is by no means the only domain of cognition affected by AD. Expressive language difficulties are common and often manifest as anomia and a vacuous speech quality, empty of word content (Bayles, Boone, Tomoeda, Slauson, & Kaszniak, 1989). Verbal flexibility becomes deficient, leading to selective disturbances on semantic fluency procedures (Troster et al., 1998). Behavioral patterns emerge to compensate for this problem in expression, typified by circumlocution (e.g., describing the object) during the moderate stages of AD. Receptive speech, such as aural comprehension, is relatively better preserved early in the disorder but is affected later as cognition continues to erode. Essentially, the language disturbance of early- to middle-stage AD resembles a transcortical sensory aphasia; by late stages it may be more akin to a frank Wernicke-type aphasia (Cummings, Benson, Hill, & Reed, 1985; Hier, Hagenlocker, & Shindler, 1985; Murdoch, Chenery, Wilks, & Boyle, 1987).

Rather classic visuospatial disturbances also occur in AD (Benke, 1993). Apraxia is common in the middle stages of the disorder, often manifesting in everyday life as difficulty in initiating and organizing previously known motor tasks (e.g., dressing, manipulating hand tools). Other problems can occur in spatial navigation, judgment of distances, and correct perception of objects (Damasio, Tranel, & Rizzo, 2000; Rizzo, Reinach, McGhee, & Dawson, 1997; Rizzo, Anderson, Dawson, & Nawrot, 2000). Constructional tasks, such as drawing tests or block assembly, are commonly used to assess apraxia, whereas spatial perception is commonly assessed with any of a number of procedures, such as the Judgement of Line Orientation test (Benton, Hamsher, Varney, & Spreen, 1983). Spatial integration may be determined by using tests such as the Hooper Visual Organization Test or other similar procedures (Lezak, 1995) that require the individual to determine the likely identity of an object when presented with fragments or deconstructed component parts, akin to puzzle pieces. Form perception can be determined with visual matching procedures (e.g., Facial Recognition Test; Benton et al., 1983), and spatial navigation can be measured with computerized tests or with simple paper-and-pencil tests of maze completion (Lezak, 1995).

Intelligence, or what might be termed "higher-order conceptualization," is uniformly affected in the early to middle stages of AD. This problem can be assessed with tests of intelligence (Wechsler Adult Intelligence Scale or its revisions [WAIS-R, WAIS-III]; see Wechsler, 1987, 1997), or by administering selected subtests from these batteries, such as measures of abstraction (e.g., Similarities) or tests of reasoning and judgment (e.g., Comprehension). Related to intelligence is executive function, an ability to think flexibly and creatively. Executive function is perhaps best conceptualized as a global "processing control function" that is imposed over the basic perceptual-, memory-, and language-based functions of thought and behavior. Executive function involves the shifting, adjusting, or withholding of behavioral responses in problem-solving situations. Discussed previously, working memory, an ability to hold one idea in mind while attending to other new information, may be considered a process that has both executive and memory demands (e.g., Baddeley, 1986). Executive functions are among the earliest cognitive domains affected by AD. Though perhaps subtler than the prominent memory problems, difficulties in conceptualizing, behavioral regulation, and/or novel problem solving can be detected using tests such as the Trail Making Test, Wisconsin Card Sorting Test, or the Stroop Neuropsychological Screening Test. Other control processes affected by AD include different aspects of attention and concentration. Both the ability to shift visual attention when required and the capacity to divide attention across competing tasks are affected early in the AD process (Baddeley, Baddeley, Bucks, & Wilcock, 2001; Greenwood, Parasuraman, & Alexander, 1997; Parasuraman, Greenwood, & Sunderland, 2002), as described below.

Neuropsychological Profile

Early-Stage AD Dementia

As discussed, memory disorder characterized by rapid forgetting is the typical early manifestation of AD. On formal neuropsychological testing, this difficulty is easily discerned using formal memory tests in which delay intervals are imposed to assess retention under cued and uncued procedures. Delayed memory is a particularly powerful discriminator between early AD and normal aging. In one study, delayed word-list recall correctly distinguished 91% of subjects diagnosed as very-mild-stage AD (CDR 0.5, MMSE > 24) from controls. Naming also is a significant early predictor when combined with delayed memory, but does not increase the overall correct classification rate (Welsh et al., 1992). In community-based samples the same finding holds, underscoring the importance of memory assessment. However, other measures of expressive language and executive control also appear to be important. In one study (Cahn et al., 1995) immediate and delayed recall on the Benton Visual Retention Test and delayed recall on the CERAD Word-List Memory Test showed good sensitivity and specificity in distinguishing patients with AD from controls. Equally important was performance on lexical fluency and executive function, measured through Trails B. Together, the combination of measures was particularly powerful, leading to a correct classification of 98% of the cognitively normal individuals and 82% of the AD-affected subjects in the sample. Other population-based studies also underscore the relevance of impairment profiles. For example, Tschanz et al., 2000 applied strict cut-points for impairment (< 7% percentile on any test) and suggested that neuropsychological algorithms of dementia may fare as well as more extensive clinical diagnostic procedures in correctly classifying individuals into broad categories (e.g., dementia vs. not demented; Tschanz et al., 2000).

This same cognitive profile demonstrated in early AD (i.e., profound memory impairment, executive disturbances, and difficulties in expressive language) is also characteristic of the early preclinical phase of the disorder, albeit of a lesser magnitude overall. Most of the studies that have demonstrated this effect include population-based investigations or community-based samples that focus attention on large unselected groups and then follow the cognitively normal individuals forward in time to prospectively determine the cognitive changes that were predictive of early symptomatic disease, years before diagnosis. Using this approach, analyses from the Framingham study (Elias et al., 2000; Linn et al., 1995) have shown distinctive differences in baseline test performances in the subsample of individuals who later develop AD over a 5-year observation interval. Specific deficits were reported in baseline measures of delayed memory (Logical Memory II from the Wechsler Memory Scale—Revised [WMS-R]), memory tests involving novel associations and retention (verbal paired associates, WMS-R) and on tests of abstraction (WAIS-R Similarities subtests; Elias et al., 2000). Other approaches to determine early preclinical cognitive changes have used smaller, more select samples that are at risk for developing AD over a shorter interval than most unaffected individuals. These samples included older unaffected family members in "AD-enriched" families—families in which there is multigenerational evidence of AD transmission (Almkvist, Axelman, Basun, Wahlund, & Lannfelt, 2002). Another enrichment procedure is to oversample older individuals who carry the AD risk-promoting gene, apolipoprotein E4 (Baxter, Caselli, Johnson, Reiman, & Osborne, 1996; Bondi, Salmon, Galasko, Thomas, & Thal, 1999; Tierney et al., 1996). Using this latter approach, one study has demonstrated memory deficits on the California Verbal Learning Test 1–2 years before an AD diagnosis could be made (Bondi et al., 1994).

These prospective investigations have repeatedly provided evidence that there are detectable and characteristic cognitive disorders that precede AD dementia onset (Elias et al., 2000), an observation that bolsters the notion that there is a continuum of cognitive change in AD that spans normal cognition to a transition zone, as noted, now referred to as mild cognitive impairment (MCI; Reisberg, Ferris, de Leon, & Crook, 1988), before finally developing into fully manifest symptoms of AD dementia (see Figure 3.1). Although not technically considered the prodrome to AD (Petersen et al., 1999), there is no clear consensus on this point, with some arguing that when properly diagnosed so as to exclude other possible explanations, MCI is, in point of fact, early-stage AD (Morris et al., 2001). Additional longitudinal studies will be needed to fully resolve the issue. Regardless, it is clear that individuals with these so-called "borderzone disorders" such as MCI are at 5–10 times increased risk of developing dementia when compared to cognitively healthy individuals (Tuokko et al., 2003). In general, studies of MCI report conversion

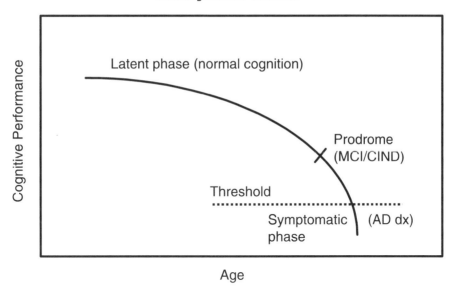

FIGURE 3.1. Trajectory of cognitive change in AD.

rates of 12–15% per year to AD compared to a base rate of 1–2% in age-matched, cognitively normal individuals (Petersen et al., 2001). More broadly defined syndromes may have even higher rates of conversion to dementia outcomes (Ritchie & Touchon, 2001; Ritchie et al., 2001; Unverzagt et al., 2001). Cognitive impairment no dementia (CIND), proposed by the Canadian Study of Health and Aging (CHSA; Ebly, Hogan, & Parhad, 1995), is one of the more broadly defined transitional conditions. In contrast to MCI, it is a broad heterogeneous category of conditions with more liberal exclusion criteria; no assumptions are made regarding the role of age-associated disease comorbidities such as depression, vascular disease, or medications (Graham et al., 1997). Aging-associated cognitive decline (AACD), proposed by the World Health Association (Levy, 1994), has broad inclusion criteria for cognitive decline, permitting any domain to be affected (akin to multiple-domain MCI). Both of these more broadly defined conditions have rates of overall conversion to dementia approaching 20–29% in some studies (Ritchie et al., 2001; Unverzagt et al., 2001). For further discussion of normal aging and mild cognitive disorders, see Smith and Rush (Chapter 2, this volume).

Moderate Stages of AD

With progression of AD into the moderate to more severe stages of the illness, other predictable aspects of cognitive decline begin to emerge that parallel the neuropathological trajectory of the illness (Locascio, Growdon, & Corkin, 1995; Welsh et al., 1992), resulting ultimately in global and pervasive cognitive impairments. By the end stages of the illness, the dementia of AD can be virtually indistinguishable from other similar neurodegenerative conditions, including VaD, PD-D, or FTD; however, some distinctions are present even in moderate stages of illness (Binetti, Locascio, Corkin, Vonsattel, & Growdon, 2000; Graham, Emery, & Hodges, 2004). Throughout the moderate stages of AD, episodic memory remains profoundly affected, bottoming out quickly on formal testing and providing little useful information when staging the progression of illness. Likewise, reasoning ability and higher-order conceptualization as might be assessed with tests of executive function or set shifting (e.g., Trail Making Test, Part B), are profoundly affected and of little utility in tracking disease progression or responsiveness to therapies.

Typically, deficits emerging in the moderate stages of illness include more pronounced difficulties in expressive speech, language comprehension, and praxis (Welsh et al., 1992). Errors in memory recognition performance, both for previous target items and for correctly discerning foil items, are common at this stage of illness. Intrusional tendencies are characteristic, which, with the other recognition memory difficulties, suggest that the memory problem has progressed beyond consolidation deficits to more defective encoding and temporal tagging of events from past stored experiences. The temporal profile of change can be very useful in distinguishing AD from other neurodegenerative conditions (Storey, Slavin, & Kinsella, 2002). The unfolding of symptoms across a longitudinal time frame provides a rich definition of the disease, and is characteristically different in AD, PD-D, and frontotemporal disorders. As described later in the text, Pick's disease and FTD commonly present in the initial stages with profound personality disorders and/or rather isolated language and semantic memory disorders; AD, by contrast, is characterized initially by memory disorders, and the personality changes similar to those of frontal-lobe disorders emerge much later, usually at the moderate stages of the disease. Language declines in the moderate stages of AD are likewise less precipitous than in frontal dementias, suggesting a rather slow and gradual erosion of function over time in AD (Binetti et al., 2000). When compared to dementias with motor-neuron involvement (e.g., Lewy body dementia or PD-D), the disturbances in visuospatial processing are less profound in AD and the memory problems more severe when the groups are adequately matched for demographic variables, overall dementia severity, and stage of illness (Aarsland, Andersen, Larsen, Lolk, & Kragh-Sorenson, 2003; Heyman et al., 1999).

There have been some attempts to quantify the average deterioration on neuropsychological measures for purposes of facilitating estimates of transitional probabilities or conversion rates in untreated patients between stages of dementia, and for purposes of determining effect sizes in pharmaceutical and other interventional studies (Morris et al., 1993). For simple metrics such as the Mini-Mental State Examination (MMSE), there is approximately a 10% change in score per year (e.g., 3 points on the MMSE per year) in AD, although the relationship is curvilinear with dementia severity, and cognitive decline in the moderate stage tends to be faster than in the early or late stage (Morris et al., 1993). Modeling average change on other domains is a bit trickier than on global assessment measures. Despite typical profiles of cognition in AD, there is tremendous variability in disease progression across patients due to a host of intervening variables, such as age, education, gender, premorbid abilities, area of brain affected by disease, presence and absence of disease comorbidities, and other factors. More rapid decline has been suggested in some AD variants, underscoring the potential influence of genes and gene–gene and gene–environment interactions on disease expression and variability over time (Farrer et al., 1995).

Also affecting rate of change are neuropsychiatric symptoms that can lead to "excess disability" both cognitively, on neuropsychological tests, and in functioning. Depressive symptoms are common early in the illness (Lykestos et al., 2002) and may even precede detection of cognitive impairment, perhaps reflecting the individual's own awareness of subtle deficits (Moore, Sandman, McGrady, & Kesslak, 2001). Later in the disorder, patients frequently develop significant behavioral disturbances, including agitation, hallucinations, and delusions (Steinberg et al., 2003). All of these problems, when untreated, can lead to what appears to be a more pronounced loss in ability.

Neurobiology

AD is defined not only by its well-recognized neuropsychological manifestations but also by its distinctive neuropathological features, first described by Alzheimer in 1907 (see Alzheimer et al., 1995). These changes, easily visualized under the microscope, include the amyloid plaque, an extracellular accumulation of a viscous transmembrane protein (amyloid; 39-42 amino acid derivative) at the core of the plaque, surrounded by cellular debris from dead and dying neurites, inflammatory markers, and glia. The second common neuropathological feature is the appearance of neurofibrillary tangles within neurons. This intraneuronal abnormality consists of paired helical filaments resulting from an abnormally hyperphosporylated microtubular protein, tau. The abnormal cross-linking of these proteins results in a massively disturbed microtubular array, leading to a contorted cytoskeletal structure, unable to support the normal intracellular transport of proteins, and eventually, neuronal death.

Plaques and tangles are not unique to AD; each individual feature can be seen in other neuronal disorders. Amyloid plaques occur in some prion diseases, in dementia pugilistica, and in a vascular disorder termed *amyloid angiopathy*. Tangles in isolation can be seen in FTD, progressive supranuclear palsy, corticobasal degeneration, and are also seen in some elderly patients without dementia. It is the abundance of the pathology and the characteristic distribution of the features that distinguish AD (Hyman et al., 1984). The pathology is largely confined to the hippocampus and entorhinal areas of the medial temporal lobe, but as the disease progresses, expands to include association areas of the neocortex (Arnold et al., 1991; Braak & Braak, 1991).

Genetics

The causes that precipitate the neuropathological cascade of events in the brain, leading ultimately to the cognitive demise of the patient with AD, are not entirely clear. However, determining the triggers and events that regulate or contribute to AD onset is of critical importance in effecting a treatment and in eventually eradicating the disease altogether. There can be little dispute that genes play a pivotal role in both AD risk and pathogenesis (see Pericak-Vance et al., 2000, for review). Three gene loci, on chromosomes 21, 14, and 1, have been identified as causal in the majority of early-onset AD cases: APP (Goate et al., 1991), presenilin 2 (PS2; Levy-Lahad et al., 1995), and presenilin 1 (PS1; St.-George Hyslop et al., 1992). These genes account for only 1–2% of all AD cases. Another gene, apolipoprotein E (apoE), has also been identified as a genetic risk factor for AD. Unlike the other genes, it is not causal for AD but rather influences disease susceptibility and symptom onset (Corder et al., 1993; Saunders et al., 1993a, 1993b; Strittmatter et al., 1993). ApoE is a common gene that regulates the transport of lipids and appears to play a role in neuronal repair. Polymorphisms, or common variations, in this gene appear to play a role in modifying AD risk and symptom onset. There are seven allele types (E1–E7) of the apoE gene, although some forms vary by only a couple of amino acids; the three allele types—E2, E3, and E4—are, for the most part, the only forms seen commonly, with 99% of the population having at least one copy of these three isoforms. The E4 genotype, although relatively infrequent in the population (14% of European Americans), is associated with approximately 15–50% of the late-onset forms of AD (Evans et al., 1997; Plassman & Breitner, 1996) in a dose-dependent fashion, so that the E4/E4 genotype is at highest risk of AD, followed by E4/E3, and then E3/E3.

Several lines of evidence suggest that apoE does not account for all the genetic variation of AD (see Pericak-Vance et al., 2000 for review). Combined together, the various genes identified only account for 55% of the genetic risk for the disease (see Plassman & Steffens, 2004, for review). Continued study suggests that there are likely several more "risk" genes operating in AD and that in all likelihood, there are complex interactions among multiple genes from different causal pathways giving risk to AD. Using association methods, a number of other genes has been suggested in late-onset AD. Early studies using genetic linkage suggest that there is at least one gene on chromosome 12 associated with late-onset AD (Pericak-Vance & Haines, 1998), a finding later confirmed with expanded datasets and enhanced genetic models that control for potential gene–gene interactions (Scott et al., 2000). Myriad other gene associations with AD has been reported, although many of these findings have not been consistently replicated. Among the most interesting and secure of the recent findings include reports of genetic loci of interest on chromosome 10 (Bertram et al., 2000; Ertekin-Taner, et al., 2000; Myers, Holmans, Marshall, Hardy, & Goate, 2000) and chromosome 9 (Pericak-Vance et al., 2000).

Diagnosis of AD Dementia

The clinical diagnosis of AD can be made with a high degree of accuracy (85% accuracy or more at major medical centers) if the clinician is proficient in recognizing the disorder and adheres to standard accepted clinical criteria (McKhann et al., 1984). These criteria, summarized in Table 3.1, draw heavily on what is now understood about the clinical symptomatology as specified through neuropsychological study. The syndrome of rapid memory impairment, accompanied by other deficits in at least one area of cognition, is required. The neurocognitive problem must be acquired in adulthood (not a longstanding, static problem from development), represent a change from a previous level of function, and must be causing impairments in the individual's ability to perform everyday functions. Finally, other potential contributing medical or psychiatric conditions must be excluded as the primary cause of the cognitive disorder.

Neurocognitive and Functional Assessment

The neuropsychological evaluation plays a central role in establishing the presence of the required inclusionary features of AD dementia. The evaluation is not required in all cases of dementia, when the syndrome is evident. A diagnosis will require more than neuropsychological testing, however. To establish the presence of functional loss, interview with a knowledgeable informant (e.g., spouse, adult child) may be needed to verify this information, because a loss of insight is common in AD and may result in the affected individual being unable to reliably report his or her functional abilities accurately. Commonly used for this purpose are interview tools developed for the Clinical Dementia Rating Scale, a metric with which to gauge the functional impairment in AD (Hughes, Berg, Danziger, Cohen, & Martin, 1982). This scale rates patients across 6 different functional domains (orientation, memory, language, home, social activities, personal care) and results in an overall cumulative score that can range from 0 (normal) to 0.5 (questionable dementia) to 1.0 (mild dementia), 2.0 (moderate), 3.0 (severe), 4.0 (profound), and 5.0

TABLE 3.1. NINCDS–ADRDA Criteria for Alzheimer's Disease

Probable Alzheimer's disease

1. Dementia established by clinical examination and documented by mental status testing. Defined as
   • Disturbance in intellectual function that significantly interferes with work or usual social activities or relationships with others.
   • Demonstrable impairment in memory.
2. Dementia confirmed by neuropsychological assessment.
3. Deficits in two or more areas of cognition (can include memory, abstract thinking, constructional ability, language, and orientation).
4. Progression in symptoms over time.
5. No disturbances in consciousness (no delirium).
6. Late onset and not developmentally acquired; onset between ages 40–90.
7. Absence of other conditions that are capable of producing dementia.

Possible Alzheimer's disease

1. Atypical onset, presentation or progression of dementia symptoms, and/or
2. Presence of another systemic or other brain disease capable of producing dementia but not thought to be the cause in the case under consideration.
3. Meets criteria for dementia, as confirmed by clinical examination and neuropsychological testing.
4. Progressive decline in symptoms over time.
5. No disturbances in consciousness.
6. Absence of other identifiable causes.

Definite Alzheimer's disease

1. Clinical criteria for probable Alzheimer's disease are fulfilled.
2. Histopathological evidence of Alzheimer's disease by biopsy or postmortem examination.

(terminal stage). An informant version of the scale has been developed (Dementia Severity Rating Scale) and can be employed in clinical settings as a useful screening tool; informants then can be queried in more detail to clarify the nature, extent, and onset of reported difficulties (Clark & Ewbank, 1996).

Interpreting neurocognitive test results and observed functional impairments requires consideration of competing causes for the observed problems. Developmental history must be considered and weighed in the clinical decision making. Learning disabilities, such as attention deficit disorder or dyslexia, may result in learning and memory difficulties that can confound the interpretation of newly acquired problems. Furthermore, the clinician needs to consider other related modifying variables: Level of schooling, familiarity with cognitive testing, age, and cultural variables can all influence testing performance and potentially lead to erroneous decisions regarding the presence and severity of cognitive losses (Anthony, LeResche, Niaz, von Korff, & Folstein, 1982). To this end, education level has been shown repeatedly to be directly related to cognitive performance on neuropsychological measures and must be taken into account before interpreting test performance (see Lezak, 1995, for review). In the absence of age and educational allowances, false-positive errors for dementia diagnosis are more likely in the sample of individuals that is older or has low formal education (8 years or less; Welsh et al., 1994). Similarly, differences in cognitive performance are commonly reported on the neuropsychological measures that are used for clinical diagnosis in some minority groups; these differences are related to levels of acculturation and educational experiences. As an example, a number of studies contrasting neurocognitive performance of elderly African American samples and European American groups has shown differences even after educational correction (Manly et al., 1998; Welsh et al., 1995); these changes appear to be related to cultural variables and educational inequities, because the group differences virtually disappear when premorbid ability and quality of schooling are controlled (Manly, Jacobs, Touradji, Small, & Stern, 2002, 2003).

Excluding Medical Comorbidities

A necessary part of the clinical diagnosis of AD is to rule out other medical explanations for the cognitive loss. Perhaps the single most important component of the dementia evaluation is obtaining a thorough medical history, which allows the review of symptoms, their evolution of time, and the presence or absence of other medical problems that coincide with symptom onset or may potentially explain the problems described. A diagnosis of AD can be made with a great degree of certainty based solely on the report of functional and cognitive loss, described above. With a history of a slowly evolving, gradually progressive cognitive decline, characterized by memory impairment and leading to functional losses, a diagnosis of AD would be prime consideration. The absence of competing causes for the loss would make the diagnosis an "almost certainty." Studies investigating the influence of different sources of information in the diagnosis suggest high prediction of the AD diagnosis with medical history information and cognitive test scores (Steffens et al., 1996).

However, it is recognized that phenocopies of AD do occur; that is, disorders with virtually identical symptoms but other provoking etiologies. Some of these disorders are treatable, such as VaD (see Table 3.2), whereas others are not and are due to neurological disorders such as FTD, vascular disease, and other progressive dementias described later in this chapter or in other parts of the text. Very similar patterns of neurocognitive change (e.g., recent-onset memory loss, attentional disorders) can result from diverse medical causes, including but not limited to thyroid disorders, perturbations in B_{12} or folate levels, cardiovascular disease, stroke, and other neurological conditions. Some of these disorders are reversible if treated early, before significant neurological injury has occurred (Eastley, Wilcock, & Bucks, 2000; Goebels & Soyka, 2000; Lehmann, Regland, Blennow, & Gottfries, 2003). A careful history and laboratory tests are needed to fully rule out the potential contributions of these causes in the cognitive syndrome. Typically,

TABLE 3.2. Criteria for Vascular Dementia

1. Meets criteria for dementia, as described previously.
2. Presence of clinical syndrome of stroke with:
   a. CT or MRI findings consistent with clinical focal deficits, or
   b. In the absence of consistent CT or MRI findings, clinical syndrome cannot be explained by any other cause.
3. Onset of dementia within 3 months of the onset of stroke, with evidence (by history or previous evaluation) of intact function prior to stroke.
4. In the assessment of cognitive ability to evaluate the presence of criteria for dementia, both of the following are required:
   a. Memory impairment cannot be directly attributable to the focal deficit associated with the site of lesion.
   b. Two other cognitive deficits are required. One of these must be in a domain that is not attributable to focal deficit associated with the site of the stroke lesion.

Note. Based on Tatemichi et al. (1994) criteria; essentially a revision of the Roman et al. (1993) criteria.

the laboratory studies order include a complete blood count, thyroid panel, serum levels of B_{12}, other vitamins, and homocysteine, as well as other blood studies of kidney, liver, and endocrine function (Clark & Karlawish, 2003).

Psychiatric Factors

In the medical history and clinical examination, attention must also be directed to current and past psychiatric health. Depression and other psychiatric factors can result in cognitive disorders that are difficult to distinguish from dementia. Additionally, these problems can co-occur with dementia and exacerbate the underlying memory disorders. Identification and treatment of psychiatric comorbidities may reduce, or entirely reverse, the cognitive and functional symptoms. For more detailed discussion of the cognitive effects of depression, see Houston and Bondi (Chapter 5, this volume).

Diagnostic Procedures

Structural Imaging. The diagnostic evaluation of dementia includes structural imaging of the brain, primarily to rule out space-occupying lesions (e.g., tumors), stroke, or other types of neurological conditions that might be treated. Typically in the early stages of AD, results of the computed tomography (CT) or magnetic resonance imaging (MRI) are normal on visual inspection. However, quantification of regional changes and comparisons to either normative standards (for cross-sectional analysis) or to images obtained from the affected individual over a previous 2-year interval or more reveal selective atrophy of the temporal lobe, hippocampus, and amygdala (Moore et al., 2001). This technique shows purpose as an early, surrogate marker of AD but is considered experimental at this point. Structural variability across individuals normally makes any routine clinical assessment difficult and prone to error. As the disease progresses, diffuse cortical atrophy and ventricular enlargement become prominent. There is cortical cell loss, with typical sparing of the occipital cortices.

Functional Imaging. New imaging methods targeting brain neuropathology show particularly encouraging diagnostic potential but are not yet a routinely accepted method for AD diagnosis. Positron emission tomography (PET) studies using the radioligand fluorodeoxyglucose have shown particular utility in the early AD stages or in atypical presentations, serving to support diagnostic suspicions (e.g., Silverman et al., 2001). A pattern of bilateral or asymmetric temporoparietal hypometabolism is seen in AD and is detectable even in the early stages of the disorder, perhaps even before the symptoms are clearly manifest (Reiman et al., 1999; Small et al., 2000). The imaging pattern has been validated in autopsy-confirmed AD cases and is considered fairly prototypical of the disorder (Hoffman et al., 2000). However, the use of fluorodeoxyglucon positron emission tomography (FDG-PET) studies or related methods (such as single photon emission tomography [SPECT]) remains controversial in diagnostic settings from both health economic and basic clinical practice perspectives (Kulasingam et al., 2003). In the absence of effective treatments for AD, the radiation exposure and the fact that care decisions will be essentially unchanged by the results make the merit of pursing SPECT or PET imaging low compared to the potential risks and costs.

Recently, selective markers that bind with high affinity to brain amyloid have been used in conjunction with PET (Klunk et al., 2003). If such methods can be safely and effectively used in patients with AD, they may permit a method for analyzing the in-life amyloid burden in key brain areas of the medial temporal lobe affected by AD. The advantage of this approach would be in its ability to directly monitor any changes in the underlying disease response to treatment over time. It may even allow a strategy for direct treatment delivery, if therapeutic molecules could be attached to the ligands, permitting targeted delivery to cells with high amyloid burden.

Genetics and Family History Information

When diagnosing AD and other neurodegenerative dementias, it is important to secure a good family history of any related illnesses. Each of the disorders under consideration in this chapter—AD, FTD, PD-D, and Lewy body dementia—carry some genetic risk. Familial forms and sporadic forms exist for each of the disorders; and even in sporadic forms of illness, genetic predisposition may play a role in an individual's risk of disease.

FRONTOTEMPORAL DEMENTIA

FTD, like AD, is a slowly progressive neurodegenerative condition with onset in middle to late adulthood. Unlike AD, where severe memory problems dominate the clinical picture, FTD is generally characterized by prominent personality change and expressive language problems. Memory complaints, although present, are more variable in nature and are more commonly attributed to impaired attentional focus. The typical onset of symptoms in FTD occurs relatively early compared to AD, occurring primarily in the fifth or sixth decade of life. The condition evolves over the course of 5–10 years and results in significant social and occupational impairments and, ultimately, death. Impairments in judgment, behavioral regulation, and diminished insight throughout the illness render the condition particularly challenging to the family and other caregivers, who must accommodate for the affected individual in society. As FTD progresses, severe impairments occur in emotional and behavioral regulation, resulting in a spectrum of abnormal behaviors from disinhibition, perseveration, lability, to severe akinesia and mutism. Ultimately, the disorder culminates in complete functional dependence and, ultimately, a vegetative state, indistinguishable clinically from AD and other end-stage dementias. In the early stages, however, because of its insidious onset, progressive nature, and similarity in some of the clinical symptoms to those of AD (e.g., forgetfulness, language disorder), FTD can be clinically confused with AD. Even so, on closer inspection an astute clinician can usually distinguish between the two disorders. It is now clear that FTDs are a unique clinical entity, separable from AD in terms of underlying neuropathology, anatomical specificity of damaged brain circuitry, genetic loci, and clinical presentation (see McKhann et al., 2001, for review). These characteristics are reviewed in the following text.

Epidemiology

Population- and community-based studies of dementia in the United States and abroad are shedding light on the public health significance of FTD in the context of aging and other dementias. Historically, FTD was considered relatively rare, with Pick's disease, a form of frontal dementia, representing the prototype (see Rossor, 2001, for a historical overview). The original six cases described by Arnold Pick were characterized by a relatively circumscribed language impairment (amnesic aphasia), which progressed over time and corresponded to temporal lobe atrophy at postmortem examination (Alzheimer et. al., 1995). The neuropathological correlates of the illness were later described by Alzheimer et al. (1995) and underscored the absence of senile plaques and the relative sparing of the hippocampus—pathological features characterizing Alzheimer's disease. Two histopathological features were thought to be the gold standard for the condition—argyrophilic inclusions and swollen achromatic cells—and were termed Pick bodies and Pick cells, respectively. These histopathological features were certainly correlated with the dementia but were only rarely observed, leading to the conclusion that the frontal dementia, or Pick's disease, was an infrequent condition. This perception of its relative prevalence has also been influenced by imperfect clinical recognition.

The importance of FTD as a much more common family of neurodegenerative disorders is a more recent concept. Over the last 25 years a number of case series and epidemiological reports have described patients with very similar clinical symptoms to Pick's disease, who were lacking the classic lobar atrophy and histopathological signatures of the condition on postmortem examination. These disorders have carried descriptive names, characterizing the uniqueness in the cellular pathological features (e.g., frontal-lobe dementia of the non-Alzheimer's type; dementia lacking distinctive histopathology), or in the unique clustering of clinical symptomatology (e.g., semantic dementia, primary progressive aphasia). It is now believed that rather than a rare phenomenon, the disorder may be a fairly common cause of dementia in middle adulthood (ages 45–65). Neuropathological series suggest that it accounts for nearly 10% of the dementia cases that come to postmortem examination (Neary & Snowdon, 1996). Clinic-based series and epidemiological studies place the prevalence as high as 20% in the general population (Snowden, Neary, & Mann, 2002). The condition has been pathologically verified in individuals as young as 21 years of age (Snowden, Neary, & Mann, 2004), and although it is unusual to find cases of the disorder in carefully examined populations over age 75 (Breitner et al., 1999), one study reports a prevalence as high as 3% in a Swedish population over age 85 (Gislason, Sjogren, Larsson, & Skoog, 2003). Men and women appear to be affected equally by the disorder, and there is some familial aggregation suggesting a role of genetic factors.

Genetics

FTD is likely not a single disorder with a single cause but a family of conditions arising from a complex interaction of genetic and environmental factors, resulting in a final common pathway of selective neurodegeneration confined initially to the frontal cortex and its efferent connections. As noted previously, familial aggregation is common in FTD, with evidence of genetic transmission across generations. A history of similar dementia is present in approximately half the cases of FTD that come to clinical attention (McKhann et al., 2001), and mutations in the tau gene on chromosome 17 has been verified in some familial forms of the condition (see Spillantini & Goedert, 2001, for review). These tau mutations account for only about 5–6% of the cases of FTD (Poorkaj et al., 2001). In all likelihood other genes and environmental precipitants are important. Genetic linkages to chromosome 3 (Brown et al., 1995) and chromosome 9 (Hosler et al., 2000) have been reported, but the actual causal genes in these instances have not yet been identified. Mutations in the presenilin gene, located on chromosome 14, have also been associated with some familial forms of FTD (Raux et al., 2000) as well as some instances of autopsy-confirmed Pick's disease—the latter occurring without amyloid plaques (Dermaut et al., 2004), suggesting that FTD and AD may share common biological causal pathways.

The neuropathology of FTD is heterogeneous but differs from AD by the absence of amyloid plaques. Tangles, however, are common to both disorders. Neurofibrillary tangles are a requisite pathology in AD dementia; they are also a common feature in FTD, being found in almost half the cases (McKhann et al., 2001). At least three histopathological subtypes have been described (Knopman, Boeve, & Petersen, 2003; Snowden et al., 2002); a microvacuolar subtype accounts for approximately 60% of the cases. This subtype is characterized by spongiform degeneration or "microvacuolation" of the superficial neuropil and a loss of large cortical neurons in the frontal and temporal cortices. Gliosis is generally absent, and the limbic system and striatum can be affected, but usually only to a minimal extent. A second type, the Pick body subtype, accounts for perhaps as much as 23% of the cases and is characterized by the loss of cortical neurons, widespread gliosis, swollen, chromatic, and distended neurons (Pick cells), along with tau and ubiquitin positive inclusions in the surviving neuropil (Pick bodies). The limbic system and striatum tend to be more heavily affected in this subtype, but typically the hippocampus is spared, and spongiform changes in the cortex are absent. A third subtype, occurring in 15% of the cases, has clinical features of both FTD and motor-neuron disease during life and also has correspondingly neuropathological features of both disorders at autopsy.

Diagnosis

Diagnostic criteria that aid the clinician in identifying the disorder in its various symptom manifestations (Lund & Manchester Groups, 1994) are summarized in Table 3.3. Because the location of the pathology to frontal systems can be located to anterior, mesial, or lateral sectors of the frontal cortex, the constellation of symptoms can vary tremendously. Although histopathological subtypes are well described in FTD, the disorder is now generally conceptualized as falling into one of two distinctive clinical subtypes: *a behavioral subtype*, often heralded by changes in personality and behavioral regulation; *and a language subtype*, comprised of semantic dementia and/or progressive nonfluent aphasia (Hodges et al., 2004). Most clinical cases present with a combination of the behavioral and language problems. Additionally, motor symptoms are common to both clinical presentations (Hodges, 2001). The neurocognitive and behavioral features of each of the subtypes are described in the following text.

Neuropsychological Presentation

Behavioral Subtype. The neuropsychological presentation of FTD varies by subtype, but it almost certainly includes a combination of behavioral and neurocognitive features. In the more common behavioral form of the disorder, the neurocognitive features may be indefinite, particularly early on. It is not uncommon for affected individuals to test in the normal range on conventional tests used in dementia evaluations, such as mental status screening examinations (e.g., MMSE of 27 or higher) and tests of intelligence and recent memory function, including delayed recall (Cherrier et al., 1997; Pachana, Boone, Miller, Cummings, & Berman, 1996). However, deficits are easily discerned on tests of frontal executive function (Pachana et al., 1996). These patients have difficulty on tasks such as the Wisconsin Card Sorting Test or the Short Category Test, which involve behavioral

TABLE 3.3. Clinical Diagnostic Features of Frontotemporal Dementia

Core diagnostic features

1. *Behavioral disorder* that is insidious in onset, slowly progressive, and characterized by any of the following early features:
   a. Loss of personal awareness (e.g., neglect of personal hygiene or grooming)
   b. Loss of social awareness (e.g., loss of social tact, misdemeanors etc)
   c. Decreased insight into pathological changes in own behavior or mental state
   d. Disinhibition early in course (e.g., unrestrained sexuality)
   e. Mental inflexibility
   f. Hyperorality
   g. Sterotyped and perseverative behaviors
   h. Utilization behavior (i.e., unrestrained exploration of objects in the environment)

2. *Affective symptoms* are common and include any of the following:
   a. Depression, anxiety, sentimentality, suicidal and fixed ideation or delusions early in the disorder
   b. Hypochondriasis or bizarre somatic preoccupations early in the illness
   c. Emotional indifference or lack of empathy, sympathy, apathy
   d. Amimia (inertia, aspontaneity)

3. *Speech disturbances* characteristic of the disorder uniquely distinguish it from other common dementias. Symptoms include:
   a. Progressive reduction of speech (aspontaneity, economy of utterance)
   b. Sterotyped speech (limited repertoire of words or themes)
   c. Echolalia or perseveration
   d. Late mutism

4. *Frontal lobe* signs and other physical signs:
   a. Early primitive reflexes
   b. Early incontinence
   c. Late akinesia, rigidity, tremor
   d. Low and labile blood pressure

5. *Perceptual spatial disorders* are absent; intact abilities to negotiate the environment.

6. *Investigative findings* include:
   a. Normal EEG, despite clinically evident dementia
   b. Brain imaging (structural or functional or both) that shows predominantly frontal or anterior temporal lobe abnormalities.
   c. Neuropsychology findings of profound failure on frontal lobe tests; absence of severe memory impairments, aphasic disorder, or perceptual spatial disturbance

Supportive diagnostic features

1. Onset before age 65
2. Positive family history of similar disorder in first-degree relative (i.e., parent, sibling)
3. Bulbar palsy, muscular weakness, wasting, fasciculations (e.g., motor-neuron disease)

Exclusionary features

Abrupt onset with ictal events	Head trauma related to the onset
Early severe amnesia	Early spatial disorientation or other signs of agnosia
Early severe apraxia	Logoclonic speech with rapid loss of train of thought
Myoclonus	Corticobulbar and spinal deficits
Cerebellar ataxia	Choreoathetosis
Early, severe pathological EEG	Laboratory tests indicating brain inflammatory process

Brain imaging with either predominant postcentral structural
   or functional defect or multifocal cerebral lesions (CT/MRI)

Relative diagnostic exclusions

1. Typical history of chronic alcoholism
2. Sustained hypertension
3. History of vascular disease

Note. Summarized from Brun et al. (1994).

regulation, flexibility, higher-order conceptualization, and multitasking. Additionally, expressive language may appear normal in casual conversation but is typically characterized by difficulty in word generation, as can be discerned on tests of either confrontation naming or verbal fluency.

More notably in the behavioral form of FTD is the character change. Central to the disorder is difficulty in behavioral regulation, which can lead to excessive irritability, volatility, or emotional lability that is described by family members as uncharacteristic of the patient's normal baseline behavior. At the other extreme, some individuals display severe apathy and behavioral inertia that can progress to mutism. Personality changes accompanying the disorder include early signs of declining social judgment, impulsivity, disinhibition of thought and action, and difficulty in maintaining personal boundaries (e.g., a normally reserved person starting inappropriate conversations with strangers). Unusual behaviors, including components of the Kluver–Bucy syndrome such as hyperorality or hypersexuality, are also noted in some cases. In diagnosing the disorder, it is absolutely essential to obtain a thorough history of behavioral change, neurocognitive observations, and psychiatric symptoms from a knowledgeable informant to complement the objective neurocognitive testing and assessment of function. Patients themselves are often unable to self-reflect on their own difficulties; and early on the neurocognitive profile may appear relatively unremarkable, despite enormous changes in everyday functioning.

Language Subtype. The language subtype of FTD can be subdivided into two distinctive entities in which the symptom manifestations, at least in the early phases of the illness, are almost entirely confined to the language domain. The symptom complex differs in the two language variants of FTD, and there is some indication that the differing phenotypes may share different pathogenesis (Hodges et al., 2004). One form of language disorder in FTD involves impaired language expression and is termed nonfluent "primary progressive aphasia" (Mesulam, 2001), also discussed in Clare (Chapter 13, this volume; Johnson, 2005). The less common form of language disorder in FTD involves selective difficulty in understanding word meaning and has been designated as "semantic dementia" (Hodges, 2001; Hodges & Miller, 2001).

The early manifestations in primary progressive aphasia (PPA) include rather isolated and distressing difficulties in word retrieval leading to labored speech, articulation problems, reduction in output, circumlocution, and anomia on formal assessment. Comprehension is generally intact at this stage of illness, as are many other aspects of neurocognitive function, including general intelligence and visuospatial functioning. The impairment is not usually accompanied by problems in new learning or memory; however, performance on verbally based memory tests may suggest deficiencies due to the aphasic element. When memory problems are evident, they are less severe overall than those of AD. When patients present with prominent language disorders and memory impairments, the diagnosis of AD with prominent language disturbances may be more appropriate (Knopman, Boeve, & Petersen 2003). As the condition of PPA progresses, language decline becomes much more pronounced and generalized, resulting in comprehension impairments, severe reduction in verbal output, and eventually mutism. Other aspects of cognition are almost invariable impaired at the later stages of the disorder, making clinical differentiation from AD difficult in the absence of reliable historical information of symptom manifestation and progression.

Semantic dementia, by contrast, is characterized by fluent speech but substantial impairments in word comprehension. Word-finding difficulty is common across the two subtypes and can be elicited on clinical examination by tests of naming. Characteristically, these patients have difficulty on semantic memory tests that assess their verbal and nonverbal knowledge of object relations and categorical membership (Hodges et al., 2004). In addition, there are often a number of behavioral or psychiatric features in semantic dementia. Depending on the area of focal brain involvement, different neuro-cognitive and behavioral features emerge. In left anterior temporal cases, language problems, as described, are accompanied commonly by depression. In many instances there are also reported changes in dietary habits and development of food fads (Thompson, Patterson, & Hodges, 2003). In cases where the neuronal degeneration is more lateralized to the right temporal lobe, word finding is a common complaint, comprehension is generally unaffected, but there is often poor facial identification. This pattern is coupled with behavioral changes that include bizarre affect and impaired social conduct; patients are often described as rude, disinhibited, socially awkward, and lacking insight.

Attendant Data

Beyond neuropsychological testing, a diagnosis of FTD requires a complete medical history, similar to evaluation of any other neuropsychological disorder. Differential diagnostic considerations in FTD include prior serious head injury, cerebrovascular events, brain tumor, metastic illness, or other progressive neurodegenerative disorders, such as AD or progressive supranuclear palsy. Because FTD shows a heritable component in nearly 50% of the cases, a good family history of mid- to late-life neurological and psychiatric disorders can be helpful and provide useful supportive information for the diagnosis. Genetic testing for mutations in the tau gene is not commonly done in the clinical evaluation of FTD and is generally only appropriate in instances where chromosome 17 FTD is suspected by virtue of proven multigenerational evidence of FTD in the family kindred (Knopman et al., 2001).

Perhaps the most useful attendant information to secure a diagnosis of FTD comes from structural and functional neuroimaging studies. To exclude focal lesions in the frontal and anterior temporal areas, MRI studies are generally preferred over CT for the evaluation of suspected FTD. Although these studies may be unremarkable initially in symptom manifestation, the presence of focal atrophy confined either to the prefrontal cortex or the anterior temporal areas provides confirmatory evidence of the FTD diagnosis. Functional studies using either PET or SPECT also can provide direct evidence of focal frontotemporal dysfunction. The metabolic patterns associated with FTD and AD are very different, with hypometabolism confined largely to the frontal and temporoparietal cortices in the respective disorders. This contrasting pattern allows the disorders to be reliably identified by a skilled neuroradiologist or other dementia specialist trained and qualified to interpret neuroimaging scans using standard visual inspection methods (Higdon et al., 2004).

DEMENTIA OF PARKINSON'S DISEASE AND LEWY BODY DEMENTIA

Parkinson's disease (PD) has attendant changes in cognition that may evolve over time into a full dementia syndrome in about a third of affected patients (Jacobs et al., 1995; Janvin, Aarsland, Larsen, & Hugdahl, 2003). Current estimates place the rates of dementia between 19 and 40% in PD patients, compared to elderly adults unaffected by the disorder (Aarsland et al., 2001, 2003; Marder, Tang, Cote, Stern, & Mayeux, 1995; Tison et al., 1995). Risk factors for the development of dementia in PD include older age, late-onset age of PD, family history of dementia, longer disease duration, greater motor symptom severity, depression, hypertension, limited education, low socioeconomic status, and confusion or psychosis associated with treatment with levodopa or related agents (Emre, 2003).

Lewy body disease is a spectrum of disorders, with onset in the 60s and 70s typically, which overlaps substantially with both PD and AD (Ballard et al., 1999). The dementia associated with cortical Lewy bodies is characterized by attentional disturbances, parkinsonism, and cognitive impairment. As noted it is often referred to as Lewy body dementia (LBD); other common terms include dementia with Parkinsonism, dementia with Lewy bodies—DLB—or DLB with Parkinsonism. For this discussion we use the term Lewy body dementia—LBD—to describe the clinical syndrome, because the presence of Lewy body neuropathology requires postmortem examination, and this information is not always available in many clinical reports describing the neurocognitive characteristics. The diagnostic criteria for the disorder are summarized in Table 3.4 and are elaborated in the text that follows.

The prevalence of PD-D and LBD in the population over 60 is not completely understood. Currently, the frequency of PD alone in the elderly is estimated at approximately 1% (Baldereschi et al., 2003; Strickland & Bertoni, 2004). Most studies estimate that the PD-D spectrum disorders (PD-D and LBD combined) may account for nearly 15–22% of the cases of late-onset dementias, making it roughly as common as VaD and about half as common as AD (Campbell, Stephens, & Ballard, 2001; Lennox, 1998; Rahkonen et al., 2003). Some studies suggest that the rates may be even higher if combinations of pathology are considered. One community-based study, confirming the diagnosis with postmortem examinations, suggests that Lewy body neuropathology is very common in normal aging, with approximately 22.5% showing these changes on postmortem examination. In the demented subgroup, LBD dementia accounted for nearly 41% of the cases (Wakisaka et al., 2003).

Genetics

The etiological causes of PD-D and LBD are not at all understood but appear to be multifactorial and more than likely involve a complex interplay of genetic factors with environmental exposures, as is true in the related conditions of AD and PD more generally. The evidence for genetic causes is supported first by observations of genetic heritability in both early and late onset PD (Marder et al., 2003; Payami, Zareparsi, James, & Nutt, 2002; see also Cato & Crosson, Chapter 4, this volume). These studies suggest that in some instances, PD follows patterns of genetic transmission and accounts for approximately 10% of the cases (Dawson & Dawson, 2003). In these familial forms, causal mutations have been identified in the gene "parkin" that codes for the protein alpha-synuclein, a known protein that aggregates within the Lewy bodies and the Lewy neurites of PD and LBD. Genetic linkage has also been reported on chromosome 2, on the short arm of chromosome 4, and at three different loci on chromosome 1 (see Gwinn-Hardy, 2002; Dawson & Dawson, 2003 for reviews).

The role of environmental exposures and lifestyle factors in PD-D–LBD is even more tenuous. In PD there is some support for environmental exposures playing a role in the more common sporadic (nonfamilial) form of the disorder; whether this finding extends to LBD remains to be seen. At least 20 different studies report smoking as a protective factor in PD, suggesting a possible role of the cholinergic pathway and its demise in PD (see Fratiglioni & Wang, 2000, for review). In addition, PD appears to be more common

TABLE 3.4. Clinical Diagnostic Features of Lewy Body Dementia

1. Central feature of LBD is a progressive dementia of sufficient magnitude to interfere with normal social and occupational function. Prominent or persistent memory impairment may not occur in early stages but is evident with progression. Deficits on tests of attention and frontal-subcortical skills and visuospatial ability may be particularly prominent.

2. Probable and possible LBD: Two of the following core features are essential for the diagnosis of *probable LBD*. One of the features is necessary for designation of *possible LBD*.
   a. Fluctuating cognition with pronounced variations in attention and alertness
   b. Recurrent visual hallucinations that are typically well formed and detailed
   c. Spontaneous motor features of parkinsonism

3. Features supportive of the diagnosis
   a. Repeated falls
   b. Syncope
   c. Transient loss of consciousness
   d. Neuroleptic sensitivity
   e. Systematized delusions
   f. Hallucinations in other modalities

Note. Summarized from McKeith et al. (1996).

in men, leading some to posit that estrogen may be neuroprotective (Baldereschi et al., 2003). Herbicide and pesticide exposure has been linked to an enhanced risk of the condition (Seidler, et al., 1996), with some studies providing evidence of a genetic interaction that serves to provoke symptoms (Hubble et al., 1998). It is not clear that exposure to any of these agents plays a role in LBD.

The clinical similarity between PD-D–DLB and AD has suggested that these disorders may be linked etiologically. However, evidence for the same genetic causes in AD and PD spectrum conditions has not yet been definitely demonstrated. It is posited that if the same genetic mechanisms underlie the conditions, then AD and PD disorders should co-occur with high frequency within the same families. This co-occurrence has not been found. In recent work examining the risk of AD in familial PD, no increased susceptibility was found for AD when compared to control families (Levy et al., 2004). However, in this study probands with PD-D were not included, which may have biased the findings toward the null result. Other studies suggest that genes with overlapping susceptibility to brain neurodegenerative conditions may act in concert with specific AD or PD etiological factors, which then act to trigger one disorder or the other (Li et al., 2002, 2004).

Whatever the genetic or environmental triggers of PD, the ultimate etiological factor underlying both PD-D and LBD appears to be the aggregation of cortical Lewy bodies and not AD cortical changes. A series of investigations has examined the neuropathological correlates of these dementias. And, although alpha-synuclein aggregates occur in PD, LBD, and AD (Lippa, Schmidt, Lee, Trojanowski, 2001), the dementia associated with PD and LBD appears to be more strongly related to cortical Lewy bodies than to the plaques and tangles of AD (Hurtig et al., 2000; Mattila, Rinne, Helenius, Dickson, & Roytta, 2000).

Diagnosis

The diagnosis of PD-D dementia or LBD rests, in large part, on the relative occurrence of dementia with regard to extrapyramidal motor symptoms. A diagnosis of PD-D is made when global cognitive and functional impairments emerge in patients who have already been diagnosed and treated for PD. The diagnosis of LBD is made when the symptoms of dementia either predate or follow the onset of parkinsonism within a 1-year time interval; however, frequently, the dementia and motor symptoms coincide. Three key features define the LBD disorder: (1) arousal disturbances characterized by sleepiness, altered arousal, and fluctuations in attention; (2) motor problems, which typically include gait and balance problems, rigidity, and akinesia; and (3) a cognitive disorder, similar to AD, with characteristic prominent memory impairments. As described later, the neurocognitive profile is actually readily distinguishable from that typical of AD. Rapid eye movement (REM) sleep disorders commonly precede LBD and are reportedly present in nearly half of the cases (Boeve et al., 2003). Patients also typically experience fully formed visual hallucinations early in the disorder; some researchers have suggested that there may be intrusions of REM sleep into the wakefulness cycle (Knopman et al., 2003). LBD tends to have a faster progression rate than AD and generally poorer prognosis with shorter survival intervals (Olichney et al., 1998). However, with pharmacological interventions for management of the sleep disorder and neuropsychiatric disturbances, this situation may be changing.

Neuropsychological Profile of PD

The cognitive problems typically associated with the PD process are described in detail in Chapter 4 of this volume. However, to fully understand the presentation of PD-D–LBD it is important to be clear on the neurocognitive distinctions between PD and AD. We briefly review key features of PD here, but refer the reader to Cato and Crosson (Chapter 4, this volume) for a more comprehensive discussion.

The disorder of PD is characterized by forgetfulness, a slowing in the thought process, attentional problems, and difficulty in spontaneous word retrieval, particularly in the absence of structural support or cuing (Janvin et al., 2003). These changes in cognition are not generally disabling, and patients frequently develop adaptive strategies to accommodate for some of these problems. Qualitatively, PD patient examinations are dominated by the extrapyramidal features associated with this disease; hypophonic speech is common, along with bradykinesia, bradyphrenia, and poor graphic motor skills such as micrographia (Hodges, 2001). Typically, this constellation of behaviors, along with the cognitive profile of PD (described in Chapter 4), has been labeled by neuropsychologists as "subcortical" in nature, and the disorder seen as distinguishable from AD by the absence of rapid forgetting (Noe et al., 2004). Although the cognitive problems are not likely all based on the subcortical brain changes associated with PD, the "subcortical" descriptor has been a useful construct with which clinician refer to the central processing problem of PD and related conditions of the basal ganglia and nigrostriatal system, which all share problems in retrieval mechanisms and flexible behavior and benefit from structural support strategies.

The key features of the neuropsychological profile of PD are mild executive and attentional problems (Woods & Troster, 2003), which can be discerned on tests of sustained attention and concentration, such as digit span or other simple span tasks. Memory impairment is also commonly reported in PD; however, when investigations carefully control for age, education, and other confounding variables, PD patients generally have less severe memory deficits than matched groups with AD (Heyman et al., 1999). In contrast to AD, recognition memory is either intact or generally less affected in PD when compared to AD, and PD patients also benefit more from cues in paragraph recall tasks. Verbal fluency is almost always impaired in PD, but naming is not. Visual constructional abilities are characteristically affected by PD and not entirely due to the motor symptoms. Some have suggested that an underlying fundamental defect in organizational ability and executive function is responsible for the cognitive deficits described in speech, memory, and visuoconstruction. In one study, in which executive function was controlled by covarying the results of individual performance on the Wisconsin Card Sorting Test, the deficiencies in learning, memory, visual perception, and visuoconstruction were no longer significant in the PD-affected groups (Bondi, Salmon, Galasko, Thomas, & Thal, 1999).

Neuropsychological Profile of LBD

LBD can be difficult to distinguish from PD-D, but can be discerned from other conditions such as AD and progressive supranuclear palsy (PSP) fairly readily (Aarsland et al., 2003; Hamilton et al., 2004). LBD is characterized by the presence of marked deficits in attention and executive function, visuospatial impairments, and constructional difficulties early within the process (Connor et al., 1998; Galasko, Katzman, Salmon, & Hansen, 1996; Hansen et al., 1990; Salmon et al., 1996). Selective impairments often occur very early in the disorder within attentional allocation and working memory (Ballard et al., 1999; Emre, 2003). Patients with LBD have anterograde memory problems similar to those of AD, although these deficits appear less severe in LBD (Hamilton et al., 2004; Stern et al., 1998). Both AD and LBD show impaired acquisition scores on tests such as the California Verbal Learning Test CVLT), the Logical Memory subtest of the Wechsler Memory Scale, and the Buschke Selective Reminding Test, but delayed recall, savings scores, and recognition performances are all comparatively better retained in the LBD group. The memory problems of LBD are accompanied by better naming skills but poorer executive and visuospatial functions in contrast to AD (Ballard et al., 1999; Heyman et al., 1999). Qualitatively, when matched by stage these patients may appear more apathetic than patients with AD, and they may show more distractibility and greater tendencies toward perseveration, confabulations, and intrusions (Doubleday, Snowden, Varma, & Neary, 2002). In the latter regard, although both groups make intrusional errors, LBD patients show a propensity toward environmentally triggered errors (e.g., upon seeing a trash can in the testing room, and LBD patient would be inclined to volunteer *trash can* as a word on a memory test). The intrusions in AD tend to be more semantically related to target stimuli or derive from previously administered tests.

Because of the overlap between the neurocognitive and behavioral features of LBD with AD, the reliability of the diagnosis based on neuropsychological profile alone is imperfect. Clinical pathological studies have shown limits in both sensitivity and specificity of the diagnosis, even when adhering to the published criteria, which include much more than neuropsychological data (Holmes, Cairns, Lantos, & Mann, 1999; Mega et al., 1996). Improving the diagnosis will require further understanding of the causal mechanisms underlying each of the disorders: AD, PD, and LBD. Until that time, the clinical diagnosis at present can be enhanced by the clinician's careful attention to the prominent defining characteristics of the LBD disorder: the arousal and motor disturbances (Knopman, Boeve, et al., 2003). Other neurodegenerative conditions that can mimic the disorder need to be carefully considered in the differential diagnosis, including progressive supranuclear palsy (PSP) and corticobasal degeneration (CBD). These conditions can usually be distinguished clinically, based on the presentation of the motor findings. PSP generally has ocular and brain stem abnormalities, along with Parkinsonian signs, mild subcortical cognitive profile, and balance problems (Litvan et al., 1996). CBD is often, but not invariably, characterized by focal motor apraxia along with other similar parkinsonism and cognitive features (Grimes, Lang, & Bergeron, 1999).

Attendant Data

The diagnosis of PD-D and LBD requires a careful consideration of current and past history variables regarding the relative onset of motor signs and dementia. The crux of the differential diagnosis rests on the relative occurrence of dementia in the context of PD symptoms. LBD diagnosis requires that the dementia did not occur within 1 year of PD symptoms. Some have argued that this distinction is arbitrary and not supported on clinical grounds (e.g., Ballard et al., 2002). It remains to be seen if the two disorders are indeed separate entities. At present, subtyping is useful in the event that the disorders show different responsiveness to pharmacological treatments. Both disorders appear responsive to cholinergic therapies, but differential responsiveness to levodopa therapy can distinguish PD from LBD. Presence of visual hallucinations, not associated with treatment, can also help distinguish LBD from PD-D. In the future, the differential diagnosis of the conditions from other dementias may be facilitated by consideration of biological markers, neurological findings, laboratory, test results, and functional and structural imaging data. No reliable diagnostic test for either PD-D or LBD is yet available.

Ultimately the firm diagnosis of PD, LBD, and AD rests on neuropathological verification of these illnesses. The typical neuropathology of PD includes depigmentation of the substantia nigra and locus coeruleus, along with neuronal loss in the nucleus basalis of Meynert, the dorsal raphe nucleus, the dorsal motor nucleus of the vagus, and thalamic nuclei. The remaining neurons within these areas show the characteristic presence of Lewy bodies—round eosinophilic inclusions that are composed of a halo of fibrils surrounding a less defined core. These cellular inclusions are classic for the illness, along with dystrophic neuritis (Lewy neuritis). LBD contrasts with PD in that the distribution of Lewy bodies (intracytoplasmic eosinophilic inclusion bodies) in LBD is diffuse and widespread across the cortex, nucleus basalis of Meynert, and substantia nigra. It should be noted that there is considerable overlap in the neuropathology of these different entities, however; most cases of LBD also show senile plaques and may also have neurofibrillary tangles (Lennox, 1998). The overlap likely underscores shared etiological mechanisms. Coming to a further understanding of this continuum of pathological presentations and its correspondence to the unfolding of clinical features will be important in ultimately identifying causal pathways.

CONCLUSIONS

AD and its prodrome, MCI, are easily detected and distinguished from other cognitive disorders of late life through clinical methods, a cornerstone of which is detailed neuropsychological testing (Grundman et al., 2004). There is overlap in the clinical features of related dementias of late life, including PD-D, LBD, FTD, and vascular disorders (not reviewed here). In part this clinical overlap reflects the overlap in the pathogenic features that underlie the conditions, and the presence of mixed etiologies for the cognitive disorders (Bird et al., 2003; Knopman et al., 2003). Distinguishing between disorders and determining the relative contributions of various disease comorbidities is facilitated by the advances in biotechnology, genetics, and functional imaging (Cacabelos, 2002;

Machulda et al., 2003). These methods already have produced useful biomarkers (such as apoE) that assist in early and reliable AD detection. The advent of surrogate markers for tracking disease course and responsiveness to therapy, in conjunction with effective pharmacotherapies, may allow streamlined treatment of patients in the future in a way that is tailored to their specific diagnosis (e.g., AD vs. LBD) and other variables related to drug responsiveness (e.g., genotype). The field is exploding at present, with huge private industry and government-supported investments in the pharmacogenetics, proteomics, and metabolomics of dementia (Butterfield, Boyd-Kimball, & Castegna, 2003). Although no "cures" for late-life dementias are immediately forthcoming, the potential for effective treatment in the future is evident and appears not only strategically possible but encouraging.

REFERENCES

Aarsland, D., Andersen, K., Larsen, J. P., Lolk, A., & Kragh-Sorensen, P. (2003). Prevalence and characteristics of dementia in Parkinson disease: An 8-year prospective study. *Archives of Neurology, 60*, 387–392.

Aarsland, D., Andersen, K., Larsen, J. P., Lolk, A., Nielsen, H., & Kragh-Sorensen, P. (2001). Risk of dementia in Parkinson's disease: A community-based, prospective study. *Neurology, 56*, 730–736.

Almkvist, O., Axelman, K., Basun, H., Wahlund, L. O., & Lannfelt, L. (2002). Conversion from preclinical to clinical stage of Alzheimer's disease as shown by decline of cognitive function in carriers of the Swedish APP-mutation. *Journal of Neural Transmission Supplementum, 62*, 117–125.

Alzheimer, A., Stelzmann, R. A., Schnitzlein, H. N., & Murtagh, F. R. (1995). An English translation of Alzheimer's 1907 paper, "*Uber eine eigenartige Erkankung der Hirnrinde.*" *Clinical Anatomy, 8*, 429–431.

Anthony, J. C., LeResche, L., Niaz, U., von Korff, M. R., & Folstein, M. F. (1982). Limits of the "Mini-Mental State" as a screening test for dementia and delirium among hospital patients. *Psychological Medicine, 12*, 397–408.

Arnold, S. E., Hyman, B. T., Damasio, A. R., & Van Hoesen, G. W. (1991). The topographical and neuroanatomical distribution of neurofibrillary tangles and neuritic plaques in the cerebral cortex of patients with Alzheimer's disease. *Cerebral Cortex, 1*, 103–116.

Baddeley, A. D. (1986). *Working memory.* Oxford, UK: Oxford University Press.

Baddeley, A. D., Baddeley, H. A., Bucks, R. S., & Wilcock, G. K. (2001). Attentional control in Alzheimer's disease. *Brain, 124*, 1492–1508.

Baldereschi, M., Di Carlo, A., Vanni, P., Ghetti, A., Carbonin, P., Amaducci, L., et al. (2003). Lifestyle-related risk factors for Parkinson's disease: A population-based study. Italian Longitudinal Study on Aging Working Group. *Acta Neurologica Scandinavica, 108*, 239–244.

Ballard, C. G., Ayre, G., O'Brien, J., Sahgal, A., McKeith, I. G., Ince, P.G., et al. (1999). Simple standardized neuropsychological assessments aid in the differential diagnosis of dementia with Lewy bodies from Alzheimer's disease and vascular dementia. *Dementia and Other Geriatric Cognitive Disorders, 10*, 104–108.

Baxter, L. C., Caselli, R. J., Johnson, S. C., Reiman, E., & Osborne, D. (2003). Apolipoprotein E epsilon 4 affects new learning in cognitively normal individuals at risk for Alzheimer's disease. *Neurobiology of Aging, 24*, 947–952.

Bayles, K. A., Boone, D. R., Tomoeda, C. K., Slauson, T. J., & Kaszniak, A. W. (1989). Differentiating Alzheimer's patients from the normal elderly and stroke patients with aphasia. *Journal of Speech and Hearing Disorders, 54*, 74–87.

Becker, J. T. (1988). Working memory and secondary memory deficits in Alzheimer's disease. *Journal of Clinical and Experimental Neuropsychology, 10*(6), 739–753.

Benke, T. (1993). Two forms of apraxia in Alzheimer's disease. *Cortex, 29*, 715–725.

Benton, A. L., Hamsher, K., Varney, N., & Spreen, O. (1983). *Contributions to neuropsychological assessment*. New York: Oxford University Press.

Bertram, L., Blacker, D., Mullin, K., et al. (2000). Evidence for the Genetic linkage of Alzheimer's disease to chromosome 10q. *Science, 290*, 2302–2303.

Binetti, G., Locascio, J. J., Corkin, S., Vonsattel, J. P., & Growdon, J. H. (2000). Differences between Pick disease and Alzheimer's disease in clinical appearance and rate of cognitive decline. *Archives of Neurology, 57*(2), 225–232.

Bird, T., Knopman, D., VanSwieten, J., Rosso, S., Feldman, H., Tanabe, H., et al. (2003). Epidemiology and genetics of frontotemporal dementia/Pick's disease. *Annals of Neurology, 54*(Suppl. 5), S29–S31.

Boeve, B. F., Silber, M. H., Parisi, J. E., et al. (2003). Synucleinopathy pathology and REM sleep behavior disorder plus dementia or parkinsonism. *Neurology, 61*, 40–45.

Bondi, M. W., Salmon, D. P., Galasko, D., Thomas, R. G., & Thal, L. J. (1999). Neuropsychological function and apolipoprotein E genotype in the preclinical detection of Alzheimer's disease. *Psychology and Aging, 14*(2), 295–303.

Bowen, J., Teri, L., Kukull, W., McCormick, W., McCurry, S. M., & Larson E. B. (1997). Progression to dementia in patients with isolated memory loss. *Lancet, 349*, 763–765.

Bowler, J. V. (2002). The concept of vascular cognitive impairment. *Journal of the Neurological Sciences, 204*, 11–15.

Braak, H., & Braak, E. (1991). Neuropathological staging of Alzheimer-related changes. *Acta Neuropathologica, 82*, 239–259.

Breitner, J. C. S., Wyse, B., Anthony, J., Welsh-Bohmer, K., Steffens, D., Norton, M., et al. (1999). APOE E4 count predicts age when prevalence of AD increases, then declines. The Cache County Study. *Neurology, 53*, 321–331

Brown, J., Ashworth, A., Gydesen, S., et al. (1995). Familial non-specific dementia maps to chromosome 3. *Human Molecular Genetics, 4*, 1625–1628.

Brookmeyer, R., Gray, S., & Kawas, C. (1998). Projections of Alzheimer's disease in the United States and the public health impact of delaying disease onset. *American Journal of Public Health, 88*(9), 1337–1342.

Brun, A., Englund, B., Gustafson, L., et al. (1994). Clinical and neuropathological criteria for frontotemporal dementia. *Journal of Neurology, Neurosurgery, and Psychiatry, 57*, 416–418.

Butterfield, D. A., Boyd-Kimball, D., & Castegna, A. (2003). Proteomics in Alzheimer's disease: Insights into potential mechanisms of neurodegeneration. *Journal of Neurochemistry, 86*, 1313–1327.

Cacabelos, R. (2002). Pharmacogenomics for the treatment of dementia. *Annals of Medicine, 34*, 357–379.

Cahn, D. A., Salmon, D. P., Butters, N., Weiderholt, W. C., Corey-Bloom, J., Edelstein, S. L., et al. (1995). Detection of dementia of the Alzheimer type in a popular-based sample: Neuropsychological test performance. *Journal of the International Neuropsychological Society, 1*(3), 252–260.

Campbell, S., Stephens, S., & Ballard, C. (2001). Dementia with Lewy bodies: Clinical features and treatment. *Drugs and Aging, 18*, 397–407.

Cherrier, M. M., Mendez, M. F., Perryman, K. M., Pachana, N. A., Miller, B. L., & Cummings, J. L. (1997). Frontotemporal dementia versus vascular dementia: Differential features on mental status examination. *Journal of the American Geriatrics Society, 45*, 579–583.

Chertkow, H., & Bub, D. (1990). Semantic memory loss in dementia of Alzheimer's type: What do various measures measure? *Brain, 113*, 397–417.

Clark, C. M., & Ewbank, D. C. (1996). Performance of the Dementia Severity Rating Scale: A caregiver questionnaire for rating severity in Alzheimer Disease. *Alzheimer Disease and Associated Disorders, 10*, 31–39.

Clark, C. M., & Karlawish, J. H. T. (2003). Alzheimer disease: Current concepts and emerging diagnostic and therapeutic strategies. *Annals of Internal Medicine, 138*, 400–410.

Connor, D. J., Salmon, D. P., Sandy, T. J., Galasko, D., Hansen, L. A., & Thal, L. J. (1998). Cognitive profiles of autopsy-confirmed Lewy body variant versus pure Alzheimer disease. *Archives of Neurology, 55*, 994–1000.

Corder, E. H., Saunders, A. M., Strittmatter, W. J., et al. (1993). Gene dose of apolipoprotein E type 4 and the risk of Alzheimer's disease in late onset families. *Science, 261*, 921–923.

Cummings, J. L., & Benson, D. (1992). *Dementia: A clinical approach.* Stoneham, MA: Butterworth–Heinemann.

Cummings, J. L., Benson, F., Hill, M. A., & Read, S. (1985). Aphasia in dementia of the Alzheimer type. *Neurology, 35*(3), 394–397.

Damasio, A. R., Tranel, D., & Rizzo, M. (2000). Disorders of complex visual processing. In M. M. Mesulam (Ed.), *Principles of behavioral and cognitive neurology* (2nd ed.). New York: Oxford University Press.

Dawson, T. M., & Dawson, V. L. (2003). Rare genetic mutations shed light on the pathogenesis of Parkinson's disease. *Journal of Clinical Investigation, 111*, 145–151.

DeKosky, S. T., & Orgogozo, J. M. (2001). Alzheimer disease: Diagnosis, costs, and dimensions of treatment. *Alzheimer Disease and Associated Disorders, 15*(Suppl. 1), S3–S7.

Dermaut, B., Kumar-Singh, S., Engelborghs, S., et al. (2004). A novel presenilin 1 mutation associated with Pick's disease but not beta-amyloid plaques. *Annals of Neurology, 55*, 617–626.

Doubleday, E. K., Snowden, J. S., Varma, A. R., & Neary, D. (2002). Qualitative performance characteristics differentiate dementia with Lewy bodies and Alzheimer's disease. *Journal of Neurology, Neurosurgery, and Psychiatry, 72*, 602–607.

Eastley, R., Wilcock, G. K., & Bucks, R. S. (2000). Vitamin B_{12} deficiency in dementia and cognitive impairment: The effects of treatment on neuropsychological function. *International Journal of Geriatric Psychiatry, 15*, 226–233.

Ebly, E. M., Hogan, D. B., & Parhad, I. M. (1995). Cognitive impairment in the nondemented elderly: Results from the Canadian Study of Health and Aging. *Archives of Neurology, 52*, 612–619.

Elias, M. F., Beiser, A., Wolf, P. A., Au, R., White, R. F., & D'Agostino, R. B. (2000). The preclinical phase of Alzheimer's disease: A 22-year prospective study of the Framingham cohort. *Archives of Neurology, 57*, 808–813.

Emre, M. (2003). Dementia associated with Parkinson's disease. *Lancet Neurology, 2*, 229–237.

Ertekin-Taner, N., Graff-Radford, N., Younkin, L. H., et al. (2000). Linkage of plasma Abeta42 to quantitative locus on chromosome 10 in late onset AD pedigrees. *Science, 290*, 2303–2404.

Evans, D. A., Beckett, L. A., Field, T. S., et al. (1997). Apolipoprotein E epsilon 4 and evidence of Alzheimer's disease in a community population of older persons. *Journal of American Medical Association, 277*(10), 822–824.

Farrer, L. A., Cupples, L. A., van Duijn, C. M., Connor-Lacke, L., Kiely, D. K., & Growdon, J. H. (1995). Rate of progression of Alzheimer's disease is associated with genetic risk. *Archives of Neurology, 52*, 918–923.

Fillit, H., & Hill, J. (2002). The costs of vascular dementia: A comparison with Alzheimer's disease. *Journal of the Neurological Sciences, 203–204*, 35–39.

Flicker, C., Ferris, S. H., & Reisberg, B. (1991). Mild cognitive impairment in the elderly: Predictors of dementia. *Neurology, 41*, 1006–1009.

Fox, P. J., Kohatsu, N., Max, W., & Arnsberger, P. (2001). Estimating the costs of caring for people with Alzheimer disease in California: 2000–2040. *Journal of Public Health Policy, 22*(1), 88–97.

Fratiglioni, L., De Ronchi, D., & Aguero-Torres, H. (1999). Worldwide prevalence and incidence of dementia. *Drugs and Aging, 15*, 365–75.

Fratiglioni, L., & Wang, H. X. (2000). Smoking and Parkinson's and Alzheimer's disease: Review of the epidemiological studies. *Behavioral Brain Research, 113*, 117–120.

Galasko, D., Katzman, R., Salmon, D. P., & Hansen, L. (1996). Clinical and neuropathological findings in Lewy body dementias. *Brain and Cognition, 31*, 166–175.

Geldmacher, D. S., & Whitehouse, P. J., Jr. (1997). Differential diagnosis of Alzheimer's disease. *Neurology, 48*(5 Suppl. 6), S2–S9.

Gislason, T. B., Sjogren, M., Larsson, L., & Skoog, I. (2003). The prevalence of frontal variant frontotemporal dementia and the frontal lobe syndrome in a population based sample of 85 year olds. *Journal of Neurology, Neurosurgery, and Psychiatry, 74*, 867–871.

Goate, A. M., Chartier, M. C., Mullin, M. C., et al. (1991). Segregation of a missense mutation in the amyloid precursor protein gene with familial Alzheimer's disease. *Nature, 33*, 53–56.

Goebels, N., & Soyka, M. (2000). Dementia associated with vitamin B(12) deficiency: Presentation of two cases and review of the literature. *Journal of Neuropsychiatry and Clinical Neurosciences, 12*, 389–394.

Graham, J. E., Rockwood, K., Beattie, B. L., Eastwood, R., Gauthier, S., Tuokko, H., et al. (1997). Prevalence and severity of cognitive impairment with and without dementia in an elderly population. *Lancet, 349*, 1793–1796.

Graham, N. L., & Hodges, J. R. (2004). Distinctive cognitive profiles in Alzheimer's disease and subcortical vascular dementia. *Journal of Neurology, Neurosurgery, and Psychiatry, 75*(1), 61–71.

Graves, A. B., Larson, E. B., Edland, S. D., Bowen, J. D., McCormick, W. C., McCurry, S. M., et al. (1996). Prevalence of dementia and its subtypes in the Japanese American population of King County, Washington state: The Kame Project. *American Journal of Epidemiology, 144*, 760–771.

Greenwood, P. M., Parasuraman, R., & Alexander, G. E. (1997). Controlling the focus of spatial attention during visual search: Effects of advanced aging and Alzheimer disease. *Neuropsychology, 11*, 3–12.

Grimes, D. A., Lang, A. E., & Bergeron, C. B. (1999). Dementia as the most common presentation of cortical-basal ganglionic degeneration. *Neurology, 53*, 1969–1974.

Grundman, M., Petersen, R. C., Ferris, S. H., Thomas, R. G., Aisen, P. S., Bennett, D. A., et al. (2004). Mild cognitive impairment can be distinguished from Alzheimer disease and normal aging for clinical trials. *Archives of Neurology, 61*, 59–66.

Gwinn-Hardy, K. (2002). Genetics of Parkinsonism. *Movement Disorders, 17*, 645–656.

Hamilton, J. M., Salmon, D. P., Galasko, D., Delis, D. C., Hansen, L. A., Masliah, E., et al. (2004). A comparison of episodic memory deficits in neuropathologically-confirmed dementia with Lewy bodies and Alzheimer's disease. *Journal of the International Neuropsychological Society, 10*, 689–697.

Hansen, L., Salmon, D., Galasko, D., Masliah, E., Katzman, R., DeTeresa, T., et al. (1990). The Lewy body variant of Alzheimer's disease: a clinical and pathologic entity. *Neurology, 40*(1), 1–8.

Hanson, L., Salmon, D., Galasko, D., et al. (1990). The Lewy body variant of Alzheimer's disease: A clinical and pathological entity. *Neurology, 40*, 1–8.

Hart, R. P., Kwentos, J. A., Harkins, S. W., et al. (1988). Rate of forgetting in mild Alzheimer's type dementia. *Brain and Cognition, 7*, 31–38.

Hart, R. P., Kwentus, J. A., Taylor, J. R., & Harkins, S. W. (1987). Rate of forgetting in dementia and depression. *Journal of Consulting and Clinical Psychology, 55*, 101–105.

Hebert, L. E., Scherr, P. A., Bienias, J. L., Bennett, D. A., & Evans, D. A. (2003). Alzheimer disease in the U.S. population: Prevalence estimates using the 2000 census. *Archives of Neurology, 60*, 1119–1122.

Heyman, A., Fillenbaum, G. G., Gearing, M., Mirra, S. S., Welsh-Bohmer, K. A., Peterson, B., et al. (1999). Comparison of Lewy body variant of Alzheimer's disease with pure Alzheimer's disease: Consortium to Establish a Registry for Alzheimer's Disease, Part XIX. *Neurology, 52*, 1839–1844.

Hier, D. B., Hagenlocker, K., & Shindler, A. G. (1985). Language disintegration in dementia: Effects of etiology and severity. *Brain and Language, 25*, 117–133.

Higdon, R., Foster, N. L., Koeppe, R. A., DeCarli, C. S., Jagust, W. J., Clark, C. M., et al. (2004). A comparison of classification methods for differentiating fronto-temporal dementia from Alzheimer's disease using FDG-PET imaging. *Statistics in Medicine, 23*, 315–326.

Hodges, J. R. (2001). Frontotemporal dementia (Pick's disease). Clinical features and assessment. *Neurology, 56*, S6–S10.

Hodges, J. R., Davies, R. R., Xuereb, J. H., Casey, B., Broe, M., Bak, T. H., et al. (2004). Clinicopathological correlates in frontotemporal dementia. *Annals of Neurology, 56*, 399–406.

Hodges, J. R., & Miller, B. (2001). The classification, genetics, and neuropathology of frontotemporal dementia. Introduction to the special topic papers: Part 1. *Neurocase, 7*(1), 31–35.

Hoffman, J. M., Welsh-Bohmer, K. A., Hanson, M., Crain, B., Hulette, C., Earl, N., et al. (2000). Fluorodeoxyglucose (FDG) and positron emission tomography (PET) in pathologically verified dementia. *Journal of Nuclear Medicine, 41*, 1920–1928.

Holmes, C., Cairns, N., Lantos, P., & Mann, A. (1999). Validity of current clinical criteria for Alzheimer's disease, vascular dementia and dementia with Lewy bodies. *British Journal of Psychiatry, 174*, 45–50.

Hosler, B. A., Siddique, T., Sapp, P. C., Sailor, W., Huang, M. C., Hossain, A., et al. (2000). Linkage of familial amyotrophic lateral sclerosis with frontotemporal dementia to chromosome 9q21–q22. *Journal of the American Medical Association, 284*, 1664–1669.

Hubble, J. P., Kurth, J. H., Glatt, S. L., Kurth, M. C., Schellenberg, G. D., Hassanein, R. E., et al. (1998). Gene–toxin interaction as a putative risk factor for Parkinson's disease with dementia. *Neuroepidemiology, 17*, 96–104.

Hughes, C. P., Berg, L., Danziger, W. I., Coben, L. A., & Martin, R. L. (1982). A new clinical scale for the staging of dementia. *British Journal of Psychiatry, 140*, 566–572.

Hurtig, H. I., Trojanowski, J. Q., Galvin, J., Ewbank, D., Schmidt, M. L., Lee, V. M., et al. (2000). Alpha-synuclein cortical Lewy bodies correlate with dementia in Parkinson's disease. *Neurology, 54*, 1916–1921.

Hyman, B. T., Van Hoesen, G. W., Damasio, A. R., & Barnes, C. L. (1984). Alzheimer's disease: Cell-specific pathology isolates the hippocampal formation. *Science, 225*, 1168–1170.

Jacobs, D. M., Marder, K., Cote, L. J., Sano, M., Stern, Y., & Mayeux, R. (1995). Neuropsychological characteristics of preclinical dementia in Parkinson's disease. *Neurology, 45*, 1691–1696.

Janvin, C., Aarsland, D., Larsen, J. P., & Hugdahl, K. (2003). Neuropsychological profile of patients with Parkinson's disease without dementia. *Dementia and Geriatric Cognitive Disorders, 15*, 126–131.

Klunk, W. F., Engler, H., Nordberg, A., Bacskai, B. J., Wang, Y., Price, J. C., et al. (2003). Imaging the pathology of Alzheimer's disease: Amyloid-imaging with positron emission tomography. *Neuroimaging Clinics of North America, 13*(4), 781–789.

Knopman, D. S., Boeve, B. F., & Petersen, R. C. (2003). Essentials of the proper diagnoses of mild cognitive impairment, dementia, and major subtypes of dementia. *Mayo Clinic Proceedings, 78*, 1290–1308.

Knopman, D. S., DeKosky, S. T., Cummings, J. L., Corey-Bloom, J., Relkin, N., Small, G. W., et al. (2001). Practice parameter: Diagnosis of dementia (an evidence based review). Report of the Quality Standards Subcommittee of the American Academy of Neurology. *Neurology, 56*, 1143–1153.

Knopman, D. S., Parisi, J. E., Boeve, B. F., Cha, R. H., Apaydin, H., Salviati, A., et al. (2003). Vascular dementia in a population-based autopsy study. *Archives of Neurology, 60*, 569–575.

Kulasingam, S. L., Samsa, G. P., Zarin, D. A., Rutschmann, O. T., Patwardhan, M. B., McCrory, D. C., et al. (2003). When should functional neuroimaging techniques be used in the diagnosis and management of Alzheimer's dementia? A decision analysis. *Value in Health, 6*, 542–50.

Lehmann, M., Regland, B., Blennow, K., & Gottfries, C. G. (2003). Vitamin B_{12}–B_6–folate treatment improves blood–brain barrier function in patients with hyperhomocysteinaemia and mild cognitive impairment. *Dementia and Geriatric Cognitive Disorders, 16*, 145–150.

Lennox, G. G. (1998). Dementia with Lewy bodies. In J. H. Growdon & M. N. Rossor (Eds.), *The dementias* (pp. 67–79). Boston: Butterworth–Heinemann.

Levy, G., Louis, E. D., Mejia-Santana, H., Cote, L., Andrews, H., Harris, J., et al. (2004). Lack of familial aggregation of Parkinson's disease and Alzheimer's disease. *Archives of Neurology, 61*, 1033–1039.

Levy-Lahad, E., Wasco, W., Poorkaj, P., Romano, D. M., Oshima, J., & Pettingell, W. H. (1995). Candidate gene for the chromosome 1 familial Alzheimer's disease locus. *Science, 269*(5226), 973–977.

Levy, R. (1994). Aging-associated cognitive decline. *International Psychogeriatrics, 6*, 63–68.

Lezak, M. D. (1995). *Neuropsychological assessment* (3rd ed.). New York: Oxford University Press.

Li, Y. J., Oliveira, A., Xu, P., Martin, E. R., Stenger, J. E., Scherzer, C. R., et al. (2003). Glutathione S-transferase, omega-1 (GSTO1) modifies age at onset of Alzheimer's disease and Parkinson's disease. *Human Molecular Genetics, 12*, 3259–3267.

Li, Y. J., Scott, W. K., Hedges, D. J., Zhang, F., Gaskell, P. C., Nance, M. A., et al. (2002). Onset in neurodegenerative diseases is genetically controlled. *American Journal of Human Genetics, 70*, 985–993.

Linn, R. T., Wolf, P. A., Bachman, D. L., Knoefel, J. E., Cobb, J. L., Belanger, A. J., et al. (1995). The 'preclinical phase' of probable Alzheimer's disease: A 13-year prospective study of the Framingham cohort. *Archives of Neurology, 52*(5), 485–490.

Lippa, C. F., Schmidt, M. L., Lee, V. M., & Trojanowski, J. Q. (2001). Alpha-synuclein in familial Alzheimer disease: Epitope mapping parallels dementia with Lewy bodies and Parkinson disease. *Archives of Neurology, 58*, 1817–1120.

Litvan, I., Agid, Y., Jankovic, J., et al. (1996). Accuracy of clinical criteria for the diagnosis of progressive supranuclear palsy (Steele–Richardson–Olszewski syndrome). *Neurology, 46*, 922–930.

Lobo, A., Launer, L. J., Fratiglioni, L., Andersen, K., Di Carlo, A., Breteler, M. M., et al. (2000). Prevalence of dementia and major subtypes in Europe: A collaborative study of population-based cohorts. Neurologic Diseases in the Elderly Research Group. *Neurology, 54*(11 Suppl. 5), S4–S9.

Locascio, J. J., Growdon, J. H., & Corkin, S. (1995). Cognitive test performance in detecting, staging, and tracking Alzheimer's disease. *Archives of Neurology, 52*, 1087–1099.

Looi, J., & Sachdev, P. S. (1999). Differentiation of vascular dementia from AD on neuropsychological tests. *Neurology, 53*, 670–678.

Lund and Manchester Groups. (1994). Clinical and neuropathological criteria for frontotemporal dementia. *Journal of Neurology, Neurosurgery, and Psychiatry, 57*, 416–418.

Lyketsos, C. G., Lopez, O., Jones, B., Fitzpatrick, A. L., Breitner, J., & DeKosky S. (2002). Prevalence of neuropsychiatric symptoms in dementia and mild cognitive impairment: Results from the cardiovascular health study. *Journal of American Medical Association, 288*, 1475–1483.

Manly, J. J., Jacobs, D. M., Sano, M., Bell, K., Merchant, C. A., Small, S. A., et al. (1998). Cognitive test performance among nondemented elderly African Americans and whites. *Neurology, 50*, 1238–45.

Manly, J. J., Jacobs, D. M., Touradji, P., Small, S. A., & Stern, Y. (2002). Reading level attenuates differences in neuropsychological test performance between African American and white elders. *Journal of the International Neuropsychological Society, 8*, 341–348.

Manly, J. J., Touradji, P., Tang, M. X., & Stern Y. (2003). Literacy and memory decline among ethnically diverse elders. *Journal of Clinical and Experimental Neuropsychology, 25*, 680–690.

Marder, K., Levy, G., Louis, E. D., Mejia-Santana, H., Cote, L., Andrews, H., et al. (2003). Familial aggregation of early- and late-onsct Parkinson's disease. *Annals of Neurology, 54*, 507–513.

Marder, K., Tang, M. X., Cote, L., Stern, Y., & Mayeux, R. (1995). The frequency and associated risk factors for dementia in patients with Parkinson's disease. *Archives of Neurology, 52*, 695–701.

Matsuda, O., Saito, M., & Sugishita, M. (1998). Cognitive deficits of mild dementia: A comparison between dementia of the Alzheimer's type and vascular dementia. *Psychiatry and Clinical Neurosciences, 52*, 87–91.

Mattila, P. M., Rinne, J. O., Helenius, H., Dickson, D. W., & Roytta, M. (2000). Alpha-synuclein-immunoreactive cortical Lewy bodies are associated with cognitive impairment in Parkinson's disease. *Acta Neuropathologica, 100*, 285–290.

Mayeux, R. (2003). Epidemiology of neurodegeneration. *Annual Review of Neurosciences*, *26*, 81–104.

McKeith, I. G., Galasko, D., Kosaka, K., Perry, E. K., Dickson, D. W., Hansen, L. A., et al. (1996). Clinical and pathological diagnosis of dementia with Lewy bodies (DLB): Report to the Consortium on Dementia with Lewy Bodies International Workshop. *Neurology*, *47*, 1113–1124.

McKhann, G. M., Albert, M. S., Grossman, M., Miller, B., Dickson, D., & Trojanowski, J. Q. (2001). Clinical and pathological diagnosis of frontotemporal dementia: Report of the Work Group on Frontotemporal Dementia and Pick's Disease. *Archives of Neurology*, *58*, 1803–1809.

McKhann, G. M., Drachman, D., Folstein, M., Katzman, R., Price, D., & Stadlan, E. M. (1984). Clinical diagnosis of Alzheimer's disease: Report of the NINCDS–ADRDA Work Group. *Neurology*, *34*, 939–944.

Mega, M. S., Masterman, D. L., Benson, D. F., Vinters, H. V., Tomiyasu, U., Craig, A. H., et al. (1996). Dementia with Lewy bodies: Reliability and validity of clinical and pathologic criteria. *Neurology*, *47*, 1403–1409.

Mesulam, M. M. (2001). Primary progressive aphasia. *Annals of Neurology*, *49*, 425–432.

Moore, S., Sandman, C. A., McGrady, K., & Kesslak, J. P. (2001). Memory training improves cognitive ability in patients with dementia. *Neuropsychological Rehabilitation*, *11*, 245–261.

Morris, J. C., Edland, S., Clark. C., Galasko, D., Koss, E., Mohs, R., et al. (1993). The Consortium to Establish a Registry for Alzheimer's Disease (CERAD): Part IV. Rates of cognitive change in the longitudinal assessment of probable Alzheimer's disease. *Neurology*, *43*, 2457–2465.

Morris, J. C., Storandt, M., Miller, J. P., McKeel, D. W., Price, J. L., Rubin, E. H., et al. (2001). Mild cognitive impairment represents early-stage Alzheimer disease. *Archives of Neurology*, *58*, 397–405.

Murdoch, B. E., Chenery, H. J., Wilks, V., & Boyle, R. S. (1987). Language disorders in dementia of the Alzheimer type. *Brain and Language*, *31*, 122–137.

Myers, A., Holmans, P. Marshall, H., Hardy, J., & Goate, A. M. (2000). Susceptibility locus for Alzheimer's disease on chromosomes 10. *Science*, *290*, 2304–2305.

Neary, D., & Snowden, J. S. (1996). Fronto-temporal dementia: Nosology, neuropsychology, and neuropathology. *Brain and Cognition*, *31*, 176–187.

Nebes, R. D., & Madden, D. J. (1988). Different patterns of cognitive slowing produced by Alzheimer's disease and normal aging. *Psychology and Aging*, *3*(1), 102–104.

Noe, E., Marder, K., Bell, K. L., Jacobs, D. M., Manly, J. J., & Stern Y. (2004). Comparison of dementia with Lewy bodies to Alzheimer's disease and Parkinson's disease with dementia. *Movement Disorders*, *19*, 60–67.

Olichney, J. M., Galasko, D., Salmon, D. P., Hofstetter, C. R., Hansen, L. A., Katzman, R., et al. (1998). Cognitive decline is faster in Lewy body variant than in Alzheimer's disease. *Neurology*, *51*, 351–357.

Pachana, N. A., Boone, K. B., Miller, B. L., Cummings, J. L., & Berman, N. (1996). Comparison of neuropsychological functioning in Alzheimer's disease and frontotemporal dementia. *Journal of the International Neuropsychological Society*, *2*, 505–510.

Parasuraman, R., Greenwood, P. M., & Sunderland, T. (2002). The apolipoprotein E gene, attention, and brain function. *Neuropsychology*, *16*(2), 254–274.

Payami, H., Zareparsi, S., James, D., & Nutt, J. (2002). Familial aggregation of Parkinson disease: A comparative study of early-onset and late-onset disease. *Archives of Neurology*, *59*, 848–850.

Pericak, Vance, M. A., Grubber, J., Bailey, L. R., Hedges, D., West, S., Santoro, L., et al. (2000). Identification of novel genes in late-onset Alzheimer's disease. *Experimental Gerontology*, *25*, 1343–1352.

Pericak, Vance, M. A., & Haines, J. L. (1998). Potential chromosome 12 locus for late-onset Alzheimer's disease. *Journal of American Medical Association*, *279*, 433.

Petersen, R. C., Doody, R., Kurz, A., Mohs, R. C., Morris, J. C., Rabins, P. V., et al. (2001). Current concepts in mild cognitive impairment. *Archives of Neurology*, *58*, 1985–1992.

Petersen, R. C., Smith, G. E., Waring, S. C., Ivnik, R. J., Tangalos, E. G., & Kokmen, E. (1999). Mild cognitive impairment: Clinical characterization and outcome. *Archives of Neurology*, *56*, 303–308 & erratum, 760.

Petersen, R. C., Stevens, J. C., Ganguli, M., Tangalos, E. G., Cummings, J. L., & DeKosky, S. T. (2001). Practice parameter: Early detection of dementia—mild cognitive impairment (an evidence-based review). Report of the Quality Standards Subcommittee of the American Academy of Neurology. *Neurology*, *56*, 1133–1142.

Plassman, B. L., & Breitner, J. C. S. (1996). Apolipoprotein E and cognitive decline in Alzheimer's disease. *Neurology*, *47*, 917–920.

Plassman, B. L., & Steffens, D. C. (2004). Genetics. In D. G. Blazer, D. C. Steffens, & E. Busse (Eds.), *Textbook of geriatric psychiatry* (3rd ed., pp. 109–120). Washington, DC: American Psychiatric Publishing.

Poorkaj, P., Grossman, M., Steinbart, E., Payami, H., Sadovnick, A., Nochlin, D., et al. (2001). Frequency of tau gene mutations in familial and sporadic cases of non-Alzheimer dementia. *Archives of Neurology*, *58*, 383–377.

Rahkonen, T., Eloniemi-Sulkava, U., Rissanen, S., Vatanen, A., Viramo, P., & Sulkava, R. (2003). Dementia with Lewy bodies according to the consensus criteria in a general population aged 75 years or older. *Journal of Neurology, Neurosurgery, and Psychiatry*, *74*, 720–724.

Raux, G., Gantier, R., Thomas-Anterion, C., Bouiliat, J., Verpillat, P., Hannequin, D., et al. (2000). Dementia with prominent frontotemporal features associated with L113P presenilin 1 mutation. *Neurology*, *55*, 1577–1578.

Reid, W. G. (1992). The evolution of dementia in idiopathic Parkinson's disease: Neuropsychological and clinical evidence in support of subtypes. *International Psychogeriatrics*, *4*(Suppl. 2), 147–160.

Reiman, E. M., Caseli, R. J., Yun, L. S., et al. (1996). Preclinical evidence of Alzheimer's disease in persons in homozygous for the e4 allele for apolipoprotein E. *New England Journal of Medicine*, *334*, 725–758.

Reisberg, B., Ferris, S. H., de Leon, M. J., & Crook T. (1988). Global Deterioration Scale (GDS). *Psychopharmacology Bulletin*, *24*, 661–663.

Ritchie, K., Artero, S., & Touchon, J. (2001). Classification criteria for mild cognitive impairment: A population-based validation study. *Neurology*, *56*, 37–42.

Ritchie, K., & Touchon, J. (2001). Mild cognitive impairment: conceptual basis and current nosological status. *Lancet*, *355*, 225–228.

Rizzo, M., Anderson, S. W., Dawson, J., & Nawrot, M. (2000). Vision and cognition in Alzheimer's disease. *Neuropsychologia*, *38*, 1157–1169.

Rizzo, M., Reinach, S., McGhee, D., & Dawson, J. (1997). Simulated car crashes and crash predictors in drivers with Alzheimer disease. *Archives of Neurology*, *54*, 545–551.

Rockwood, K., Wentzel, C., Hachinski, V., Hogan, D. B., MacKnight, C., & McDowell, I. (2000). Prevalence and outcomes of vascular and cognitive impairment: Vascular cognitive impairment investigators of the Canadian Study of Health and Aging. *Neurology*, *54*(2), 447–451.

Roman, G. C., Tatemichi, T. K., Erkinjuntti, T., et al. (1993). Vascular dementia: Diagnostic criteria for research studies. Report of the NINDA–AIREN International workshop. *Neurology*, *43*, 250–260.

Rossor, M. N. (2001). Pick's disease: A clinical overview. *Neurology*, *56*(Suppl. 4), S3–S5.

Salmon, D. P., Galasko, D., Hansen, L. A., Masliah, E., Butters, N., Thal, L. J., et al. (1996). Neuropsychological deficits associated with diffuse Lewy body disease. *Brain and Cognition*, *31*, 148–165.

Salmon, D. P., Thomas, R. G., Pay, M. M., Booth, A., Hofstetter, C. R., Thal, L. J., et al. (2002). Alzheimer's disease can be accurately diagnosed in very mildly impaired individuals. *Neurology*, *59*, 1022–1028.

Saunders, A. M., Schmader, K., Breitner, J. C. S., et al. (1993a). Apolipoprotein E e4 allele distributions in late onset Alzheimer's disease and in other amyloid forming disease. *Lancet*, *342*, 710–711.

Saunders, A. M., Strittmatter, W. J., Schmechel, D., et al. (1993b). Association of apolipoprotein E allele e4 with late onset of familial and sporadic Alzheimer's disease. *Neurology, 43,* 1467–1472.

Scott, W. K., Grubber, J. M., Conneally, P. M., Small, G. W., Hulette, C. M., et al. (2000). Fine mapping of the chromosome 12 late-onset Alzheimer disease locus: Potential genetic and phenotypic heterogeneity. *American Journal of Human Genetics, 66*(3), 922–932.

Seidler, A., Hellenbrand, W., Robra, B. P., Vieregge, P., Nischan, P., Joerg, J., et al. (1996). Possible environmental, occupational, and other etiologic factors for Parkinson's disease: A case-control study in Germany. *Neurology, 46,* 1275–1284.

Silverman, D. H. S., Small, G. W., Chang, C. Y., Lu, C. S., Kung de Aburto, M. A., Chen, W., et al. (2001). Neuroimaging in evaluation of dementia: Regional brain metabolism and long-term outcome. *Journal of the American Medical Association, 286,* 2120–7.

Small, G. W., Ercoli, L. M., Silverman, D. H. S., et al. (2000). Cerebral metabolic and cognitive decline in persons at genetic risk for Alzheimer's disease. *Proceedings of the National Academy of Sciences, 97,* 6037–6042.

Snowden, J. S., Neary, D., & Mann, D. M. (2002). Frontotemporal dementia. *British Journal of Psychiatry, 180,* 140–143.

Snowden, J. S., Neary, D., & Mann, D. M. (2004). Autopsy proven sporadic frontotemporal dementia due to microvacoular-type histology, with onset of 21 years of age. *Journal of Neurology, Neurosurgery, and Psychiatry, 75*(9), 1337–1339.

Spillantini, M. G., & Goedert, M. (2001). Tau gene mutations and tau pathology in frontotemporal dementia and parkinsonism linked to chromosome 17. *Advances in Experimental Medicine and Biology, 487,* 21–37.

Steffens, D. C., Welsh, K. A., Burke, J. R., Helms, M. J., Folstein, M. F., Brandt, J., et al. (1996). Diagnosis of Alzheimer's disease in epidemiological studies by staged review of clinical data. *Neuropsychiatry, Neuropsychology, and Behavioral Neurology, 9,* 107–113.

Steinberg, M., Sheppard, J.M., Tschanz, J. T., Norton, M. C., Steffens, D. C., Breitner, J. C., et al. (2003). The incidence of mental and behavioral disturbances in dementia: The Cache County Study. *Journal of Neuropsychiatry and Clinical Neurosciences, 15,* 340–345.

Stern, Y., Tang, M. X., Jacobs, D. M., Sano, M., Marder, K., Bell, K., et al. (1998). Prospective comparative study of the evolution of probable Alzheimer's disease and Parkinson's disease dementia. *Journal of the International Neuropsychological Society, 4,* 279–284.

St. George-Hyslop, P., Haines, J., Rogeeav, E., et al. (1992). Genetic evidence for a novel familial Alzheimer's disease locus on chromosome 14. *Nature Genetics, 2,* 330–334.

Storey, E., Slavin, M. J., & Kinsella, G. J. (2002). Patterns of cognitive impairment in Alzheimer's disease: Assessment and differential diagnosis. *Frontiers in Bioscience, 7,* e155–e184.

Strickland, D., & Bertoni, J. M. (2004). Parkinson's prevalence estimated by a state registry. *Movement Disorders, 19,* 318–323.

Strittmatter, W. J., Saunders, A. M., Schmechel, D., et al. (1993). Apolipoprotein E: High affinity binding to beta amyloid and increased frequency of type 4 allele in late onset familial Alzheimer's. *Proceedings of the National Academy of Sciences, 90,* 1977–1981.

Tatemichi, T., Sacktor, N., & Mayeux, R. (1994). Vascular dementia. In R. Katzman (Ed.), *Alzheimer's disease* (pp. 123–166). New York: Raven Press.

Thompson, S. A., Patterson, K., & Hodges, J. R. (2003). Left/right asymmetry of atrophy in semantic dementia: Behavioral–cognitive implications. *Neurology, 61,* 1196–1203.

Tierney, M. C., Black, S. E., Szalai, J. P., Snow, W. G., Fisher, R. H., Nadon, G., et al. (2001). Recognition memory and verbal fluency differentiate probable Alzheimer disease from subcortical ischemic vascular dementia. *Archives of Neurology, 58,* 1654–1659.

Tierney, M. C., Szalai, J. P., Snow, W. G., Fisher, R. H., Nores, A., Nadon, G., et al. (1996). Prediction of probable Alzheimer's disease in memory impaired patients: A prospective longitudinal study. *Neurology, 46,* 661–665.

Tison, F., Dartigues, J. F., Auriacombe, S., Letenneur, L., Boller, F., & Alperovitch, A. (1995). Dementia in Parkinson's disease: A population-based study in ambulatory and institutionalized individuals. *Neurology, 45,* 705–708.

Troster, A. I., Fields, J. A., Testa, J. A., Paul, R. H., Blanco, C. R., Hames, K. A., et al. (1998). Cortical and subcortical influences on clustering and switching in the performance of verbal fluency tasks. *Neuropsychologia, 36,* 295–304.

Tschanz, J. T., Corcoran, C., Skoog, I., Khachaturian, A. S., Herrick, J., & Hayden, K. M. (2004). Dementia: The leading predictor of death in a defined elderly population. The Cache County Study. *Neurology, 62*(7), 1156–1162.

Tschanz, J., Welsh-Bohmer, K., Norton, M., Corcoran, C., & Breitner, J. (2003). Progression to dementia in diverse types of mild cognitive impairments of aging. *Journal of the International Neuropsychological Society, 9*(2), 225.

Tschanz, J. T., Welsh-Bohmer, K. A., West, N., Norton, M. C., Wyse, B. W., Breitner, J. C. S., et al. (2000). Identification of dementia cases derived from a neuropsychological algorithm: Comparisons with clinically derived diagnoses. *Neurology, 54,* 1290–1296.

Tuokko, H., Frerichs, R., Graham, J., Rockwood, K., Kristjansson, B., Fisk, J., et al. (2003). Five-year follow-up of cognitive impairment with no dementia. *Archives of Neurology, 60,* 577–582.

Unverzagt, F. W., Gao, S., Baiyewu, O., Ogunniyi, A. O., Gureje, O., Perkins, A., et al. (2001). Prevalence of cognitive impairment: Data from the Indianapolis Study of Health and Aging. *Neurology, 57,* 1655–1662.

Wakisaka, Y., Furuta, A., Tanizaki, Y., Kiyohara, Y., Iida, M., & Iwaki, T. (2003). Age-associated prevalence and risk factors of Lewy body pathology in a general population: The Hisayama study. *Acta Neuropathology, 106,* 374–382.

Wechsler, D. (1987). *Wechsler Memory Scale—Revised Manual.* New York: Psychological Corporation.

Wechsler, D. (1997). *Wechsler Adult Intelligence Scale—III.* New York: Psychological Corporation.

Welsh, K. A., Butters, N., Hughes, J. P., Mohs, R. C., & Heyman, A. (1991). Detection of abnormal memory decline in mild Alzheimer's disease using CERAD neuropsychological measures. *Archives of Neurology, 48,* 278–281.

Welsh, K. A., Butters, N., Hughes, J. P., Mohs, R. C., & Heyman, A. (1992). Detection and staging of dementia in Alzheimer's disease: Use of the neuropsychological measures developed for the Consortium to Establish a Registry for Alzheimer's Disease (CERAD). *Archives of Neurology, 49,* 448–452.

Welsh, K. A., Butters, N., Mohs, R. C., Beekly, D., Edland, S., Fillenbaum, G., et al. (1994). The Consortium to Establish a Registry for Alzheimer's Disease (CERAD): Part V. A normative study of the neuropsychological battery. *Neurology, 44,* 609–614.

Welsh, K. A., Fillenbaum, G., Wilkinson, W., Heyman, A., Mohs, R. C., Stern, Y., et al. (1995). Neuropsychological performance of black and white patients with Alzheimer's disease. *Neurology, 45,* 2207–2211.

Woods, S. P., & Troster, A. I. (2003). Prodromal frontal/executive dysfunction predicts incident dementia in Parkinson's disease. *Journal of the International Neuropsychological Society, 9,* 17–24.

4

Stable and Slowly Progressive Dementias

M. ALLISON CATO
BRUCE A. CROSSON

In this chapter we review neurological, epidemiological, pathophysiological, and neuropsychological characteristics of a number of slowly progressive dementias. Many of the dementias presented in this chapter share a frontosubcortical presentation in contrast to that of the more "cortical" profile associated with Alzheimer's disease (AD). Whereas the dementias reviewed by Welsh-Bohmer and Warren (Chapter 3, this volume) are invariably progressive, the dementias presented in this chapter often progress slowly, and in some cases, are even stable in course. We do not cover all slowly progressive dementias, however. The etiologies covered here (Parkinson's disease, vascular, alcohol use, and head trauma) were selected, in part, because of their relevance to the aging population.

Because the purpose of this discussion of dementias is to review information pertinent to geriatric neuropsychological assessment, a few introductory remarks regarding current definitions of, and classifications among, slowly progressive dementias are warranted. The neurocognitive profile associated with AD has greatly influenced conceptualization of dementia as a construct (Looi & Sachdev, 1999). Historically speaking, the cornerstone criterion for dementia was memory dysfunction. In frontosubcortical dementias, perhaps more devastating than the memory impairment (which is primarily one of retrieval rather than encoding) are deficits in executive functions as well as debilitating slowness in movement and thinking. Thus the following questions arise. Does the broad term of *dementia* connote the same neuropsychological and functional disability in cortical and frontosubcortical dementias? What level of cognitive impairment and what level of functional decline are necessary and sufficient for a diagnosis of dementia? It is not clear that a consensus has been reached, even among health care professionals, about this boundary line for the dementias. We will return to this important issue at the conclusion of the chapter. We now present Parkinson's disease dementia, considered a prototype among the fronto-subcortical dementias.

89

PARKINSON'S DISEASE DEMENTIA

Illness Characterization

Idiopathic Parkinson's disease (PD) is a neurodegenerative disorder identified clinically by a classic motor-symptom triad consisting of (1) a resting "pill-rolling" tremor that disappears during intentional movement, (2) muscular rigidity, and (3) bradykinesia (slowness of movement) (Jankovic, 1987). Cognitive slowing, or bradyphrenia, is another primary feature of PD (Brown & Marsden, 1991). An obvious and sustained response to levodopa or dopamine agonists is characteristic of PD. Other common clinical symptoms related to muscular rigidity include gait disturbances (shuffling, short-stepped gait; diminished arm swing; turn en bloc); stooped posture (with flexion of hips, knees, elbows, and neck); mask-like facial expression; hypophonia; and dysarthria. Muscular rigidity can present in the form of a cogwheel (superimposed ratchety motion) or a plastic (smooth increase in resistance) subtype. Other motor symptoms may include akinesia (a difficulty initiating and paucity of movements), as well as a difficulty stopping movements once in motion. Hypokinesia, or small movements, is observable in micrographia (small, constricted handwriting). Postural instability secondary to loss of righting reflexes and poor prosody (monotoned speech) are also commonly observed (Levy & Cummings, 2000). The clinical manifestations of PD can be highly variable. Two clinical subtypes, the akinetic-rigid and the tremor-dominant, have been characterized in the literature and have been associated with slightly different patterns of cell loss in the substantia nigra (Jellinger, 2002).

Onset of the disease is typically asymmetrical with unilateral onset of tremor. Mean age of onset occurs between 58 and 62 years of age (range 40–70 years), with peak onset in the sixth decade (Duvoisin, 1984; Martilla, 1987). In terms of course, this disease tends to follow a two-stage trajectory as dopamine levels are nearly depleted before motor symptoms become manifest. Thus a prodromal phase occurs during the two or more decades prior to the obvious motor symptoms. During this prodromal phase, the degeneration of substantia nigra cells is slow and insidious. Following onset of clinical symptoms, this second stage can be further divided into early (1–5 years), middle (6–10 years), and advanced (11–20+ years) stages. Cognitive decline is characteristically slow. Once clinical symptoms become manifest, average time to death in PD if untreated is 8 years (range 1–30 years). With medications, 50% of patients are alive 16 years after onset (Levy & Cummings, 2000).

PD is observed in 150–200 out of every 100,000 individuals in the general population (0.12–0.2%), and prevalence increases with age (Lezak, 1995). Parkinson's disease affects men more than women, but with no differences between sexes in age at disease onset, duration, or severity. Estimates of prevalence of dementia in PD (PD-D) have varied widely in the past, ranging from 4 to 93%, depending on the diagnostic criteria used (Mindham et al., 1993; Woods & Tröster, 2003). Currently accepted prevalence of PD-D is between 25 and 40% (Hughes, Daniel, Blankson, & Lees, 1993).

Attendant Data

The pathophysiological hallmark of PD is the progressive depigmentation and loss of dopamine-containing neurons in the compact zone of the substantia nigra (SNpc) and other brain stem nuclei, leading to a loss of dopaminergic input to the neostriatum (the putamen, especially posterior portions, is more severely affected than the caudate) and neocortex (Levy & Cummings, 2000). Once dopamine levels drop below 30%, motor symptoms become apparent (Lezak, 1995). Regarding the mechanism by which the loss of dopamine leads to the clinical syndrome of PD, a number of theoretical explanations have been offered (e.g., Mink, 1996; Penney & Young, 1986). Briefly, between the basal ganglia and the thalamus, two normally dynamically balanced circuits, commonly referred to as the direct and indirect loops, decrease and increase (respectively) inhibitory inputs to the thalamic nuclei. The thalamic nuclei, in turn, project to the neocortex. The direct motor loop, via disinhibition of specific regions within the motor nuclei of the thalamus (i.e., ventrolateral or VL nuclei), is thought to mediate desired motor programs, whereas the indirect motor loop, via increased inhibition of specific regions within VL nuclei of the thalamus, is thought to mediate the suppression of unwanted motor behaviors.

More recently, the role of direct corticosubthalamic connections in the initiation of behavior has been explored (Nambu et al., 2000; Nambu, Tokuno, & Takada, 2002); however, this route is not directly affected by PD because it bypasses the neostriatum (caudate nucleus and putamen), where the loss of dopaminergic input has its impact. In brief, the loss of dopaminergic input from the SNpc to the putamen results in a disruption of the usual harmony between the two dynamic loops that pass through it, resulting in unopposed inhibition of the thalamus. This inhibition of the thalamus leads to insufficient glutamatergic thalamocortical input and resultant parkinsonism. Presumably, the loss of SNpc dopamine may affect other frontosubcortical loops (Alexander, Delong, & Strick, 1986) in addition to the motor loop leading to other components of the disease, such as bradyphrenia, executive dysfunction, and personality/mood changes.

It should be noted that the loss of dopamine in PD is not the sole pathophysiological mechanism, and further, that PD is heterogeneous in its pathophysiology and resultant clinical presentation. In frankly demented PD patients, pathophysiological mechanisms include comorbid AD pathology, diffuse Lewy body disease, degeneration of other subcortical projection nuclei (locus coeruleus, nucleus basalis of Meynert) or any combination of the above. Obviously, the dementia syndrome is not always the same in PD-D patients, given the heterogeneity of the underlying neuropathology. In fact, approximately one third of all PD patients develop a dementia of the AD type or AD-D (Levy & Cummings, 2000; Salmon, Heindel, & Hamilton, 2001). Whereas approximately 33% of patients with PD have Alzheimer's pathology, a greater number of patients with PD-D have dementia that is not attributable to Alzheimer pathology. The prototypical neuropsychological profile of PD-D without AD differs from AD and is the focus of the next section.

The frequency of depression in PD is high and is more common in patients diagnosed with PD-D. Thirty to fifty percent of PD patients will develop symptoms of depression. Diagnosis of depression in PD is complicated by the fact that anergia, motor retardation, and early awakening can occur in PD patients with or without depression. Anxiety disorders are present in 30–40% of PD patients, with simple phobia the most common subtype, then panic disorder, and then social phobia. These mood and anxiety disorders may be due to neuronal cell loss in noradrenergic and serotonergic nuclei. Another hypothesized mechanism is reduced dopaminergic stimulation of the orbitofrontal cortex, the primary source of cortical input to brain stem serotonergic nuclei (Levy & Cummings, 2000).

Family history of PD or essential tremor and increasing age are two risk factors for PD. Exposure to pesticides or heavy metals is another postulated risk factor. Conversely, cigarette smoking and diets rich in vitamin E have been associated with reduced risk of

PD (Tanner & Goldman, 1996). Risk factors for dementia in PD include older age at on-set, longer disease duration, and greater severity of motor symptoms (Glatt et al., 1996; Marder, Tang, Cote, Stern, & Mayeux, 1995).

Neuropsychological Profile

With the caveat that mild cognitive compromise is more common than dementia in PD, deficits are typically observed in the broad domains of frontal or executive functions and memory retrieval. In addition, bradykinesia (psychomotor slowing) and bradyphrenia (slowed thinking), as evidenced by slowed psychomotor speed and reaction times, are the most common aspects of cognitive dysfunction present even in nondemented PD patients (PD-ND).

Executive Functions

Problems with self-directed generation (e.g., verbal/design fluency), maintenance of set (e.g., Wisconsin Card Sorting Test [WCST]), slowness in set shifting (e.g., WCST; alter-nating motor programs; serial hand sequences), concept formation (e.g., Matrices; WCST, Category Test), and cognitive tracking and flexibility are often seen in PD (Duke & Kaszniak, 2000). With regard to attentional functioning, there is evidence that the def-icit in attention observed in PD patients differs from that of patients with frontal pathol-ogy alone: Patients with frontal-lobe lesions may have relatively greater difficulty with disengaging attention, whereas PD patients may show greater difficulty in maintaining and reengaging a cognitive set (Partiot et al., 1996).

Memory

The typical memory profile in PD involves a deficit in short-term memory for novel, supraspan information across verbal and visual domains. This deficit is observed in mini-mal recall of units of information, but without the commission of intrusions during re-call. Delayed recognition performances are better, indicative of some level of intact en-coding and long-term storage. Semantic memory tends to remain intact (Brown & Marsden, 1990; Dubois, Boller, Pillon, & Agid, 1991; Raskin, Borod, & Tweedy, 1990; Taylor & Saint-Cyr, 1995).

Language

Language deficits may include reduced phrase length and output. Word-finding problems are also common. Reduced word-list generation is often observed, the most common pat-tern of findings reports better performance generating items from semantic categories than words beginning with a specific letter. However, this pattern of better semantic than lexical generation continues to be debated in the literature (Piatt, Fields, Paolo, Koller, & Tröster, 1999). Presumably, an underlying retrieval deficit contributes to difficulties in word generation.

Other Neurocognitive Deficits

Visuospatial deficits observed in patients with PD are shown to worsen with severity of rigidity and bradykinesia. Some argue that underlying problems of motor and executive dysfunction contribute to visuospatial deficits. This multifactorial view of visuospatial deficits in PD has been discussed elsewhere (Lezak, 1995).

Variants

Variants of the pattern of neuropsychological deficits associated with PD have been reported. For example, the scope of cognitive deficits in some PD patients includes such "cortical" features as aphasia, amnesia, agnosia, and apraxia. In these cases, the presence of cortical Lewy bodies, Alzheimer pathology, or both may contribute to a dementia with mixed "cortical" and "subcortical" features (Levy & Cummings, 2000).

Course of Cognitive Decline

A limited number of studies has begun to disentangle the type and severity of cognitive deficits in patients with clinical manifestations consistent with PD who do not have dementia (PD-ND) versus those associated with PD-D. First, sustained and selective attention is intact in early stages (Duke & Kaszniak, 2000; Pillon, Dubois, Ploska, & Agid, 1991) but impaired in PD-D. Second, performance on tests of novel problem solving declines as a function of disease progression (Duke & Kaszniak, 2000). Piatt et al. (1999) found that whereas a PD-D group of patients performed more poorly on three verbal fluency tasks (lexical, semantic, and action), compared to normal controls and a PD-ND group, the disparity between the PD-ND and PD-D groups was largest for the measure of action fluency. Thus impaired action fluency may be an especially sensitive indicator of the conversion from PD-ND to PD-D. This finding is certainly of interest in light of the action semantics literature that ascribes specificity of the frontal lobes in semantic processing of action information (e.g., Damasio & Tranel, 1993; Hauk, Johnsrude, & Pulvermüller, 2004; Pulvermüller, 2001). Finally, in a longitudinal study Woods and Tröster (2003) found that patients with PD who were classified with PD-D the following year performed consistently worse on some neurocognitive measures than patients who retained a diagnosis of PD-ND the following year. The measures that discriminated between these two groups were Digits Backward from the Wechsler Memory Scale—Revised; word-list learning (trials 1–5) and delayed recognition discriminability from the California Verbal Learning Test; and perseverative errors on the Wisconsin Card Sorting Test. These differences among PD patients with and without dementia suggest a gradual decline of neurocognitive functioning predictive of the onset of dementia.

VASCULAR DEMENTIA

Illness Characterization

Until recently, the heterogeneity of pathology leading to vascular dementia (VaD) was less well recognized, and VaD was thought to be caused by multiple large-vessel ischemic damage. It is now recognized that different forms of VaD can arise from a variety of vascular events involving large and/or small vessels and hemorrhagic or ischemic damage. The magnitude and type of cognitive impairment that follows a neurovascular event generally are associated with the location and amount of affected tissue. Findings consistent with focal brain lesion are often seen early in the course of VaD, such as mild motor or sensory deficits, visual field cut, bulbar signs such as dysarthria and dysphagia, extrapyramidal signs such as rigidity and akinesia, or gait disorder (Roman et al., 1993). Manifestation of neurological signs is, of course, dependent on location and extent of tissue affected.

VaD can be further categorized by the extent of cortical versus subcortical involvement. In cortical VaD, sensorimotor changes often occur, along with abrupt onset of cognitive impairment, including aphasia if the language-dominant hemisphere is affected. In subcortical VaD, pure motor hemiparesis may occur, along with bulbar signs and dysarthria. Some small infarcts remain clinically "silent," especially in the case of subcortical white matter ischemic events. An accumulation of subcortical white matter events can lead to dementia, referred to as subcortical ischemic vascular disease (SIVD). SIVD follows from occlusion of the deep penetrating arteries and arterioles that feed the basal ganglia, the thalamus, the internal capsule, and subcortical white matter. Overall, in most cases of vascular origin, size of impacted tissue relates to severity of overall cognitive impairment (Paul et al., 2000).

Typically, VaD is characterized by a relative abrupt onset (days to weeks), stepwise deterioration (some recovery after worsening), and fluctuating course of cognitive functions. Notably, this pattern can be seen with repeated lesions that affect cortical and corticosubcortical brain structures, with large vessel multi-infarct VaD, and with watershed infarcts. In contrast, in patients with small-vessel dementia, such as SIVD, onset is relatively insidious and the course is more slowly progressive (Chui et al., 1992; Leys, Englund, & Erkinjuntti, 2002; Roman et al., 1993).

VaD is second only to AD in prevalence: from 10 to 50% of all dementia cases, depending on geographic location, population, and criteria used (Leys et al., 2002). Among the subtypes of VaD, SIVD may represent the most common form (Paul et al., 2001). In the United States, the reported prevalence of VaD in people 65 years and older is 2.8%. Generally, with increasing age the prevalence doubles every 5 years. Stroke patients have increased risk of dementia: 1 year after stroke the probability of new-onset dementia is 5.4% in patients over 60 years and 10.4% in patients over 90 years (Leys et al., 2002). Incidence rates of dementia among patients with cerebrovascular disease are complicated by vastly different rates of sensitivity and specificity for the diagnosis of VaD among the common diagnostic criteria used (Gold et al., 2002).

Several sources of diagnostic criteria are widely used to diagnose VaD, all developed by consensus: the DSM-IV (American Psychiatric Association, 1994), the International Classification of Diseases (ICD-10; World Health Organization, 1992), the State of California Alzheimer's Disease Diagnostic and Treatment Centers (ADDTC; Chui et al., 1992), and the National Institute of Neurological and Communicative Disorders and Stroke–Association Internationale pour la Recherche et l'Enseignement en Neurosciences (NINCDS–AIREN) criteria (Roman et al., 1993). The literature abounds with articles on the inconsistency in the diagnosis of VaD (e.g., Chui et al., 2000; Wetterling, Kanitz, & Borgis, 1996). Contributing factors include different criteria for dementia among the major classification systems, different conceptualizations of how to establish a vascular etiology for dementia, and the heterogeneity of possible etiologies within VaD. Recently, Gold et al. (2002) compared the sensitivity and specificity of these most commonly used diagnostic criteria against the "gold standard" of neuropathological diagnosis with autopsy. Their findings indicated that the criteria are not interchangeable due to their different emphases and levels of sensitivity and specificity. They found that the ADDTC criteria for possible VaD are the most sensitive for detection (.70), whereas the DSM-IV and the NINDS–AIREN criteria for possible VaD are more effective in excluding mixed dementia. The NINDS–AIREN criteria are currently the most widely used in clinical drug trials on VaD. In general, criteria for VaD must recognize the heterogeneity of the syndrome and the variability in clinical course. Also important is the relationship between lesion and cognition, as well as the temporal relationship between vascular event(s) and dementia onset.

Attendant Data

Focal brain infarcts visible by computed tomography (CT) or magnetic resonance imaging (MRI) are found in 70–100% of VaD cases (Leys et al., 2002). MRI, although more costly, is the preferred imaging modality due to greater sensitivity. T_1-weighted images provide sharper anatomic resolution. However, T_1-weighted images can underestimate the extent of damage relative to T_2-weighted, or FLAIR, images, which reveal changes in water content, provide good visualization of white matter lesions and smaller infarcts, and allow visualization of perilesional tissue. Single-photon emission computed tomography (SPECT) and positron emission tomography (PET) can also be beneficial in characterizing tissue affected by vascular events. For example, a patchy, multifocal reduction of regional cerebral blood flow and metabolism is often seen in VaD. In addition, cortical infarcts are visible by areas of absent blood flow, and diffuse white matter change can be inferred with either generalized cortical reduction in blood flow or, in the case of subcortical white matter changes at the level of the basal ganglia, reduced cortical blood flow primarily to the frontal lobes (O'Brien & Barber, 2000). Finally, diffusion-weighted MRI can reveal ischemia of recent onset and can differentiate chronic from acute infarcts (Choi et al., 2000).

Most classification criteria require (ADDTC, NINDS–AIREN) or recommend (ICD-10, DSM-IV) evidence of relevant cerebrovascular disease by brain imaging in order to classify dementia etiology as vascular. Visible by structural neuroimaging are large-vessel strokes, single strategically placed infarcts (e.g., in the angular gyrus, thalamus, basal forebrain, posterior cerebral arteries (PCA), or anterior cerebral arteries (ACA) territories), multiple basal ganglia and white matter lacunes, and extensive periventricular white matter lesions. Any of the latter observations (or combination of some of the latter) provides evidence that could be consistent with an etiological basis of VaD (Choi et al., 2000). Risk factors for VaD include hyperlipidemia, hypertension, diabetes mellitus, cardiac abnormality or disorder, carotid bruit, and hematocrit level over 45%. Psychiatric comorbidity with VaD can include depression, anxiety, and emotional lability, among other psychiatric symptoms. Depression, emotional lability, and psychomotor retardation frequently accompany subcortical VaD (Leys et al., 2002).

Neuropsychological Profile

Second only to AD, the movement to provide a diagnostic label for mild cognitive changes below the threshold of dementia is underway for VaD (e.g., Bowler, 2000; Bowler & Hachinski, 1995; Hachinski, 1994; Hachinski & Bowler, 1993; Meyer, Xu, Thornby, Chowdhury, & Quach, 2002). In fact, in a recent Canadian study examining epidemiology of vascular cognitive impairment, vascular cognitive impairment without dementia (sometimes referred to as vascular CIND) was found to be the most prevalent form compared to VaD and AD with a vascular component (Rockwood et al., 2000). Some even argue that the term *dementia* never aptly describes the cognitive sequelae associated with vascular changes in the brain (Bowler, 2000). A basis for this argument is that the memory deficits associated with VaD are different qualitatively and quantitatively from those that characterize AD. Because cerebrovascular disease does not preferentially affect the mesial temporal lobe, as is the case with AD, encoding problems, a hallmark of AD, are usually absent in VaD, as evidenced by normal delayed recognition discriminability for verbal and nonverbal material (for review of cognitive impairments in AD vs. VaD, see Looi & Sachdev, 1999). Although the VaD memory profile generally conforms to a frontosubcortical pattern, the neuropsychological sequelae vary by size and location of lesion. Thus a neurocognitive profile similar to AD can follow from vascular etiology.

Much work has been done in describing the syndromes that accompany large-vessel cortical strokes (such as aphasias, apraxias, and neglect). A growing but more recent literature is beginning to characterize the neuropsychological profile associated with SIVD. The neuropsychological profile associated with SIVD has been likened to that of the frontosubcortical dementia profile (for review, see Libon et al., 2001; see also Moser et al., 2001; Yuspeh, Vanderploeg, Crowell, & Mullan, 2002). Overall, the pattern of cognitive difficulties resulting from subcortical ischemic change includes memory impairment (retrieval rather than encoding deficits), prominent psychomotor slowing, and executive deficits. This pattern of cognitive difficulties presumably arises in response to a disruption of frontosubcortical circuits; and this pattern is quite similar to that of PD (Paul et al., 2001).

ALCOHOLIC DEMENTIA

Illness Characterization

Alcoholic dementia refers to a profound and global cognitive decline following long-term alcoholism. Alcoholic dementia bears many similarities to the Wernicke–Korsakoff syndrome. Briefly, the Wernicke–Korsakoff syndrome is a two-phase disease that begins with Wernicke encephalopathy involving a triad of acute symptoms: global confusion, gait ataxia, and ocular abnormalities. This encephalopathy results from thiamine deficiency secondary to malnutrition associated with prolonged alcohol use (Victor, Adams, & Collins, 1989). Subsequent to this encephalopathy, 84% of patients develop alcoholic Korsakoff (AK) syndrome. The hallmarks of the AK syndrome include severe anterograde amnesia of declarative knowledge (Butters & Cermak, 1980) and a temporally graded retrograde amnesia, with better recall for remote than for recent events (Squire & Cohen, 1984). Another clinical feature is marked confabulation, exhibited often during memory testing (Delis, 1989).

Prevalence rates of alcoholic dementia vary greatly due to difficulty with differentiation between alcoholic dementia and individuals with the AK syndrome. Furthermore, it has been demonstrated that continued abstinence after chronic alcohol abuse can lead to at least a partial reversal of neuropsychological (e.g., Brandt, Butters, Ryan, & Bayog, 1983; Fabian & Parsons, 1983; Grant, Adams, & Reed, 1986) and even neuropathological changes (e.g., Artmann, Gall, Hacker, & Herrlich, 1981; Carlen, Wortzman, Holgate, Wilkinson, & Rankin, 1978). Many call into question the validity of an "alcoholic dementia" classification. For example, the ICD-10 does not include a category for alcoholic dementia. Many recent studies that examine alcohol abuse and the prevalence of dementia have not included alcoholic dementia as one of the primary subtypes (e.g., Ruitenberg et al., 2002; Truelsen, Thudium, & Grønbæk, 2002), but rather report prevalence of AD, VaD, and "other dementia" as primary subtypes of dementias that occur in chronic alcoholics.

Some studies do include a subtype of "cognitive impairment no dementia" (CIND) secondary to chronic alcohol use (e.g., Thomas & Rockwood, 2001). One study that specifically examined the prevalence of alcoholic dementia reported rates of 7.6% of alcoholic men and 14.3% of alcoholic women based on 1,000 alcoholic patients examined in Melbourne, Australia (Wilkinson, Kornaczewski, Rankin, & Santamaria, 1971).

Attendant Data

Potential pathophysiological mechanisms for alcoholic dementia include a direct toxic effect of ethanol (Mann et al., 2001) leading to cortical atrophy (especially reduced white matter volume). Signs of cortical atrophy include ventricular enlargement and sulcal widening as well as atrophy of the cerebellum. Punctate hemorrhagic lesions at the level of the diencephalon and brain stem may also be present (e.g., Jernigan et al., 1991; Kril, Halliday, Svoboda, & Cartwright, 1997). Affected subcortical structures implicated in the amnesia of the AK syndrome and of alcoholic dementia include the basal forebrain nuclei, the mammillary bodies, and the dorsomedial nucleus of the thalamus (Salmon, Butters, & Heindel, 1993).

Neuropsychological Profile

Alcoholic dementia consists of an anterograde amnesia as severe as that associated with the AK syndrome (Longmore & Knight, 1988). In addition to the memory deficit, in contrast to the AK syndrome, are more global neurocognitive deficits, including conceptual and problem-solving impairments, and deficits of visuospatial abilities and visuoconstruction. Furthermore, blunted affect, apathy, inertia, impaired judgment, and bradykinesia are associated with alcoholic dementia.

DEMENTIA DUE TO HEAD TRAUMA AND DEMENTIA PUGILISTICA

According to a consensus development panel on rehabilitation (National Institutes of Health, 1999), approximately 70,000–90,000 individuals incur traumatic brain injury (TBI) each year at a severity level resulting in long-term significant loss in physical and mental functioning. The DSM-IV-TR criteria for dementia due to head trauma, which requires the presence of memory impairment and/or other cognitive disturbances that cause significant impairment in social or occupational functioning, can apply to many individuals who have had TBIs. On the other hand, many TBI patients eventually return to gainful employment. Recently León-Carrión (2002) argued that dementia secondary to TBI should be differentiated from moderate or severe TBI because the severity and functional impact of the deficits may be rehabilitated in the latter cases. On the other hand, a longitudinal study of long-term outcomes of individuals following severe TBI 10–20 years postinjury (Hoofien, Gilboa, Vakil, & Donovick, 2001) revealed that the impact of this level of injury is chronic. Among the most frequent long-term sequelae of severe traumatic brain injury are high rates of depression and other psychiatric symptoms, psychomotor slowness, slowed processing speed, and loneliness/social withdrawal. Thus, although it is still debated how often even severe TBI should be conceptualized as dementia, most cases of severe TBI do sustain long-term sequelae that require ongoing treatment and caregiver support.

Dementia due to head trauma is considered stable, or nonprogressive; the possibility of a slowly progressive dementia due to repeated head injury is also recognized and referred to as dementia pugilistica (DP). DP, caused by repeated blows to the head, is most frequently studied with regard to sports-related injuries; however, DP could conceivably occur from other circumstances (e.g., chronic physical abuse). A recent review of findings regarding DP in sports (Erlanger, Kutner, Barth, & Barnes, 1999) revealed that mild cognitive deficits exist far more frequently than dementia following sports-related head injuries. Risk factors for DP include level of exposure to head injuries (e.g., length of professional boxing career; amateur vs. professional) and number of concussions. Early detection of DP is critical for better outcomes in this population. Clinical use of neuropsychological data to advise professional boxers, for example, should be considered because this group is at great risk for DP.

Historically, DP has been associated with a "Parkinsonian" pattern of decline, with noted clinical observations of tremor in the head and/or upper extremities. Cognitive impairments affect memory performances and result in reduced psychomotor speed, dysarthria, and behavioral or personality changes. Underlying brain damage includes diffuse axonal injuries, shearing, intra- and extracerebral hemorrhages, and edema. Neuropathological characteristics associated with DP include cerebral atrophy, the presence of neurofibrillary tangles in cortical and subcortical areas, reduced cholinergic activity in the basal forebrain, and diffuse presence of beta-amyloid plaques. Presence of the apolipoprotein E epsilon-4 allele has been identified as a potential genetic risk factor for developing DP during a career of boxing (Jordon et al., 1997). Conversely, Lye and Shores (2000), in a review article, cite a great deal of convergent evidence that TBI increases risk for AD.

CONCLUSIONS

This review of current information about the clinical and neuropsychological characteristics of a number of stable and slowly progressive dementias highlights several future directions in geriatric neuropsychological assessment. First, our current classification system does not adequately take advantage of the sensitivity of neuropsychological assessment measures. Neuropsychological assessment provides domain-specific (e.g., verbal memory, visual memory, executive functions, language) information about relative strengths and weaknesses in neurocognition. In addition, a neuropsychological assessment provides information about the *level* of impairment within each domain. Although neuropsychological assessments already provide both types of information, current classification systems do not adequately take into account level of neurocognitive impairment. Level of deficit severity within and across cognitive domains should be systematically considered to make an empirically valid determination about whether that level is more consistent with dementia or a designation of MCI. Creating a modified classification system in which severity designations are operationalized (e.g., in MCI, by standard deviation from the average performance in a normative group) would be one giant step toward more accurate identification of neurocognitive status and improved diagnostic accuracy in geriatric populations. The work of broadening MCI to dementias other than Alzheimer's is already underway (e.g., Petersen, 2004).

Study and better characterization of the course of these slowly progressive dementias would provide an excellent service to patients and clinicians. Development of diagnostic labels to capture prodromal stages of neurocognitive decline in slowly progressive dementias could lead to a variety of benefits to the patient, including early detection and intervention. Furthermore, classification of cognitive deficits as mild in patients whose deficits do not yet meet criteria for dementia will foster increased well-being and autonomy. Conversely, the diagnosis of, for example, MCI secondary to PD or SIVD would alert the clinician to the possibility of future cognitive decline to a severity level that may later merit a diagnosis of dementia.

An interest in improved classification of stages of neurocognitive decline will lead to better characterization of the prodromal phase of each dementing illness, increasing our accuracy in detection at ever earlier stages. Of great importance, earlier detection provides a greater window of opportunity for rehabilitative treatments, the focus of the second half of this volume.

REFERENCES

Alexander, G. E., DeLong, M. R., & Strick, P. L. (1986). Parallel organization of segregated circuits linking basal ganglia and cortex. *Annual Review of Neuroscience, 9,* 357–381.

American Psychiatric Association. (2000). *Diagnostic and Statistical Manual of Mental Disorders* (4th ed., text rev.). Washington DC: Author.

Artmann, H., Gall, M. V., Hacker, H., & Herrlich, J. (1981). Reversible enlargement of cerebral spinal fluid spaces in chronic alcoholics. *American Journal of Neuroradiology, 2,* 23–27.

Bowler, J. V. (2000). Criteria for vascular dementia: Replacing dogma with data. *Archives of Neurology, 57,* 170–171.

Bowler, J. V., & Hachinski, V. (1995). Vascular cognitive impairment: A new approach to vascular dementia. *Baillieres Clinical Neurology, 4,* 357–376.

Brandt, J., Butters, N., Ryan, C., & Bayog, R. (1983). Cognitive loss and recovery in long-term alcohol abusers. *Archives of General Psychiatry, 40,* 435–442.

Brown, R. G., & Marsden, C. D. (1990). Cognitive function in Parkinson's disease. *Trends in Neurosciences, 13,* 21–29.

Brown, R. G., & Marsden, C. D. (1991). Dual task performance and processing resources in normal subjects and patients with Parkinson's disease. *Brain, 114,* 215–231.

Butters, N., & Cermak, L. S. (1980). *Alcoholic Korsakoff's syndrome.* New York: Academic Press.

Carlen, P. L., Wortzman, G., Holgate, R. C., Wilkinson, D. A., & Rankin, J. C. (1978). Reversible cerebral atrophy in recently abstinent chronic alcoholics measured by computed tomography scans. *Science, 200,* 1076–1078.

Choi, S. H., Na, D. L., Chung, C. S., Lee, K. H., Na, D. G., & Adair, J. C. (2000). Diffusion-weighted MRI in vascular dementia. *Neurology, 54,* 83–89.

Chui, H. C., Mack, W., Jackson, J. E., Mungas, D., Reed, B. R., Tinklenberg, J., et al. (2000). Clinical criteria for the diagnosis of vascular dementia: A multicenter study of comparability and interrater reliability. *Archives of Neurology, 57,* 191–196.

Chui, H. C., Victoroff, J. I., Margolin, D., Jagust, W., Shankle, R., & Katzman, R. (1992). Criteria for the diagnosis of ischemic vascular dementia proposed by the State of California Alzheimer's Disease Diagnostic and Treatment Centers. *Neurology, 42,* 473–480.

Damasio, A. R., & Tranel, D. (1993). Nouns and verbs are retrieved with differently distributed neural systems. *Proceedings of the National Academy of Science, 90,* 4957–4960.

Delis, D. C. (1989). Neuropsychological assessment of learning and memory. In F. Boller & J. Grafman (Eds.), *Handbook of neuropsychology* (Vol. 3, pp. 3–33). New York: Elsevier.

Dubois, B., Boller, F., Pillon, B., & Agid, Y. (1991). Cognitive deficits in Parkinson's disease. In F. Boller & J. Grafman (Eds.), *Handboodk of neuropsychology* (Vol. 5, pp. 195–240). New York: Elsevier.

Duke, L. M., & Kaszniak, A. W. (2000). Executive control functions in degenerative dementias: A comparative review. *Neuropsychology Review, 10,* 75–99.

Duvoisin, R. C. (1984). *Parkinson's disease: A guide for patient and family.* New York: Raven Press.

Erlanger, D. M., Kutner, K. C., Barth, J. T., & Barnes, R. (1999). Neuropsychology of sports-related injury: Dementia pugilistica to post concussion syndrome. *Clinical Neuropsychologist, 13,* 193–209.

Fabian, M. S., & Parsons, O. A. (1983). Differential improvements of cognitive functions in recovering alcoholic women. *Journal of Abnormal Psychology, 92,* 87–95.

Glatt, S. L., Hubble, J. P., Lyons, K., Paolo, A., Tröster, A. I., Hassanein, R. E., et al. (1996). Risk factors for dementia in Parkinson's disease: Effect of education. *Neuroepidemiology, 15,* 20–25.

Gold, G., Bouras, C., Canuto, A., Bergallo, M. F., Herrmann, F. R., Partick, R. H., et al. (2002). Clinicopathological validation study of four sets of clinical criteria for vascular dementia. *American Journal of Psychiatry, 159,* 82–87.

Grant, I., Adams, K. M., & Reed, R. (1986). Intermediate-duration (subacute) organic mental disorder of alcoholism. In I. Grant (Ed.), *Neuropsychiatric correlates of alcoholism* (pp. 38–60). Washington, DC: American Psychiatric Press.

Hachinski, V. C. (1994). Vascular dementia: A radical redefinition. *Dementia, 5,* 130–132.

Hachinski, V. C., & Bowler, J. V. (1993). Vascular dementia. *Neurology, 43,* 2159–2160.

Hauk, O., Johnsrude, I., & Pulvermüller, F. (2004). Somatotopic representation of action words in human motor and premotor cortex. *Neuron, 41,* 301–307.

Hoofien, D., Gilboa, A., Vakil, E., & Donovick, P. J. (2001). Traumatic brain injury (TBI) 10–20 years later: A comprehensive outcome study of psychiatric symptomatology, cognitive abilities and psychosocial functioning. *Brain Injury, 15,* 189–209.

Hughes, A. J., Daniel, S. E., Blankson, S., & Lees, A. J. (1993). A clinicopathologic study of 100 cases of Parkinson's disease. *Archives of Neurology, 50,* 140–148.

Jankovic, J. (1987). Pathophysiology and clinical assessment of motor symptoms in Parkinson's disease. In W. C. Koller (Ed.), *Neurology: Vol. 7. Movement disorders 2* (pp. 124–165). London: Butterworths.

Jellinger, K. A. (2002). Recent developments in the pathology of Parkinson's disease. *Journal of Neural Transmission, Supplementum, 62,* 347–376.

Jernigan, T. L., Butters, N., DiTraglia, G., Schafer, K., Smith, T., Irwin, M., et al. (1991). Reduced cerebral gray matter observed in alcoholics using magnetic resonance imaging. *Alcohol Clinical and Experimental Research, 15,* 418–427.

Jordon, B. D., Relkin, N. R., Ravin, L. D., Jacobs, A. R., Bennett, A., & Gandy, S. (1997). Apolipoprotein E associated with chronic traumatic brain injury in boxing. *Journal of the American Medical Association, 278,* 136–140.

Kril, J. J., Halliday, G. M., Svoboda, M. D., & Cartwright, H. (1997). The cerebral cortex is damaged in chronic alcoholics. *Neuroscience, 79,* 983–998.

León-Carrión, J. (2002). Dementia due to head trauma: An obscure name for a clear neurocognitive syndrome. *NeuroRehabilitation, 17,* 115–122.

Levy, M. L., & Cummings, J. L. (2000). Parkinson's disease. In E. C. Lauterbach (Ed.), *Psychiatric management in neurological disease* (pp. 41–70). Washington, DC: American Psychiatric Press.

Leys, D., Englund, E., & Erkinjuntti, T. (2002). Vascular dementia. In N. Qizilbash, L. S. Schneider, H. Chui, P. Tariot, H. Brodaty, J. Kaye, & T. Erkinjuntti (Eds.), *Evidence-based dementia practice* (pp. 260–287). Oxford, UK: Blackwell.

Lezak, M. D. (1995). *Neuropsychological assessment.* Oxford: Oxford University Press.

Libon, D. J., Bogdanoff, B., Leopold, N., Hurka, R., Bonavita, J., Skalina, S., et al. (2001). Neuropsychological profiles associated with subcortical white matter alterations and Parkinson's disease: Implications for the diagnosis of dementia. *Archives of Clinical Neuropsychology, 16*, 19–32.

Longmore, B. E., & Knight, R. G. (1988). The effect of intellectual deterioration on retention deficits in amnesic alcoholics. *Journal of Abnormal Psychology, 97*, 448–454.

Looi, J. C. L., & Sachdev, P. S. (1999). Differentiation of vascular dementia from AD on neuro-psychological tests. *Neurology, 53*, 670–678.

Lye, T. C., & Shores, E. A. (2000). Traumatic brain injury as a risk factor for Alzheimer's disease: A review. *Neuropsychology Review, 10*, 115–129.

Mann, K., Agartz, I., Harper, C., Shoaf, S., Rawlings, R. R., Momenan, R., et al. (2001). Neuro imaging in alcoholism: Ethanol and brain damage. *Alcoholism: Clinical and Experimental Research, 25*, 104S-109S.

Marder, K., Tang, M.-X., Cote, L., Stern, Y., & Mayeux, R. (1995). The frequency and associated risk factors for dementia in patients with Parkinson's disease. *Archives of Neurology, 52*, 695–701.

Martilla, R. J. (1987). Epidemiology. In W. C. Koller (Ed.), *Handbook of Parkinson's disease* (pp. 35–50). New York: Dekker.

Meyer, J. S., Xu, G., Thornby, J., Chowdhury, M. H., & Quach, M. (2002). Is mild cognitive impairment prodromal for vascular dementia like Alzheimer's disease? *Stroke, 33*, 1981–1985.

Mindham, R. II. S., Biggins, C. A., Boyd, J. L, Harrop, F. M., Madeley, P., Randall, J. I., et al. (1993). A controlled study of dementia in Parkinson's disease over 54 months. *Advances in Neurology, 60*, 470–474.

Mink, J. W. (1996). The basal ganglia: Focused selection and inhibition of competing motor programs. *Progress in Neurobiology, 50*, 381–425.

Moser, D. J., Cohen, R. A., Paul, R. H., Paulsen, J. S., Ott, B. R., Gordon, N. M., Bell, S., & Stone, W. M. (2001). Executive function and magnetic resonance imaging subcortical hyperintensities in vascular dementia. *Neuropsychiatry, Neuropsychology, and Behavioral Neurology, 14*, 89–92.

Nambu, A., Tokuno, H., Hamada, I., Kita, H., Imanishi, M., Akazawa, T., et al. (2000). Excitatory cortical inputs to pallidal neurons via the subthalamic nucleus in the monkey. *Journal of Neurophysiology, 84*, 289–300.

Nambu, A., Tokuno, H., & Takada, M. (2002). Functional significance of the cortico-subthalamo–pallidal "hyperdirect" pathway. *Neuroscience Research, 43*, 111–117.

National Institutes of Health. (1999). Consensus development panel on rehabilitation of persons with traumatic brain injury. *Journal of the American Medical Association, 282*, 974–983.

O'Brien, J., & Barber, B. (2000). Neuroimaging in dementia and depression. *Advances in Psychiatric Treatment, 6*, 109–119.

Partiot, A., Verin, M., Pillon, B., Teixeira-Ferreira, C., Agid, Y., & Dubois, B. (1996). Delayed response tasks in basal ganglia lesions in man: Further evidence for a striato-frontal cooperation in behavioural adaptation. *Neuropsychologia, 34*, 709–721.

Paul, R. H., Cohen, R. A., Ott, B. R., Zawacki, T., Moser, D. J., Davis, J., et al. (2000). Cognitive and functional status in two subtypes of vascular dementia. *NeuroRehabilitation, 15*, 199–205.

Paul, R. H., Moser, D., Cohen, R., Browndyke, J., Zawacki, T., & Gordon, N. (2001). Dementia severity and pattern of cognitive performance in vascular dementia. *Applied Neuropsychology, 8*, 211–217.

Penney, J. B., & Young, A. B. (1986) Striatal inhomogeneities and basal ganglia function. *Movement Disorders, 1*, 3–15.

Petersen, R. C. (2004). Mild cognitive impairment as a diagnostic entity. *Journal of Internal Medicine, 256*, 183–194.

Piatt, A. L., Fields, J. A., Paolo, A. M., Koller, W. C., & Tröster, A. I. (1999). Lexical, semantic, and action verbal fluency in Parkinson's disease with and without dementia. *Journal of Clinical and Experimental Neuropsychology, 21*, 435–443.

Pillon, B., Dubois, B., Ploska, A., & Agid, Y. (1991). Severity and specificity of cognitive impairment in Alzheimer's, Huntington's, and Parkinson's diseases and progressive supranuclear palsy. *Neurology, 41*, 634–643.

Pulvermüller, F. (2001). Brain reflections of words and their meaning. *Trends in Cognitive Sciences*, *5*, 517–524.

Raskin, S. A., Borod, J. C., & Tweedy, J. (1990). Neuropsychological aspects of Parkinson's disease. *Neuropsychology Review*, *1*, 185–221.

Rockwood, K., Wentzel, C., Hachinski, V., Hogan, D. B., MacKnight, C., & McDowell, I. (2000). Prevalence and outcomes of vascular cognitive impairment. *Neurology*, *54*, 447–451.

Roman, G. C., Tatemmichi, T. K., Erkinjuntti, T., Cummings, J. L., Masteu, J. C., Garcia, J. H., et al. (1993). Vascular dementia: Diagnostic criteria for research studies: Report of the NINDS–AIREN International Workshop. *Neurology*, *43*, 250–260.

Ruitenberg, A., van Sweiten, J. C., Witteman, J. C. M., Mehta, K. M., van Duijn, C. M., Hofman, A., et al. (2002). Alcohol consumption and risk of dementia: The Rotterdam study. *Lancet*, *359*, 281–286.

Salmon, D. P., Butters, N., & Heindel, W. C. (1993). Alcoholic dementia and related disorders. In R. W. Parks & R. F. Zec (Eds.), *Neuropsychology of Alzheimer's disease and other dementias* (pp. 186–209). New York: Oxford University Press.

Salmon, D. P., Heindel, W. C., & Hamilton, J. M. (2001). Cognitive abilities mediated by frontal–subcortical circuits. In D. G. Lichter & J. L. Cummings (Eds.), *Frontal–subcortical circuits in psychiatric and neurological disorders* (pp. 114–150). New York: Guilford Press.

Squire, L. R., & Cohen, N. J. (1984). Human memory and amnesia. In G. Lynch, J. L. McGaugh, & N. M. Weinberger (Eds.), *Neurobiology of learning and memory* (pp. 3–64). New York: Guilford Press.

Tanner, C. M., & Goldman, S. M. (1996). Epidemiology of Parkinson's disease. *Neurological Clinics*, *14*, 317–335.

Taylor, A. E., & Saint-Cyr, J. A. (1995). The neuropsychology of Parkinson's disease. *Brain and Cognition*, *28*, 281–296.

Thomas, V. S., & Rockwood, K. J. (2001). Alcohol abuse, cognitive impairment, and mortality among older people. *Journal of the American Geriatrics Society*, *49*, 415–420.

Truelsen, T., Thudium, D., & Grønbæk, M. (2002). Amount and type of alcohol and risk of dementia: The Copenhagen city heart study. *Neurology*, *59*, 1313–1319.

Victor, M., Adams, R. D., & Collins, G. H. (1989). *The Wernicke–Korsakoff Syndrome*. Philadelphia: Davis.

Wetterling, T., Kanitz, R.-D., & Borgis, K.-J. (1996). Comparison of different diagnostic criteria for vascular dementia (ADDTC, DSM-IV, ICD-10, NINDS–AIREN). *Stroke*, *27*, 30–36.

Wilkinson, P., Kornaczewski, A., Rankin, J. G., & Santamaria, J. N. (1971). Physical disease in alcoholism: Initial survey of 1,000 patients. *Medical Journal of Australia*, *1*, 1217–1223.

Woods, S. P., & Tröster, A. I. (2003). Prodromal frontal/executive dysfunction predicts incident dementia in Parkinson's disease. *Journal of International Neuropsychological Society*, *9*, 17–24.

World Health Organization. (1992). *International statistical classification of diseases and related health problems. Tenth Revision*. Geneva, Switzerland: Author.

Yuspeh, R. L., Vanderploeg, R. D., Crowell, T. A., & Mullan, M. (2002). Differences in executive functioning between Alzheimer's disease and subcortical ischemic vascular dementia. *Journal of Clinical and Experimental Neuropsychology*, *24*, 745–754.

Potentially Reversible Cognitive Symptoms in Older Adults

WES S. HOUSTON
MARK W. BONDI

The identification of "reversible" or "treatable" causes of dementia is a common part of any clinical and/or medical investigation. As such, the practice of "ruling out" reversible cognitive decline is routine in the various neuropsychological and neurology practica and/or supervision settings. But how common are reversible dementias? To what extent do they actually reverse? Which dementing disorders are most likely to reverse, given the appropriate treatment? The primary focus of this chapter is to review the literature on various medical conditions with neurological and cognitive consequences that are commonly identified as being reversible or treatable.

For the past three to four decades researchers and clinicians alike have sought to identify medical conditions that are potentially reversible causes of intellectual and general cognitive decline (Freemon & Rudd, 1982; Ovsiew, 2003). Widely differing results (ranging from less than 1% to approximately 30%) have emerged from the numerous studies examining the frequency with which dementing conditions have been shown to be treatable. For example, an early paper by Marsden and Harrison (1972) reported that, of 84 patients admitted to the hospital with a diagnosis of dementia, a treatable condition was found in approximately 15% of patients. Another investigation by Freemon (1976) found that approximately 30% of patients with progressive intellectual decline had potentially reversible symptoms. This finding of a high prevalence in the treatability of dementia was commonplace in the 1970s and 1980s (see also Smith, Kiloh, Ratnavale, & Grant, 1976; Larson, Reifler, Featherstone, & English, 1984).

However, more recently—in the 1990s and 2000s—studies have generally reported a dramatic decrease in the prevalence of reversible or treatable dementias. Most investigations on the topic have concluded that the rate of reversibility of dementia is very low, ranging from less than 1% to about 4% (Burke, Sengoz, & Schwartz, 2000; Freter, Bergman, Gold, Chertkow, & Clarield, 1998; Walstra, Teunisse, van Gool, & van Crevel,

1997). These more recent studies tended to examine a sample of consecutive referrals to memory disorder clinics, then retrospectively identify and treat those who had potentially treatable conditions (e.g., vitamin B_{12} deficiency, depression, normal-pressure hydrocephalus) and judge, either clinically or with standardized tests, the level of improvement in cognitive and functional status. As an example, Walstra, Teunisse, van Gool, and van Crevel (1997) found that 45 of 176 demented patients referred to their clinic were viewed as having potentially reversible conditions, but none had a complete remittance and only one was determined to show substantial functional improvement (i.e., an individual who had depression with epilepsy). Five other individuals were regarded as improved based on clinical follow-up examination after treatment, but formal assessment did not confirm this subjective improvement. Thus Walstra et al. (1997) found a reversibility rate of approximately 0.6%. This low rate among clinic-based samples does not appear to be an unusual finding in the literature.

There are a number of potential reasons for the vastly different findings in dementia reversibility rates over the past few decades. One reason is the broad heterogeneity in the patient populations included in the literature. Of particular import may be the variability in cognitive impairment, ranging from mild deficits to severe intellectual decline. Accordingly, some studies have included only outpatients—with presumably milder disorders—whereas others have examined only severely impaired hospitalized patients. The wide-ranging level of impairment across studies leads to another related methodological difference: the use of different diagnostic criteria for dementia. The term *dementia* has been applied quite loosely across studies; some studies included individuals with depression and nutritional deficiencies, whereas other investigations evaluated patients with primary progressive dementias such as Alzheimer's disease (AD). We should expect to find different rates of treatment success when examining such heterogeneous patient groups. Important methodological differences have also extended to the specific cognitive assessment instruments utilized to evaluate patients' cognitive status. Although some studies administered only a brief general cognitive screening measure (e.g., the Mini-Mental State Examination [MMSE]) to estimate gross functional status, others employed formal, comprehensive, neuropsychological assessment batteries that are aimed at evaluating disparate cognitive functions. It could be argued that broad-based, relatively easy measures might be insensitive to changes following treatment, whereas very specific tests may have an increased likelihood of identifying a cognitive change.

Other factors also may have led to the contrasting findings in the rates of reversibility of cognitive decline, such as the use of individual case studies versus well-controlled clinical trials. Furthermore, there may be critical periods in the progression of some of the medical conditions, such that once a threshold has been crossed all attempts at reversibility are futile. In addition, the rates of treatment likely depend on the specific disorder being treated. Thus different medical conditions should not be lumped together in studies. Finally, as noted by Ovsiew (2003), perhaps the findings of abnormal laboratory tests are incidental. That is, some individuals may have had AD as well as an inconsequentially low vitamin deficiency or hypothyroidism. In such cases, treatment of the ancillary condition should have little effect on patients' overall cognitive functioning.

Given the myriad factors that cloud our ability to identify the true rate of reversibility of various medical conditions, we limited the scope of this chapter in the following two ways. First, because this volume is dedicated to the assessment and management of geriatric disorders, we confined our discussion of disorders to those which older adults are prone, despite the fact that many of the following conditions/diseases also occur in younger individuals (e.g., congenital hypothyroidism, normal-pressure hydrocephalus from secondary causes, medication side effects). Second, because many of the conditions discussed below do not frequently lead to dementia, as defined either by the National Institute of Neurological and Communicative Disorders and Stroke–Alzheimer's Disease Related Disorders Association (NINCDS–ADRDA) criteria (McKhann et al., 1984) or DSM-IV criteria (American Psychiatric Association, 1994), rather than refer to the conditions as reversible or treatable *dementias*, we prefer to discuss them in terms of potential amelioration of the cognitive symptoms that are commonly associated with the particular treatable conditions.

What follows is a review of the research on the neuropsychological effects of a variety of medical conditions often described as being reversible following proper treatment, including normal-pressure hydrocephalus, hypothyroidism, vitamin deficiencies (B_{12} and thiamine), depression, sleep-disordered breathing (obstructive sleep apnea), and medication effects. These are only a subset of the many conditions with potential cognitive consequences in older adults; however, they represent some of the more commonly occurring conditions as well as those that are discussed most frequently as being "reversible."

NORMAL-PRESSURE HYDROCEPHALUS

Description and Prevalence

Normal-pressure hydrocephalus (NPH), first described by Hakim and Adams (1965), is among the most commonly reported neurological syndromes to be referred to as a treatable or reversible form of cognitive decline. Although NPH has been observed in young adults and even children, it most typically affects adults over age 60 (Vanneste, 2000). However, it accounts for only a small fraction (less than 5%) of dementia cases, and the majority of cases are a result of secondary known sources such as subarachnoid hemorrhage and head trauma (Heidebrink, 2003; Katzman, 1977). A review 914 cases of NPH by Katzman (1977) found that only 34% were idiopathic.

Etiology

The specific cause of NPH remains unclear, although it is commonly believed that the condition results from impaired cerebrospinal fluid (CSF) absorption at the arachnoid villi (Miller & Adams, 1992). This explanation, however, has been challenged by the finding that such stagnation in the villi would not lead to the pressure gradient between the intra- and extraventricular spaces that is necessary to produce the ventricular dilatation characteristically observed in NPH (Ekstedt & Fridén, 1984). A more recent explanation for the pathophysiology of NPH refers to a "suprasylvian subarachnoid block" that suggests impaired CSF flow within the subarachnoid space over the convexity and medial hemisphere surface (Adams, Victor, & Ropper, 1997).

Cognition

The most common characteristic features of NPH include the triad of impaired (magnetic) gait, sphincter dysfunction, and mental deterioration. The gait disturbance, typically the first symptom to appear, can be quite variable, ranging from ataxic and wide-based to difficulties in initiation of walking and shuffling with frequent falls (Vanneste,

2000). Urinary incontinence tends to occur only late in the course of NPH, but urinary urgency is often present throughout the disorder (Corkill & Cadoux-Hudson, 1999).

The cognitive features of NPH are quite variable and can advance to meet the diagnostic criteria of dementia, but the course of mental decline is usually slowly progressive over months to years, with more severe deficits being likely with a longer duration. Relatively few studies have investigated cognitive patterns of functioning using a standardized and quantitative method. Memory complaints appear common, although a review of the literature suggests that a "subcortical" pattern of deficits is associated with NPH. That is, NPH patients tend to show relatively mild inattentiveness and poor initiation, with slowed mental processes as well as apathy and emotional indifference (Heidebrink, 2003). In addition, a number of studies have found evidence of deficits on measures typically associated with frontal-lobe functioning as well as relatively better recognition memory compared with rather poor delayed recall (Caltagirone, Gainotti, & Masullo, 1982; Gustafson & Hagberg, 1978; Heidebrink, 2003; Iddon et al., 1999; Thomsen, Borgeson, Bruhn, & Gjerris, 1986). In another study, Stambrook et al. (1988) noted more severe dementia, with deficits occurring in most areas measured, including motor speed, attention/concentration, immediate and delayed recall for verbal and visual material, and visuomotor sequencing/set shifting.

Treatment

The typical method of managing NPH involves the periventricular shunt procedure, and successful procedures have been documented (Bech-Azeddine et al., 2001; Sekhar, Moody, & Guthkeich, 1982). However, numerous significant risks are associated with shunting, including subarachnoid hemorrhage, infections (e.g., meningitis), aqueductal stenosis, blocked shunts, and mechanical shunt failures. Thus physicians (and patients) must strike a balance between monitoring the progression of the cognitive effects associated with NPH and risking complications from the surgical procedure. In general, good candidates for shunting include those who show gait disturbance predating mental decline, a brief history of cognitive decline, and substantial clinical improvement following CSF taps. Factors that appear to be suggestive of poor clinical outcome following shunting include severe dementia, presence of dementia predating the gait disturbance, and significant cerebral atrophy or white matter lesions (Heidebrink, 2003; Vanneste, 2000).

Assessing the actual reversibility of the cognitive impairment in NPH has been problematic, given that the surgical literature often does not utilize standardized neuropsychological tests (either preshunting or following the procedure). Often only physicians' ratings of change and/or quality of life indicators are employed (Stambrook et al., 1988). However, in general the literature suggests that there is broad variability (ranging from 30 to 80%) in the extent to which an individual will improve significantly, let alone show complete recovery, following surgical treatment (Alexander & Geshwind, 1984; Thomsen et al., 1986; Vanneste, 2000). It appears that some of the variability in postshunting improvement rate is explained by the etiology of the NPH—with secondary NPH patients having a better chance of significant cognitive improvement compared to those with idiopathic NPH (Stambrook et al., 1988; Thomsen et al., 1986; Vanneste, 2000).

Klinge et al. (2002) examined the neuropsychological profiles of NPH patients preshunting as well as at 1 week and 7 months following a shunting procedure. They found that early outcome scores on measures of visual attention and visuomotor precision (i.e., line tracing) were most predictive of long-term improvement after shunting. Nonresponsiveness to the shunt procedure was associated with no improvement (actually, a decline) in verbal (word-list) recall early after the surgery. In another neuropsychological study, Thomsen et al. (1986) measured a variety of cognitive abilities both prior to and following shunting. An examination of pre–post cognitive functioning found that 40% of the sample of 40 patients showed improved cognition, whereas 48% were unchanged and 12% actually deteriorated.

To summarize, although the cognitive and behavioral pattern of NPH can be variable, in general, the most common findings are gait disturbance, urinary urgency/incontinence, and mental decline. Specific areas of cognitive decrement include retrieval, executive skills, attention, and visuomotor sequencing abilities. With regard to other neuropsychological skills, it is rare to see memory consolidation, language, and visuospatial deficits. The rate of improvement also varies widely, but, not surprisingly, better outcome is associated with a shorter duration of illness, milder cognitive deficits, prominence of gait disturbance over cognitive decline, and less cortical atrophy on imaging studies.

HYPOTHYROIDISM

Description and Prevalence

Although many of the endocrine disorders can have noteworthy effects on cognitive abilities, hypothyroidism is one of the more commonly observed that leads to impaired cognition. Hypothyroidism can occur at any time during the lifespan; however, for this chapter, we are interested in adult-onset hypothyroidism, particularly in older adults, in whom the symptoms could possibly be mistaken for a progressive dementing disorder. In terms of prevalence of this disorder, Luboshitzky, Oberman, Kaufman, Reichman, and Flatau (1996) reported that hypothyroidism increases with age to around 14% in older adults. Because of its prevalence, recent practice parameter recommendations suggest routine screening for hypothyroidism in any dementia workup (Knopman et al., 2001)

Etiology

Thyroid-stimulating hormone (TSH) is secreted by the pituitary gland, which regulates the thyroid gland. In response to levels of TSH the thyroid gland releases thyroxine (T_4), among other hormones. TSH and T_4 operate as a negative feedback system such that increases in T_4, in response to secreted TSH, decreases pituitary secretion of TSH, and vice versa. However, in hypothyroidism, malfunction of this system occurs for any number of reasons. If blood levels of TSH are elevated but T_4 is in the normal range, the condition is referred to as subclinical hypothyroidism. If T_4 is abnormally low, the condition is referred to as overt hypothyroidism or primary hypothyroidism caused by dysfunction of the thyroid gland (Smith & Granger, 1992).

Cognition

Hypothyroidism is most well known for its associated features of depression, lethargy, dry skin, and feeling cold (Dugbartey, 1998); however, it is the related cognitive symptoms that are of import here. Many clinical case reports and well-controlled experimental studies have sought to elucidate the specific pattern of cognitive impairments that has been linked to hypothyroidism. The variety of different causes and ranges of severity of the disorder lead to wide variability in reported cognitive symptoms. Whereas most studies of this disorder have assessed limited cognitive domains, taken together, studies generally report deficits in memory, visuomotor processing, and visuospatial and visuoconstructional skills (Dugbartey, 1998; Haggerty, Evans, & Prange, 1986; Mennemeier, Garner, & Heilman, 1993; Osterweil et al., 1992; Whybrow, Prange, & Treadway, 1969). In contrast, neurocognitive skills such as sustained attention, language, and verbal fluency as well as gross motor abilities have been consistently reported as being intact (Mennemeier et al., 1993; Osterweil et al., 1992).

Some research on subclinical hypothyroidism suggests that cognitive deficits may also be present in this milder form of the disorder. For example, Baldini et al. (1997) found that control subjects outperformed subclinical patients on a measure of verbal memory. Conversely, Luboshitzky et al. (1996) did not find evidence of cognitive deficits (on the MMSE) in their sample of mild, untreated hypothyroidism patients. Still, it has been pointed out that this variant of the disorder may show the same clinical picture as overt or primary hypothyroidism (Morganti et al., 2002). Furthermore, a recent investigation suggested that subclinical hypothyroidism in women may be associated with an increased risk of future cognitive decline (Volpato et al., 2002).

Treatment

With regard to the reversibility of cognitive difficulties associated with hypothyroidism, the literature appears to be quite mixed. Clarnette (1994) found only one case of reversible dementia (followed for 3 months) due to the disorder. In his review of 32 studies, only 18 of 2,781 cases of dementia were specifically documented as being due to hypothyroidism. Five of the 18 cases were lost to follow-up, six cases showed improvement or partial recovery, and six either did not improve or continued to deteriorate. In contrast to these findings, a more recent study by Baldini et al. (1997) found that a sample of 19 subclinical hypothyroid women showed improvements in verbal story memory, visual memory, and attention over controls following 3 months of thyroxine treatment. In addition, Smith and Granger (1992) reported on two cases of hypothyroidism (one subclinical) that demonstrated some improvement, though perhaps not to baseline levels, on a gross cognitive screen.

Thus, although there are fairly consistent patterns of cognitive impairments in patients with overt hypothyroidism and, perhaps to a lesser degree, the subclinical variety of this disorder, studies on the remediation of deficits are less clear. It appears that subclinical hypothyroidism may be more likely to resolve with thyroxine treatment than the overt form. This resolution may be due to the decreased severity of the subclinical disorder and the duration of thyroid malfunction. Complete recovery, however, appears to be rare.

VITAMIN B_{12} DEFICIENCY

Description and Prevalence

Vitamin B_{12} (also known as cobalamin) deficiency is one of the most common nutritional disorders that occurs in older adults (Dharmarajan, Adiga, Pitchumoni, & Norkus, 2003; Dharmarajan & Norkus, 2001). Levels of B_{12} appear to be reduced as a function of increasing age (Robins Wahlin, Wahlin, Winblad, & Bäckman, 2001). Deficiency in B_{12} levels occurs commonly in both community-dwelling older adults as well as those in nursing homes or hospitals, with estimates of the prevalence of low serum B_{12} being 26% and 17%, respectively (Dharmarajan, Adiga, Pitchumoni, & Norkus, 2003). Because of its relatively high prevalence, routine vitamin B_{12} screening has been recommended in dementia evaluations (Knopman et al., 2001).

Etiology

The most common cause of vitamin B_{12} deficiency is food-B_{12} malabsorption, which accounts for up to 50% of the cases (Dharmarajan, Adiga, Pitchumoni, et al., 2003). Other causes include pernicious anemia, atrophic gastritis, exocrine pancreas insufficiency, small intestinal bacterial overgrowth (SIBO), and malabsorption due to drug interactions (Dharmarajan, Adiga, & Norkus, 2003; Robins Wahlin et al., 2001). Foods that are high in vitamin B_{12} content include organ meats, dairy products, some seafood, meats, and egg yolks. Because the U.S. recommended daily amount of B_{12} consumption is relatively small, and the content in foods is far greater than daily recommendations, is it rare that an individual will become deficient due to dietary restrictions (although strict vegetarians are an exception), and it often takes years to develop significant B_{12} deficiency (Dharmarajan, Adiga, Pitchumoni, et al., 2003).

Cognition

For several decades researchers and clinicians have examined the relationship between cognitive impairment and low serum B_{12} levels. The findings of cognitive (and psychiatric) disturbances, potentially leading to dementia, that are associated with low vitamin B_{12} levels have been well documented in the nutrition research literature (Garry, Goodwin, & Hunt, 1984; Goodwin, Goodwin, & Garry, 1983; Robins Wahlin et al., 2001). The appearance of clinical manifestations of vitamin B_{12} deficiency tends not to occur until the later stages of the disorder but can be wide ranging, including physical complaints such as lethargy, fatigue, and weakness; hematological features such as leukopenia and thrombobocytopenia; and/or a variety of cognitive deficits. The believed mechanism of the neurological and neuropsychological symptoms associated with deficient vitamin B_{12} is demyelination and axonal degeneration, ultimately leading to cell death (Babior & Bunn, 1998). The clinical and cognitive presentation can vary depending on the extent of degeneration to the peripheral nervous system, the spinal cord, and/or the cerebrum.

Well-controlled neuropsychological studies of the cognitive profiles of patients with vitamin B_{12} deficiency have very rarely been investigated. Many of the reported findings tend to be either case studies or they lack detailed descriptions of specific cognitive functions. However, given that demyelination and axonal degeneration occur with vitamin B_{12} deficiency, it is not surprising that numerous reports of the neuropsychological sequelae associated with this disorder have described a "subcortical-type" pattern of deficits. For example, several studies have suggested that the cognitive deficit profile includes impairments in abstraction, problem solving, complex visual perceptual skills, memory, letter fluency, constructional apraxia, psychomotor retardation, and apathy (Meadows, Kaplan, & Bromfield, 1994; Riggs, Spiro, Tucker, & Rush, 1996; Robins Wahlin et al., 2001; Saracaceanu, Tramoni, & Henry, 1997). Some studies have found more severe impairment, including deficits in visual and verbal memory (recall and recognition), naming and word finding, but these tend to be case studies (cf. Larner, Janssen, Cipolotti, & Rossor, 1999).

It is noteworthy that some findings have noted that subclinically low levels of vitamin B_{12} may also be associated with subtle cognitive deficits. That is, generally healthy individuals with no significant medical history but with serum B_{12} levels slightly above the established cutoff for deficiency, have been shown to exhibit lower verbal memory and problem-solving scores than individuals with optimal serum B_{12} levels (Goodwin et al., 1983; Wahlin, Hill, Winblad, & Backman, 1996). In addition, a recent study by Bunce, Kivipelto, and Wahlin (2004) demonstrated an intriguing gene–environment interaction between the apolipoprotein E (apoE) epsilon-4 (ε4) allele (i.e., a susceptibility gene for AD) and low vitamin B_{12} on episodic memory. Given that the apoE gene may play a general role in neural support and repair mechanisms, and that possession of the ε4 allele results in a poorer capacity than does the ε2 or ε3 allele in this regard, the authors suggest that brain reserve may vary as a function of the apoE genotype and that ε4 carriers may be particularly vulnerable to cognitive impairment in the presence of an additional factor (i.e., low vitamin B_{12}) that deleteriously influences neuroanatomical structures and processes.

Treatment

The standard treatment regimen for individuals with low serum B_{12} is administration of the deficient vitamin. Traditionally, treatment has been intramuscular administration in doses from 100 to 1000 micrograms per day for up to 1 week. This is typically followed by monthly to quarterly injections for the rest of the patient's life (Dharmarajan, Adiga, Pitchumoni, et al., 2003). Preparations of oral, intranasal, and sublingual administrations are also available.

Although laboratory tests are likely to show rapid improvement following supplementation, the pattern of recovery for neurological and cognitive functions is not quite as clear. Neurological symptoms may recover rapidly and completely if treatment is begun quickly and the disorder has not gone untreated for a long period. In general, studies of the reversibility of cognitive impairments associated with deficient vitamin B_{12} have not been positive. Clarfield (1988) found only one case of dementia (out of 3,000) that reversed completely with supplementation. Also, Hector and Burton (1988) reviewed studies between 1959 and 1986 and found only three cases of dementia that improved with vitamin B_{12} administration. Meadows et al. (1994) presented a case report with mixed results. That is, the patient demonstrated improved memory performances, but abstraction and visuomotor scanning/sequencing remained impaired. Finally, a review paper by Chiu (1996) found that 14 studies (totaling 69 patients) reported in the literature (from 1966 to 1995) identified cases of cognitive impairment that were attributable to deficient B_{12} levels. Twenty-five of the patients were judged to have cognitive deficits severe enough to be diagnosed with dementia. Of those 25, 10 patients demonstrated marked improvement following treatment with vitamin B_{12}.

In summary, there are numerous studies supportive of the notion that there are significant cognitive effects associated with vitamin B_{12} deficiency, though individuals often demonstrate a few scattered or isolated mild deficits rather than a global dementia. The severity of deficits appears to be related to the duration of the disorder. It has been suggested that the "window of opportunity" for treating and reversing complications due to deficiency is brief, being only a few months before neurological symptoms become irreversible (Dharmarajan, Adiga, Pitchumoni, et al., 2003). Though some investigations, primarily case studies, have reported improvement in cognitive functions following vitamin B_{12} supplementation, most reviews of the literature suggest that complete recovery is rare.

THIAMINE DEFICIENCY

Description and Prevalence

Celik and Kaya (2004) describe vitamin B_1 (or thiamine) as a coenzyme in carbohydrate metabolism that has a role in the maintenance of osmotic gradients between cellular membranes. Although inadequate oral thiamine intake still accounts for the majority of cases of thiamine deficiency (TD) in people in underdeveloped countries, approximately 95% of cases seen in people living in developed countries are associated with alcohol use (Thomson, 2000). Although rare, TD is also sometimes seen in people with cancer, AIDS, eating disorders, excessive vomiting caused by chemotherapy, diarrheal disorders, or any condition where there is poor oral intake (Celik & Kaya, 2004). There are also a relatively high number of older adults with TD, in particular, those living in hospitals or institutions (Johnson, Bernard, & Funderburg, 2002).

Etiology

Common consequences of TD include the Wernicke–Korsakoff syndrome (WKS) as well as maple syrup urinary disease, heart failure (wet beriberi), and peripheral neuropathy (Johnson, Bernard, & Funderburg, 2002; O'Keeffe, Tormey, Glasgow, & Lavan, 1994). TD often occurs in individuals who have consumed large quantities of alcohol for a prolonged period of time. This occurrence is due, in part, to the fact that some individuals dependent on alcohol obtain much of their caloric intake from alcohol and are often malnourished. However, according to Gastaldi, Casirola, Ferrari, and Rindi (1989), alcohol itself may cause TD by inhibiting the intestinal absorption of thiamine. Ciccia and Langlais (2000) suggest that, when TD interacts with alcohol, there is a synergistic effect. The period of time needed to become deficient in thiamine is subject to individual differences but can occur quite quickly, leading to serious medical complications in as short a time as 2–3 weeks (Ambrose, Bowden, & Whelan, 2001).

Cognition

Prolonged and heavy use of alcohol has been associated with a wide variety of cognitive and neurological impairments (Ciccia &Langlais, 2000; see also Salmon, Butters, & Heindel, 1993, for review). These can range from very subtle or no deficits to the severe amnesia that accompanies WKS. Mild deficiencies in thiamine can cause a number of cognitive symptoms, including perceptual–motor difficulties, visuospatial problems, decreased abstraction/problem solving, and learning and memory deficits (Parsons & Nixon, 1993). When TD progresses to a more severe state, Wernicke's encephalopathy can occur, presenting as a clinical triad of confusion, ataxia, and nystagmus (Johnson et al., 2002). Worsening of the neuropsychological profile to include both retrograde and anterograde amnesia constitutes WKS (Ambrose et al., 2001; Johnson et al., 2002; Kopelman, 1995).

Treatment

Treatment requires daily administration of thiamine hydrochloride in adequate doses for repletion of brain thiamine levels (Ambrose et al., 2001; Thomson, 2000). The probability of recovery from WKS is not high. Thiamine treatment of Wernicke's encephalopathy often results in a reduction of confusion in addition to improving the ataxia and eye movement abnormalities, but not in all studies (Ambrose et al., 2001; Todd & Butterworth, 1999, but see Johnson et al., 2002). The severe memory impairment associated with WKS does not show improvement in the majority of cases (Parsons & Nixon, 1993), and Victor, Adams, and Collins (1989) estimate that less than 25% of those patients who survive a Wernicke's encephalopathy show a complete return to their premorbid personality or intellectual state, especially if their medical history includes long-term alcoholism. However, a recent study examined thiamine treatment on working memory deficits in people with alcoholism without the clinical signs of WKS (Ambrose et al., 2001) and found a dose-related (up to 200 mg) improvement in performance on a delayed alternation task in this sample of 107 detoxifying patients.

Thus there appears to be some evidence of neuropsychological improvement with thiamine treatment in a small percentage of patients with thiamine deficiency and alcoholism, although in those with WKS, prognosis for recovery is poor (Johnson et al., 2002). Bowden (1990), however, suggested a more optimistic outlook: that patients with WKS who completely abstain from alcohol use for a significant period of time show improvement in cognitive function.

Given the mixed results from the various investigators and research designs (Bowden, 1990; Martin, McCool, & Singleton, 1993), it is important to continue to investigate the benefits of thiamine treatment on those detoxifying from ethanol as well as examining the effects of long-term abstinence from chronic alcohol consumption as a way of alleviating the deleterious effects of TD. An inexpensive and relatively harmless treatment, it is wise to begin thiamine supplementation at the earliest signs (Morcos, Kerns, & Shapiro, 2004). Important considerations include the appropriate dosage, duration, and the method of administration (Bowden, Bardenhagen, Ambrose, & Whelan, 1994).

DEPRESSION-RELATED COGNITIVE DYSFUNCTION

Description and Prevalence

There are a number of terms that refer to the presence of potentially reversible cognitive impairments associated with depression in older adults. Terms such as *pseudodementia* (Kiloh, 1961) and *dementia syndrome of depression* (Folstein & McHugh, 1978) are commonly used but may not be the most appropriate. The cognitive effects of depression can be variable in scope and severity, often not meeting the specific criteria for dementia. Thus the term selected for use here is *depression-related cognitive dysfunction* (Stoudemire, Hill, Gulley, & Morris, 1989), because it refers to depression and is general enough to cover a range of deficit severity.

The prevalence of major depressive disorder in adults age 65 and older has been reported to be approximately 2% (Myers et al., 1984). However, the rate jumps to about 20% if those with significant depressive symptoms, but not meeting the formal DSM-IV criteria for major depression, are included (Blazer, Hughes, & George, 1987). Further complicating the situation is the rather high comorbidity of depression in dementia. For example, although major depression in AD is considered rare, dysphoric affect and demoralization are more common and thought to occur in as many as 50% of AD patients (see Kaszniak & DiTraglia Christenson, 1994, for discussion). Given the high frequency of depressive symptoms in older adults, there is a clear need to evaluate the potential cognitive effects of this disorder.

Cognition

Interest in the neuropsychological features of late-life depression is a relatively new and incompletely understood area of research. Although numerous studies have examined the cognitive effects of depression in older adults, many have utilized only limited test batteries (see Butters et al. 2000, for discussion). Still, when summarized, studies have shown a relatively consistent pattern of cognitive deficits in visuospatial skills, executive functioning, and psychomotor speed (see Boone et al., 1995; Hart, Kwentus, Taylor, & Harkins, 1987; Lesser et al., 1996; Palmer, Boone, Lesser, & Wohl, 1996).

It has been argued that depressed individuals with significant cognitive deficits represent a heterogeneous group, with some patients being in the early stages of a dementia, such as AD or a vascular dementia (Kaszniak & DiTraglia Christenson, 1994). In support of this notion is a study by Paterniti, Verdier-Taillefer, Dufouil, and Alpérovitch (2002) that found that the presence of cognitive deficits in depressed individuals predicted future decline at follow-up approximately 4 years later. This finding has been reported previously in the literature as well (see Bassuk, Berkman, & Wypij, 1998; Chen et al., 1999; Geerlings et al., 2000).

However, not all depressed patients have significant cognitive deficits. Often older adults may show only mild neuropsychological deficits, but they continue to report memory and concentration difficulties. On cognitive tests, these milder cases tend to have lower scores on more effortful tests, such as those that require a free recall compared with recognition (see review by La Rue, 1992). Historically, subjective memory complaints have been shown to be more highly associated with depression in late life than with objective memory impairments (see discussion by Kaszniak & DiTraglia Christenson, 1994). However, most of these studies have been cross-sectional and few, if any, have specifically addressed whether subjective memory deterioration predicts future dementia. Toward that end, Wang et al. (2004) conducted a community-based longitudinal study of over 1,800 older adults, investigating the temporal relationship between subjective memory decline and future dementia. In short, they found that subjective memory deterioration significantly predicted the development of dementia. They also demonstrated consistencies with previous findings, such as cross-sectional associations between subjective memory decline and depression as well as important modifying relationships. For example, they showed that advancing age diminished the strength of prediction of future dementia. They concluded by suggesting that subjective memory decline provides additional information about future dementia at a time when objective cognitive impairment is not observed.

The implications of this study highlight that, in addition to depression assessments, evaluation of subjective memory decline in older adults may be an important additional component to both screening as well as comprehensive cognitive assessments. Moreover, there appears to be poorer utility of this information with increasing age, perhaps due to increasing executive or self-monitoring deficits with advancing age or the possibility that memory problems are more common among very old adults (≥ 80). Thus distinguishing between subjective memory decline as an early indicator of dementia or a concomitant aspect of normal aging is more difficult in those who are very old. Nevertheless, the findings of Wang et al. (2004) provide important information on the prediction of future dementia from subjective estimations of memory decline, aside from their overlap with depression.

In addition, Kaszniak and DiTraglia Christenson (1994) offered a variety of qualitative features in cognitive assessments that might be helpful in differentiating AD from depression. Compared to patients with AD, one would expect depressed individuals to show relatively intact recognition memory, fewer false-positive errors on recognition memory testing, more "don't know" errors, poorer effort in attempting to perform tasks, more variability in performance on tasks of similar difficulty, buttressed performance with semantic organization and prompting, and an intact awareness of impairment. Of course, longitudinal assessment, with treatment of depression, affords the greatest degree of precision in determining whether cognitive impairments abate.

Treatment

Regarding the ameliorative effects of antidepressant medication on the cognitive impairments in older adults with depression, studies tend to be somewhat inconsistent. Butters et al. (2000) found that those who demonstrated cognitive impairments showed improvement in executive functions following remission of depressive symptoms. In contrast, Dahabra et al. (1998) reported that cognitive impairments persisted after recovery from depression, whereas Nebes et al. (2000) found that measures of processing speed and working memory improved following remission, but no more than that observed in control participants with repeat testing.

These contradictory findings suggest that there are different subgroups of depressed older patients that influence the extent to which these patients will demonstrate cognitive improvement. The findings that (1) only a portion of depressed patients actually demonstrates cognitive deficits and (2) that some depressed patients with cognitive impairments are a greater risk for future decline support the subgroup hypothesis. Also supportive is the finding by Taylor, Wagner, and Steffens (2002) who reported that more severely depressed patients were less likely to show cognitive improvement following treatment. Finally, there does seem to be a fairly consistent finding that, if cognitive improvement occurs following remission of depressive symptoms, it tends not to improve to baseline levels on retesting (Butters et al., 2000; Nebes et al., 2000).

SLEEP-DISORDERED BREATHING

Description and Prevalence

The most common health condition associated with sleep-disordered breathing is the syndrome of obstructive sleep apnea (OSA; Adams, Strauss, Schluchter, & Redline 2000). This breathing disorder is usually caused by repetitive upper airway obstruction; its primary symptoms are loud snoring and breathing stoppage during sleep (Dealberto, Pajot, Courbon, Alpérovitch, 1996; Shochat & Pillar, 2003). OSA occurs more commonly in men, increases with age, and is strongly correlated with body mass index. Its prevalence in the general population is estimated to be between 2 and 5%, but it increases dramatically to more than 25% for individuals over age 65 (Dealberto et al., 1996; Naegele et al., 1995).

Etiology

The obstruction of the upper airway in affected individuals may involve compromised pharyngeal airway anatomy (e.g., macroglossia, hypertrophy of tonsils, increased uvula size, or long soft palate), leading investigators to surmise that an anatomical abnormality of the pharynx eventually causes the collapse of the upper airway during sleep. Other risk factors include smoking, alcohol consumption, use of sedative medications, lying in the supine position, sleep deprivation, and several medical conditions, including hypothyroidism and acromegaly (Shochat & Pillar, 2003).

As a consequence of OSA, many patients experience daytime sleepiness, irritability, impatience, and depressive symptoms. In addition, OSA has been associated with hypertension, cardiovascular and pulmonary disease, and increased mortality. Finally, a significant consequence of the disorder is cognitive impairment that may resemble dementia in older adults (Bliwise, 2002; Shochat & Pillar, 2003).

Cognition

Specific cognitive deficits include executive dysfunction, psychomotor slowing, inattentiveness and memory impairment (Bedard, Montplaisir, Richer, Rouleau, & Malo, 1991; Bliwise, 2002; Kales, Caldwell, Cadieux, Vela-Bueno, Ruch, & Mayes, 1985; Naegele et al., 1995; Naegele et al., 1998; Shochat & Pillar 2003). Although some researchers have related these impairments to the transient but repeated hypoxemia that accompanies OSA, others have suggested that the impairments have more to do with the sleep disruption and subsequent daytime sleepiness (Findley et al., 1986; Redline et al., 1997). This controversy has led to the suggestion that cognitive impairments are due to multiple causes in OSA. That is, perhaps the cognitive deficits associated with executive functioning and psychomotor slowing are related to the hypoxemia, whereas the memory and attention difficulties may be due to decreased vigilance (Bedard et al., 1991). Regardless of the specific causes of the cognitive impairments, Bliwise (2002) suggested that there is little doubt that sleep apnea leads to a complex neurobehavioral syndrome in old age (i.e., motor slowing, memory impairment, apathy, and dysphoric mood) that resembles dementia, if left untreated.

Treatment

Treatments of OSA include continuous positive airway pressure (CPAP), bilevel positive airway pressure (BiPAP), the avoidance of lying in a supine position, weight loss, nasal reconstruction, pharyngeal reconstruction, and in some cases, tracheostomy. Medications have been found to be largely unsuccessful due to tolerance effects and adverse effects. CPAP is the treatment of choice due to its low risk and noninvasive nature (Bassetti & Gugger, 2002; Schochat & Pillar 2003), although it must be worn indefinitely, and this necessity could lead to compliance problems.

There is a growing interest in preventing or reversing the cognitive effects of OSA. Bliwise (1996) suggests that preventing OSA by use of a CPAP or BiPAP may improve cognitive function or mood, particularly if alertness improves. Naegele et al. (1998) re-evaluated OSA patients after 4–6 months of CPAP treatment and found that their scores on measures of visual memory and executive functions were significantly improved and returned to normal. However, tests of attention and working memory remained impaired.

Bliwise (2002) also reported two cases in which treatment with a CPAP resulted in improved immediate visual memory and psychomotor speed.

In summary, the functional level of OSA patients appears to deteriorate in direct relationship to the severity and chronicity of their sleep apnea (Kales et al., 1985). Preventing sleep apnea may lead to reversibility of symptoms in at least some cases of cognitive decline, although more clinical trials are needed to test this hypothesis further.

MEDICATION EFFECTS

Neuropsychologists and other clinicians are often confronted with estimating the degree to which an individual's cognitive impairment is related to medication effects versus a dementing disease. Given that most drugs administered in sufficient dosages can cause cognitive impairment, especially in susceptible individuals, careful interviewing regarding patients' medication regimen and ability to manage their medications appropriately is necessary to determine the likelihood that drugs may be causing cognitive alterations. In addition, being informed about the typical side effect profiles of different classes of medications, as well as the specific drugs that are most likely to cause cognitive impairment, is becoming increasingly important.

Over the past decade clinicians have increased their study of the effects of psychotropic medication on cognitive functioning (Stein & Strickland, 1998). A comprehensive examination of the effects of medications on cognition is beyond the scope of this chapter; however, there are a number of detailed reviews on the topic to which the reader is referred (Amado-Boccara, Gougoulis, Poirier Littré, Galinowski, & Lôo, 1995; Gray, Lai, & Larson, 1999; Muldoon, Waldstein, & Jennings, 1995; Stein & Strickland, 1998). In this section, we briefly summarize the most common cognitive effects of some of the more frequently prescribed classes of medication in older adults, including antidepressants, sedative-hynotics/anxiolytics, antihypertensives, anticonvulants, and antihistamines. As is the case with most of the other medical conditions described in this chapter, the cognitive consequences associated with medication use are not typically so severe that they lead to diagnoses of dementia per se. More often, the effects are characterized as leading to deficits in attention, concentration, memory and/or psychomotor speed.

Antidepressants

The widespread use of antidepressants among older persons necessitates that clinicians keep abreast of the potential cognitive deficits associated with these medications. Numerous studies have examined the cognitive effects of the different classes of antidepressant medications (tricyclic antidepressants, monoamine oxidase inhibitors [MAOIs], selective serotonin reuptake inhibitors [SSRIs]). However, studies of the effects of these drugs are confounded by a number of important issues, including the fact that many of the antidepressant medications are prescribed for medical conditions other than depression, including chronic pain (tricyclics), Parkinson's disease (MAOIs) and obsessive–compulsive symptoms (SSRIs), among others. Also, the effects appear to differ depending on the population being studied (e.g., depressed individuals, healthy control groups, young adults, older adults) and the methodology (e.g., single dose, short-term, long-term administration).

Despite these relevant variables, in general it appears that tricyclic antidepressants, particularly amitriptyline, have been shown to have negative cognitive effects, including slowed reaction time, slowed information processing, decreased attention, and lowered verbal recall (but not recognition; Amado-Boccara et al., 1995; Branconnier, DeVitt, Cole, & Spera, 1982; Sakulsripong, Curran, & Lader, 1991; & Stein & Strickland, 1998). Fewer studies have examined the cognitive profiles of SSRIs, and many of these studies, often industry sponsored, utilitzed few neuropsychological tests; typically psychomotor speed and verbal memory are tested on relatively small sample sizes (Stein & Strickland, 1998). The results have varied from mostly minimal cognitive effects to improved effects on some tests such as perceptual function and reaction time (Kerr, Fairweather, & Hindmarch, 1993). MAOIs also appear to be superior to tricyclic antidepressants regarding cognitive effects and may be comparable to the SSRIs (Stein & Strickland, 1998).

Sedatives/Hypnotics

Most sedative/hypnotic medications (e.g., benzodiazepines, barbiturates) have wide-ranging cognitive effects. These medications are commonly used for anxiety reduction, as sleep aids, to combat irritability and agitation, and for seizure control; by definition, they cause sedation and drowsiness that can affect cognitive abilities in older adults.

Benzodiazepines are the most frequently prescribed antianxiety drugs in older adults (Madhusoodanan & Bogunovic, 2004). Although tolerance to the effects of benzodiazepines often develops after multiple doses, older adults may develop tolerance more slowly than younger individuals and thus be at risk for continued cognitive impairment. In general, studies have documented cognitive effects with both short-term and long-term use, such as slowed psychomotor speed, impaired verbal and visual learning, and impaired vigilance (Morrison & Katz, 1989; Nikaido, Ellinwood, Heatherly, & Gupta, 1990; Pomara, Deptula, Medel, Block, & Greenblatt, 1989). Basic attentional skills do not appear to be significantly affected by benzodiazepines (Mac, Kumar, & Goodwin, 1985). These drugs are also associated with increased risk of delirium in older adults (Gray et al., 1999). Support for benzodiazepine-related cognitive effects was found in a study by Larson, Kukull, Buchner, and Reifler (1987), which showed that cognition improved following the withdrawal of this class of drug.

Nonbenzodiazepine anxiolytic medications such as zolpidem and buspirone are viewed as safer alternatives to benzodiazepines with regard to adverse neuropsychological impairment (Barbee, Black, & Todorov, 1992; DeClerk & Bisserbe, 1997).

Antihypertensives

Hypertension is a common disorder in older adults, and it is a well-known risk factor for cognitive impairment due to cerebrovascular disease. Concerns about the cognitive effects of the medications used in the treatment of this condition, especially the beta-adrenergic blockers, has led to many studies of cognitive functioning during and following withdrawal of antihypertensive medications. Although it was initially thought that some beta-blockers (e.g., propranolol) were more likely to cause cognitive impairment, reports from multiple reviews of the literature have disputed this early claim (Dimsdale, Newton, & Joist, 1989; Gray et al., 1999; Stein & Strickland, 1998). A number of studies have examined cognitive functioning with both relatively short-term (e.g., 16 weeks) and long-term (e.g., 54 months) use (see Applegate et al., 1991; Prince, Bird, Blizard, & Mann, 1996;

Skinner et al., 1992). The cognitive abilities most commonly examined included aspects of attention, memory, and psychomotor functioning.

In general, it appears that there are no consistent neuropsychological changes due to taking antihypertensive medications, including diuretics, angiotension-converting enzyme (ACE) inhibitors, beta-blockers, and calcium channel blockers, although less is known about the effects of this latter class of drugs. Interestingly, psychomotor speed actually improved in a few studies of treatment with ACE inhibitors (see Stein & Strickland, 1998).

Anticonvulsants

Assessment of the neuropsychological effects of anticonvulsants is confounded by the fact that very few studies have examined older adults, and they often do not include healthy volunteers. According to Bergey (2004), the incidence of new-onset seizure disorders is higher in older adults, and anticonvulsants are increasingly being used in psychiatric patients (e.g., for bipolar disorder); thus evaluation of potential cognitive side effects from antiepileptic drugs (AEDs) remains important. Basically, all AEDs are associated with dose-related effects on cognition and/or delirium. However, when administered in therapeutic doses, most of the major AEDs have little or no significant cognitive effects (Devinsky, 1995). One study of first-generation AEDs in older adults found that valproate had relatively worse effects on attention than did phenytoin, although the overall cognitive effects over 1 year were similarly minimal (Craig & Tallis, 1994).

Overall, it appears that first-generation AEDs (e.g., valproate, phenytoin, carbamazepine, phenobarbital, primidone) have a greater side effect profile than the newer second-generation AEDs (e.g., oxcarbazepine, topiramate, zonisamide, levetiracetam). Also, monotherapy tends to result in fewer cognitive problems (Gray et al., 1999). Of the older AEDs, phenobarbital appears to produce the greatest negative neuropsychological effects on psychomotor skills, attention/concentration, and memory, but phenytoin also may have significant dose-related cognitive effects on memory and motor speed (Stein & Strickland, 1998). At any rate, there is wide variability in the tolerability of AEDs among older adults.

Antihistamines

It appears that the older, sedating antihistamines have effects on psychomotor speed, attention and, to a lesser degree, memory (Stein & Strickland, 1998). In older adults, diphenhydramine has been shown to be associated with impairments in attention, vigilance, reaction time, and short-term verbal memory (Katz et al., 1998; Kay et al., 1997). The second-generation antihistamines (e.g., loratadine, astemizole) generally cause less sedation and cognitive problems (Kay et al., 1997).

In conclusion, many medications that are frequently prescribed to older adults can cause cognitive impairment, particularly tricyclic antidepressants, benzodiazepines, first-generation anticonvulsants, and older, highly sedating antihistamines, among many others. Certainly, there is evidence for dose-dependent cognitive effects for many medications. Older adults may also be particularly sensitive to the effects of medications, perhaps due to factors such as decline in renal function and metabolic clearance differences. As clinicians charged with assessing cognitive functioning, it is necessary that we remain aware of potential medication side effects in older adults in order differentiate permanent cognitive impairments from potentially reversible conditions.

CONCLUSIONS

This chapter reviewed literature relevant to some of the more commonly reported causes of "reversible dementia." There is significant variability in the findings, both across disorders and within the literature specific to each condition, as highlighted in Table 5.1. However, there are several general conclusions that can be drawn from the literature. A summary of the general findings from the broad literature covered in this review follows.

1. Although a severe dementia can result from some of the above disorders, most of them do not typically present as a global dementia. More commonly, we find a few isolated deficits, many of which are often mild rather than severe.

2. When dementia does result, the modal pattern or profile of deficits is consistent with a "subcortical" dementia syndrome with deficits in memory retrieval, executive functions, and psychomotor and cognitive processing speed.

3. Differentiating between the representative cognitive symptoms associated with these disorders and normal aging can be quite difficult. The symptoms of slowed psychomotor speed, slowed mental processing, and retrieval problems, particularly when they are mild in these disorders, are consistent with the typical profile of age-related cognitive decline.

4. Complete reversal of the symptoms associated with the reviewed conditions appears to be very rare. Even when improvement does occur, cognitive functioning usually does not return to premorbid levels. Patients are often left with residual deficits.

5. In general, a shorter duration of illness is desirable for a better prognosis. Early treatment tends to lead to greater recovery. Also, the less the severity of the medical condition, the more likely there will be cognitive improvement when treatment is provided.

6. For each of the conditions discussed in this review, the literature is fraught with methodological limitations that constrain our ability to draw hard conclusions from the data. Pertinent methodological issues include heterogeneous patient samples, lack of follow-up data, few prospective investigations, limited comprehensiveness of neuropsychological assessments, limited standardization in assessment procedures, use of varying criteria in diagnosing conditions, and a heavy reliance on case studies. These limitations interfere with our ability to identify reliable percentages of patients who are likely to improve with treatment or the degree to which they will improve with treatment.

Given that most of the above conditions do not commonly present as a "full-blown" dementia syndrome but often result in scattered, isolated, and/or mild cognitive dysfunction, it may not be accurate to refer to the cognitive consequences from these conditions as a "dementia." Furthermore, the extent of cognitive recovery is dependent upon many factors but does not typically result in a complete return to previous levels of functioning. Thus the appropriateness of the term "reversible" could also be questioned. As such, based on the findings in the literature, it seems that the comment by Byrne (1987) that the term *reversible dementia* is a misnomer has merit.

The material presented in this chapter was provided as a starting point for those in-

TABLE 5.1. Summary of the General Findings Regarding Treatable Medical Conditions

Condition	Prevalence	Etiology	Clinical features	Cognitive profile	Treatment	Reversibility
Normal-pressure hydrocephalus	• Most commonly occurs over age 60 • Accounts for < 5% of dementia cases • Most cases are secondary to another condition (e.g., SAH, TBI)	• Unclear; perhaps impaired CSF absorption at the arachnoid villi, or "suprasylvian subarachnoid block"	• Impaired gait, mental deterioration, and sphincter dysfunction • Slow progression	• "Subcortical" pattern • Mild inattention • Poor initiation • Slowed mental processes • Recogniton > recall	Periventrucular shunt	• Variable (30–80%) • Secondary NPH • Gait disturbance prior to mental decline • Improvement following CSF tap
Hypothyroidism	• Increases with age • Approximately 14% in older adults (Luboshitzky et al., 1996)	• Malfunction in the negative feedback system between TSH from the pituitary gland and T_4 from the thyroid gland • Subclinical hypothyroidism (high TSH but normal T_4) • Primary hypothyroidism (T_4 abnormally low)	• Depression • Lethargy • Dry skin • Feeling cold	Impaired • Memory • Visuomotor processing • Visuospatial/visuoconstruction Commonly intact • Sustained attention • Language skills (including fluency) • Gross motor abilities	Supplementation of T_4	• Literature mixed • Symptoms associated with subclinical versus primary (overt) hypothyroidism appear to be more amenable to improvement
Vitamin B_{12} deficiency	• 26% in community-dwelling older adults • 17% in hospitalized and/or nursing home patients	• B_{12} levels reduced with age • Food-B_{12} malabsorption (50% of cases) • Pernicious anemia • Other causes: atropic gastritis, pancreas insufficiency, SIBO, malabsorption due to drug interactions • Results in demyelination and axonal degeneration	• Fatigue • Weakness • Loss of appetite • Sore mouth/tongue • Diarrhea • Tingling of hands/feet	• "Subcortical" pattern • Severity of symptoms related to duration of disorder • Typically a few scattered deficits Common impairments • Abstraction/problem solving • Complex visual perceptual skills • Visuoconstruction • Letter fluency • Verbal memory impairment • Psychomotor slowing	Prescription (intramuscular) and OTC (oral) B_{12} supplements	Lab tests show rapid recovery of B_{12} levels following supplementation • Neurological symptoms may completely resolve if treatment is begun quickly ("window of opportunity" only a few months) • Otherwise, results of studies are not optimistic • Complete recovery appears to be rare

Condition	Epidemiology	Etiology	Clinical presentation	Cognitive findings	Treatment	Outcome/prognosis
Thiamine deficiency	• Oral thiamine intake deficiency is common in underdeveloped countries • 95% of cases in developed countries is associated with alcohol use	• Malnourishment, often due to high-caloric intake of alcohol rather than food • Alcohol may also inhibit the intestinal absorption of thiamine • Deficiency can occur rather quickly, in as little as 2–3 weeks	• Acute presentation of thiamine deficiency • Gait and truncal ataxia • Ophthalmic disorders (nystagmus, lateral rectus palsy, conjugate gaze palsy), progressing to ophthalmoplegia • Confusional state • Tachycardia	Mild deficiencies • Perceptual–motor difficulties • Visuospatial problems • Learning and memory • Abstraction/problem solving Severe deficiencies • Wernicke–Korsakoff syndrome • Severe anterograde amnesia • Retrograde amnesia • Possibly confabulation	Daily administration of thiamine hydrochloride	Wernicke's encephalopathy • Reduced confusion • Decreased ataxia • Improved eye movements Wernicke–Korsakoff syndrome • Prognosis is poor • Memory deficit stable • Abstinence may help
Depression-related cognitive dysfunction	• MDD in those 65+: 2% • Significant depressive symptoms: 20% • Complication: Dysphoria in AD is about 50%	Likely multiple etiologies	• Depression • Subjective concentration and memory complaints • Decreased energy, fatigue • Appetite and sleep problems	Variable findings, often no cognitive deficits Most common deficits cited • Psychomotor speed • Executive functioning • Visuospatial skills Other findings • Intact memory recognition • Few false-positive recognition errors • More "don't know" responses • Variability on tests of similar cognitive abilities	• Antidepressant medications • Psychotherapy	• Study results are inconsistent, possibly due to heterogeneous subgroups of depressed patients Possibly improvement in: • Executive functions • Processing speed • Working memory • If improvement does occur, it tends to fall short of baseline abilities

(continued)

TABLE 5.1. (continued)

Condition	Prevalence	Etiology	Clinical features	Cognitive profile	Treatment	Reversibility
Sleep-disordered breathing	• Most common associated health condition: obstructive sleep apnea • General population: 2–5% • More than 25% in those 65 and older • More common in men • Correlated with body mass index	Repetitive upper airway obstruction Risk factors • Smoking • Weight gain • Alcohol/sedative consumption • Lying in supine position • Sleep deprivation • Hypothyroidism • Acromegaly	• Loud snoring • Breathing stoppage during sleep • Daytime sleepiness • Irritability/impatience • Depression • Associated with high blood pressure, cardiovascular, and pulmonary diseases	Unclear if deficits are due to transient, repeated hypoxemia or sleep disruption and subsequent sleepiness, or perhaps both Impaired • Psychomotor slowing • Executive dysfunction • Inattentiveness • Memory	• CPAP/BiPAP • Avoidance of lying in supine position • Weight loss • Nasal/ pharyngeal reconstruction • Tracheostomy	• Some suggestion that preventing OSA can lead to improved cognitive symptoms • More studies are needed • Appears to be some improvement in visual memory, psychomotor speed, and executive functions • Attention deficits may remain

Note. NPH, normal-pressure hydrocephalus; SAH, subarachnoid hemorrhage; TBI, traumatic brain injury; CSF, cerebrospinal fluid; TSH, thyroid-stimulating hormone; SIBO, small intestinal bacterial overgrowth' MDD, major depressive disorder; CPAP, continuous positive airway pressure; BiPAP, bilevel positive airway pressure; OSA, obstructive sleep apnea.

terested in this topic, who are further referred to additional sources for more detail on conditions discussed.

REFERENCES

Adams, N., Strauss, M., Schluchter, M., & Redline, S. (2000). Relation of measures of sleep-disordered breathing to neuropsychological functioning. *American Journal of Respiratory and Critical Care Medicine, 163*, 1626–1631.

Adams, R. D., Victor, M., & Ropper, A. D. (1997). *Principles of neurology* (6th ed.). New York: McGraw-Hill.

Alexander, M. P., & Geshwind, N. (1984). Dementia in the elderly. In M. L. Albert (Ed.), *Clinical neurology of aging* (pp. 254–276). New York: Oxford University Press.

Amado-Boccara, I., Gougoulis, N., Poirier Littré, M. F., Galinowski, A., & Lôo, H. (1995). Effects of antidepressants on cognitive functions: A review. *Neuroscience and Biobehavioral Reviews, 19*(3), 479–493.

Ambrose, M. L., Bowden, S. C., & Whelan, G. (2001). Thiamin treatment and working memory function of alcohol-dependent people: Preliminary findings. *Alcoholism: Clinical and Experimental Research, 25*, 112–116.

American Psychiatric Association. (1994). *Diagnostic and statistical manual of mental disorders* (4th ed.). Washington, DC: Author.

Applegate, W. B., Phillips, H. L., Schnaper, H., Shepherd, A. M., Schocken, D., Luhr, J. C., et al. (1991). A randomized controlled trial of the effects of three antihypertensive agents on blood pressure control and quality of life in older women. *Archives of Internal Medicine, 151*, 1817–1823.

Babior, B. M., & Bunn, F. H. (1998). Megalobiastic anemias. In A. S. Fauci, E. Braunwald, & K. J. Isselbacher (Eds.), *Harrison's principles of internal medicine* (pp. 653–659). New York: McGraw-Hill.

Baldini, I. M., Vita, A., Mauri, M. C., Amodei, V., Carrisi, M., Bravin, S., et al. (1997). Psychopathological and cognitive features in subclinical hypothyroidism. *Progress in Neuro-Psychopharmacology and Biological Psychiatry, 21*, 925–935.

Barbee, J. G., Black, T. W., & Todorov, A. A. (1992). Differential effects of alprazolam and buspirone upon acquisition, retention, and retrieval processes in memory. *Journal of Neuropsychiatry and Clinical Neuroscience, 4*, 308–314.

Bassetti, C. L., & Gugger, M. (2002). Sleep disordered breathing in neurologic diseases. *Swiss Medicine Weekly, 132*, 109–115.

Bassuk, S., Berkman, L., & Wypij, D. (1998). Depressive symptomatology and incident cognitive decline in an elderly community sample. *Archives of General Psychiatry, 55*, 1073–1081.

Bech-Azeddine, R., Waldemar, G., Knudsen, G. M., Hogh, P., Bruhn, P., Wildschiodtz, G., et al. (2001). Idiopathic normal-pressure hydrocephalus: Evaluation and findings in a multidisciplinary memory clinic. *European Journal of Neurology, 8*, 601–611.

Bedard, M. A., Montplaisir, J., Richer, F., Rouleau, I., & Malo, J. (1991). Obstructive sleep apnea syndrome: Pathogenesis of neuropsychological deficits. *Journal of Clinical and Experimental Neuropsychology, 1991*, 950–964.

Bergey, G. K. (2004). Initial treatment of epilepsy. *Neurology, 63*, S40–S48.

Blazer, D., Hughes, D. C., & George, L. K. (1987). The epidemiology of depression in an elderly community population. *Gerontologist, 27*, 281–287.

Bliwise, D. L. (1996). Is sleep apnea a cause of reversible dementia in old age? *Journal of the American Geriatrics Society, 44*, 1407–1409.

Bliwise, D. L. (2002). Sleep apnea, APOE4 and Alzheimer's disease 20 years and counting? *Journal of Psychosomatic Research, 53*, 539–546.

Boone, K. B., Lesser, I. M., Miller, B. L., Wohl, M., Berman, N., Lee, A. B. P., et al. (1995). Cognitive functioning in older depressed outpatients: Relationship of presence and severity of depression to neuropsychological test scores. *Neuropsychology, 9*, 390–398.

Bowden, S. C. (1990). Separating cognitive impairment in neurologically asymptomatic alcoholism from Wernicke–Korsakoff syndrome: Is the neuropsychological distinction justified? *Psychological Bulletin, 107*, 355–366.

Bowden, S. C., Bardenhagen, F., Ambrose, M., & Whelan, G. (1994). Alcohol, thiamin deficiency, and neuropsychological disorders. *Alcohol and Alcoholism* (Suppl. 2), 267–272.

Branconnier, R. J., DeVitt, D. R., Cole, J. O., & Spera, K. F. (1982). Amitriptyline selectively disrupts verbal recall from secondary memory of the normal aged. *Neurobiology of Aging, 3*(1), 55–59.

Bunce, D., Kivipelto, M., & Wahlin, A. (2004). Utilization of cognitive support in episodic free recall as a function of apolipoprotein E and vitamin B_{12} or folate among adults aged 75 years and older. *Neuropsychology, 18*, 362–370.

Burke, D., Sengoz, A., & Schwartz, R. (2000). Potentially reversible cognitive impairment in patients presenting to a memory disorders clinic. *Journal of Clinical Neurosciences, 7*, 120–123.

Butters, M. A., Becker, J. T., Nebes, R. D., Zmuda, M. D., Mulsant, B. H., Pollock, B. G., et al. (2000). Changes in cognitive functioning following treatment of late-life depression. *American Journal of Psychiatry, 157*, 1949–1954.

Byrne, E. (1987). Reversible dementia. *International Journal of Geriatric Psychiatry, 2*, 73–81.

Caltagirone, C., Gainotti, G., Masullo, C., & Villa, G. (1982). Neuropsychological study of normal pressure hydrocephalus, *Acta Psychiatria Scandinavia, 63*, 93–100.

Celik, Y., & Kaya, M. (2004). Brain SPECT findings in Wernicke's encephalopathy. *Neurological Sciences, 25*, 23–26.

Chen, P., Ganguli, M., Mulsant, B. H., & DeKosky, S. T. (1999). The temporal relationship between depressive symptoms and dementia: A community-based prospective study. *Archives of General Psychiatry, 56*, 261–266.

Chiu, H. F. K. (1996). Vitamin B_{12} deficiency and dementia. *International Journal of Geriatric Psychiatry, 11*, 851–858.

Ciccia, R. M., & Langlais, P. J. (2000). An examination of the synergistic interaction of ethanol and thiamine deficiency in the development of neurological signs of long-term cognition and memory impairments. *Alcoholism: Clinical and Experimental Research, 24*, 622–634.

Clarfield, A. M. (1988). The reversible dementias: Do they reverse? *Annals of Internal Medicine, 109*, 476–486.

Clarnette, R. M. (1994). Hypothyroidism: Does treatment cure dementia? *Journal of Geriatric Psychiatry and Neurology, 7*, 23–27.

Corkill, R., & Cadoux-Hudson, T. A. D. (1999). Normal pressure hydrocephalus: Developments in determining surgical prognosis. *Current Opinion in Neurology, 12*(6), 671–677.

Craig, I., & Tallis, R. (1994). Impact of valproate and phenytoin on cognitive function in elderly patients: Results of a single-blind randomized comparative study. *Epilepsia, 35*, 381–390.

Cummings, J., Benson, F., & Stephen, L. (1980). Reversible dementia: Illustrative cases, definition and review. *Journal of the American Medical Association, 243*, 2434–2439.

Dahabra, S., Ashton, C. H., Bahrainian, M., Britton, P. G., Ferrier, I. N., McAllister, V. A., et al. (1998). Structural and functional abnormalities in elderly patients clinically recovered from early- and late-onset depression. *Biological Psychiatry, 44*, 34–46.

Dealberto, M.-J., Pajot, N., Courbon, D., & Alpérovitch, A. (1996). Breathing disorders during sleep and cognitive performance in an older community sample: The EVA study. *Journal of the American Geriatrics Society, 44*, 1287–1294.

DeClerk, A. C., & Bisserbe, J. C. (1997). Short-term safety profile of zolpidem: Objective measures of cognitive effects. *European Journal of Psychiatry, 12*(Suppl.), 15s–20s.

Devinsky, O. (1995). Cognitive and behavioral effects of antiepileptic drugs. *Epilepsia, 36*(Suppl. 2), S46–S65.

Dharmarajan, T. S., Adiga, G. U., & Norkus, E. P. (2003). Vitamin B$_{12}$ deficiency: Recognizing subtle symptoms in older adults. *Geriatrics, 58*(3), 30–38.

Dharmarajan, T. S., Adiga, G. U., Pitchumoni, S., & Norkus, E. P. (2003). Vitamin B$_{12}$ deficiency. In T. S. Dharmarajan & R. A. Norman (Eds.), *Clinical geriatrics* (pp. 625–634). Boca Raton, FL: CRC Press/Parthenon.

Dharmarajan, T. S., & Norkus, E. P. (2001). Approaches to vitamin B$_{12}$ deficiency. *Postgraduate Medicine, 110*, 99–105.

Dimsdale, J. E., Newton, R. P., & Joist, T. (1989). Neuropsychological side effects of beta-blockers. *Archives of Internal Medicine, 149*, 514–525.

Dugbartey, A. T. (1998). Neurocognitive aspects of hypothyroidism. *Archives of Internal Medicine, 158*, 1413–1418.

Ekstedt, J., & Fridén, H. (1984). CSF hydrodynamics for the study of the adult hydrocephalus syndrome. In K. Shapiro, A. Marmarou, & H. Portnoy (Eds.), *Hydrocephalus* (pp. 363–382). New York: Raven Press.

Findley, L. J., Barth, J. T., Powers, D. C., Wilhoit, S. C., Boyd, D. G., & Suratt, P. M. (1986). Cognitive impairment in patients with obstructive sleep apnea and associated hypoxemia. *Chest, 90*, 686–690.

Folstein, M. F., & McHugh, P. R. (1978). Dementia syndrome of depression. *Aging, 7*, 87–93.

Freemon, F. R. (1976). Evaluation of patients with progressive intellectual deterioration. *Archives of Neurology, 33*, 658–659.

Freemon, F. R., & Rudd, S. M. (1982). Clinical features that predict potentially reversible progressive intellectual deterioration. *American Geriatrics Society, 30*, 449–451.

Freter, S., Bergman, H., Gold, S., Chertkow, H., & Clarfield, A. M. (1998). Prevalence of potentially reversible dementias and actual reversibility in a memory clinic cohort. *Canadian Medical Associations Journal, 159*, 657–662.

Garry, P. J., Goodwin, J. S., & Hunt, W. C. (1984). Folate and vitamin B$_{12}$ status in a healthy elderly population. *Journal of the American Geriatrics Society, 32*, 719–726.

Gastaldi, G., Casirola, D., Ferrari, G., & Rindi, G. (1989). Effects of chronic ethanol administration on thiamine transport in microvillus vesicles of rat small intestine. *Alcohol and Alcoholism, 24*, 83–89.

Geerlings, M., Schoevers, R., Beekman, A., et al. (2000). Depression and risk of cognitive decline and Alzheimer's disease: Results of two prospective community-based studies in the Netherlands. *British Journal of Psychiatry, 176*, 568–575.

Goodwin, J. S., Goodwin, J. M., & Garry, P. J. (1983). Association between nutritional status and cognitive functioning in a healthy elderly population. *Journal of the American Medical Association, 249*, 2917–2921.

Gray, S. L., Lai, K. V., & Larson, E. B. (1999). Drug-Induced cognition disorders in the elderly: Incidence, prevention and management. *Drug Safety, 21*, 101–122.

Gustafson, L., & Hagberg, B. (1978). Recovery in hydrocephalic dementia after shunt operation. *Journal of Neurology, Neurosurgery and Psychiatry, 41*, 940–947.

Haggerty, J. J., Evans, D. L., & Prange, A. J. (1986). Organic brain syndrome associated with marginal hypothyroidism. *American Journal of Psychiatry, 143*, 785–786.

Hakim, S., & Adams, R. D. (1965). The special clinical problems of symptomatic children with normal cerebrospinal fluid pressure: Observations on cerebrospinal fluid hydrodynamics. *Journal of Neurological Science, 2*, 307–327.

Hart, R. P., Kwentus, J. A., Taylor, J. R., & Harkins, S. W. (1987). Rate of forgetting in dementia and depression. *Journal of Consulting and Clinical Psychology, 55*, 101–105.

Hector, M., & Burton, J. R. (1988). What are the psychiatric manifestations of vitamin B$_{12}$ deficiency? *Journal of the American Geriatrics Society, 36*, 1105–1112.

Heidebrink, J. L. (2003). Neurologic aspects of nondegenerative, nonvascular dementias. In P. A. Lichtenberg, D. L. Murman, & A. M. Mellow (Eds.), *Handbook of dementia: Psychological, neurological, and psychiatric perspectives* (pp. 197–227). Hoboken, NJ: Wiley.

Iddon, J. L., Pickard, J. D., Cross, J. J. L., Griffiths, P. D., Czosnyka, M., & Sahakian, B. J. (1999). Specific patterns of cognitive impairment in patients with idiopathic normal pressure hydrocephalus and Alzheimer's disease: A pilot study. *Journal of Neurology, Neurosurgery, and Psychiatry*, 67, 723–732.

Johnson, K. A., Bernard, M. A., & Funderburg, K. (2002). Vitamin nutrition in older adults. *Clinical Geriatric Medicine*, 18, 773–799.

Kales, A., Caldwell, A. B., Cadieux, R. J., Vela-Bueno, A., Ruch, L. G., & Mayes, S. D. (1985). Severe obstructive sleep apnea: II. Associated psychopathology and psychosocial consequences. *Journal of Chronic Diseases*, 38, 427–434.

Kaszniak, A. W., & Ditraglia Christenson, G. (1994). In M. Storandt & G. R. VandenBos (Eds.), *Neuropsychological assessment of dementia and depression in older adults: A clinician's guide* (pp. 81–117). Washington, DC: American Psychological Association.

Katz, I. R., Sands, L. P., Bilker, W., DiFilippo, S., Boyce, A., & D'Angelo, K. (1998). Identification of medications that cause cognitive impairment in older people: The case of oxybutynin chloride. *Journal of the American Geriatrics Society*, 46, 8–13.

Katzman, R. (1977). Normal pressure hydrocephalus. In C. E. Wells (Ed.), *Dementia* (2nd ed., pp. 69–92). Philadelphia: Davis.

Kay, G. G., Berman, B., Mockoviak, S. H., Morris, C. E., Reeves, D., Starbuck, V., et al. (1997). Initial and steady-state effects of diphenhydramine and loratadine on sedation, cognition, mood, and psychomotor performance. *Archives of Internal Medicine*, 157, 2350–2356.

Kerr, J. S., Fairweather, D. B., & Hindmarch, I. (1993). Effects of fluoxetine on psychomotor performance, cognitive function and sleep in depressed patients. *International Clinical Psychopharmacology*, 8, 341–343.

Kiloh, L. G. (1961). Pseudo-dementia. *Acta Psychiatrica Scandinavica*, 37, 336–351.

Klinge, P., Ruckert, N., Schuhmann, M., Dorner, L., Brinker, T., & Samii, M. (2002). Neuropsychological testing to improve surgical management of patients with chronic hydrocephalus after shunt treatment. *Acta Neurochirurgica*, 81(Suppl.), 51–53.

Knopman, D. S., DeKosky, S. T., Cummings, J. L., Chui, H., Corey-Bloom, J., Relkin, N., et al. (2001). Practice parameter: Diagnosis of dementia (an evidence-based review). *Neurology*, 56, 1143–1153.

Kopelman, M. D. (1995). The Korsakoff syndrome. *British Journal of Psychiatry*, 166, 154–173.

Larner, A. J., Janssen, J. C., Cipolotti, L., & Rossor, M. N. (1999). Cognitive profile in dementia associated with vitamin B12 deficiency due to pernicious anaemia. *Journal of Neurology*, 246, 317–319.

La Rue, A. (1992). *Aging and neuropsychological assessment*. New York: Plenum Press.

Larner, A. J., Janssen, J. C., Cipolotti, L., & Rossor, M. N. (1999). *Journal of Neurology*, 246, 317–319.

Larson, E. B., Kukull, W. A., Buchner, D., & Reifler, B. V. (1987). Adverse drug reactions associated with global cognitive impairment in elderly persons. *Annals of Internal Medicine*, 107, 169–173.

Larson, E. B., Reifler, B. V., Featherstone, H. J., & English, D. R. (1984). Dementia in elderly outpatients: A prospective study. *Annals of Internal Medicine*, 100, 417–423.

Lesser, I. M., Boone, K. B., Mehringer, C. M., Wohl, M. A., Miller, B. L., & Berman, N. G. (1996). Cognition and white matter hyperintensities in older depressed patients. *American Journal of Psychiatry*, 153, 1280–1287.

Luboshitzky, R., Oberman, A. S., Kaufman, N., Reichman, N., & Flatau, E. (1996). Prevalence of cognitive dysfunction and hypothyroidism in an elderly community population. *Israeli Journal of Medical Science*, 32, 60–65.

Mac, D. S., Kumar, R., & Goodwin, D. W. (1985). Anterograde amnesia with oral lorazepam. *Journal of Clinical Psychiatry*, 46, 137–138.

Madhusoodanan, S., & Bogunovic, O. J. (2004). Safety of benzodiazepines in the geriatric population. *Expert Opinion on Drug Safety*, 3(5), 485–493.

Marsden, C. D., & Harrison, M. J. G. (1972). Outcome of investigation of patients with presenile dementia. *British Medical Journal, 2,* 249–252.

Martin, P., McCool, B., & Singleton, C. (1993). Genetic sensitivity to thiamine deficiency and development of alcoholic organic brain disease. *Alcoholism: Clinical and Experimental Research, 17,* 31–37.

McKhann, G., Drachman, D., Folstein, M., Katzman, R., Price, D., & Stadlin, E. M. (1984). Clinical diagnosis of Alzheimer's disease: Report of the NINCDS–ADRDA work group under the auspices of the Department of Health and Human Services Task Force on Alzheimer's disease. *Neurology, 34,* 939–944.

Meadows, M-E., Kaplan, R. F., & Bromfield, E. B. (1994). Cognitive recovery with vitamin B_{12} therapy: A longitudinal neuropsychiatric assessment. *Neurology, 44,* 1764–1765.

Mennemeier, M., Graner, R. D., & Heilman, K. M. (1993). Memory, mood and measurement in hypothyroidism. *Journal of Clinical and Experimental Neuropsychology, 15,* 822–831.

Miller, J. D., & Adams, J. H. (1992). The pathophysiology of raised intracranial pressure. In J. H. Adams & L. W. Duchen (Eds.), *Greenfield's neuropathology* (5th ed., pp. 69–105). London: Arnold.

Morcos, Z., Kerns, S. C., & Shapiro, B. E. (2004). Wernicke encephalopathy. *Archives of Neurology, 61,* 775–776.

Morganti, S., Ceresini, G., Nonis, E., Regbecchi, I., Bertone, L., Montanari, I., et al. (2002). Evaluation of thyroid function in outpatients affected by dementia. *Journal of Endocrinology Investigation, 25,* 69–70.

Morrison, R. L., & Katz, I. R. (1989). Drug-related cognitive impairment: Current progress and recurrent problems. *Annual Review of Gerontology and Geriatrics, 9,* 232–279.

Muldoon, M. F., Waldstein, S. R., & Jennings, J. R. (1995). Neuropsychological consequences of antihypertensive medication use. *Experimental Aging Research, 21,* 353–368.

Myers, J. K., Weissman, M. M., Tischler, G. L., Holzer, C. E., III, Leaf, P. J., Orvaschel, H., et al. (1984). Six-month prevalence of psychiatric disorders in three communities. *Archives of General Psychiatry, 41,* 959–967.

Naegele, B., Pepin, J.-L., Levy, P., Bonnet, C., Pellat, J., & Feuerstein, C. (1998). Cognitive executive dysfunction in patients with obstructive sleep apnea syndrome (OSAS) after CPAP treatment. *Sleep, 21,* 392–397.

Naegele, B., Thouvard, V., Pepin, J.-L., Levy, P., Bonnet, C., Perret, J. E., et al. (1995). Deficits of cognitive executive functions in patients with sleep apnea syndrome. *Sleep, 18,* 43–52.

Nebes, R. D., Butters, M. A., Mulsant, B. H., Pollock, B. G., Zmuda, M. D., Houck, P. R., et al. (2000). *Psychological Mediciene, 30,* 679–691.

Nikaido, A. M., Ellinwood, E. H., Heatherly, D. G., & Gupta, S. K. (1990). Age-related increases in CNS sensitivity to benzodiazepines as assessed by task difficulty. *Psychopharmacology* (Berl.), *100,* 90–97.

O'Keeffe, S. T., Tormey, W. P., Glasgow, R., & Lavan, J. N. (1994). Thiamine deficiency in hospitalized elderly patients. *Gerontology, 40,* 18–24.

Osterweil, D., Syndulko, K., Cohen, S. N., Pettler-Jennings, P., Hershman, J., Cummings, J., et al. (1992). Cognitive function in non-demented older adults with hypothyroidism. *Journal of the American Geriatrics Society, 40,* 325–335.

Ovsiew, F. (2003). Seeking reversibility and treatability in dementia. *Seminars in Clinical Neuropsychiatry, 8,* 3–11.

Palmer, B. W., Boone, K. B., Lesser, I. M., & Wohl, M. A. (1996). Neuropsychological deficits among older depressed patients with predominantly psychological or vegetative symptoms. *Journal of Affective Disorders, 41,* 17–24.

Parsons, O. A., & Nixon, S. J. (1993). Neurobehavioral sequelae of alcoholism. *Behavioral Neurology, 11,* 205–218.

Paterniti, S., Verdier Taillefer, M.-H., Dufouil, C., & Alpérovitch, A. (2002). Depressive symptoms and cognitive decline in elderly people. *British Journal of Psychiatry, 181,* 406–410.

Pomara, N., Deptula, D., Medel, M., Block, R. I., & Greenblatt, D. J. (1989). Effects of diazepam on recall memory: Relationship to aging, dose and duration of treatment. *Psychopharmacology Bulletin*, 25, 144–148.

Prince, M. J., Bird, A. S., Blizard, R. A., & Mann, A. H. (1996). Is the cognitive function in older patients affected by antihypertensive treatment? Results from 54 months of the Medical Research Council's treatment trial of hypertension in older adults. *British Medical Journal*, 312, 801–805.

Redline, S., Strauss, M. E., Adams, N., Winters, M., Roebuck, T., Spry, K., et al. (1997). Neuropsychological function in mild sleep disordered breathing. *Sleep*, 20, 160–167.

Riggs, K. M., Spiro, A., III, Tucker, K., & Rush, D. (1996). Relations of vitamin B-12 vitamin B-6, folate, and homocysteine to cognitive performance in the normative aging study. *American Journal of Clinical Nutrition*, 63, 306–314.

Robins Wahlin, T.-B., Wahlin, A., Winblad, B., & Bäckman, L. (2001). The influence of serum vitamin B_{12} and folate status on cognitive functioning in very old age. *Biological Psychology*, 56, 247–265.

Sakulsripong, M., Curran, H. V., & Lader, M. (1991). Does tolerance develop to the sedative and amnesic effects of antidepressants? A comparison of amitriptyline, trazodone and placebo. *European Journal of Clinical Pharmacology*, 40(1), 43–48.

Salmon, D. P., Butters, N., & Heindel, W. C. (1993). Alcoholic dementia and related disorders. In R. W. Parks, R. F. Zec, & R. S. Wilson (Eds.), *Neuropsychology of Alzheimer's disease and other dementias* (pp. 186–209). New York: Oxford University Press.

Saracaceanu, E., Tramoni, A. V., & Henry, J. M. (1997). An association between subcortical dementia and pernicious anaemia: A psychiatric mask. *Comprehensive Psychiatry*, 38, 349–351.

Sekhar, L. N., Moody, J., & Guthkeich, A. N. (1982). Malfunctioning ventriculoperitoneal shunts: Clinical and pathological features. *Journal of Neurosurgery*, 56, 411–416.

Shochat, T., & Pillar, G. (2003). Sleep apnea in the older adult. *Drugs and Aging*, 20, 551–560.

Skinner, M. H., Futterman, A., Morrissette, D., Thompson, L. W., Hoffman, B. B., & Blaschke, T. F. (1992). Atenolol compared with nifedipine: Effect on cognitive function and mood in elderly hypertensive patients. *Annals of Internal Medicine*, 116, 615–623.

Smith, C. L., & Granger, C. V. (1992). Hypothyroidism producing reversible dementia: A challenge for medical rehabilitation. *American Journal of Physical Medicine and Rehabilitation*, 71, 28–30.

Smith, J. S., Kiloh, L. G., Ratnavale, G. S., & Grant, D. A. (1976). The investigation of dementia: The results in 100 consecutive admissions. *Medical Journal of Australia*, 63, 403–405.

Stambrook, M., Cardoso, E., Hawryluk, G. A., Eirikson, P., Piatek, D., & Sicz, G. (1988). Neuropsychological changes following the neurosurgical treatment of normal pressure hydrocephalus. *Archives of Clinical Neuropsychology*, 3, 323–330.

Stein, R. A., & Strickland, T. L. (1998). A review of the neuropsychological effects of commonly used prescription medications. *Archives of Clinical Neuropsychology*, 13(3), 259–284.

Stoudemire, A., Hill, C., Gulley, L. R., & Morris, R. (1989). Neuropsychological and biomedical assessment of depression—dementia syndromes. *Journal of Neuropsychiatry and Clinical Neurosciences*, 1, 347–361.

Taylor, W. D., Wagner, H. R., & Steffens, D. C. (2002). Greater depression severity associated with less improvement in depression-associated cognitive deficits in older adults. *American Journal of Geriatric Psychiatry*, 10, 632–635.

Thomsen, A. M., Borgesen, S. E., Bruhn, P., & Gjerris, F. (1986). Prognosis of dementia in normal-pressure hydrocephalus after a shunt operation. *Annals of Neurology*, 20, 304–310

Thomson, A. D. (2000). Mechanisms of vitamin deficiency in chronic alcohol misusers and the development of the Wernicke–Korsakoff syndrome. *Alcohol and Alcoholism*, 35(Suppl.), 2–7.

Todd, K. G., & Butterworth, R. F. (1999). Mechanisms of selective neuronal cell death due to thiamine deficiency. *Annals of the New York Academy of Sciences*, 893, 404–411.

Vanneste, J. A. L. (2000). Diagnosis and management of normal-pressure hydrocephalus. *Journal of Neurology*, 247, 5–14.

Victor, M., Adams, R. D., & Collins, G. H. (1989). *The Wernicke–Korsakoff syndrome*. Philadelphia, PA: Davis.

Volpato, S., Guralnik, J. M., Fried, L. P., Remaley, A. T., Cappola, A. R., & Launer, L. J. (2002). Serum thyroxine level and cognitive decline in euthyroid older women. *Neurology, 58,* 1055–1061.

Wahlin, A., Hill, R. D., Winblad, B., & Backman, L. (1996). Effects of serum B_{12} and folate status on episodic memory performance in very old age: A population-based study. *Psychology and Aging, 11,* 487–496.

Walstra, G. J. M., Teunisse, S., van Gool, W. A., & van Crevel, H. (1997). Reversible dementia in elderly patients referred to a memory clinic. *Journal of Neurology, 244,* 17–22.

Wang, L., van Bell, G., Crane, P. K., Kukull, W. A., Bowen, J. D., McMormick, W. C., et al. (2004). Subjective memory deterioration and future dementia in people aged 65 and older. *Journal of the American Geriatrics Society, 52,* 2045–2051.

Whybrow, P. C., Prange, A. J., & Treadway, C. R. (1969). Mental changes accompanying thyroid gland dysfunction: A reappraisal using objective psychological measurement. *Archives of General Psychiatry, 20,* 48–63.

Specific Considerations

Section B of the assessment portion of the text includes chapters that draw attention to specific considerations that are essential in the assessment of elders. Indeed, the integrity of our evaluations often rests upon the issues highlighted: the use of appropriate normative data, the application of our data instrumentation to functional concerns, and sensitivity to multicultural issues.

Chapter 6 begins this section with a critical review of the current available norms for tests commonly used in the neuropsychological evaluation of the elderly. Most importantly, this chapter highlights the appropriate conceptualization of data, given the source of normative comparisons. Many of the insights of this chapter are aptly applied to the interpretation of any neuropsychological data, regardless of the age of the patient. However, they are unmistakably critical in regard to elders, because norms in the higher age ranges are often vulnerable in key methodological areas affecting the normative product. This chapter also addresses the importance of normative methods when utilizing longitudinal data, which is often central to establishing or confirming diagnosis, tracking progression or treatment outcomes, and staging symptom severity in elderly groups.

Chapter 7 offers a review of the role of neuropsychology in the assessment of everyday functional abilities, with information about the relationship of our traditional tests to meaningful life-event outcomes and the importance of newer instruments in enhancing our skills in assessing these functional areas. Innovative perspectives regarding the conceptualization and measurement of competencies and capacities are eloquently presented.

Chapter 8 discusses factors critical to the assessment of elders from minority cultural backgrounds. The current prevalence rates for dementia in African Americans are presented with a discussion of the sociocultural factors contributing to the accuracy of case identification and symptom measurement. Methodological factors and patient variables that affect clinical evaluations and programs of research are reviewed, offering a conceptual context within which to evaluate and conduct relevant work.

Finally, we encourage our readers to carefully consider the importance of feedback, as outlined in Chapter 9. This chapter presents the feedback session as the primary method of communicating assessment results and recommendations. The opportunity for the provision of education through this process is inherently understood. However, this potentially pivotal meeting also offers an opportunity to introduce the concept of intervention; often this is the only time when the option of such work is considered, given that our field and allied health practitioners are only now becoming versed in such approaches as favorable reports emerge.

Not surprisingly, given the nature of these special considerations, none of these chapters offers definitive solutions in the areas they cover. Any such "solution" would likely lack depth and would become quickly antiquated, given our continual efforts to expand our understanding in these areas. Instead, these chapters present the reader with a much more valuable conceptual framework within which to consider the relevant issues as we move forward with our daily clinical and research efforts.

6

Using Norms in Neuropsychological Assessment of the Elderly

ROBYN M. BUSCH
GORDON J. CHELUNE
YANA SUCHY

The practice of clinical neuropsychology in the United States is heavily rooted in psychometric assessment and the use of normative information (Davison, 1974). Despite this emphasis, test users frequently focus on issues of interpretation, with little consideration given to how norms are developed and how this factor affects the interpretive statements that can be made about a patient's test performance. This problem is especially evident in neuropsychological evaluation of the elderly, where test development and age-appropriate norms have been slow to emerge, despite growing interest in elder populations.

GENERAL CONSIDERATIONS

Assessment of older adults presents a unique set of considerations for the clinical neuropsychologist. One of the first areas that must be considered is the life context of the aging individual. The transition from middle to old age is accompanied by a number of "normal" life changes. Not only are elders adjusting to new roles and social expectations as they enter retirement, but they must also cope with the physical (e.g., reduced visual acuity, hearing loss, motor slowing) and cognitive (e.g., cognitive slowing, memory difficulties, decline in executive skills) changes that accompany normal aging (Cullum, Butters, Troster, & Salmon, 1990; Erkinjuntti, Laaksonen, Sulkava, Syrjalainen, & Palo, 1986; Howieson, Holm, Kaye, Oken, & Howieson, 1993; Van Gorp, Satz, & Mitrushina, 1990). In addition to the inevitable changes associated with advancing age, elderly individuals are also at increased risk to develop a host of medical conditions, including heart disease, cancer, stroke, chronic obstructive pulmonary disorders, pneumonia, influenza, diabetes, and arthritis, which may require multiple medical treatments and behavioral interventions. These health problems are also often associated with depression (Koltai & Branch, 1999).

All of these age-related factors can adversely affect cognitive functioning and the ability to perform activities of daily living (ADLs). The contribution of each of these factors to current cognitive functioning can be difficult to tease apart, and neuropsychologists are frequently called upon for assistance in this regard. Neuropsychological evaluation can be recommended for a variety of reasons, including assistance with diagnostic issues (e.g., differentiation between depression, dementia, and delirium; see Section A of Part I of this volume), determination of competency or functional capacity (e.g., decisional capacity, ADLs, driving, living alone, etc.; see Marson & Hebert, Chapter 7, this volume), and/or assessment of change in cognitive functioning over time (e.g., to track the course of a dementing process; see Albert & Moss, 1988).

Historically, there has been a paucity of neuropsychological tests specifically designed to address the issues unique to older adults, as well as a lack of normative data for the oldest old. Advances in test development and research over the last decade have started to fill some of these gaps. There is a growing body of literature designed to assist neuropsychologists with the assessment of this population (Albert & Moss, 1988; Koltai & Welsh-Bohmer, 2000; Nussbaum, 1998; Tuokko & Hadjistavropoulos, 1998). This literature includes recommendations for the selection of appropriate testing instruments and alterations in test administration protocols to control for factors unique to older adults that may confound test results (e.g., large print to compensate for visual difficulties). Many researchers also highlight issues related to specific referral questions and the interpretation of test data for older adults. All of these recommendations are important in assuring that the test user obtains accurate and reliable test results and gives important consideration to issues unique to the population of older adults.

Selection of the appropriate normative data with which to compare a patient's test results is another very important, and often neglected, issue in neuropsychological assessment of older adults. Although great efforts have been made in recent years to develop normative data for elderly individuals (Ivnik, Malec, Tangalos, et al., 1992; Ivnik, Tangalos, Petersen, Kokmen, & Kurland, 1992; Malec et al., 1992; Morris et al., 1989), not many texts provide guidance on how to select the most suitable norms for a particular patient based on his or her unique history and presentation. Norms provide an objective reference or standard against which to compare an individual's current test performance and weigh heavily into the interpretations made about a patient's cognitive abilities or deficits. Therefore, selection of the appropriate normative comparison group is one of the most important aspects of neuropsychological assessment, particularly as it pertains to older adults.

This chapter provides a guide for evaluating the nature and adequacy of available norms for use with elderly populations. We begin with a discussion of the nature and purpose of normative data as well as a summary of how normative samples are obtained and the various methods by which norms are developed. This overview is followed by a discussion of what constitutes a "representative" normative sample and the key factors one should consider in selecting a normative comparison group. Finally, we identify specific considerations for assessing cognitive change in elderly individuals over time.

THE NATURE AND PURPOSE OF NORMS

Norms describe the distribution of performances on a given test that can be considered the standard for the group concerned. In addition, norms provide the context within which the performances of an individual external to the reference group can be interpreted (Mitrushina, Boone, & D'Elia, 1999). Although not specific to the evaluation of older adults, there are some fundamental issues about norms that need to be considered. At a macro level, there are two very different ways in which test norms can be used to answer clinically relevant questions, and they both influence, and are influenced by, the composition of the normative standard. Neuropsychological assessments are used to answer a wide range of questions about patients; these questions can be grouped into those that are *descriptive* in nature and those that are *diagnostic*. Depending on the nature of the question to be addressed, different normative standards are necessary.

As the following sections indicate, when used for descriptive purposes, norms allow the test user to address a fundamental question: "How is this individual functioning relative to the reference population?" The emphasis is on determining *where* the individual's performance on a test falls among the range of performances observed in the reference population. The reference standard is the *general population* within which the patient is believed to be a member. A patient's scores can be characterized as "below average," "average," "high average," and so on.

In contrast, when used for diagnostic purposes, norms aid the test user in answering the question, "Is the functioning of this patient impaired or not? That is, does my patient's score *deviate* from premorbid expectations (i.e., the score that would have been obtained in the absence of an intervening illness or injury)?" The reference standard is the premorbid status of the individual, and the deviations of interest from this *individual comparison standard* are typically unidirectional. Thus performances are characterized as "normal" or "within normal limits" versus "mildly impaired," "moderately impaired," etc. The key point here is that population-based descriptive norms cannot be directly used to make diagnostic statements about normality versus abnormality unless the test user employs a different normative approach that infers a *discrepancy* between the patient's observed performance and presumed premorbid functioning. Let us further consider the distinction between the descriptive and the diagnostic use of norms.

Descriptive Use of Norms

Norms intended for descriptive purposes are inherently *population-based* and are grounded in principles of central tendency (Mitrushina et al., 1999). They assume that the construct measured by the test procedure is normally distributed and that all potential test scores fall under a *normal curve*. This curve has basic psychometric properties; that is, there is a true midpoint or population mean, with half of the normative sample falling above and half below this mean, and the distribution of scores is characterized by the standard deviation of the mean. Using such population-based descriptive norms, the test user can determine where a given person is functioning within the reference group. This norm-based *position* can be expressed as a percentile, *z*-score, standard score, or *T*-score, and labels such as "borderline," "low average," "average," "high average," etc., can be used to describe ranges of performance around the mean. Many tests commonly used in the evaluation of older adults employ descriptive population-based norms. The norms for the Wechsler tests (Psychological Corporation, 1997) are classic exemplars.

Although the foregoing material may appear quite elementary, the astute reader will discern at least three key issues that are particularly relevant when evaluating elders. First, norms for tests that are primarily used for descriptive purposes are designed to measure abilities that are presumed normally distributed in the reference group. That is, a person's cognitive ability, as reflected by his or her test performance, can be below the average, average, or above the average. This is quite different from tests that are *deficit-*

oriented. For example, performances on popular mental status measures such as the Dementia Rating Scale (DRS; Mattis, 1988) or the Mini-Mental State Examination (MMSE; Folstein, Folstein, & McHugh, 1975) are not normally distributed and tend to be highly skewed and prone to ceiling effects. Rather than invoking concepts related to central tendency when describing performances on these measures, it is more appropriate to think of test performances in terms of normality and use unidirectional descriptors such as "normal," "mildly impaired," "moderately impaired," and so on. It is easy to appreciate this point when considering a construct such as mental status; that is, it makes sense to speak of an elder as having a normal versus abnormal or "impaired" mental status rather than describing the elder as having an above-average versus a below-average mental status. However, this distinction is less apparent when considering performances on a measure such as the Boston Naming Test (BNT; Goodglass & Kaplan, 1983), especially when large descriptive datasets have been published (Heaton, Miller, Taylor, & Grant, 2004; Ivnik, Malec, Smith, Tangalos, & Petersen, 1996; Tombaugh & Hubley, 1997). Still, the careful test user will note that naming ability, as assessed by the BNT, is not normally distributed, even among older adults, for whom test performance becomes more variable around the mean with increasing age (Tombaugh & Hubley, 1997). Norms for tests such as these are best considered for diagnostic rather than descriptive purposes.

Second, it should be apparent that population-based descriptive norms cannot, in themselves, be used to identify abnormal or impaired performances without inferring a discrepancy between the observed score and the estimated premorbid score. By definition, descriptive norms describe normally distributed test scores, and all potential test scores fall under the normal curve. Because decrements in normal cognitive ability are age-related, descriptive test norms are stratified by age to normalize the distribution of scores within a given age group. Thus descriptive norms assume that a person's position within the reference group is invariant across the age span. A Wechsler Adult Intelligence Scale–III (WAIS-III; Wechsler, 1997a) IQ of 75 is relatively rare, occurring in only 5% of the standardization sample for a given age group, and can be described as being in the "borderline" range. However, it is not necessarily "abnormal," unless the test user infers that this score deviates from a premorbid level as the result of an abnormal condition.

The final and most fundamentally important issue to consider when using descriptive norms is the composition of the normative sample itself. Because descriptive norms allow us to address questions about how our patient is performing *relative* to the normative sample, it is imperative to know what kind of individuals actually make up the reference group to which the patient is to be compared. For example, is our patient being compared to a U.S. Census-matched sample of elders (Randolph, 1998; Psychological Corporation, 1997) or those from a specific geographical area (Ivnik et al., 1996; Ivnik, Malec, Smith, et al., 1992; Ivnik et al., 1990; Ivnik, Malec, Tangalos, et al., 1992; Ivnik, Tangalos, et al., 1992; Lucas et al., 1998) or specific ethnic group (Friedman, Schinka, Mortimer, & Borenstein Graves, 2002; Heaton et al., 2004)? Is the reference group screened for neurological and psychiatric illnesses (Randolph, 1998; Psychological Corporation, 1997), or does it include elders regardless of their physical and mental health status (Crum, Anthony, Bassett, & Folstein, 1993) in an attempt to increase its representativeness? Our inferences about a patient's level of performance are context-specific and limit what we can say about the patient's abilities. The nature and composition of the reference group is especially important in the case of norms for elder populations and is addressed in detail later in this chapter.

Diagnostic Use of Norms

Unlike descriptive norms that employ traditional psychometric methods and principles of central tendency, diagnostic norms use *individual comparison standards* (Crawford, Johnson, Mychalkiw, & Moore, 1997) and follow more of the medical, pathognomonic sign approach (Davison, 1974), in which it is assumed that normal individuals will show little variability in the performance of a task and that deviations are due to abnormal conditions. For example, the presence of a visual field defect can be considered pathognomonic of an abnormality in the visual system, because such defects do not otherwise occur among individuals who are neurologically intact. Errorless or near errorless performance on a measure of cognitive ability is the *comparison standard* against which an individual is compared, with deviations from this expectation representing degrees of abnormality. Many of our widely used neuropsychological tests are patterned after the pathognomonic model and can be described as *deficit-oriented* rather than *population-based* tests. Many global measures of cognitive functioning commonly used in the evaluation of mental status with elders fall into this category (e.g., MMSE [Folstein et al., 1975]; DRS [Mattis, 1988]; Telephone Interview for Cognitive Status [Brandt & Folstein, 2003]; and the Repeatable Battery for the Assessment of Neuropsychological Status [RBANS; Randolph, 1998]).

The use of individual comparison standards (Crawford et al., 1997) is even fundamental to the common practice of pattern analysis in neuropsychological assessment (Hawkins & Tulsky, 2003; Lezak, Howieson, & Loring, 2004). When analyzing patterns of individual performance, the focus is not so much on the magnitude of either of the scores being compared but on the use of one test score to establish expectations regarding the other score. Since the seminal publication of the "Base rate data for the WAIS-R" (Matarazzo & Herman, 1984), there has also been a growing appreciation that it is not enough for the discrepancy between two scores to be statistically significant (reliable), but the base rate of the difference must also be sufficiently rare to signify an abnormality or impairment (Chelune, 2002b; Ivnik et al., 2001; Smith, 2002).

It should be clear that the use of diagnostic norms requires a different conceptual framework and a different set of statistical concepts. We are not so much interested in how much of an ability a patient has or where the patient falls within the reference group; rather we seek to know whether a performance is more likely to be characteristic of the reference group or one that is outside of it (i.e., abnormal; see Chelune, 2002b; Smith, 2002). The utility of diagnostic norms depends heavily on cutoff scores; test-operating characteristics such as sensitivity, specificity, and positive and negative predictive power; and statistics such odds ratios, likelihood ratios, and receiver-operating characteristics (Ivnik et al., 2001; Ivnik et al., 2000).

Because many neuropsychological evaluations are diagnostic in nature, there has been considerable interest in developing diagnostic norms for tests that are largely population-based and primarily designed for descriptive purposes. The approach generally takes one of two forms, both of which are based on a discrepancy model (Hawkins & Tulsky, 2003). In some cases a predicted difference method is used in which performance on one measure is used to predict the *expected* performance on a second measure, based on the correlation between these tests in a population-based normative sample. The significance of the *difference* between what is observed and what is expected is then interpreted in terms of the frequency of the discrepancy score in the normative sample. The larger and less frequent a discrepancy between the observed and expected score, the greater the likelihood that it is clinically meaningful. For example, predicted difference tables have been provided for the Wechsler Memory Scale–III (WMS-III) for identifying potentially meaningful memory deficits (Psychological Corporation, 1997). A patient's Full Scale IQ score (FSIQ) is used to predict an *expected* WMS-III performance, and the discrepancy between the *observed* and *expected* memory scores can then be compared to statistical tables to determine whether the discrepancy is statistically reliable and relatively rare in the standardization sample. This method often mirrors what practitioners do clinically; that is, they attempt to determine a patient's premorbid level of functioning and then look for test scores that appear to deviate from this expected level. This latter approach is highly subjective and prone to potential errors, but it can be enhanced by using objective test measures that are assumed to be relatively unaffected by brain dysfunction. For example, oral reading tests such as the Wechsler Test of Adult Reading (WTAR; Psychological Corporation, 2001) are often used to assist the clinician in estimating the patient's premorbid level of functioning.

The second and most widely used discrepancy approach for translating population-based norms into those with potential diagnostic value involves the use of demographic corrections to predict the *individual comparison standard* for the individual. Because it is well established that age is inversely correlated with performance on many neuropsychological measures, it is common to correct test performances for the effects of age so as to avoid misclassifying elders as impaired. However, there is overwhelming evidence that cognitive test performances in normal adults are also affected by other demographic factors such as education, sex, and ethnicity (Heaton, Taylor, & Manly, 2003). By adjusting population-based test norms for demographic factors that are known to affect test performance, we can increase the specificity or probability of the test to correctly classify a normal performance as "normal," while conversely increasing the sensitivity or probability of the test to correctly classify an abnormal performance as "abnormal" (Taylor & Heaton, 2001).

By adjusting norms for relevant demographic factors, we essentially create a *predicted* standard against which the individual's *observed* performance can be compared. Deviations from this individual comparison standard can be normally distributed and may be expressed by *T*-scores or scaled scores, but they should be interpreted in a unidirectional manner when used diagnostically. Extensive diagnostic norms based on demographically adjusted individual comparison standards covering the elder age range have been developed for both population-based tests (e.g., WAIS-III and WMS-III—Psychological Corporation, 2002; California Verbal Learning Test—Delis, Kramer, Kaplan, & Ober, 2000; Hopkins Verbal Learning Test—Vanderploeg et al., 2000; MicroCog—Powell, Kaplan, Whitla, Catlin, & Funkenstein, 1993) and deficit-oriented tests and test batteries (e.g., DRS—Lucas et al., 1998; Schmidt et al., 1994; Wisconsin Card Sorting Test [WCST]—Heaton, Chelune, Talley, Kay, & Curtiss, 1993; Mayo Older Americans Normative Studies [MOANS]—Ivnik et al., 1996; Ivnik, Malec, Smith, et al., 1992; Ivnik et al., 1990; Ivnik, Malec, Tangalos, et al., 1992; Ivnik et al., 1997; Ivnik et al., 1991; Ivnik, Tangalos, Petersen, et al., 1992; Lucas et al., 1998; Malec et al., 1992; Schmidt et al., 1994; Expanded Halstead–Reitan Battery—Heaton et al., 2004).

APPROACHES TO NORMS DEVELOPMENT

A number of different procedures has been employed to develop normative data for use with older populations. The most common approach to norms development is the *strati-*

fied normative procedure. Although tabled norms can be stratified by using any number of descriptive variables of import, the most common form of stratification is on the basis of age: The sample is simply divided into non-overlapping consecutive age bands, with norms reported for each of the specified age ranges (e.g., 50–59, 60–69; Tombaugh & Hubley, 1997). Variations of this method have attempted to increase the "representativeness" of norms by selecting samples of individuals that closely match the demographic characteristics of the overall population to which they intend to generalize. For example, the norms for the WAIS-III and the WMS-III (Wechsler, 1997b) were created using an age-stratified sampling method in which adults in the sample were selected to match the U.S. Census data on a number of identified demographic variables (i.e., age, sex, race/ethnicity, education level, and geographic location). Still other studies using a simple age-stratification method have recognized the importance of comparing a patient with specific demographic characteristics that are underrepresented in the general population to a specialized population-based normative sample concordant on those demographic features. For example, specific age-stratified normative data for the tests in the Consortium to Establish a Registry for Alzheimer's Disease (CERAD; Morris et al., 1989) have been collected for African Americans (Unverzagt et al., 1996), Indians (Ganguli et al., 1996), and Koreans (Lee et al., 2004).

One of the major limitations of the age-stratification method is that it is often very difficult to find equal numbers of participants within each age band, unless the study is conducted in a prospective manner. Hence, the mean for each age block (e.g., 50–59, 60–69) is unlikely to be truly reflective of the midpoint of that age band. As a result, the distribution of scores around these age means is not as equidistant as the age bands imply. Therefore, it is quite possible that the patient one is attempting to evaluate is actually closer in age to the mean of the adjacent category than to the mean of the age band within which his or her age actually falls. It is also often the case with this procedure that the data may not be normally distributed within each non-overlapping age category, which could result in improper interpretations of a patient's performance. In addition, if adjustments must be made to account for significant modifying variables, such as age, education, or sex, the stratification method will require a diverse normative sample as well as a large number of tables to cover all possible modifier subgroupings (Pauker, 1988).

In order to address some of the limitations inherent in the simple stratification method, two alternate methods have been suggested: *overlapping cell tables* (Pauker, 1988) and *continuous norming* (Gorsuch, 1983; Roid, 1983; Zachary & Gorsuch, 1985). The former method has been employed in normative studies published out of the MOANS (Ivnik et al., 1996; Ivnik, Malec, Smith, et al., 1992; Ivnik, Malec, Tangalos, et al., 1992; Ivnik et al., 1991; Ivnik, Tangalos, et al., 1992). In this method, first proposed by Pauker (1988), overlapping cell norm tables are created at specified age midpoints. Hence, cells that are adjacent to one another differ in midpoint means but overlap in range, allowing any one particular subject to appear in one or more of the adjacent cells. Although there are redundant cases within each age block, the group means are more stable, resulting in less abrupt mean shifts between age blocks. This technique maximizes the amount of useful information that can be gleaned from a sample and is particularly appropriate when sample sizes are relatively small (Pauker, 1988).

Continuous norming, the other alternative to simple stratification, involves a procedure based on the use of polynomial regression-based models in which standard scores or percentile ranks are predicted rather than calculated (Angoff & Robertson, 1987; Zachary & Gorsuch, 1985). The norms for tests such as the WCST (Heaton et al., 1993), those in the Expanded Halstead–Reitan Battery (Heaton et al., 2004), and the demographically corrected WAIS-III and WMS-III (Psychological Corporation, 2002) are based on this procedure. Continuous norming first involves derivation of polynomial regression (linear lines or nonlinear curves) equations that best fit the progression of means and standard deviations across small age subgroups. Combined with estimates of the mean, standard deviation, skewness, and kurtosis of the distribution of the test variable, percentile scores and standard scores are then generated. Because the estimators are continuously based, there are no abrupt shifts between cells, as is often the case when simple stratification methods are used. As Zachary and Gorsuch (1985) point out, this procedure likely results in better estimates for each age level, because the descriptive statistics from the *entire* normative group are used to calculate the normalized distributions within each age band, whereas the stratification method only makes use of data in each individual cell in the stratification table. This procedure also helps to correct for irregularities that may exist within individual age bands, especially when the sample size is small within a given age band.

Regardless of the method employed, it is important to be mindful of how the normative sample was selected, how representative the normative data are with regard to a particular patient, and which approach was used to develop the normative data. Only then can a test user make an informed decision about the usefulness and applicability of a particular set of norms for the individual patient being evaluated.

CHALLENGES IN NORMS DEVELOPMENT

Availability of high-quality norms is essential to high-quality clinical practice and research. Although most clinicians and researchers are likely to endorse this statement, few are likely to be aware of the scope of challenges faced by test developers. Table 6.1 summarizes many of these challenges, which include problems with obtaining funding, the conceptual conundrums of defining normative populations, and the difficulty of recruiting participants.

Funding and the Origin of Normative Samples

As pointed out by Mitrushina et al. (1999), norms development has traditionally not been viewed as particularly "scientific" due to the inherently descriptive nature of the work; therefore, it has not been deemed worthy of research funding or academic support (p. 5). Consequently, funding and resources available for norms development vary widely. Psychological tests such as the WAIS-III and WMS-III, which have a broad-based market or promise of considerable commercial value, are acquired and/or developed by publishing companies that have considerable resources available for norms development. In contrast, most neuropsychological measures do not appeal to a large enough audience to afford funding of large-scale, prospective norms development. Many normative studies in neuropsychology rely on relatively small samples or on samples that do not match national Census data. For example, five out of eight published normative studies of phonemic fluency that employed age stratification or circumscribed age groups had fewer than 45 participants in at least some of their age groups (Axelrod & Henry, 1992; Boone, Miller, Lesser, Hill, & D'Elia, 1990; Kozora & Cullum, 1995; Norris, Blankenship-Reuter, Snow-Turek, & Finch, 1995; Yeudall, Fromm, Reddon, & Stefanyk, 1986), and the remaining three normative studies had between 90 and 100 participants per group (Gladsjo et al., 1999; Ruff, Light, & Parker, 1996; Selnes et al., 1991). In contrast, the

TABLE 6.1. Challenges to Norms Development

Challenges	Issues to consider	Effect on norms
Funding of normative studies and origin of normative samples	• Normative studies not viewed as scientific enough to secure research funding • Neuropsychological instruments not having broad enough market base to secure funding from publishing companies • Instruments in public domain not attracting publishing companies	• Norms as byproduct of research projects • Small samples • Local samples • Constricted samples (control groups for studies)
Defining the normative standard	• For a single normative study, participants of different ages are sampled from different segments of population	• Intranorm incompatibilities
	• Different instruments have different purposes and different normative standards	• Intertest incompatibilities
	• Screening for cognitive impairment is often defined by absence of dementia (e.g., MMSE > 24)	• Mild cognitive impairment (MCI) individuals included in normative samples
Subject recruitment	• Methods of recruitment vary	• Unknown effects on sample composition
	• Difficulties recruiting elderly participants	• Smaller cells at higher age brackets

WAIS-III norms are comprised of a national sample of 2,450 adults, with 200 participants in each of 11 age bands from 16–79 years, 150 participants in the 80- to 84-year-old band, and 100 in the 85- to 89-year-old age band (Wechsler, 1997a).

To complicate matters further, many neuropsychological tests first appear in the research literature and are in the public domain. Because such measures do not initially attract funding from publishing companies, norms for these tests are often the by-product of research projects that are conducted for purposes other than norms development. As a result, such norms are generally comprised of samples that come from local, rather than national, populations. The Trail Making Test (TMT; Reitan & Wolfson, 1985) is a classic example of these measures. In fact, all but two (Heaton, Grant, & Matthews, 1991; Heaton, Ryan, Grant, & Matthews, 1996) of 16 TMT normative studies listed in the *Handbook of Normative Data for Neuropsychological Assessment* (Mitrushina et al., 1999) collected data from a single location.

In some cases normative samples for tests originally in the public domain later become commercially available. For example, normative samples from different research studies with the WCST (Heaton et al., 1993) and the Expanded Halstead–Reitan Battery (Heaton et al., 2004) have been compiled by investigators and secondarily have been made commercially available by publishing companies. Because the elders included in these norms were recruited as controls to match specific parameters of patient groups in these research projects, they represent a narrow segment of the general population of elders. Although economical, this approach has several potentially serious limitations. For example, some of the original research studies may have excluded individuals who were above or below a certain educational level, or only examined those who came from a particular geographical region or particular socioeconomic group. As a result, the variability of performance among these normative control groups is apt to be somewhat restricted, compared to the population as a whole. Although this is not a problem if one is interested only in a comparison of the experimental (or quasi-experimental) group and the control group, it may lead to serious misinterpretations of results, should one use such a control group as a reference for clinical decision making. Test users should therefore be cautious when comparing an elder patient to these norms, and remember that norms are context specific.

Defining the Normative Standard

The term *norm* implies something that is common, standard, and *normal*. This statement begs the question, "Normal or standard for what?" There are potentially as many *normal* populations as there are assessment questions. For example, the Graduate Record Examination (GRE; Educational Testing Service, 2004) is designed to aid in the selection of future graduate students, and as such its norms were developed on a narrowly defined group of graduate school applicants. On the other hand, the WAIS-III (Wechsler, 1997a) is designed for placing individuals' intellectual performance on the continuum that theoretically encompasses the entire U.S. population. As such, this instrument was normed on a much broader and inclusive sample.

As can be seen from these illustrations, the intended assessment purposes and client/patient characteristics provide the conceptual framework for the composition of comparison populations. This framework must then be operationalized by clearly stated and well-defined inclusion and exclusion criteria. Inclusion criteria are typically generous and include points such as being of the appropriate age and able to comprehend instructions. Greater emphasis is generally placed on exclusion criteria in normative studies of older adults, and these typically include points such as evidence of recent cognitive decline, history of central nervous system illnesses or injury, history of medical illnesses or disorders that are reported to have compromised cognition, and presence of psychiatric disorders, substance abuse, psychoactive medications, and sensory or motor difficulties (Malec, Ivnik, & Smith, 1993; Randolph, Tierney, Mohr, & Chase, 1998; Psychological Corporation, 1997). However, one population-based normative study of the MMSE, involving the National Institute of Mental Health (NIMH) Epidemiologic Catchment Area Program, included individuals regardless of their physical or mental health status (Crum et al., 1993).

It is important to recognize that any given set of exclusion criteria may or may *not* be successful at capturing the intended population of interest. Yet, once in place, exclusion criteria define not only the composition of a given normative sample but also the specific decisions that can be made about patients. Thus, defining the exclusion criteria may well represent the single most important decision a test developer makes.

Issues that need to be considered when selecting specific exclusion criteria for normative studies with older adults include (1) intranorm incompatibilities, (2) intertest incompatibilities, and (3) inadvertent inclusion of individuals with incipient dementia or mild cognitive impairment.

Intranorm Incompatibilities

Intranorm incompatibilities arise when a single set of norms spans a wide range of cohorts ranging from young adults through older adults. When this happens, differential exclusion rates within the normative sample may result simply due to the fact that older adults often have a higher prevalence of many of the typical exclusion criteria. In particular, the elderly tend to experience declines in cognitive functioning, health status, sensory acuity, motor control, and functional independence much more frequently than their younger counterparts (Albert & Moss, 1988; Koltai & Chelune, 1996; Koltai & Welsh-Bohmer, 2000; Nussbaum, 1995). Consider, for example, the WAIS-III and WMS-III exclusion criterion of "seeing a doctor or other professional for memory problems" (Psychological Corporation, 1997). Although the exact prevalence of voiced memory complaints in a doctor's office is not known, as many as 25% of those ages 65 and over do complain of memory difficulties in other settings (Tobiansky, Blizard, Livingston, & Mann, 1995). Thus, by combining exclusion criteria that have high prevalence among the elderly, normative samples may end up recruiting individuals from only the highest ranks of successfully aging older adults, especially when sampling those of the category of oldest old.

Although selection of only the healthiest individuals for a normative comparison is not a problem in itself, it becomes problematic when an application of the same exclusion criteria results in the selection of much more *normal* or average individuals from the younger groups. Thus, when norms are developed for a given test on truly *normal* 40-year-olds but only *superior* 80-year-olds, the net result is that any average 40-year-old is bound to exhibit a spurious *normative* decline by the age of 80.

Intertest Incompatibilities

Intertest incompatibilities arise when multiple tests designed for different purposes are used in the same evaluation. Tests that are designed specifically for the elderly do not face as large a problem with differential exclusion rates among cohorts as do those designed for populations throughout the lifespan. However, because tests for older adults tend to be designed for fairly specific purposes (e.g., screening for dementia, screening for mild cognitive impairment, competency assessment, prediction of functional independence), they often rely on somewhat disparate normative samples, causing comparisons between standard scores from different tests to be problematic.

As an example, consider the potential intertest incompatibility between the CERAD (Morris et al., 1989) battery and the Behavioral Dyscontrol Scale (BDS; Grigsby & Kaye, 1992). The CERAD battery was developed specifically for the purpose of identifying Alzheimer's disease in individuals age 50 and over. As such, its norms were developed on a group of healthy community-dwelling individuals who were deemed to be cognitively intact, based on obtaining a score above 24 on either the MMSE (Folstein et al., 1975) or the Short Blessed Test (Katzman et al., 1983). In contrast, the BDS was developed for the purpose of predicting functional independence among elderly patients who may have suffered a stroke or who may even be in the early stages of dementia. As such, norms for this instrument were developed on a heterogeneous sample that included both inpatients and outpatients; only individuals with severe sensory deficits or a history of psychosis were excluded.

The reader should note that intertest incompatibilities between normative standards can arise in any comprehensive evaluation, regardless of the age of the patient, and they have important implications for interpretation. The problem may be particularly acute in the evaluation of an elder, because each set of norms may define impairment quite differently. Consider, for example, a 55-year-old patient with early-onset dementia who may be exhibiting mild cognitive deficit on the CERAD battery. If this patient's deficit is not substantial enough to be reflected in the more permissive BDS norms, one might appropriately conclude that the patient may still be safe to live independently. However, although the results from each of the two tests have their own interpretive value, the two sets of data cannot be compared side by side. In particular, it would be a mistake for a clinician to suggest that the above-described patient has experienced a greater decline on the domains assessed by the CERAD battery than on those assessed by the BDS.

Mild Cognitive Impairment

Mild cognitive impairment (MCI) has received considerable attention in recent years (see Smith & Rush, Chapter 2, this volume) as there has been a growing interest in the early detection and prevention of cognitive decline (Brandt, 2001; Petersen et al., 1999). These efforts foreshadow the need for the development of norms that are based on only the most cognitively intact older adults. However, the definition of *cognitively intact* appears to be a moving target. Whereas a number of older normative studies excluded individuals with MMSE scores below 24 (Bolla-Wilson & Bleecker, 1986; Kozora & Cullum, 1995; Mitrushina, Satz, Chervinsky, & D'Elia, 1991; Morris et al., 1989), 23 (Ardila & Rosselli, 1989), or even 20 (Norris et al., 1995), none of these standards may be adequate for future normative efforts. In particular, MCI patients, by definition, have MMSE scores above 23 (Petersen et al., 1999), and thus much higher standards need to be employed if such individuals are to be excluded from normative samples. Of course, this also means that individuals with MCI have traditionally been included in many older sets of norms.

Because the main interest in MCI is the identification of individuals with incipient dementia (Petersen et al., 1999), one possible way of dealing with this issue is to exclude anyone with either known physical (e.g., hypertension, diabetes, heart disease) or familial (i.e., family histories of dementia) risk factors for various dementing processes. However, such norms might exclude normal individuals who are characterized by levels of functioning that are normally low rather than abnormally declining.

As a clever way of excluding individuals with incipient dementia from a normative sample, Marcopulos, McLain, and Giuliano (1997) conducted a follow-up with a group of elders who had participated in a normative study 4 years earlier. By reexamining the normative data after removing those participants who had converted to dementia in the course of the 4 years, these researchers were able to determine to what degree early dementia participants skewed the norms. Interestingly, the results showed that these individuals did not appreciably affect the norms. Although studies such as this one lend credence to our current normative procedures, more work is needed.

Subject Recruitment

Various strategies have been used to attract and recruit participants, including random telephone calls, advertising in the media, and approaching various community organizations (e.g., the WAIS-III/WMS-III; Psychological Corporation, 1997), as well as approaching relatives of patients (e.g., the CERAD battery; Morris et al., 1989). Any of these methods may be associated with varying amounts of reimbursement for time and effort and varying degrees of initiative required on the part of the participant (e.g., requiring that participants travel to the place where testing takes place versus conducting testing near or in participants' homes).

Unfortunately, it is not fully known to what extent different methods of recruitment affect the final composition of the normative sample. However, one might speculate that relatives of patients may be particularly conscientious in their performance, if they believe that the research in which they are participating will ultimately help their loved ones, for example. On the other hand, participants who are primarily interested in a financial reward may not be motivated to do more than simply put it the time. And finally, participants who do not receive any financial reward for participation (e.g., the MOANS project; Malec et al., 1993) may represent the most prosocially motivated and intellectually curious from among their cohort.

In addition to potential confounds introduced by different recruitment methods, simply finding elderly participants who are both free of all exclusion characteristics and willing to participate represents a challenge. In fact, it is not uncommon for normative samples to shrink in size with increasing age bands. For example, the WAIS-III (Psychological Corporation, 1997) normative samples for the two highest age groups (80–84 and 85–89) were only 100 and 75, respectively, as compared to 200 per age group for younger participants. As an even more dramatic illustration, the MOANS normative sample for the TMT (Ivnik et al., 1996) drops from over 50 participants among the 56- to 79-year-olds to only five in the 90- to 95-year age group.

Such decreases in sample size have detrimental effects on the validity of any norms, but even more so when norms are developed for the elderly. In particular, as people grow older, the random cumulative effects of education, life experience, illness, medications, and neurological insults lead to a progressively greater normal variability in cognitive functioning among individuals, with successfully aging older adults on the one end of the normal distribution and those exhibiting MCI on the other. As a result, accurately capturing the range of performances among the elderly necessarily requires larger normative samples. It is unfortunate, then, that it is often the highest age ranges where normative sample sizes drop off considerably.

USING TEST NORMS WISELY

Even when norms are thoughtfully constructed based on clearly defined populations, clinicians still face challenges when applying normative data to specific patients. Some of these challenges include (1) selecting from among many different sets of norms available in the literature, (2) determining the construct validity of different measures at different ages, (3) dealing with decreases in test discriminability with an increase in age, and (4) understanding the complexities of interactions of various moderating factors.

Multiple Norms

Given the difficulties of funding norms development, selecting appropriate populations, and recruiting representative participants, it is sometimes the case that norms published in test manuals may not fully meet the needs of clinicians. To address this issue, supplementary norms have been developed and made available for many tests that are particularly popular among clinicians. Multiple sets of norms are especially common for measures that are in the public domain, such as the TMT (Reitan & Wolfson, 1985) or measures that have multiple versions such as the Stroop (Dodrill, 1978; Golden, 1978;

Spreen & Strauss, 1991; Trenerry, Crosson, DeBoe, & Leber, 1989). Thus, for example, 16 normative studies for the TMT have been published between 1968 and 1996, together spanning ages 15–91 and education from 5 to more than 16 years (Mitrushina et al., 1999). Similarly, 21 Stroop norms have been developed between 1962 and 1997, together spanning ages 15–94 and from 8 to more than 18 years (Mitrushina et al., 1999) of education.

Because different sets of norms are best suited for different patient populations, test users need to be thoughtful in selecting the norms that are both psychometrically sound and most comparable to the characteristics of a given patient. Additionally, different norms are organized in different formats. For example, whereas some studies use years of education as a stratification variable (Heaton et al., 1991), others stratify participants according to their FSIQ (Dodrill, 1978). This distinction may be important for patients for whom FSIQ is known and who have been deprived of educational opportunities or have educationally underachieved for other reasons. Finally, some normative studies may be characterized by fairly narrow sampling procedures but may nevertheless be of interest when assessing patients from special groups, such as gay and bisexual men (Miller et al., 1990) or elderly depressed patients (Boone et al., 1995).

Construct Validity

As previously mentioned, many tests are developed specifically for use with the elderly. Such tests tend to assess constructs that are relevant for, and have been validated with, elderly populations, such as functional independence or the presence of a particular type of dementia. However, at other times test developers attempt to take a test that was originally developed for younger adults and make it applicable to elders by simply extending upward the age range of the normative sample (Heaton et al., 1993; Psychological Corporation, 1997), assuming that the construct being measured remains the same. For pediatric neuropsychologists, this is akin to test developers assuming that norms for a test originally developed for adults can simply be extended downward for children. When this is attempted, even the best normative data will not address potential problems with the validity of the constructs measured.

It is well recognized that qualitative aspects of cognition, and thus the constructs we measure, change with age (Sattler, 2001). Evidence for such change can be gleaned from results of factor analytic research, wherein different factor structures may be identified with different age groups. For example, an examination of factor loadings reported in the *WAIS-III/WMS-III Technical Manual* (Psychological Corporation, 1997) reveals that the Picture Arrangement, Block Design, and Picture Completion subtests all load on the Perceptual Organization factor for individuals under the age of 75 but on the Processing Speed factor for individuals 75 and over. Direct statistical examination of longitudinal and cross-sectional invariance in the factor structure of many tests has repeatedly demonstrated that the factor structures of the youngest and the oldest groups tend to differ from each other (Schaie, Maitland, Willis, & Intrieri, 1998), whereas a reasonably stable factor structure is present in the middle age groups. Thus test users need to exercise care in how they interpret poor performances on a variety of indices among very old adults, because the construct for which the index is named may be somewhat different. Furthermore, careful consideration also needs to be given to a variety of possible intervening variables that may contribute to changes in constructs, such as peripheral motor and sensory problems or alteration in insight and motivation.

Discriminability and Floor Effects

Problems with limited discriminability due to floor effects tend to arise when norms for a test developed for younger populations are simply extended upward for application to the elderly. An example of this problem is the Logical Memory subtest of the WMS-III (Wechsler, 1997c). An 85-year-old who only recalls one story detail after a delay receives a scaled score of 5. However, another 85-year-old who, after a delay, does not recall having heard any stories, let alone recalling specific details, also receives a scaled score of 5. A naïve clinician may interpret both performances as being in the borderline range if he or she relies on scaled scores alone, although in reality the latter case more likely represents a significant impairment of memory. An even more dramatic example of floor effects can be seen with the Verbal Paired Associates subtest of the WMS-III (Wechsler, 1997c). Here, an 85-year-old can recall anywhere between zero and two words to receive a scaled score of 6, a score that falls in the low end of the low-average range.

To address this problem test users need to examine raw scores as well as carefully consider behavioral observations and pathognomonic signs; in addition, they should supplement their batteries with tasks that are more appropriate for elders. However, it should be noted that reasonably interpretable scores can be achieved on Logical Memory II of the WMS-III up to the age of 74, where recall of zero or one story detail results in scaled scores of 1 and 2, respectively.

Interaction of Age with Other Moderator Variables

Another complication in casually using norms when evaluating older adults arises from the fact that some exclusion criteria may interact with demographic factors. For example, consider how dementia screening may interact with ethnicity at different age ranges (see Manly, Chapter 8, this volume). At the younger age range, it is unlikely that many individuals would be found to be demented. With increasing age, some volunteers would be screened out due to suspected dementia. However, the gap between the educational opportunities of the ethnic minority and the ethnic majority also increases with age, simply as a function of changing historical and political milieu. In other words, ethnic differences in cognitive performance increase with age, resulting in an overexclusion of many ethnic minority volunteers due to suspected dementia (Baker, 1996).

A similar situation arises when the MMSE cutting score of 24 is applied across the board with the goal of screening out volunteers with cognitive difficulties. In particular, the work of Crum and colleagues (1993) has shown that the combined effects of age and education can account for as many as 11 points on this instrument. For example, individuals with fewer than 4 years of formal education perform at 24 or below at all but two age groups, and as such, would virtually always be screened out of normative studies. On the other hand, individuals with 5–8 years of education perform above 26 at all but the highest age bracket (i.e., > 84), possibly resulting in underrepresentation of this particular age group in the normative sample. Because such interaction effects are not always fully outlined in test manuals or studies reporting normative data for the elderly, test users need to use their own judgment when considering the particular demographic characteristics of their patients and how well or poorly these might be represented in a given normative sample.

As these challenges demonstrate, test users need to exercise careful judgment when selecting norms for their patients. Not only is it important to consider whether a given set of norms matches the characteristics of a patient, it is equally important to think carefully about the purpose of the assessment and the questions one is attempting to answer. For example, if the question concerns an 84-year-old patient's ability to live independently, then such a patient should best be compared to a sample of 84-year-old independent community-dwellers. On the other hand, if the question is whether or not the patient is suffering from dementia, the use of norms that are based on nondemented 84-year-olds, regardless of their functional status, may be more appropriate.

SERIAL ASSESSMENT WITH THE ELDERLY

Evaluation of an elder's cognitive status not only requires appropriate test procedures but normative data that are also appropriate. As we have seen, there are many factors to consider when applying normative information to older adults. There are additional issues to consider when cognitive tests are used serially.

Neuropsychological tests are typically designed only to assess the current capacity or state of the individual. Still, there are many situations in which neuropsychological procedures are administered serially to monitor changes in cognitive status or function over time. This is especially the case in relation to elders, for whom the accurate diagnosis of dementia is better characterized by a pattern of test–retest change than cognitive performance at any one point in time (Desmond, Moroney, Bagiella, Sano, & Stern, 1998; Sawrie, Marson, Boothe, & Harrell, 1999). Cognitive rehabilitation programs for the elderly and clinical trials research aimed at identifying meaningful cognitive change after an intervention or treatment also rely on serial assessments (Gonzalez-Torrecillas, Mendelwicz, & Lobo, 1995; Koltai & Chelune, 1996; Koltai & Welsh-Bohmer, 2000; Yesavage, 1985). Until recently, test users have simply attempted to deduce meaningful change by comparing a patient's current test scores against his or her baseline scores, often with only superficial attention to factors such as practice effects, measurement error, or regression to the mean (Chelune, 2002a, 2002b; Lineweaver & Chelune, 2003). Fortunately, pressures from the emerging evidence-based medicine movement (Sackett, Straus, Richardson, Rosenberg, & Haynes, 2000) have led to a growing body of empirical methods for assessing reliable change; these methods can be used in both research and clinical practice at the level of the individual (Chelune, 2002a; Maassen, 2000, 2004; Murkin, 2001; Timken, Heaton, Grant, & Dikmen, 1999).

Basic Considerations: Bias and Error

In the absence of a significant intervening event, a person's test performance should be the same at retest as it was at the time of original administration. However, tests do not have perfect stability and reliability, and we must deal with their statistical counterparts—bias and error. Bias represents a systematic change in performance; for a cognitive test given two or more times, the most common cause of change is a positive *practice effect*, in which performance is enhanced by previous exposure to the test materials. When large practice effects are the norm, the absence of change may actually reflect a decrement in performance (Chelune, 2002a). Simply lengthening the test–retest interval does not necessarily eliminate the effects of practice because significant retest gains have been noted among the elderly tested over even 1- to 2-year test–retest intervals (Ivnik et al., 1999; Sawrie et al., 1999). As is discussed later in this section, normal aging itself is a form of systematic bias that may interact with practice (Barrett, Chelune, Naugle, Tulsky, & Ledbetter, 2000; Chelune et al., 1999; Lineweaver & Chelune, 2003). Failure to take into account expected practice effects could lead to serious errors in interpretation. For example, the absence of an expected test–retest change in an elder suspected of early dementia could be seen as signifying stability and delay early intervention, when, in fact, the elder's cognitive function may have deteriorated from expected retest levels. Conversely, the presence of an increase in test performance following a cognitive intervention might be interpreted as a positive treatment outcome when, in fact, the change may be merely the result of practice.

In addition to the systematic bias introduced by practice effects, cognitive tests themselves are imperfect tools and can introduce an element of error across serial administrations. For our discussion here, we consider two sources of imprecision in measurement, both of which are inversely related to a test's reliability (Chelune, 2002a). The first is the *standard error measurement*—that is, the distribution of random variations in a test score around the true score. The second source of error is *regression to the mean*—that is, the susceptibility of retest scores to regress toward the population mean. The more a baseline score deviates from the population mean, the more it is likely to regress toward the mean on retest as a function of the test's reliability. Retest performances on measures with less than what is typically considered good test–retest reliability (e.g., $\geq .80$) can vary widely simply on the basis of error, possibly obscuring or exaggerating true change.

Solutions

Our ability to detect meaningful test–retest changes as the result of disease progression, recovery of function, intervention, or treatment requires us to separate the effects of bias and error on test performance from the effects of the variable of interest. Use of *alternate test forms* has been suggested as an effective means for avoiding or minimizing practice effects. Although well-constructed alternate forms may attenuate the effects of content-specific practice effects for some measures (Benedict & Zgaljardic, 1998; Delis et al., 2000), research still demonstrates significant practice gains (Franzen, Paul, & Iverson, 1996; Goldstein et al., 1990; Ruff et al., 1996) because alternate forms do not control for procedural or skill-based learning (i.e., test-taking strategies) and other factors (e.g., familiarity with the testing context and examiner, performance anxiety) that contribute to the overall practice effect. Furthermore, alternate forms do not address the issues of reliability and error. Thus alternate forms do not necessarily remedy the psychometric challenges inherent in serial assessments, prompting the development of methods of reliable change that better account for test–retest bias and error.

Reliable change methods are statistical procedures (Basso, Bornstein, & Lang, 1999; Chelune, Naugle, Luders, Sedlak, & Awad, 1993; Dikman, Heaton, Grant, & Timken, 1999; Hermann et al., 1996; Iverson, 2001; Jacobson & Truax, 1991; McSweeny, Naugle, Chelune, & Luders, 1993; Sawrie, Chelune, Naugle, & Luders, 1996) that attempt to describe the spread or distribution of test–retest change scores that would be expected to occur in the absence of true change. It is beyond the scope of this chapter to detail these methods here, but the interested reader can refer to Chelune (2002a) for a detailed discussion on how to calculate many of these reliable change measures. In their simplest form (Chelune et al., 1993; Iverson, 2001; Ivnik et al., 1999; Jacobson & Truax, 1991; Timken et al., 1999), reliable change indices focus on the observed or estimated mean and standard deviation of the *difference (change) scores* between time 1 and time 2 rather than the actual obtained test scores. These approaches are univariate and can take into account mean practice effects and measurement error, but not regression to the mean, and can define the magnitude of change necessary to be considered sufficiently rare so as to be meaningful (e.g., a change that would be expected to occur by chance in only 5% of a given test–retest population). In more complex models (Barrett et al., 2000; Chelune et al., 1999; Hermann et al., 1996; Lineweaver & Chelune, 2003; McSweeny et al., 1993; Sawrie et al., 1996; Sawrie et al., 1999), multivariate regression procedures are used to create standardized regression-based norms for change that build into the regression equation (1) the effects of practice, measurement error, and regression to the mean; (2) differences in baseline scores between subjects, and (3) demographic variables that can differentially affect the magnitude of test–retest change.

Although the use of reliable change methods is increasingly being used in outcome research (Hermann et al., 1996; Kneebone, Andrew, Baker, & Knight, 1998; Sawrie et al., 1996; Timken et al., 1999), only a few studies have been explicitly conducted among elders. Ivnik and colleagues (1999) present data and univariate reliable change index scores for the Mayo Cognitive Factor Scale scores on a sample of elders that was tested three or four times at 1- to 2-year intervals. These data clearly demonstrate statistically significant retest gains among the elders from time 1 to time 2, with performances beginning to plateau between times 2 and 3. Reliable change indices are also presented for defining the upper and lower cutoff scores for deciding whether a cognitive factor has shown a reliable change over the test–retest interval. Sawrie and associates (1999) developed standardized regression-based norms for a small group of normal elders tested twice over a 1-year interval on measures such as the DRS, subtests from the WAIS-R (Wechsler, 1981) and WMS-R (Wechsler, 1987), and common language measures such as the BNT. The multiple Rs for these equations were generally high (> .81), with sex and ethnicity entering, along with baseline scores, to predict expected retest scores.

Standardized regression-based norms have been also developed for the WAIS-III and WMS-III (Barrett et al., 2000; Chelune et al., 1999; Lineweaver & Chelune, 2003), albeit from standardization data covering the adult lifespan (ages 16–89) and with very short test–retest intervals (2–12 weeks; Psychological Corporation, 1997). Whereas baseline scores were the primary predictor of retest performance in all of the equations, age, education, and sex also entered into many of the equations, suggesting that test–retest changes in cognitive performance are moderated by demographic factors. It is important for test users to note that age was an important predictor of test–retest change in many of these equations, even though the Wechsler scores themselves are age-corrected at time 1 and time 2; that is, age appears to moderate the amount of score inflation that can be expected from repeated exposure to the Wechsler test materials. Examination of the beta weights for age in these equations indicates that the magnitude of score inflation decreases with increasing age. Thus application of simple reliable change methods that treat practice as a constant may be especially inappropriate in an aging population, where increasing age may offset expected gains due to repeated exposures to the test material (Chelune, 1998).

CONCLUSIONS

With the growing numbers of elders in the United States, neuropsychologists will undoubtedly be called upon increasingly to perform evaluations to answer diagnostic issues and questions concerning functional capacity. In the last decade there has been an influx of tests and normative data for use with even the oldest of the old. However, the accuracy and utility of our evaluations will depend on the capacity of test users to skillfully interpret their test results within the context of available normative information.

In this chapter we have not attempted to provide a survey of available tests for use with elders or to provide an encyclopedic critique of available normative samples. Rather, by presenting a discussion of the nature and purpose of norms, how norms are obtained and developed, the nuances of defining the normative standard, and issues inherent in serial assessment among the elderly, we have attempted to provide a conceptual guide for evaluating the nature and adequacy of available norms for use with elder populations. We may be limited to the tests and norms currently available, but we can nonetheless practice in a more informed manner by better understanding and recognizing the nature of our normative information.

REFERENCES

Albert, M. S., & Moss, M. B. (Eds.). (1988). *Geriatric neuropsychology*. New York: Guilford Press.

Angoff, W. H., & Robertson, G. J. (1987). A procedure for standardizing individually administered tests, normed by age or grade level. *Applied Psychological Measurement, 11*(1), 33–46.

Ardilla, A., & Rosselli, M. (1989). Neuropsychological characteristics of normal aging. *Developmental Neuropsychology, 5*(4), 307–320.

Axelrod, B. N., & Henry, R. R. (1992). Age-related performance on the Wisconsin Card Sorting, Similarities, and Controlled Oral Word Association Tests. *Clinical Neuropsychologist, 6*(1), 16–26.

Baker, F. M. (1996). Issues in assessing dementia in African American elders. In G. Yeo & D. Gallagher-Thompson (Eds.), *Ethnicity and the dementias* (pp. 59–76). Washington, DC: Taylor & Francis.

Barrett, J., Chelune, G., Naugle, R., Tulsky, D., & Ledbetter, M. (2000). Test–retest characteristics and measures of meaningful change for the Wechsler Adult Intelligence Scale–III. *Journal of the International Neuropsychological Society, 6*, 147–148.

Basso, M. R., Bornstein, R. A., & Lang, J. M. (1999). Practice effects on commonly used measures of executive function across twelve months. *Clinical Neuropsychologist, 13*(3), 283–292.

Benedict, R. H. B., & Zgaljardic, D. J. (1998). Practice effects during repeated administrations of memory tests with and without alternate forms. *Journal of Clinical and Experimental Neuropsychology, 20*, 339–352.

Bolla-Wilson, K., & Bleecker, M. L. (1986). Influence of verbal intelligence, sex, age, and education on the Rey Auditory Verbal Learning Test. *Developmental Neuropsychology, 2*(3), 203–211.

Boone, K. B., Lesser, I. M., Miller, B. L., Wohl, M., Berman, N., Lee A., et al. (1995). Cognitive functioning in older depressed outpatients: Relationship of presence and severity of depression to neuropsychological test scores. *Neuropsychology, 9*(3), 390–398.

Boone, K. B., Miller, B. L., Lesser, I. M., Hill, E., & D'Elia, L. (1990). Performance on frontal lobe tests in healthy, older individuals. *Developmental Neuropsychology, 6*(3), 215–223.

Brandt, J. (2001). Mild cognitive impairment in the elderly. *American Family Physician, 63*(4), 620–626.

Brandt, J., & Folstein, M. F. (2003). *Telephone Interview of Cognitive Status*. Odessa, FL: Psychological Assessment Resources.

Chelune, G. J. (1998, February). *Reliable neuropsychological change: An elaboration of methods for assessing meaningful change*. Paper presented at the International Neuropsychological Society, Honolulu, HI.

Chelune, G. J. (2002a). Assessing reliable neuropsychological change. In R. Franklin (Ed.), *Prediction *in forensic and neuropsychology: New approaches to psychometrically sound assessment* (pp. 123–148). Mahwah, NJ: Erlbaum.

Chelune, G. J. (2002b). Making neuropsychological outcomes research consumer friendly: A commentary on Keith et al. (2002). *Neuropsychology, 16*(3), 422–425.

Chelune, G. J., Naugle, R. I., Luders, H., Sedlak, J., & Awad, I. A. (1993). Individual change after epilepsy surgery: Practice effects and base-rate information. *Neuropsychology, 7*, 41–52.

Chelune, G. J., Sands, K., Barrett, J., Naugle, R. I., Ledbetter, M., & Tulsky, D. (1999). Test–retest characteristics and measures of meaningful change for the Wechsler Memory Scale–III. *Journal of the International Neuropsychological Society, 5*, 109.

Crawford, J. R., Johnson, D. A., Mychalkiw, B., & Moore, J. W. (1997). WAIS-R performance following closed-head injury: A comparison of the clinical utility of summary IQs, factor scores, and subtest scatter indices. *Clinical Neuropsychologist, 11*, 345–355.

Crum, R. M., Anthony, J. C., Bassett, S. S., & Folstein, M. F. (1993). Population-based norms for the Mini-Mental State Examination by age and educational level. *Journal of the American Medical Association, 269*, 2386–2391.

Cullum, C. M., Butters, N., Troster, A. I., & Salmon, D. P. (1990). Normal aging and forgetting rates on the Wechsler Memory Scale—Revised. *Archives of Clinical Neuropsychology, 5*(1), 23–30.

Davison, L. A. (1974). Introduction. In R. M. Reitan & L. A. Davison (Eds.), *Clinical neuropsychology: Current status and applications* (pp. 1–18). New York: Wiley.

Delis, D. C., Kramer, J. H., Kaplan, E. F., & Ober, B. A. (2000). *California Verbal Learning Test—Second Edition.* San Antonio, TX: Psychological Corporation.

Desmond, D. W., Moroney, J. T., Bagiella, E., Sano, M., & Stern, Y. (1998). Dementia as a predictor of adverse outcomes following stroke: An evaluation of diagnostic methods. *Stroke, 29*, 69–74.

Dikman, S. S., Heaton, R. K., Grant, I., & Timken, N. R. (1999). Test–retest reliability and practice effects of Expanded Halstead–Reitan Neuropsychological Test Battery. *Journal of the International Neuropsychological Society, 5*, 346–356.

Dodrill, C. B. (1978). A neuropsychological battery for epilepsy. *Epilepsia, 19*(6), 611–623.

Educational Testing Service. (2004). *Graduate Record Exam.* Princeton, NJ: Author.

Erkinjuntti, T., Laaksonen, R., Sulkava, R., Syrjalainen, R., & Palo, J. (1986). Neuropsychological differentiation between normal aging, Alzheimer's disease and vascular dementia. *Acta Neurologica Scandinavica, 74*(5), 393–403.

Folstein, M. F., Folstein, S. E., & McHugh, P. R. (1975). Mini-Mental State: A practical method for grading the cognitive state of patients for the clinician. *Journal of Psychiatric Research, 12*(3), 189–198.

Franzen, M. D., Paul, D., & Iverson, G. L. (1996). Reliability of alternate forms of the Trail Making Test. *Clinical Neuropsychologist, 10*, 125–129.

Friedman, M. A., Schinka, J. A., Mortimer, J. A., & Borenstein Graves, A. (2002). Hopkins Verbal Learning Test—Revised: Norms for elderly African Americans. *Clinical Neuropsychologist, 16*(3), 356–372.

Ganguli, M., Chandra, V., Gilby, J. E., Ratcliff, G., Sharma, S. D., Pandav, R., et al. (1996). Cognitive test performance in a community-based nondemented elderly sample in rural India: The Indo–U.S. Cross-National Dementia Epidemiology Study. *International Psychogeriatrics, 8*, 507–524.

Gladsjo, J. A., Schuman, C. C., Evans, J. D., Peavy, G. M., Miller, S. W., & Heaton, R. K. (1999). Norms for letter and category fluency: Demographic corrections for age, education, and ethnicity. *Assessment, 6*(2), 147–178.

Golden, C. J. (1978). *The Stroop Color and Words Test (Manual).* Chicago: Stoetling.

Goldstein, G., Materson, B. J., Cushman, W. C., Reda, D. J., Freis, E. D., Ramirez, E. A., et al. (1990). Treatment of hypertension in the elderly: II. Cognitive and behavioral function. *Hypertension, 15*, 361–369.

Gonzalez-Torrecillas, J. L., Mendelwicz, J., & Lobo, A. (1995). Effects of early treatment of poststroke depression on neuropsychological rehabilitation. *International Psychogeriatrics, 7*, 547–560.

Goodglass, H., & Kaplan, E. F. (1983). *The assessment of aphasia and related disorders* (2nd ed.). Philadelphia: Lea & Febiger.

Gorsuch, R. L. (1983, August). *Continuous norming: An alternative to tabled norms?* Paper presented at the 91st Annual Convention of the American Psychological Association, Anaheim, CA.

Grigsby, J., & Kaye, K. (1992). *The Behavioral Dyscontrol Scale: Manual.* Denver, CO: Authors.

Hawkins, K. A., & Tulsky, D. S. (2003). WAIS-III WMS-III discrepancy analysis: Six-factor model index discrepancy base rates, implications, and a preliminary consideration of utility. In D. S. Tulsky, D. H. Saklofske, G. J. Chelune, R. K. Heaton, R. J. Ivnik, R. Bornstein, et al. (Eds.), *Clinical interpretation of the WAIS-III and WMS-III* (pp. 211–272). New York: Academic Press.

Heaton, R. K., Chelune, G. J., Talley, J. L., Kay, G. G., & Curtiss, G. (1993). *Wisconsin Card Sorting Test Manual: Revised and expanded.* Odessa, FL: Psychological Assessment Resources.

Heaton, R. K., Grant, I., & Matthews, C. G. (1991). *Comprehensive norms for an expanded Halstead–Reitan Battery: Demographic corrections, research findings, and clinical applications.* Odessa, FL: Psychological Assessment Resources.

Heaton, R. K., Miller, S. M., Taylor, M. J., & Grant, I. (2004). *Revised comprehensive norms for an expanded Halstead–Reitan Battery: Demographically adjusted neuropsychological norms for African American and Caucasian adults.* Odessa, FL: Psychological Assessment Resources.

Heaton, R. K., Ryan, L., Grant, I., & Matthews, C. G. (1996). Demographic influences on neuropsychological test performance. In I. Grant & K. Adams (Eds.), *Neuropsychological assessment of neuropsychiatric disorders* (2nd ed., pp. 141–163).

Heaton, R. K., Taylor, M. J., & Manly, J. (2003). Demographic effects and use of demographically corrected norms with the WAIS-III and WMS-III. In D. S. Tulsky, D. H. Saklofske, G. J. Chelune, R. K. Heaton, R. J. Ivnik, R. Bornstein, et al. (Eds.), *Clinical interpretation of the WAIS-III and WMS-III.* New York: Academic Press.

Hermann, B. P., Seidenberg, M., Schoenfeld, J., Peterson, J., Leveroni, C., & Wyler, A. R. (1996). Empirical techniques for determining the reliability, magnitude, and pattern of neuropsychological change following epilepsy surgery. *Epilepsia, 37,* 942–950.

Howieson, D. B., Holm, L. A., Kaye, J. A., Oken, B. S., & Howieson, J. (1993). Neurologic function in the optimally healthy oldest old: Neuropsychological evaluation. *Neurology, 43*(10), 1882–1886.

Iverson, G. L. (2001). Interpreting change on the WAIS III/WMS III in clinical samples. *Archives of Clinical Neuropsychology, 16,* 183–191.

Ivnik, R. J., Malec, J. F., Smith, G. E., Tangalos, E. G., & Petersen, R. C. (1996). Neuropsychological Tests' Norms above Age 55: COWAT, BNT, MAE Token, WRAT-R Reading, AMNART, STROOP, TMT, and JLO. *Clinical Neuropsychologist, 10*(3), 262–278.

Ivnik, R. J., Malec, J. F., Smith, G. E., Tangalos, E. G., Petersen, R. C., Kokmen, E., et al. (1992). Mayo's Older Americans Normative Studies: Updated AVLT norms for ages 56 to 97. *Clinical Neuropsychologist, 6*(Suppl.), 83–104.

Ivnik, R. J., Malec, J. F., Tangalos, E. G., Petersen, R. C., Kokmen, E., & Kurland, L. T. (1990). The Auditory Verbal Learning Test (AVLT): Norms for ages 55 years and older. *Psychological Assessment, 2,* 304–312.

Ivnik, R. J., Malec, J. F., Tangalos, E. G., Petersen, R. C., Kokmen, E., & Kurland, L. T. (1992). Mayo's Older Americans Normative Studies: WMS-R norms for ages 56 to 94. *Clinical Neuropsychologist, 6*(Suppl.), 49–82.

Ivnik, R. J., Smith, G. E., Cerhan, J. H., Boeve, B. F., Tangalos, E. G., & Petersen, R. C. (2001). Understanding the diagnostic capabilities of cognitive tests. *Clinical Neuropsychologist, 15,* 114–124.

Ivnik, R. J., Smith, G. E., Lucas, J. A., Petersen, R. C., Boeve, B. F., Kokmen, E., et al. (1999). Testing normal older people three or four times at 1- to 2-year intervals: Defining normal variance. *Neuropsychology, 13*(1), 121–127.

Ivnik, R. J., Smith, G. E., Lucas, J. A., Tangalos, E. G., Petersen, R. C., & Kokmen, E. (1997). Free and cued selective reminding test: MOANS Norms. *Journal of Clinical and Experimental Neuropsychology, 19,* 676–691.

Ivnik, R. J., Smith, G. E., Peterson, R. C., Boeve, B. F., Kokmen, E., & Tangalos, E. G. (2000). Diagnostic accuracy of four approaches to interpreting neuropsychological test data. *Neuropsychology, 14*(2), 163–177.

Ivnik, R. J., Smith, G. E., Tangalos, E. G., Petersen, R. C., Kokmen, E., & Kurland, L. T. (1991). Wechsler Memory Scale (WMS): I.Q. dependent norms for persons age 65 to 97. *Psychological Assessment, 3,* 156–161.

Ivnik, R. J., Tangalos, E. G., Petersen, R. C., Kokmen, E., & Kurland, L. T. (1992). Mayo's Older Americans Normative Studies: WAIS-R norms for ages 56 to 97. *Clinical Neuropsychologist, 6*(Suppl.), 1–30.

Jacobson, N. S., & Truax, P. (1991). Clinical significance: A statistical approach to defining meaningful change in psychotherapy research. *Journal of Consulting and Clinical Psychology, 59,* 12–19.

Katzman, R., Brown, T., Fuld, P., Peck, A., Schechter, R., & Schimmel, H. (1983). Validation of a short orientation–memory–concentration test of cognitive impairment. *American Journal of Psychiatry, 140*(6), 734–739.

Kneebone, A. C., Andrew, M. J., Baker, R. A., & Knight, J. L. (1998). Neuropsychologic changes after coronary artery bypass grafting: Use of reliable change indices. *Annals of Thoracic Surgery, 65,* 1320–1325.

Koltai, D. C., & Branch, L. (1999). Cognitive and affective interventions to maximize abilities and adjustment in dementia. *Annals of Psychiatry: Basic and Clinical Neurosciences, 7,* 241–255.

Koltai, D. C., & Chelune, G. J. (1996). Geriatric neuropsychology. In D. Jahnigen & R. Schrier (Eds.), *Geriatric medicine* (pp. 41–62). Cambridge, MA: Blackwell.

Koltai, D. C., & Welsh-Bohmer, K. A. (2000). Geriatric neuropsychological assessment. In R. D. Vanderploeg (Ed.), *Clinician's guide to neuropsychological assessment* (2nd ed., pp. 383–415). Mahwah, NJ: Erlbaum.

Kozora, E., & Cullum, C. M. (1995). Generative naming in normal aging: Total output and qualitative changes using phonemic and semantic constraints. *Clinical Neuropsychologist, 9*(4), 313–320.

Lee, D. Y., Lee, K. U., Lee, J. H., Kim, K. W., Jhoo, J. H., Kim, S. Y., et al. (2004). A normative study of the CERAD neuropsychological assessment battery in the Korean elderly. *Journal of the International Neuropsychological Society, 10,* 72–81.

Lezak, M. D., Howieson, D. B., & Loring, D. W. (2004). *Neuropsychological assessment* (4th ed.). New York: Oxford University Press.

Lineweaver, T. T., & Chelune, G. J. (2003). Use of the WAIS-III and WMS-III in the context of serial assessments: Interpreting reliable and meaningful change. In D. S. Tulsky, D. H. Saklofske, G. J. Chelune, R. K. Heaton, R. J. Ivnik, R. Bornstein, et al. (Eds.), *Clinical interpretation of the WAIS-III and WMS-III* (pp. 303–337). New York: Academic Press.

Lucas, J. A., Ivnik, R. J., Smith, G. E., Bohac, D. L., Tangalos, E. G., Kokmen, E., et al. (1998). Normative data for the Mattis Dementia Rating Scale. *Journal of Clinical and Experimental Neuropsychology, 20*(4), 536–547.

Maassen, G. H. (2000). Principles of defining reliable change indices. *Journal of Clinical and Experimental Neuropsychology, 22,* 622–632.

Maassen, G. H. (2004). The standard error in the Jacobson and Truax Reliable Change Index: The classical approach to the assessment of change. *Journal of the International Neuropsychological Society, 10,* 888–893.

Malec, J. F., Ivnik, R. J., & Smith, G. E. (1993). Neuropsychology and normal aging: The clinician's perspective. In R. W. Parks, R. F. Zec, & R. S. Wilson (Eds.), *Neuropsychology of Alzheimer's disease and other dementias* (pp. 81–111). New York: Oxford University Press.

Malec, J. F., Ivnik, R. J., Smith, G. E., Tangalos, E. G., Petersen, R. C., Kokmen, E., et al. (1992). Mayo's Older Americans Normative Studies: Utility of corrections for age and education for the WAIS-R. *Clinical Neuropsychologist, 6*(Suppl.), 31–47.

Marcopulos, B. A., McLain, C. A., & Giuliano, A. J. (1997). Cognitive impairment or inadequate norms? A study of health, rural, older adults with limited education. *Clinical Neuropsychologist, 11,* 111–131.

Matarazzo, J. D., & Herman, D. O. (1984). Base rate data for the WAIS-R: Test–retest stability and VIQ–PIQ differences. *Journal of Clinical Neuropsychology*, 6, 351–366.

Mattis, S. (1988). *Dementia Rating Scale Professional Manual*. Odessa, FL: Psychological Assessment Resources.

McSweeny, A. J., Naugle, R. I., Chelune, G. J., & Luders, H. (1993). "*T*-scores for change": An illustration of a regression approach to depicting change in clinical neuropsychology. *Clinical Neuropsychologist*, 7, 300–312.

Miller, E. N., Selnes, O. A., McArthur, J. C., Satz, P., Becker, J. T., Cohen, B. A., et al. (1990). Neuropsychological performance in HIV-infected homosexual men: The Multicenter AIDS Cohort Study (MACS). *Neurology*, 40(2), 197–203.

Mitrushina, M., Boone, K. B., & D'Elia, L. F. (1999). *Handbook of normative data for neuropsychological assessment*. New York: Oxford University Press.

Mitrushina, M., Satz, P., Chervinsky, A., & D'Elia, L. (1991). Performance of four age groups of normal elderly on the Rey Auditory Verbal Learning Test. *Journal of Clinical Psychology*, 47(3), 351–357.

Morris, J. C., Heyman, A., Mohs, R. C., Hughes, M., van Belle, G., Fillenbaum, G., et al. (1989). The Consortium to Establish a Registry for Alzheimer's Disease (CERAD): Part I. Clinical and neuropsychological assessment of Alzheimer's disease. *Neurology*, 39(9), 1159–1165.

Murkin, J. M. (2001). Editorial: Perioperative neuropsychologic testing. *Journal of Cardiothoracic and Vascular Anesthesia*, 15, 1–3.

Norris, M. P., Blankenship-Reuter, L., Snow-Turek, A. L., & Finch, J. (1995). Influence of depression on verbal fluency performance. *Aging and Cognition*, 2(3), 206–215.

Nussbaum, P. D. (1995). Aging: Issues in health and neuropsychological functioning. In A. J. Goreczny (Ed.), *Handbook of health and rehabilitation psychology* (pp. 583–604). New York: Plenum Press.

Nussbaum, P. D. (1998). Neuropsychological assessment of the elderly. In G. Goldstein, P. D. Nussbaum, & S. R. Beers (Eds.), *Neuropsychology* (pp. 83–105). New York: Plenum Press.

Pauker, J. D. (1988). Constructing overlapping cell tables to maximize the clinical usefulness of normative test data: Rationale and an example from neuropsychology. *Journal of Clinical Psychology*, 44, 930–933.

Petersen, R. C., Smith, G. E., Waring, S. C., Ivnik, R. J., Tangalos, E. G., & Kokmen, E. (1999). Mild cognitive impairment: Clinical characterization and outcome. *Archives of Neurology*, 56(3), 303–308.

Powell, D. H., Kaplan, E. F., Whitla, D., Catlin, R., & Funkenstein, H. H. (1993). *MicroCog: Assessment of Cognitive Functioning*. San Antonio, TX: Psychological Corporation.

Psychological Corporation. (1997). *Updated WAIS-III WMS-III Technical Manual*. San Antonio, TX: Author.

Psychological Corporation. (2001). *Wechsler Test of Adult Reading: Manual*. San Antonio, TX: Author.

Psychological Corporation. (2002). *WAIS-III—WMS-III—WIAT-II scoring assistant* (Rev. ed.). San Antonio, TX: Author.

Randolph, C. (1998). *RBANS: Manual for the Repeatable Battery for the Assessment of Neuropsychological Status*. San Antonio, TX: Psychological Corporation.

Randolph, C., Tierney, M. C., Mohr, E., & Chase, T. N. (1998). The Repeatable Battery for the Assessment of Neuropsychological Status (RBANS): Preliminary clinical validity. *Journal of Clinical and Experimental Neuropsychology*, 20(3), 310–319.

Reitan, R. M., & Wolfson, D. (1985). *The Halstead–Reitan Neuropsychological Test Battery: Theory and clinical interpretation*. Tucson, AZ: Neuropsychological Press.

Roid, G. H. (1983, August). *Generalization of continuous norming: Cross validation of test-score mean estimates*. Paper presented at the 91st Annual Convention of the American Psychological Association, Anaheim, CA.

Ruff, R. M., Light, R. H., & Parker, S. B. (1996). Benton Controlled Oral Word Association Test: Reliability and updated norms. *Archives of Clinical Neuropsychology*, 11, 329–338.

Sackett, D. L., Straus, S. E., Richardson, W. S., Rosenberg, W., & Haynes, R. B. (2000). *Evidence-based medicine: How to practice and teach EBM* (2nd ed.). New York: Churchill Livingston.

Sattler, J. M. (2001). *Assessment of children: Cognitive applications* (4th ed.). San Diego, CA: Sattler.

Sawrie, S. M., Chelune, G. J., Naugle, R. I., & Luders, H. O. (1996). Empirical methods for assessing meaningful neuropsychological change following epilepsy surgery. *Journal of the International Neuropsychological Society, 2,* 556–564.

Sawrie, S. M., Marson, D. C., Boothe, A. L., & Harrell, L. E. (1999). A method for assessing clinically relevant individual cognitive change in older populations. *Journal of Gerontology: Psychological Sciences, 54B,* 116–124.

Schaie, K. W., Maitland, S. B., Willis, S. L., & Intrieri, R. C. (1998). Longitudinal invariance of adult psychometric ability factor structures across 7 years. *Psychology and Aging, 13*(1), 8–20.

Schmidt, R., Freidl, W., Fazekas, F., Reinhart, B., Grieshofer, P., Koch, M., et al. (1994). The Mattis Dementia Rating Scale: Normative data from 1,001 healthy volunteers. *Neurology, 44*(5), 964–966.

Selnes, O. A., Jacobson, L., Machado, A. M., Becker, J. T., Wesch, J., Miller, E. N., et al. (1991). Normative data for a brief neuropsychological screening battery. Multicenter AIDS Cohort Study. *Perceptual and Motor Skills, 73*(2), 539–550.

Smith, G. E. (2002). What is the outcome we seek? A commentary on Keith et al. (2002) "Assessing postoperative cognitive change after cardiopulmonary bypass surgery." *Neuropsychology, 16*(3), 432–433.

Spreen, O., & Strauss, E. (1991). *A compendium of neuropsychological tests: Administration, norms and commentary.* New York: Oxford University Press.

Taylor, M. J., & Heaton, R. K. (2001). Sensitivity and specificity of the WAIS-III/WMS-III demographically corrected factor scores in neuropsychological assessment. *Journal of the International Neuropsychological Society, 7,* 867–874.

Timken, N. R., Heaton, R. K., Grant, I., & Dikmen, S. S. (1999). Detecting significant change in neuropsychological test performance: A comparison of four models. *Journal of the International Neuropsychological Society, 5,* 357–369.

Tobiansky, R., Blizard, R., Livingston, G., & Mann, A. (1995). The Gospel Oak Study stage IV: The clinical relevance of subjective memory impairment in older people. *Psychological Medicine, 25*(4), 779–786.

Tombaugh, T. N., & Hubley, A. M. (1997). The 60-item Boston Naming Test: Norms for cognitively intact adults aged 25 to 88 years. *Journal of Clinical and Experimental Neuropsychology, 19*(6), 922–932.

Trenerry, M., Crosson, B., DeBoe, J., & Leber, W. (1989). *Stroop Neuropsychological Screening Test Manual.* Odessa, FL: Psychological Assessment Resources.

Tuokko, H., & Hadjistavropoulos, T. (1998). *An assessment guide to geriatric neuropsychology.* Mahwah, NJ: Erlbaum.

Unverzagt, F. W., Hall, K. S., Torke, A. M., Rediger, J. D., Mercado, N., Gureje, O., et al. (1996). Effects of age, education and gender on CERAD neuropsychological test performance in an African American sample. *Clinical Neuropsychologist, 10*(2), 180–190.

Van Gorp, W. G., Satz, P., & Mitrushina, M. (1990). Neuropsychological processes associated with normal aging. *Developmental Neuropsychology, 6*(4), 279–290.

Vanderploeg, R. D., Schinka, J. A., Jones, T., Small, B. J., Graves, A. B., & Mortimer, J. A. (2000). Elderly norms for the Hopkins Verbal Learning Test—Revised. *Clinical Neuropsychologist, 14*(3), 318–324.

Wechsler, D. (1981). *Wechsler Adult Intelligence Scale—Revised.* San Antonio, TX: Psychological Corporation.

Wechsler, D. (1987). *Wechsler Memory Scale—Revised.* San Antonio, TX: Psychological Corporation.

Wechsler, D. (1997a). *WAIS-III administration and scoring manual.* San Antonio, TX: Psychological Corporation.

Wechsler, D. (1997b). *WAIS-III WMS-III technical manual*. San Antonio, TX: Psychological Corporation.

Wechsler, D. (1997c). *WMS-III test administration and scoring manual*. San Antonio, TX: Psychological Corporation.

Yesavage, J. A. (1985). Nonpharmocologic treatments for memory losses with normal aging. *American Journal of Psychiatry, 142,* 600–605.

Yeudall, L. T., Fromm, D., Reddon, J. R., & Stefanyk, W. O. (1986). Normative data stratified by age and sex for 12 neuropsychological tests. *Journal of Clinical Psychology, 42*(6), 918–946.

Zachary, R. A., & Gorsuch, R. L. (1985). Continuous norming: Implications for the WAIS—R. *Journal of Clinical Psychology, 41*(1), 86–94.

7

Functional Assessment

DANIEL MARSON
KATINA R. HEBERT

The population of the United States is aging rapidly, with the old-old representing the fastest growing segment of the population and those at greatest risk for poor health and functional impairment (Angel & Frisco, 2001; Fitten, 1999; Fowles, 1991; Lichtenberg & Nanna, 1994). One of the most salient and growing concerns in the field of gerontology is the steep rise in prevalence rates of functional incapacity among older adults, particularly those over the age of 85 (Wiener, Hanley, Clark, & Van Nostrand, 1990). Functional capacity represents a wide range of everyday skills and abilities that are necessary for independent living within the home and community. These skills include basic, routine physical self-care activities as well as more cognitively complex behaviors such as financial management skills, use of transportation, and medication management.

Although cognition informs both the development and exercise of simple and, in particular, higher-order functional abilities, it also remains conceptually and analytically distinct from them. Functional incapacity in the elderly may occur with or without corresponding declines in cognition. Impaired sensory processes, acute or chronic medical illness, or any other physical limitation or injury affecting strength, balance, mobility, concentration, and endurance may adversely impact functional performance (Loewenstein & Mogosky, 1999). However, for both physically and cognitively impaired older adults, functional outcomes are critical to assessment of overall disability and to appropriate residential placement decisions (Royall, Chiodo, & Polk, 2000). Therefore, it is important that functional performance be defined, measured, and interpreted separately from cognitive performance.

At the same time, a large proportion of functional decline in the elderly is intimately linked to cognitive change. A major risk factor for functional decline in older adults is a progressive neurodegenerative dementia such as Alzheimer's disease (AD), whose incidence increases dramatically with age (Angel & Frisco, 2001; Demers, Oremus, Perrault, Champoux, & Wolfson, 2000; Marson & Briggs, 2001). Functional change is a key diagnostic requirement for dementia diagnosis as well as for determining conversion from mild cognitive impairment (MCI) to dementia (Griffith et al., 2003). In order to assign a diagnosis of AD, the *Diagnostic and Statistical Manual of Mental Disorders*—Fourth Edition (DSM-IV) of the American Psychiatric Association (1994) requires that an individual demonstrate a gradual decline in memory and cognition *and also* significant impairments in social and occupational functioning. Likewise, the National Institute of Neurological and Communicative Disorders and Stroke–Alzheimer's Disease Related Disorders Association (NINCDS–ADRDA) criteria for AD-type dementia require evidence of impaired functional abilities in addition to declines in memory and cognition (McKhann et al., 1984).

In the case of patients with MCI, current clinical diagnostic criteria suggest that functional capacity is essentially preserved at the outset of the condition (Petersen et al., 1999). One must consider, however, whether the absence of functional decline as an MCI criterion reflects a true preservation of functional abilities in the face of clinically significant memory loss or a lack of objective measures or expertise to detect subtle prodromal changes in functional performance. Moreover, it is increasingly clear that MCI is a dynamic transitional period during which cumulative cognitive and functional change occurs. Whereas an individual at "entry" into MCI may have only focal memory impairment and little or no impairment in instrumental activities of daily living, the same individual at MCI "departure" (conversion to early AD) will have cognitive impairments well beyond memory and also notable declines in IADLs (Griffith et al., 2003). Not surprisingly, recent studies have found mild but salient functional deficits in financial capacity and other higher-order IADLs among persons with MCI (Albert et al., 1999; Daly et al., 2000; Griffith et al., 2003; Petersen et al., 1999; Tabert et al., 2002; Touchon & Ritchie, 1999). Thus any diagnostic assessment of individuals with suspected dementia or MCI needs to incorporate a meaningful assessment of functional capacity (Loewenstein & Mogosky, 1999). Such assessments also have practical value in determining appropriate living arrangements and planning both acute and long-term health care as well as estimating life expectancy (Angel & Frisco, 2001; Loewenstein & Mogosky, 1999).

Despite its clear importance, the evaluation of functional status has been a largely neglected aspect of geriatric neuropsychological assessment and of neuropsychology generally. For reasons of history and training, neuropsychologists have tended to focus almost entirely on cognitive and personality changes in normal and abnormal aging, with far less attention paid to functional outcomes and to the interrelationships of cognitive and functional changes. In our personal experience, few neuropsychologists routinely include measures of everyday function to complement the multitude of other cognitive and personality tests employed as part of their test battery. The field's emphasis here is slowly beginning to change, as witnessed by the increasing number of functional assessment instruments available to neuropsychologists and the growing literature examining specific kinds of functional change across a range of neurocognitive disorders (Marson, 2002). In particular, over the past two decades functional assessment in the specific form of civil competency/capacity assessment has emerged as a distinct field of clinical and forensic practice and research and has engaged the attention of neuropsychologists as well as those in other professional disciplines (Grisso, 2003; Marson, 2002; Marson & Briggs, 2001; Marson & Ingram, 1996).

The time is thus appropriate for a closer examination of the role of functional assessment in geriatric neuropsychology. In this chapter we begin with a conceptual overview of functional assessment in the elderly and address the fundamental domains of activities of daily living (ADLs) and instrumental activities of daily living (IADLs). As part of this overview we discuss different approaches to assessment of these functional abilities (i.e., self- and informant report, direct psychometric assessment). We then examine literature related to cognition and everyday functioning in the elderly, organized into areas of cognitive aging, MCI, and dementia. The remainder of the chapter focuses on four specific functional capacities that geriatric neuropsychologists frequently encounter. These are medical decision-making capacity, financial capacity, testamentary capacity (i.e., capacity to make or change a will), and driving capacity. Here we review applicable conceptual models, instrument development, empirical group studies, and relevant neuropsychological predictor models. We then provide an overall summary of the chapter and indicate future directions for research. The goal of the chapter is to increase the practitioner's knowledge and appreciation of the value of functional assessment in clinical neuropsychological research and practice.

CONCEPTUAL OVERVIEW OF FUNCTIONAL ABILITIES IN DEMENTIA

Defining Functional Capacity

As our society ages and the incidence of degenerative dementias such as AD rises, clinical assessment of functional capacity has become increasingly important (Marson, Dymek, & Geyer, 2000). Functional capacity represents a range of everyday skills and abilities that enable a person to live independently within the home and community (Loewenstein & Mogosky, 1999). Functional abilities have traditionally been divided into two broad classes: ADLs and IADLs (Angel & Frisco, 2001; Lawton & Brody, 1969; Loewenstein & Mogosky, 1999). As discussed below, ADLs involve basic self-care skills such as dressing, grooming, personal hygiene, and toileting, whereas IADLs involve more cognitively complex activities such as managing finances, using transportation, doing laundry, making health care decisions, and managing one's medications (Wolinsky, Callahan, Fitzgerald, & Johnson, 1993).

ADLs and IADLs exist on a functional continuum and primarily reflect a method of categorization rather than independent constructs (Wolinsky & Tierney, 1998). At the same time, as discussed further below, IADLs are distinguishable from ADLs by their degree of cognitive complexity and their pattern of acquisition and loss (Loewenstein & Mogosky, 1999; Reisberg et al., 1984; Reisberg, Ferris, & Franssen, 1985; Spector, Katz, Murphy, & Fulton, 1978; Stern, Hesdorffer, Sano, & Mayeux, 1990). Acquisition of functional abilities mirrors stages of cognitive development, with basic ADLs being acquired before more complex IADLs (Katz & Akpom, 1976; Spector et al., 1978). Similarly, recovery of basic ADLs precedes recovery of more complex IADLs (Katz, Downs, Cash, & Gratz, 1970) in traumatic brain injury (Olver, Ponsford, & Curran, 1996; Sohlberg & Mateer, 1989), whereas complex IADLs demonstrate an earlier and faster rate of decline than ADLs in AD-type dementia (DeBettignies, Mahurin, & Pirozzolo, 1993; Reisberg et al., 1984; Reisberg et al., 1985; Stern et al., 1990; Willis, 1996). In the following section we describe ADLs and IADLs in more detail and discuss the neurocognitive basis associated with each of these functional domains.

Activities of Daily Living

ADLs comprise a limited set of basic, everyday physical self-care activities such as bathing, grooming, dressing, eating, getting from the bed to a chair, using the toilet, and walking across the room (Loewenstein & Mogosky, 1999; Wiener et al., 1990). These activities rely on procedural memory skills and basic motor programming (Patterson et al., 1992). As such, ADLs may be classified as automatic behaviors that require little conscious attention and can be performed simultaneously with other tasks (Jorm, 1986).

ADLs are acquired early in childhood and remain relatively intact until late life in normal aging (Grigsby, Kaye, Baxter, Shetterly, & Hamman, 1998; Marsiske & Willis, 1995). They are also somewhat resilient to dementia, with declines emerging only in the later stages of AD and related dementias (Cohen-Mansfield, Werner, & Reisberg, 1995; Galasko et al., 1997; Reisberg et al., 1984). Patients with mild AD may perform equivalently with age- and education-matched nondemented individuals on ADL measures (Patterson et al., 1992; Vitaliano, Breen, Albert, Russo, & Prinz, 1984; Willis et al., 1998). Frank impairment of ADLs, therefore, is thus very often a cardinal sign of probable dementia—as long as the source of the impairment is cognitive. Care must always be exercised in interpreting ADL impairment in older adults, because impairment associated with declines in *physical abilities* is not indicative of a dementia (Patterson et al., 1992). The clinician must determine if poor performance on an ADL measure reflects cognitive decline or a loss of physical ability unassociated with dementia (Patterson et al., 1992).

ADLs have proven to be an important index of disability in the elderly. Research has found that impaired ADL functioning is associated with greater caregiver burden, higher rates of institutionalization, and subsequent mortality (Goode, Haley, Roth, & Ford, 1998; Wolinsky et al., 1993). Furthermore, an increasing number of private long-term care insurance policies use ADL measures in determining qualification for benefits, and similar practices have been proposed for public insurance programs as well (Wiener et al., 1990).

Instrumental Activities of Daily Living

In addition to ADLs, individuals must acquire and use more complex skills in order to function independently within home and community settings (Loewenstein & Mogosky, 1999). These skills include managing finances, managing medications, making medical treatment decisions, and using transportation. Although IADLs and ADLs exist on the same functional continuum, IADLs are conceptually and statistically distinct from ADLs, and this distinction is directly related to the cognitive demands of these respective abilities (Loewenstein & Mogosky, 1999; Spector et al., 1978). Put differently, whereas ADLs consist of a limited set of basic, daily self-care activities that rely primarily on automatic processing and procedural memory, IADLs comprise tasks that require controlled processing and executive function as well as procedural memory (Patterson et al., 1992).

IADL skills are acquired in later stages of human development than ADLs (Spector et al., 1978) and can be linked to frontal-lobe development (Bell-McGinty, Podell, Franzen, Baird, & Williams, 2002; Cahn-Weiner, Malloy, Boyle, Marran, & Salloway, 2000; Chen, Sultzer, Hinkin, Mahler, & Cummings, 1998; Grigsby et al., 1998). In contrast to ADLs, impairments in complex IADLs are evident in the preclinical and early stages of AD (Griffith et al., 2003; Patterson et al., 1992). This pattern of functional impairment is consistent with the course of cognitive decline observed in AD, in which fluid intelligence, executive functions, and controlled processing begin to decline at an earlier and faster rate than crystallized intelligence and automatic processing (Willis, 1996).

Household Activities of Daily Living. IADLs may be further divided into the two subsets of "household" ADLs and "advanced" IADLs (Lawton, 1990). Household ADLs involve those skills that are specific to maintaining the home environment, such as shopping for food and other necessities, preparing meals, engaging in light and heavy housework, and doing laundry. Household ADLs differ from other IADLs in that performance ratings may more accurately reflect gender roles of specific age cohorts (Lawton, 1990; Rubenstein, Schairer, Wieland, & Kane, 1984; Teunisse, 1995). For example, older adults typically subscribed to traditional roles in which the husband rarely engaged in household ADLs, leaving these responsibilities to the wife. As such, measures of IADL performance that incorporate household ADLs employ different norms for men than women (Lawton & Brody, 1969; Rubenstein et al., 1984).

Advanced Independent Activities of Daily Living. Advanced IADLs differ from basic and household ADLs in that they engage higher-order cognitive abilities that require greater levels of neuropsychological organization in addition to the routine motor movements and scripts common to ADLs (Marson, 2001a; Wolinsky & Johnson, 1991). Driving or using public transportation, managing finances, managing medications, and making medical treatment decisions are examples. Recent research suggests that declines in advanced IADLs are evident in preclinical and early dementia of the AD type (Barberger-Gateau, Fabrigoule, Helmer, Rouch, & Dartigues, 1999; Griffith et al., 2003; Marson, 2001a; Marson, Sawrie, et al., 2000). Declines in advanced IADLs differentially predict the frequency of hospital contact, nursing home placement, and mortality (Wolinsky & Johnson, 1991). An assessment of an individual's ability to carry out advanced IADLs is an essential component of appropriate diagnostic judgments and opinions concerning an individual's ability to live independently.

Methods of Assessing ADL and IADL Functioning

As was previously mentioned, a diagnosis of dementia based upon both DSM-IV (American Psychiatric Association, 1994) and NINCDS–ADRDA (McKhann et al., 1984) criteria is contingent upon impairments in functional ability in addition to changes in memory and cognition. As such, reliable and valid measures of functional ability are essential to proper diagnosis of dementia. Measures of functional assessment also provide information relevant to symptom management in AD, the making of placement decisions, and the determination of the level of assistance needed for patients with AD living in the community (DeBettignies et al., 1993; Demers et al., 2000).

Numerous measures of ADL and IADL functioning have been designed. In fact, more than 40 different measures have been described in the literature (Kluger & Ferris, 1991). These measures can be organized into three types: self-report and caregiver/informant report, performance-based functional assessments, and clinician rating measures (Loewenstein & Mogosky, 1999). Specific descriptions of these measures and their advantages and limitations are available (Demers et al., 2000; Kluger & Ferris, 1991; Loewenstein & Mogosky, 1999). In the following sections, we describe self-informant report and direct assessment methods.

Self- and Informant Reports

Self- and informant reports are the most commonly used methods for assessing functional abilities of older adults. These instruments involve the patient or (more typically) a caregiver or other knowledgeable informant (i.e., proxy) to provide ratings of the patient's ability to perform basic self-care and complex instrumental activities at home and in the community. Respondents are asked to indicate whether the individual with AD can perform a series of activities with or without the help of someone or the use of a special device (Angel & Frisco, 2001). The degree of functional disability is measured by both the number of activities with which the individual needs assistance and the amount of help needed to complete each activity (Angel & Frisco, 2001). Caregivers and proxy informants are believed to be in the best position to provide such ratings, because they observe the functional behavior of patients within the home environment on a daily basis (Loewenstein & Mogosky, 1999). Furthermore, in contrast to results of performance-based measures of ADLs and IADLs, which may fluctuate as a function of patients' motivation, cognition, and behavior (DeBettignies et al., 1993), caregiver observations of patient functioning in an everyday environment across time are assumed to result in more stable estimates of functional skills and limitations (Loewenstein & Mogosky, 1999).

On the other hand, self- and caregiver judgments of functional ability suffer a number of limitations (DeBettignies et al., 1993; Rubenstein et al., 1984; Wadley, Harrell, & Marson, 2003; Wild & Cotrell, 2003). Research has shown that dementia patients, like hospitalized elders, tend to consistently overestimate their functional abilities (Rubenstein et al., 1984; Wadley et al., 2003; Wild & Cotrell, 2003). In addition, caregivers have been found to significantly misestimate the everyday functioning of individuals with AD, resulting in low to moderate correlations with performance-based functional assessment measures (Angel & Frisco, 2001; Wadley et al., 2003; Wild & Cotrell, 2003). For instance, Wadley and colleagues (2003) found that caregiver ratings of current financial abilities demonstrated low levels of stability over a 1-month period. In addition, DeBettignies and colleagues (1993) found that spousal caregivers of individuals with AD overestimated functional impairment in comparison to spouses of individuals with multiple infarcts and healthy older adult controls. Other studies have found that caregivers underestimated functional impairments of individuals with AD, specifically related to driving and handling finances (Wadley et al., 2003; Wild & Cotrell, 2003). This pattern of misestimation among caregivers has been linked not only to patient cognition but also to fluctuations in caregivers' mood, their perceived level of burden, and their use of denial as an adaptive mechanism (DeBettignies et al., 1993; Ippen, Olin, & Schneider, 1999; Sager et al., 1992). Despite these limitations, self- and caregiver/informant ratings are still commonly used because of their minimal cost and relative ease and brevity of administration and scoring (Angel & Frisco, 2001; Loewenstein & Mogosky, 1999).

Performance-Based Assessments

In contrast to self- and informant rating scales, performance-based measures require that individuals with AD actually perform a series of tasks relevant to everyday living, as administered by a trained examiner (Angel & Frisco, 2001). Performance-based functional assessment measures have several advantages over self- and informant ratings (Zimmerman & Magaziner, 1994). These measures gauge actual abilities equivalent to those performed in the home environment in a way that is psychometrically objective, quantifiable, repeatable, and norm referenced. As such, the results of these measures are generalizable across patients and assessment settings and provide objective information to the clinician. Performance-based assessment also provides information regarding the elements of specific functional tasks that can be highly relevant to the formulation of tailored recommendations and treatment strategies. Finally, performance-based measures are not affected by the reporter bias that is inherent to self- and proxy report measures. Therefore, it is recommended that performance-based measures of ADL and IADL functioning be used regularly to inform and augment self- and informant-based measures of functional decline (Loewenstein & Mogosky, 1999; Wadley et al., 2003).

A criticism of performance-based functional assessment concerns possible limited ecological validity in relation to the patient's everyday environment (DeBettignies et al., 1993; Loewenstein & Mogosky, 1999). In contrast to a laboratory setting, patients' homes and community environments provide contextual cues that may assist individuals with AD or MCI in successfully completing functional tasks (Loewenstein & Mogosky, 1999). In addition, home and community environments also present distractions and competing demands that can interfere with patients' abilities to perform everyday tasks. As such, results of performance-based measures of ADLs and IADLs may either underestimate or overestimate the actual ability of individuals with AD to perform basic self-care and more complex instrumental tasks in their home environments. Furthermore, these measures, as opposed to self- and informant rating scales, are more difficult to administer, require special equipment and training, and are both time consuming and costly (Angel & Frisco, 2001; Sager et al., 1992). Lastly, some researchers have questioned the degree to which performance-based assessments detect subtler functional deficits in MCI and very mild AD (Loewenstein & Mogosky, 1999). However, this concern is likely due, in part, to the insensitivity of some performance-based tasks to detect these subtle performance deficits (Griffith et al., 2003; Loewenstein & Mogosky, 1999; Marson & Briggs, 2001). For example, functional impairments in MCI and very mild AD have been detected using measures that assess more cognitively demanding tasks, such as financial capacity and driving (Griffith et al., 2003; Marson, Sawrie, et al., 2000; Wild & Cotrell, 2003).

Conceptualizing Independent Living Skills through a Functional Disability Framework

Functional disability, as defined by the World Health Organization (1980), is any restriction or inability to perform an activity in a manner consistent with the individual's particular stage of sociobiological or cognitive development (Demers et al., 2000). Difficulty in performing one or more physical self-care or independent daily living skills qualifies as functional disability. The degree of functional disability is contingent upon the number of activities that are impaired as well as the amount of help needed to complete the activity (Angel & Frisco, 2001; Patterson et al., 1992). Individuals who require only verbal prompting to initiate or complete a task are qualitatively different in terms of functional disability than individuals who require actual physical guidance. Furthermore, an individual's level of previous experience with a task as well as his or her past available opportunities to perform a task are other factors that may be considered during the course of functional assessments (Patterson et al., 1992). For example, should a male patient who demonstrates difficulty in balancing a checkbook be assumed to be declining in financial capacity when his wife has always been in charge of this task? However, although prior experience and opportunity should be considered when determining dementia severity or the rate of functional decline associated with AD, these factors are of little relevance when the goal of the assessment is to identify specific functional performance deficits and the level of assistance presently needed to support independent living (Patterson et al., 1992).

Implications of Functional Incapacity for Older Adults

Functional impairment has significant implications for older adults. Research has found that functionally impaired older adults are more likely to be placed in a nursing home and have higher mortality rates than individuals who continue to function independently (Angel & Frisco, 2001; Wiener et al., 1990). Using data collected from six national epidemiological surveys, Wiener and colleagues (1990) compared estimates of functional ability in community-dwelling and institutionalized persons 65 years of age and older. Estimates of disability in one or more activities of daily living ranged from 5.0 to 8.1% of community-dwelling older adults and more than 90% for institutionalized elderly (Wiener et al., 1990). Functionally impaired older adults reported greater need for assistance, poorer health status, poorer health outcomes, and poorer quality of life than individuals who were able to perform tasks independently (Angel & Frisco, 2001).

Functional impairments and losses also have significant psychological consequences for patients and families (DeBettignies et al., 1993; Marson & Hebert, 2005; Moye, 1996). Research shows that functional incapacity is associated with greater caregiver burden (Goode et al., 1998; Haley et al., 1996). Functional changes affecting the capacity to manage finances ("taking away the checkbook") and to drive ("taking away the car keys") appear to have particularly notable psychological consequences because they implicate core aspects of autonomy in our society. Decisions to limit or remove an individual patient's autonomy in these areas thus require careful consideration by health care professionals and families.

STUDIES OF COGNITION AND FUNCTION IN THE ELDERLY

In recent years a considerable body of research has examined the relationship between cognitive abilities and ADL/IADL functional performance, with particular reference to older adult populations. Performance on various standardized psychometric measures of intelligence, attention, executive function, memory, and global cognitive functioning has been found to be significantly correlated with functional capacities of basic self-care, IADLs, and academic achievement as well as vocational attainment and performance (Heaton & Pendleton, 1981; Matarazzo, 1972). Cognitive aging studies have addressed the relationship of functional performance to verbal versus nonverbal abilities, fluid versus crystallized intelligence, and declarative versus procedural knowledge in normal aging (Leckey & Beatty, 2002; Mortimer, Ebbitt, Jun, & Finch, 1992; Willis et al., 1998). More recently, cognitive models have been developed for specific IADLs such as financial management, medical decision making, and testamentary capacity (Griffith et al., 2003; Marson, Cody, Ingram, & Harrell, 1995; Marson, Ingram, Cody, & Harrell, 1995). Despite considerable research into the cognitive abilities associated with driving performance, no neurocognitive model of driving capacity has yet been proposed. Below we discuss representative studies in these areas, using the dementia continuum of cognitive aging, MCI, and dementia as our organizing framework.

Studies of Functional Change in Cognitive Aging

Many cognitive abilities that decline with age are linked to complex tasks of daily living (Bell-McGinty et al., 2002; Cahn-Weiner et al., 2000; Willis et al., 1998). Normative age-related declines in fluid abilities such as abstract reasoning, working memory, spatial orientation, and information-processing speed have been observed to begin as early as the sixth decade of life, with the rate of cognitive decline increasing in the 70s and 80s (Schaie, 1996). In contrast, crystallized abilities such as vocabulary demonstrate later onset and slower rate of decline relative to fluid abilities, among older adults (Diehl, Willis, & Schaie, 1995; Willis, Jay, Diehl, & Marsiske, 1992).

A number of research studies has examined the association between cognitive and functional decline in normal older adults (Barberger-Gateau et al., 1999; Mortimer et al., 1992; Willis et al., 1992). In a longitudinal study of 102 community-dwelling older adults conducted by Willis and colleagues (1992), performance on measures of fluid intelligence, crystallized intelligence, and processing speed declined significantly over a 7-year interval, as did performance on a measure of everyday task competence. Fluid reasoning ability emerged as the strongest longitudinal predictor of everyday task competence (accounting for 52% of the variance), as compared to crystallized intelligence (11%), processing speed (6%), memory (less than 1%), age (5%), and education (6%). Interestingly, only 38% of the study sample demonstrated significant longitudinal declines in everyday task competence, and this percentage was equivalent to the proportion of individuals who demonstrated significantly reduced fluid reasoning ability (37%). Based on these findings, the authors concluded that changes in functional performance are not the direct result of advancing age, per se, but instead are linked to a concurrent decline in those cognitive abilities that underlie everyday task competence.

Studies of Functional Change in Mild Cognitive Impairment

It is well accepted that declines in functional as well as cognitive abilities are hallmark features of dementing illnesses. What is less appreciated is that such functional changes usually first emerge in MCI or the preclinical phase of dementia (Barberger-Gateau et al., 1999; Griffith et al., 2003; Marson, Dymek, & Geyer, 2000; Willis, 1996). According to currently accepted diagnostic criteria, individuals with MCI do not experience significant changes in their ADLs (Petersen et al., 1999). This is a critical diagnostic aspect of MCI, because once decline in ADLs is detected, the diagnostic impression under DSM-IV (American Psychiatric Association, 1994) and NINCDS–ADRDA (McKhann et al., 1984) criteria begins to shift from MCI to dementia. Thus under the "Mayo criteria," MCI individuals have been described in the literature as having "usually intact" ADLs (Ritchie, Artero, & Touchon, 2001) or "only slightly abnormal" ADLs (Petersen et al., 1999). These guidelines for functional change in MCI are vague and unsatisfactory as diagnostic criteria (Ritchie et al., 2001), and probably reflect our currently limited empirical knowledge concerning the types and extent of functional change that occur in MCI.

There is emerging evidence that individuals with MCI do experience changes in everyday function prior to dementia diagnosis (Daly et al., 2000; Morris, 2002; Ritchie et al., 2001; Touchon & Ritchie, 1999). Barberger-Gateau and colleagues (1999) found that baseline scores on a four-item IADL scale (telephone use, mode of transportation, medication management, and handling finances) predicted 3-year incident dementia in a sample of 1,582 community-dwelling older adults, even after adjusting for the Mini-Mental State Examination (MMSE) score. Touchon and Ritchie (1999) found that 2 years prior to AD diagnosis, individuals with MCI demonstrated subtle but salient declines in everyday activities such as using the telephone, dental hygiene, and dressing (Touchon & Ritchie, 1999). These changes were identified through interviews of subjects and family member proxies. The behavioral changes did not involve dramatic failures but rather occasional lapses, carelessness, task slowing, and the need for cuing (Touchon & Ritchie, 1999). Thus MCI individuals could still carry out the activities in question, but changes in qualitative performance were observed. Other recent studies using informant report have also indicated functional changes in MCI. Using a standardized clinical interview, Albert and her group (1999) identified functional changes (in financial skills, driving, hobbies, and personal care) that were associated with MCI and conversion to AD. More recently, a study using ADL report forms found that informant report of functional change in MCI subjects, and the discrepancy between MCI patient self-report and informant report, both predicted subsequent conversion to AD within a 2-year period (Tabert et al., 2002). As discussed further in the section below on specific capacities, our own group has used a direct assessment approach to show that amnestic MCI patients demonstrate mild impairments in higher-order financial skills in comparison to older controls (Griffith et al., 2003).

Studies of Functional Change in Alzheimer's Disease and Related Dementias

There is a more substantial literature that has demonstrated functional impairments in patients with AD and related dementias. This is a critical area of study because, as noted above, functional change is integral to a dementia diagnosis.

Cognitive and functional change in dementia are closely linked but also probably distinct processes. In a longitudinal study of 65 patients with probable AD (Mortimer et al., 1992), rates of cognitive and functional decline over a 4-year period were moderately correlated ($r = .63$, $p < .001$). However, only 40% of the variance in functional decline was accounted for by cognitive decline, indicating that cognition and functional capacity reflect distinct yet parallel features of the disease process. Furthermore, Mortimer and colleagues (1992) found that cognitive and functional progression rates differ substantially with regard to neuropsychological predictors. Lower baseline scores on verbal neuropsychological tests of confrontation naming, learning and recall, fluency, abstraction, and immediate memory emerged as key predictors of faster cognitive decline. In contrast, lower baseline scores on nonverbal neuropsychological measures of visuospatial function and visual memory were found to predict faster rates of functional decline. The different predictor models for functional and cognitive decline again suggested that they are distinct constructs in dementia. The results of this study also supported the utility of neuropsychological assessment in predicting functional performance.

Global Cognition and Functional Change in Dementia

Studies have explored the relationship between global cognitive functioning (using tests such as the MMSE) and everyday functional performance in patients with AD. These studies have found variable correlations across different measurement approaches: clinician ratings, caregiver ratings, self-ratings, and direct assessments of functional performance (Grigsby et al., 1998; Leckey & Beatty, 2002; Mortimer et al., 1992; Perry & Hodges, 2000; Stern et al., 1990; Willis et al., 1998). For example, Mayeux, Stern, and Spanton (1985) found that scores on the modified MMSE were moderately correlated ($r = .50$, $p < .05$) with the Blessed Dementia Rating Scale (BDRS), a clinician rating of functional aspects of dementia not assessed by neuropsychological measures. Although the BDRS was later factor analyzed to control for items unrelated to ADL/IADL performance, the MMSE remained moderately correlated with both BDRS cognitive/IADL ($r = -.44$, $p < .05$) and BDRS basic self care ($r = -.51$, $p < .05$) items (Stern et al., 1990).

In a 4-year longitudinal study of 65 patients with probable AD (Mortimer et al., 1992) that employed caregiver ratings, baseline MMSE scores were weakly correlated with caregiver ratings of ADL/IADL performance at baseline ($r = -.24$) yet moderately correlated with the rate of functional decline across time ($r = .63$). Willis and colleagues (1998) also found a correlation of .24 between MMSE scores and caregiver ratings of IADL performance in 65 patients with AD, but this association failed to reach significance.

Other studies have found a stronger association between MMSE scores and caregiver ratings of ADL/IADL performance (Leckey & Beatty, 2002; Perry & Hodges, 2000). In a study of 24 patients with AD conducted by Perry and Hodges (2000), MMSE scores were strongly correlated ($r = -.73$) with overall scores on a 25-item caregiver rating scale of functional abilities. However, items assessing memory as well as attention and executive abilities were incorporated within the functional assessment scale, possibly inflating the degree of association between caregiver ratings and global cognitive function.

In a study using the Dementia Rating Scale (DRS), Lichtenberg and Nanna (1994) found that DRS total scores were the only significant predictor of both ADLs ($r = .27$, $p < .05$) and ambulation ($r = .27$, $p < .05$) in a sample of 60 older adults admitted to an inpatient rehabilitation program, accounting for 8% and 16% of the variance, respectively. Age, education, ethnicity, medical condition, length of hospital stay, and depression were unrelated to ADL performance and ambulation.

Level of dementia severity within a sample may also influence the degree of association between global cognitive functioning and caregiver-rated functional performance (Leckey & Beatty, 2002). Although moderate correlations were found between MMSE scores and caregiver ratings of ADL ($r = .51$, $p < .05$) and IADL ($r = .69$, $p < .001$) performance, the correlation between MMSE scores and IADL performance decreased to .29 ($p < .05$) when individuals with severe AD were excluded from analyses.

With respect to patients with AD self-ratings, MMSE scores were not found to contribute significantly to the prediction of ADL and IADL performance (Grigsby et al., 1998; Willis et al., 1998). This finding probably reflects the anosognosia characteristic of AD, which appears to be particularly notable in the area of everyday functioning. Research has consistently shown that patients with AD overestimate their functional and cognitive abilities to a substantial degree (Loewenstein et al., 2001; Teri, 1997; Wadley et al., 2003; Wild & Cotrell, 2003). A recent study by Wadley indicated substantial overestimation of financial skills in a sample of 20 patients with AD, relative to caregiver ratings and a direct-assessment criterion (Wadley et al., 2003).

On the other hand, direct assessments of functional performance have yielded relatively consistent moderate associations with global cognitive functioning (Burns, Mortimer, & Merchak, 1994; Grigsby et al., 1998; Willis et al., 1998). In a study of 77 patients with mild to moderate AD and 15 normal elderly controls, MMSE scores were moderately correlated ($r = .67$, $p < .001$) with overall performance of six daily living tasks, including dressing, shopping, making toast, using the telephone, washing, and following a map (Burns et al., 1994). A moderate association ($r = .55$, $p < .05$) was also observed between MMSE scores and the performance of 65 patients with AD on a direct measure of everyday problem solving involving printed materials such as medication labels and phone bills (Willis et al., 1998). In a study of treatment-consent capacity in patients with mild to moderate AD, using a direct assessment vignette methodology, the MMSE achieved a moderate univariate association with three out of five treatment-consent abilities (i.e., capacity to appreciate the consequences of a treatment choice, $r = .49$, $p = .008$; to provide rational reasons for a treatment choice, $r = .55$, $p = .002$; and to understand treatment situation and choices, $r = .62$, $p < .001$), but failed to emerge in any of the final multivariate models (Marson, Chatterjee, Ingram, & Harrell, 1996; Marson, Cody, Ingram, & Harrell, 1995).

Thus, across a variety of assessment modalities, global cognitive functioning is significantly related to everyday functional performance in patients with dementia. At the same time, global cognitive functioning is certainly not a proxy for functional change in dementia, because it accounts for only a limited portion of variance. The actual power of global cognitive measures to predict functional impairment is even more limited. Although the MMSE has been found to account for up to 48% of the variance in IADL performance, the amount of variance accounted is reduced dramatically (to 9%) when analyses are restricted to individuals with mild to moderate dementia (Leckey & Beatty, 2002). As such, MMSE scores, by themselves, are inadequate clinically for predicting functional impairment in patients with AD.

Specific Neuropsychological Predictors of Functional Capacity in Dementia

Studies have also examined the relationship of specific neuropsychological abilities to everyday functioning in patients with dementia. In contrast to global mental status measures, neuropsychological measures hold the promise of revealing specific cognitive abilities and even the neurocognitive substrates that subserve everyday functional abilities. Viewed broadly, measures of executive function have demonstrated the most consistent relationships to functional declines in older adult populations (Marson & Harrell, 1999; Royall, Cordes, & Polk, 1997). Executive functions involve those cognitive skills necessary for regulating purposeful, goal-directed behavior, including such abilities as planning, sequencing, self-monitoring, and mental flexibility (Lezak, 1995; Royall et al., 2000; Sbordone, 2000). Executive functions have been closely linked to frontal-lobe function and integrity (Cummings, 1993; Malloy & Richardson, 1994), which declines as a result of both cognitive aging (Cahn-Weiner et al., 2000; Fisk & Warr, 1996; Grigsby et al., 1998; Salthouse & Miles, 2002; West, 1996) and dementias such as AD and Parkinson's disease dementia (Marson & Harrell, 1999; Schaie, 1996). Several studies have explored the contribution of executive functioning to everyday task performance (Grigsby et al., 1998; Loewenstein et al., 1992; Marson & Harrell, 1999; Norton, Malloy, & Salloway, 2001; Willis et al., 1998). In a sample of 1,158 community-dwelling older adults (Grigsby et al., 1998), a measure requiring attention and set shifting as well as initiation and inhibition of motor responses (Behavioral Dyscontrol Scale/BDS) was found to be significantly correlated with subjects' ability to handle money ($r = .53$, $p < .001$) and manage medications ($r = .36$, $p < .001$), as measured by the Structured Assessment of Independent Living Skills (SAILS). Furthermore, performance on the BDS accounted for more variance in functional performance than did general mental status as measured by the MMSE.

Cahn-Weiner and colleagues (2000) compared neuropsychological test scores and IADL performance in a sample of 27 community-dwelling older adults. An executive function composite score was formulated based upon performance on the Wisconsin Card Sorting Test, the Trail Making Test (TMT) Parts A & B, the Controlled Oral Word Association Test (i.e., word fluency), and Stroop test. Executive dysfunction was found to predict everyday task performance more than other cognitive measures, including memory (Hopkins Verbal Learning Test—Revised and Brief Visuospatial Memory Test—Revised), language (Boston Naming Test), visuospatial skills (Judgement of Line Orientation Test), and psychomotor speed (Grooved Pegboard Test). Furthermore, the greatest proportion of variance in IADL performance was accounted for by executive functioning.

Similarly, Willis and colleagues (1998) found moderate to strong correlations (.39–.70) between scores on measures of executive functioning (TMT; Word Fluency; Wechsler Adult Intelligence Scale—Revised/WAIS-R Digit Symbol and Block Design subtests) and performance on a direct assessment measure of everyday problem solving (Everyday Problem-Solving for the Cognitively Challenged Elderly/EPCCE). Moreover, both executive functioning and global cognitive functioning accounted for unique variance in EPCCE scores, with executive measures significantly increasing the amount of variance in EPCCE scores explained by global cognitive functioning alone (from $R^2 = .59$ to $R^2 = .69$, $p < .001$). In a sample of 22 patients with AD and 18 older adult controls (Leckey & Beatty, 2002), scores on a measure of verbal abstraction (Shipley Institute of Living Scale—Abstraction; SILS-A) were moderately correlated with caregiver ratings of both ADL ($r = .50$, $p < .05$) and IADL ($r = .57$, $p < .01$) performance, whereas tests of semantic knowledge (15-item Boston Naming Test and SILS-Vocabulary) were unrelated (Leckey & Beatty, 2002).

Performance on the executive function based Initiation/Perseveration (I/P) subscale of the DRS has been linked with everyday functioning (Lichtenberg & Nanna, 1994; Nadler, Richardson, Malloy, Marran, & Hostetler-Brinson, 1993; Norton et al., 2001). Nadler and colleagues (1993) examined the association between subscales of the DRS and subject performance on tasks involving self-care, safety, money management, cooking, medication administration, and community utilization. The DRS total score ($R^2 = .27$ to $.49$, $p < .01$) accounted for a significant amount of variance in performance for each task, with the exception of cooking. Both the I/P and Memory subscales of the DRS emerged as significant univariate predictors of everyday task performance, with the I/P subscale the most strongly correlated with five of the six performance tasks ($r = .50$ to $.68$, $p < .002$). These findings were consistent with those of Norton et al. (2001), who found that the I/P subscale accounted for 19 out of 22% of the variance in caregiver-rated IADL performance explained by the DRS. Thus existing research supports a consistent relationship of moderate strength between measures of executive function and everyday task performance.

A very interesting line of research has also suggested that visuospatial abilities may have special links to functional decline in older adults. Perry and Hodges (2000) compared neuropsychological and functional performance of 24 patients with early AD and found that caregiver ADL/IADL ratings were strongly associated with semantic memory ($r = .58$, $p < .01$) as well as global cognitive function ($r = .73$, $p < .001$), and visuospatial function ($r = .74$, $p < .001$). However, only visuospatial function emerged as a significant predictor of functional abilities, based upon multiple regression analyses. Furthermore, performance on measures of episodic memory and attention was found to be unrelated to functional performance. These results (Perry & Hodges, 2000) are consistent with those of Mortimer and colleagues (1992), who found that visuospatial function and visual memory, rather than confrontation naming, verbal recall, verbal abstraction, and immediate memory, predicted rates of functional decline over a 4-year period. The findings are also consistent with the work of Royall and his group (Royall, 1998; Royall, Chiodo, & Polk, 2000), who have found that a simple clock copy task with executive aspects (CLOX 2) has been associated with IADL impairment in the elderly. According to Royall, it is possible that right-hemisphere changes associated with aging and cerebrovascular disease foreshadow frontal-system changes that underlie diminishing task performance in older adults (Royall, 2003).

Conclusions and Implications

Research suggests that changes in functional performance occur with normal aging and are likely the result of declines in cognitive abilities that underlie everyday task performance (Willis et al., 1992). Likewise, cognitive and functional decline in MCI and AD represent related but also distinct features of the disease course (Mortimer et al., 1992). Intact cognition is thus a necessary but not sufficient condition for successful performance of everyday tasks in normal and abnormal aging (Willis et al., 1992). Global mental status measures, particularly neuropsychological measures of executive function, have been found to account for a significant portion of the variance in ADL and IADL function. In addition, deficits in higher-order cognitive abilities have been found to correspond with difficulty in performing complex tasks of everyday living even in the preclinical stages of dementia (Griffith et al., 2003). As the disease progresses, more general measures of global cognitive function emerge as significant predictors of diminished ability for basic self-care (Grigsby et al., 1998). Cognitive variables have been found to be more strongly associated with everyday living skills, as measured by direct functional assessment than caregiver or clinician rating scales of functional performance (Grigsby et al., 1998; Leckey & Beatty, 2002; Mortimer et al., 1992). In this regard, Willis and colleagues also found that functional assessment measures that require everyday problem solving of written materials (e.g., medication labels, bus schedules) are more strongly correlated with neuropsychological measures than those assessing performance of procedural tasks (e.g., using the telephone, counting money; Leckey & Beatty, 2002; Willis et al., 1998; Willis et al., 1992). Therefore, although cognitive test scores are strongly related to everyday living skills, the degree to which neuropsychological assessment can predict functional performance is contingent upon the population studied and the measures employed.

Finally, although cognitive test scores are clearly related to everyday living skills, decisions to limit autonomy in individuals with dementia should not be based solely, or even primarily, on mental status screens or neuropsychological test performance. Clinicians should rely primarily on capacity-specific information, using diagnostic and neuropsychological data as supporting evidence, in rendering clinical judgments regarding a patient's capacity or limitations in everyday living (Chelune & Moehle, 1986; Marson, 2001a; Marson & Briggs, 2001).

COMPETENCY AND CAPACITY: ASSESSING CONTEXT-SPECIFIC FUNCTIONAL ABILITIES IN OLDER ADULTS

Capacity Assessment in Clinical Neuropsychology Practice

Clinical neuropsychology is a relatively young specialty within the field of psychology that focuses on the study of brain–behavior relationships. The traditional role of neuropsychology has been threefold: (1) detecting the presence of brain lesions, (2) localizing lesions within the brain, and (3) lateralizing lesions to the right or left hemispheres of the brain (Groth-Marnat, 2000). Although these initial diagnostic and descriptive functions of neuropsychology continue to be useful, emphasis has steadily expanded to include issues of functional impairment following brain injury (Chelune & Moehle, 1986; Lemsky, 2000). In addition to assessing cognitive and personality change related to brain injury, neuropsychologists are increasingly called upon to assess important everyday functional abilities such as financial management skills, medical decision-making capacity, medication management abilities, capacity to drive, and overall capacity to live independently (Marson, 2002; Marson & Briggs, 2001; Marson, Ingram, Cody, & Harrell, 1995).

In particular, the increasing incidence of competency assessment issues in older adult patients has both expanded and complicated the practice of clinical neuropsychology (Marson, 2002). Neuropsychologists must not only assess cognitive and personality deficits, but they are also increasingly called upon to make judgments of specific medical–legal capacities. The contemporary geriatric neuropsycholoigst must be able to evaluate everyday functional changes in older adults that are frequently of paramount importance to the individual patient, his or her family, the treatment team, and the legal system. The degree to which neuropsychology as a field can successfully address these evolving clinical demands will be based upon its ability to develop conceptual models, assessment instruments, and clinical expertise relevant to capacity assessment and issues of everyday living (Chelune & Moehle, 1986; Marson, 2002; Marson et al., 1996).

In this final section we focus on four specific functional capacities relevant to community-dwelling older adults and frequently encountered by geriatric neuropsychologists: medical decision-making capacity, financial capacity, testamentary capacity (i.e., capacity to make or change a will), and driving capacity. We review conceptual models, instrument development, empirical group studies, and relevant neuropsychological predictor models for each of these capacities.

Medical Decision-Making Capacity

Background

The capacity to consent to medical treatment (hereafter referred to as "MDC," or medical decision-making capacity) is a fundamental aspect of personal autonomy, because it concerns intimate decisions regarding the care of a person's body and mind (Marson & Briggs, 2001; Marson & Hebert, 2005). *Consent capacity* refers to a patient's cognitive and emotional ability to accept a proposed treatment, to refuse treatment, or to select among treatment alternatives (Grisso, 1986; Tepper & Elwork, 1984). In the United States, consent capacity is the cornerstone of the medical–legal doctrine of informed consent, which requires that a valid consent to treatment be informed, voluntary, and competent (Kapp, 1992; Marson, Ingram, et al., 1995). From a functional standpoint, consent capacity may be viewed as an "advanced activity of daily life" (Wolinsky & Johnson, 1991) and an important component of health and independent living skills in both younger and older adults.

As a competency, MDC is distinctive for several reasons: (1) it arises in a medical and not a legal setting; (2) it generally involves a physician, psychologist, or other health care professional, and not a legal professional, as decision maker; and (3) the judgments are rarely subject to judicial review (Grisso, 1986). As discussed above, clinicians do not decide competency in a formal legal sense. However, their decisions can have the same effect as a courtroom determination insofar as the patient loses decision-making power (Appelbaum & Gutheil, 1991).

Conceptual Model

From a conceptual standpoint, MDC has been understood to consist of four different consent abilities or standards (Appelbaum & Grisso, 1988; Grisso & Appelbaum, 1995; Roth, Meisel, & Lidz, 1977). These abilities, with their underlying definitions, are:

(S1) The capacity to "evidence" a treatment choice (this standard focuses on the presence or absence of a decision, and not on the quality of the decision (Roth et al., 1977).

(S2) The capacity to make the "reasonable" treatment choice (when the alternative is unreasonable; Roth et al., 1977; Tepper & Elwork, 1984), which we reference as (S2). (S2) is not an accepted clinical standard for judging consent capacity because of concerns about arbitrariness in determining what constitutes a "reasonable choice" (Tepper & Elwork, 1984). However, it is used as an experimental variable to better understand subjects' treatment preferences (Marson, Earnst, Jamil, Bartolucci, & Harrell, 2000; Marson, Ingram, et al., 1995).

(S3) The capacity to "appreciate" emotionally and cognitively the personal consequences of a treatment choice (this standard emphasizes the patient's awareness of the consequences of a treatment decision: its emotional impact, rational requirements, and future consequences (Roth et al., 1977).

(S4) The capacity to reason about a treatment choice, or make a treatment choice based on "rational" reasons (this standard tests the capacity to use logical processes to compare risks/benefits of treatment options and weigh this information to reach a decision (Appelbaum & Grisso, 1988).

(S5) The capacity to make a treatment choice based on an "understanding" of the treatment situation and alternatives (this standard requires memory for words, phrases, ideas, and sequences of information as well as comprehension of the fundamental meaning of the treatment-related information (Appelbaum & Grisso, 1988).

These standards represent different thresholds for evaluating MDC (Marson, Schmitt, Ingram, & Harrell, 1994). For example, the first standard (evidencing a choice) requires nothing more than a subject's communication of a treatment choice to establish competency. In contrast, the fourth standard (*reasoning*) bases competency on a subject's capacity to supply rational reasoning for the treatment choice. These standards can be readily applied to other competencies to consent, such as capacity to consent to research participation and to decisional capacity, in general.

Instruments for Assessing MDC

Over the past decade several investigators have developed instruments for the assessment of decisional capacity in different patient populations (Grisso & Appelbaum, 1995; Grisso, Appelbaum, Mulvey, & Fletcher, 1995; Janofsky, McCarthy, & Folstein, 1992; Marson, Ingram, et al., 1995). In 1991 our research group used the above conceptual model to develop a psychometric instrument called the Capacity to Consent to Treatment Instrument (CCTI). The CCTI consists of two specialized clinical vignettes (Vignette A: neoplasm; Vignette B: cardiac) that tested MDC using the consent abilities detailed above (Marson, Ingram, et al., 1995). Each vignette presents a hypothetical medical problem and symptoms and two treatment alternatives with associated risks and benefits. The administration format approximates an informed consent dialogue and requires the subject to consider two different treatment options with associated risks and benefits. Vignettes are administered by having subjects simultaneously read and listen to an oral presentation of the vignette information. Subjects then answer standardized questions designed to test consent capacity under the four standards set forth above (and also [S2]). The CCTI has a detailed and well-operationalized scoring system for each vignette standard.

Empirical Studies of MDC in Dementia Populations

Study of MDC in AD. The CCTI has been used to investigate empirically the loss of competency in patients with AD (n = 29) and older controls (n = 15) (Marson, Cody, et al., 1995; Marson, Ingram, et al., 1995). Using the MMSE scores (Folstein, Folstein, & McHugh, 1975), AD subjects were divided into groups of mild dementia (MMSE $\geq$ 20; n = 15) and moderate dementia (MMSE $\geq$ 10 and < 20; n = 14). Performance on the five standards was compared across groups. As shown in Table 7.1, the CCTI discriminated the performance of the normal control, mild AD, and moderate AD subgroups on three of the five standards. Whereas the three groups performed equivalently on minimal standards requiring merely a treatment choice (S1) or the reasonable treatment choice (S2), patients with mild AD performed significantly below controls on more difficult standards requiring rational reasons (S4) and understanding treatment information (S5). Patients with moderate AD performed significantly below controls on appreciation of consequences (S3), rational reasons (S4), and understanding treatment (S5), and significantly below patients with mild AD on S4 and S5 (Marson, Ingram, et al., 1995).

Neuropsychological Models of Consent Capacity in Patients with AD. In addition to providing a standardized basis for evaluating competency performance and outcome, instruments such as the CCTI provide a psychometric criterion for investigating neurocognitive changes associated with loss of consent capacity in neurocognitive disorders such as AD. We used the CCTI and a neuropsychological test battery sensitive to dementia in the above subject sample to identify, using the four standards, cognitive predictors of declining competency performance in patients with AD (Marson et al., 1996; Marson,

TABLE 7.1. Performance on CCTI Legal Standards by Diagnostic Group

	n	LS1 0–4		[LS2] 0–1	LS3 0–10		LS4 0–12		LS5 0–70	
Older controls	15	4.0	(0.0)	.93	8.7 [a]	(1.2)	10.3 [b,c]	(3.8)	58.3 [b,d]	(6.6)
Mild AD	15	3.9	(0.4)	1.00	7.1	(2.0)	6.1 [e]	(3.4)	27.3 [e]	(9.6)
Moderate AD	14	3.6	(0.9)	.79	5.9	(2.7)	2.3	(2.4)	17.9	(10.6)

Note. No group differences emerged on [LS2], χ^2 = 4.2, p = .12. Adapted from "Assessing the competency of Alzheimer's disease patients under different legal standards: A prototype instrument" by Marson, Ingram, Cody, and Harrell (1995). Copyright 1995 by the American Medical Association. Adapted by permission.

[a] Normal mean differs significantly from moderate AD mean, p < .001.

[b] Normal means differ significantly from moderate AD mean, p < .0001.

[c] Normal mean differ significantly from mild AD mean, p < .01.

[d] Normal means differ significantly from mild AD mena, p < .0001.

[e] Mild AD mean differs significantly from moderate AD mean, p < .01.

Cody, et al., 1995). Table 7.2 presents stepwise multiple regression results for the combined AD group for these standards.

Findings from these psychometric studies suggest that multiple cognitive functions are associated with loss of consent capacity in patients with AD, as measured by the CCTI standards (Marson et al., 1996; Marson, Cody, et al., 1995; Marson & Hebert, 2005). Deficits in conceptualization, semantic memory, and probably verbal recall appear to be associated with the significantly impaired capacity of patients with mild or moderate AD to understand a treatment situation and its choices (S5). Deficits in simple executive dysfunction (word fluency) appear linked to the impaired capacity of patients with mild or moderate AD to provide rational reasons for a treatment choice (S4), and to the impaired capacity of patients with moderate AD to identify the consequences of a treatment choice (S3). Finally, receptive aphasia and semantic memory loss (severe dysnomia) may be associated with the impaired ability of patients with advanced AD to evidence a simple treatment choice (S1). The results offer insight into the relationship between different legal thresholds of competency and the progressive cognitive changes characteristic of AD, and represent an initial step toward a neurological model of competency in dementia (Marson et al., 1996; Marson, Cody, et al., 1995).

Financial Capacity

Background

In this section we discuss a second and very different civil competency: capacity to manage financial affairs (financial capacity). Financial capacity comprises a broad range of conceptual, pragmatic, and judgment abilities that are critical to the independent functioning of adults in our society (Marson & Briggs, 2001; Marson & Hebert, 2005; Marson, Sawrie, et al., 2000). As such, it differs in many respects from medical decision-making capacity. Whereas MDC is almost exclusively a verbally mediated capacity, financial capacity comprises a complex set of abilities, ranging from basic skills of identifying and counting coins/currency, to conducting cash transactions, to managing a checkbook and bank statement, to higher-level abilities of making investment decisions. Such abilities can vary enormously across individuals, depending on socioeconomic status, occupational attainment, and overall financial experience (Marson, 2001b; Marson & Briggs, 2001; Marson et al., 2000).

Loss of financial capacity (FC) has critical economic and household consequences for dementia patients and their families as well as important implications for health care

TABLE 7.2. Multivariate Cognitive Predictors of Competency Performance in the AD Group

| | LS1 | | | LS3 | | | LS4 | | | LS5 | |
	R^2	p		R^2	p		R^2	p		R^2	p
SAC	.44	.0001	CFL	58	.0001	DRS IP	.36	.0008	DRS CON	.70	.0001
									BNT	.11	.001

Note. n = 29 for the Ad group. No measures achieved univariate or multivariate significance for the control group. LS1, evidencing a choice; LS3, appreciation of situation and consequences; LS4, rational reasoning; LS5, understanding of treatment information; BNT, Boston Naming Test; CFL, Controlled Oral Word Association Test/Fluency subscale; DRS CON, Dementia Rating Scale Conceptualization subscale; DRS IP, Dementia Rating Scale Initiation/Perseveration subscale; SAC, Simple Auditory Comprehension Screen. Adapted from Marson, Chatterjee, Ingram, and Harrell (1996). Copyright 1996 by the American Academy of Neurology. Adapted by permission.

and legal professionals (Marson, 2001b; Marson & Briggs, 2001; Marson & Hebert, 2005; Marson, Sawrie, et al., 2000). Patients with AD often have difficulties paying their bills and carrying out basic financial tasks (Overman & Stoudemire, 1988). They are continually at risk for making decisions that endanger assets needed for their own long-term care or intended for testamentary distribution to family members.

Second, as discussed above, there are also important psychological consequences to FC loss. Like driving and basic mobility, FC reflects a core aspect of individual autonomy in older adults (Kane & Kane, 1981; Lawton, 1982; Marson, 1997). Much like loss of the car keys, loss of control over one's own funds represents a significant challenge to the self-concept of older adults and can lead to depression and other significant psychological consequences (Moye, 1996).

Loss of FC has important implications for health care and legal professionals as well (Marson, 2001b; Marson & Briggs, 2001; Marson, Sawrie, et al., 2000). FC assessments have diagnostic utility in that such evidence of impaired functional ability is required for a diagnosis of dementia (DMS-IV; American Psychiatric Association, 1994). Recent research has demonstrated that impairments in higher-order financial skills and judgments are often early functional changes demonstrated by AD patients (Marson, Sawrie, et al., 2000) and also patients with MCI (Griffith et al., 2003). Diminished or impaired mental capacities place an individual at increased risk of financial exploitation, an all-too-common form of elder abuse (Nerenberg, 1996). Frequent media accounts of older adults victimized in consumer fraud and other scams provide further evidence of growing public concern regarding their financial vulnerability ("Woman out $5,300 in two cons," *Birmingham News*, 1996; Walton, 2002). Furthermore, family members, professionals, and third parties may covertly exercise undue influence over the way in which older adults manage their assets (Marson, Huthwaite, & Hebert, 2004; Spar & Garb, 1992). Loss of financial capacity can also trigger important legal issues of guardianship and conservatorship (Grisso, 1986; Marson, Sawrie, et al., 2000). A disproportionately high number of older adults is subject to conservatorship proceedings each year due to high incidence of dementias and other mental and medical illnesses affecting financial competency in this vulnerable population (Grisso, 1986). These legal proceedings involve considerable time, expense, and stress for families (Marson & Briggs, 2001).

Conceptual Model of Financial Capacity

Despite the clear relationship of FC to everyday living and independence, the conceptual basis of the construct has been largely unexplored. Here we present a conceptual model of FC in older adults (Griffith et al., 2003; Marson, Sawrie, et al., 2000; Marson & Zebley, 2001). This model has been the basis for instrument development and ongoing studies of FC in adults with AD and other clinical populations.

FC represents a broad continuum of activities and specific skills (Marson & Hebert, 2005). Accordingly, it may be best conceptualized as a series of domains of activity, each of which has specific clinical relevance to independence (Marson & Briggs, 2001; Marson, Sawrie, et al., 2000). Illustrative domains include basic monetary skills, cash transactions, checkbook management, and bank statement management. This domain-based approach is clinically oriented and consistent with the presumed multidimensionality of FC and its variability across individuals. It is also consistent with the legal doctrine of limited financial competency adopted within most state legal jurisdictions, which recognizes that an individual may be competent to carry out some financial activities but not others (Grisso, 1986; Marson & Briggs, 2001; Marson, Sawrie, et al., 2000).

In addition to domains of activity, the model identifies specific financial abilities or tasks (Marson, 2001b; Marson, Sawrie, et al., 2000). Tasks reflect more basic financial skills that comprise domain level capacities. For example, the domain of "financial conceptual knowledge" might draw upon specific abilities, such as an understanding of basic concepts (e.g., a loan or savings) and the pragmatic application of such concepts in everyday life (e.g., selecting interest rates, identifying a medical deductible, making simple tax computations). The domain of financial judgment might consist of tasks related to detection/awareness of financial fraud or of making informed investment choices. Tasks represent abilities that constitute broader, clinically relevant domains of financial activity. Tasks are defined as simple or complex, depending on the level of cognitive resources they appear to require (Marson, 2001b; Marson, Sawrie, et al., 2000).

The model also includes FC at the global level (Griffith et al., 2003; Marson & Zebley, 2001). Competency assessment involves an overall categorical judgment or classification made by a clinician or legal professional. Thus the conceptual model of FC currently has three levels (Griffith et al., 2003): (1) specific financial abilities or tasks, each of which is relevant to a particular domain of financial activity; (2) general domains of financial activity, which are clinically relevant to the independent functioning of community-dwelling older adults; and (3) overall financial capacity, which reflects a global measure of capacity based on the summation of domain- and task-level performance. A current version of the conceptual model, presented in Table 7.3, comprises 9 domains, 18 tasks, and 2 global levels (Griffith et al., 2003).

Instrument for Direct Assessment of Financial Capacity

The Financial Capacity Instrument (FCI) is a psychometric instrument designed to assess performance of older adults at the task, domain, and global levels of the conceptual model. The original FCI (FCI-6) assessed 6 domains and 14 tasks (Marson, Sawrie, et al., 2000). As presented above, the current version (FCI-9) assesses 9 domains, 18 tasks, and 2 global levels. The FCI has previously demonstrated good internal, test–retest, and interrater reliabilities (Earnst et al., 2001).

Empirical Studies of Financial Capacity in Dementia Populations

Study of Financial Capacity in AD. In an initial study a sample of 23 older controls and 53 AD patients with AD (30 with mild dementia, 23 with moderate dementia) were administered the FCI-6 (Marson, Sawrie, et al., 2000). As shown in Table 7.4, we found that patients with mild AD performed equivalently with control subjects on Domain 1 (basic monetary skills), but significantly below controls on the other five domains. Patients with moderate AD performed significantly below controls and patients with mild AD on all domains. On the FCI tasks, patients with mild AD performed equivalently with controls on simple tasks such as naming coins/currency, counting coins/currency, understanding parts of a checkbook, and detecting risk of mail fraud. However, patients with mild AD performed significantly below controls on more com-

TABLE 7.3. Revised Conceptual Model of Financial Capacity

	Task description	Task difficulty
Domain 1. Basic monetary skills		
Task 1a. Naming coins/currency	Identify specific coins and currency	Simple
Task 1b. Coin/currency relationships	Indicate relative monetary values of coins/currency	Simple
Task 1c. Counting coins/currency	Accurately count groups of coins and currency	Simple
Domain 2. Financial conceptual knowledge		
Task 2a. Define financial concepts	Define a variety of simple financial concepts	Complex
Task 2b. Apply financial concepts	Demonstrate practical application/computation using concepts	Complex
Domain 3. Cash transactions		
Task 3a. One-item grocery purchase	Enter into simulated one-item transaction; verify change	Simple
Task 3b. Three-item grocery purchase	Enter into simulated three-item transaction; verify change	Complex
Task 3c. Change/vending machine	Obtain change for vending machine use; verify change	Complex
Task 3d. Tipping	Understand tipping convention; calculate/identify tips	Complex
Domain 4. Checkbook management		
Task 4a. Understand checkbook	Identify and explain parts of check and check register	Simple
Task 4b. Use checkbook/register	Enter into simulated transaction; pay by check	Complex
Domain 5. Bank statement management		
Task 5a. Understand bank statement	Identify and explain parts of a bank statement	Complex
Task 5b. Use bank statement	Identify specific transactions on bank statement	Complex
Domain 6. Financial judgment		
Task 6a. Detect mail fraud risk	Detect and explain risks in mail fraud solicitation	Simple
Task 6c. Detect telephone fraud risk	Detect and explain risks in telephone fraud solicitation	Simple
Domain 7. Bill payment		
Task 7a. Understand bills	Explain meaning and purpose of bills	Simple
Task 7b. Prioritize bills	Identify overdue utility bill	Simple
Task 7c. Prepare bills for mailing	Prepare simulated bills, checks, envelopes for mailing	Complex
Domain 8. Knowledge of assets/estate	Indicate/verify asset ownership, estate arrangements	Simple
Domain 9. Investment decision making	Understand options; determine returns; make decisions	Complex
Global 1. Sum of domains 1–7	Overall functioning across tasks and domains	Complex
Global 2. Sum of domains 1–8	Overall functioning across tasks and domains	Complex

Note. From Griffith et al. (2003). Copyright 2003 by the American Academy of Neurology. Reprinted by permission.

TABLE 7.4. FCI-6 Domain and Task Performance by Group

	Score range	Controls (n = 23)		Mild AD (n = 30)		Moderate AD (n = 20)	
Domain 1. Basic monetary skills	0–79	77.9[a]	(1.9)	75.5[c]	(3.5)	57.9	(16.3)
Task 1a. Naming coins/currency	0–30	30.0[a]	(0.0)	30.0[c]	(0.0)	26.7	(4.7)
Task 1b. Coin/currency relationships	0–37	36.0[a]	(1.8)	34.0[c]	(3.0)	22.7	(9.2)
Task 1c. Counting coins/currency	0–12	11.9[a]	(0.3)	11.5[c]	(0.8)	8.6	(3.8)
Domain 2. Financial concepts	0–41	35.5[a, b]	(2.7)	29.6[c]	(5.4)	19.1	(6.3)
Task 2a. Defining concepts	0–16	13.0[a, b]	(1.9)	9.7[c]	(2.9)	7.1	(2.7)
Task 2b. Applying concepts	0–25	22.5[a, b]	(1.4)	19.9[c]	(3.6)	12.0	(4.6)
Domain 3. Cash transactions	0–48	46.2[a, b]	(2.7)	38.6[c]	(8.5)	22.2	(10.1)
Task 3a. One-item purchase	0–16	15.3[a]	(2.5)	14.4[c]	(3.2)	8.6	(4.9)
Task 3b. Three-item purchase	0–16	15.2[a, b]	(1.3)	10.7[c]	(5.0)	4.6	(3.3)
Task 3c. Change/vending machine	0–16	15.7[a, b]	(0.6)	13.6[c]	(2.8)	9.0	(4.1)
Domain 4. Checkbook/register	0–62	60.2[a, b]	(2.1)	50.7[c]	(8.0)	33.3	(16.1)
Task 4a. Understanding checkbook	0–32	30.7[a]	(1.5)	27.9[c]	(3.1)	20.6	(7.6)
Task 4b. Using checkbook	0–30	29.5[a, b]	(1.5)	22.8[c]	(6.1)	12.2	(9.1)
Domain 5. Bank statement	0–40	37.4[a, b]	(2.2)	28.6[c]	(7.6)	14.9	(7.2)
Task 5a. Understanding bank statement	0–22	19.7[a, b]	(2.1)	15.0[c]	(4.1)	8.0	(3.6)
Task 5b. Using bank statement	0–18	17.7[a, b]	(0.9)	13.6[c]	(4.3)	6.9	(4.1)
Domain 6. Financial judgment	0–37	30.0[a, b]	(3.0)	20.8[c]	(5.4)	10.7	(5.1)
Task 6a. Detecting fraud risk	0–10	8.6[a]	(2.0)	7.8[c]	(2.2)	6.9	(2.8)
Task 6b. Investment decision	0–27	21.4[a, b]	(2.1)	13.0[c]	(4.4)	5.3	(3.5)

Note. From Marson, Sawrie, et al. (2001). Copyright 2000 by the American Medical Association. Reprinted by permission.

[a] Normal control mean differs from moderate AD mean using LSD post hoc test, $p < .01$.

[b] Normal control mean differs from mild AD mean, $p < .01$.

[c] Mild AD mean differs from moderate AD mean, $p < .01$.

plex tasks such as defining and applying financial concepts, obtaining change for vending machine use, using a checkbook, understanding and using a bank statement, and making an investment decision. Patients with moderate AD performed significantly below controls and patients with mild AD on all tasks (Marson & Briggs, 2001; Marson, Sawrie, et al., 2000).

The findings from this initial study represented the first empirical effort to investigate loss of financial capacity in patients with AD (Marson & Briggs, 2001; Marson & Hebert, 2005). The findings suggest that there is significant impairment of financial capacity early in AD. Patients with mild AD appear to experience deficits in complex financial abilities (tasks) and some level of impairment in almost all financial activities (domains). Patients with moderate AD appear to experience loss of both simple and complex financial abilities and severe impairment across all financial activities. Based on these initial findings, we proposed two preliminary clinical guidelines for assessment of financial capacity in patients with mild and moderate AD (Marson, Sawrie, et al., 2000):

(1) Mild AD patients are at significant risk for impairment in most financial activities, in particular complex activities like checkbook and bank statement management. Areas of preserved autonomous financial activity should be carefully evaluated and monitored.

(2) Moderate AD patients are at great risk for loss of all financial activities. Although each AD patient must be considered individually, it is likely that most moderate AD patients will be unable to manage their financial affairs. (p. 883)

Study of Financial Capacity in MCI. In a subsequent study our group also examined FC in patients with MCI (Griffith et al., 2003). As reflected in Table 7.5, the FCI-9 was administered to groups of older controls, patients with amnestic MCI, and patients with mild AD (Griffith et al., 2003). The groups were well-matched on demographic variables of education, gender, race, and socioeconomic status (Griffith et al., 2003). Controls performed significantly better than subjects with mild AD on all domains, with the exception of Domain 8 (knowledge of assets/estate). Controls performed significantly better than the MCI group on Domains 2 (financial concepts), 4 (checkbook management), 5 (bank statement management), 6 (financial judgment), and 7 (bill payment). In turn, the MCI group performed significantly better than patients with mild AD on Domains 1 (basic monetary skills), 2, 3 (cash transactions), 4, 5, 7, and 9 (investment decision making). There were no domains on which the MCI group performed better than controls.

Controls performed significantly better than the mild AD group on most tasks, with the exception of simple tasks of basic monetary skills, cash transactions, and telephone fraud (Griffith et al., 2003). Controls performed significantly better than the MCI group on tasks of applying financial concepts, understanding and using a bank statement, understanding bills, and preparing bills for mailing. The MCI group, in turn, demonstrated significantly higher scores than the AD group on tasks of understanding and applying financial concepts, using a vending machine, understanding and using a checkbook, understanding and using a bank statement, prioritizing bills, and preparing bills for mailing. There were no tasks on which the MCI group performed better than controls.

For overall FC (Domains 1–7), control participants performed significantly better than MCI and AD participants, and MCI participants performed significantly better than AD participants. On an experimental measure of overall FC that included knowledge of assets and estate arrangements (Domains 1–8), smaller samples of control and MCI subjects performed significantly better than patients with AD ($p < .001$) but did not differ significantly from each other.

This study represents one of the first published reports of direct assessment evidence for higher order functional decline and capacity loss in MCI (Griffith et al., 2003). We found that patients with amnestic MCI demonstrated significant, albeit mild, declines on some (but not all) financial abilities compared to age, education, gender, and racially matched normal controls. MCI patients showed a decline in overall FC (Domains 1–7) of 1.74 standard deviation units compared to control subjects. These results strongly suggested that decline in financial abilities is an aspect of functional change in MCI (Griffith et al., 2003).

Testamentary Capacity

Background

In this section we discuss conceptual and clinical aspects of a third civil competency: capacity to make a will (testamentary capacity). The right of testation, or the freedom to

TABLE 7.5. Comparisons of Group Performance on the Financial Capacity Instrument

	Score range	Controls (n = 21) Mean (SD)	MCI patients (n = 21) Mean (SD)	AD patients (n =22) Mean (SD)	p (two-tailed)	Post hoc p < .05
Domain 1. Basic monetary skills	0–48	45.2 (3.5)	44.3 (3.7)	41.0 (6.3)	.011	C M > A
Naming coins/currency	0–8	7.9 (0.3)	7.8 (0.4)	7.6 (0.7)	.050	C > A
Coins/currency relationships	0–28	24.9 (3.4)	24.8 (3.5)	22.0 (5.5)	.044	——
Counting coins/money	0–12	12.0 (0.2)	11.7 (0.5)	11.5 (1.2)	.119	——
Domain 2. Financial concepts	0–40	36.9 (3.2)	33.1 (4.7)	27.6 (7.5)	.001	C > M > A
Understanding concepts	0–15	13.8 (1.2)	12.9 (1.8)	11.2 (2.6)	.001	C M > A
Applying concepts	0–25	23.1 (2.4)	20.2 (3.6)	16.4 (5.3)	.001	C > M > A
Domain 3. Cash transactions	0–30	27.0 (3.4)	24.8 (3.6)	20.6 (5.9)	.001	C M > A
One-item transaction	0–6	6.0 (0.0)	5.8 (0.6)	5.5 (1.1)	.044	C > A
Multi-item transaction	0–7	6.1 (1.9)	5.7 (1.8)	4.5 (2.4)	.037	C > A
Vending machine	0–9	8.6 (0.9)	8.0 (1.4)	5.6 (1.9)	.001	C M > A
Tipping	0–8	6.3 (1.7)	5.4 (1.5)	5.1 (2.1)	.068	——
Domain 4. Checkbook management	0–54	53.2 (1.5)	50.6 (2.9)	42.9 (8.0)	.001	C M > A
Understanding checkbook	0–24	23.5 (0.8)	22.8 (1.5)	21.2 (2.5)	.001	C M > A
Using checkbook	0–30	29.6 (1.4)	27.9 (2.2)	21.7 (6.0)	.001	C M > A
Domain 5. Bank statement management	0–38	35.2 (2.7)	29.9 (5.6)	23.3 (8.3)	.001	C > M > A
Understanding bank statement	0–18	16.2 (1.6)	13.4 (2.7)	10.6 (3.9)	.001	C > M > A
Using bank statement	0–20	19.1 (1.5)	16.5 (4.0)	12.7 (4.9)	.001	C > M > A
Domain 6. Financial judgment	0–26	25.6 (1.2)	23.2 (3.7)	23.5 (3.5)	.029	C > M A
Mail fraud	0–8	8.0 (0.0)	7.3 (1.3)	7.1 (1.6)	.045	C > A
Telephone fraud	0–18	17.6 (1.2)	15.9 (3.0)	16.4 (2.3)	.051	——
Domain 7. Bill payment	0–46	43.7 (3.3)	38.4 (6.2)	28.3 (9.6)	.001	C > M > A
Understanding bills	0–6	5.9 (0.4)	5.1 (1.2)	4.7 (1.6)	.006	C > M A
Identifying/prioritizing bills	0–13	12.6 (0.6)	12.3 (1.1)	10.9 (1.7)	.001	C M > A
Preparing bills for mailing	0–27	25.1 (3.3)	20.4 (6.1)	12.7 (8.4)	.001	C > M > A
Domain 8. Assets and estate arrangements[a]	0–20	18.1 (1.6)	17.4 (2.6)	16.2 (2.8)	.068	——
Domain 9. Investment decision making[b]	0–17	13.9 (2.9)	12.4 (2.3)	9.2 (3.5)	.001	C M > A
FCI total score (Domains 1–7)	0–282	266.8 (13.2)	243.8 (21.7)	207.2 (38.0)	.001	C > M > A
FCI total score (Domains 1–8)[a]	0–302	282.1 (14.1)	264.0 (17.8)	223.8 (39.9)	.001	C M > A

Note. C > A, control mean is greater than AD mean; C > M > A, control mean is greater than MCI mean and AD mean, and MCI mean is greater than AD mean; C > MA, control mean is greater than MCI and AD means; CM > A, control and MCI means are greater than AD mean. Adapted from Griffith et al. (2003). Copyright 2003 by the American Academy of Neurology. Adapted by permission.

[a] Control = 15, MCI = 13, AD = 21.
[b] Control = 21, MCI = 19, AD = 18.

choose how one's property and other possessions will be disposed of following death, is a fundamental right under Anglo-American law (Frolik, 2001; Marson et al., 2004). A key requirement of the law of testation is that the person making the will (the testator) have *testamentary capacity* or *competency* (TC; Black's Law Dictionary, 1968). A will is invalid and void, in effect, if TC is lacking at the time that the will is executed (Perr, 1981).

The legal requirement of TC exists across all state jurisdictions (Marson et al., 2004). In order to make a valid will, the law across all state jurisdictions *also* requires that the testator be free from *undue influence* by another individual who may profit from a new will or a legal amendment of an existing will (i.e., a codicil) (Spar, Hankin, & Stodden, 1995). An otherwise validly executed will may be voided by the court when evidence suggests that the volition of the testator was, in effect, displaced by an individual exercising undue influence over him or her.

The current legal requirements for TC in the United States vary to some degree from state to state, but in many states four specific criteria or elements are recognized as law (Marson et al., 2004). A testator must:

1. Understand the nature of the testamentary act;
2. Understand and recollect the nature and situation of his or her property;
3. Have knowledge of the persons who are the natural objects of his or her bounty; and
4. Know the manner in which the disposition of the property is to occur.

These criteria have been detailed elsewhere (Marson et al., 2004; Spar & Garb, 1992; Walsh et al., 1997) and are described briefly in a later section.

In addition to the four legal elements of TC described above, many states require that the testator be free of delusions and hallucinations (Marson et al., 2004). However, in order for a will to be invalidated, the psychotic symptoms must cause the person to devise his or her property in such a way that he or she would not have done in the absence of the symptoms (California Probate Code). In other words, to be invalidated, the will must be the product of "insane" delusion (In re Estate of Raney, 1990).

Individuals with dementia do not lack testamentary capacity on the basis of their diagnosis alone (Becker & LeBlang, n.d.; Houts, 1985; Marson et al., 1994; Walsh et al., 1997). Although testamentary capacity may be relatively intact in the early stages of AD, as the disease course progresses, these individuals may exhibit persistent difficulty with memory for their property and potential heirs, diminished abstract reasoning ability in forming a plan for distribution of belongings after death, and a reliance on others for care and decision making, thereby increasing their susceptibility to undue influence (Becker & LeBlang, n.d.; Walsh et al., 1997). Marson (2001b) found that individuals with mild to moderate AD were impaired in their personal knowledge of assets and estate when compared with controls ($p = .001$), suggesting that cognitive decline associated with AD may hinder execution of a valid will.

Conceptual Model of Testamentary Capacity

There is currently an absence of cognitive or neuropsychological models of testamentary capacity that mental health professionals can draw upon (Marson et al., 2004). The absence of a sound scientific and theoretical base, in turn, adversely affects clinicians' conceptual knowledge and related capacity assessment practice patterns. Given the prevalence and importance of inheritance by will, testamentary capacity warrants much more research attention than it has received to date. Our capacity research group has begun work in this area and offers the following preliminary thoughts concerning the cognitive components for each of the four legal elements of testamentary capacity. These are outlined below:

Cognitive Functions Related to the Element of Understanding the Nature of a Will. This element requires a testator to understand the purposes and consequences of a will and to express these verbally or in some other adequate form to an attorney or judge. Possible cognitive functions involved may include semantic memory regarding terms such as *death*, *property*, and *inheritance*; verbal abstraction and comprehension abilities; and sufficient language abilities to express the testator's understanding. Recognition items may assist a testator with expressive language problems (Marson et al., 2004). A reply of "yes" or "no" to an attorney's queries regarding the nature of a will is unlikely to be satisfactory in this regard, because such responses do not clearly support the testator's independent understanding of the element. Similarly, a testator's signature on a legal document, by itself, does not demonstrate understanding, because a signature is an automatic procedural behavior not dependent upon higher-level cognition (Greiffenstein, 1996).

Cognitive Functions Related to Understanding the Nature and Extent of Property. The second legal element of TC requires that the testator understand the nature and extent of his or her property to be disposed (Marson et al., 2004). As reported earlier, some states differ in their interpretation of this requirement (Walsh, Brown, Kaye, & Grigsby, 1997). Possible cognitive functions involved here would include semantic memory concerning assets and ownership; historical and short-term memory enabling recall of long-term and more recently acquired assets and property; and comprehension of the value attached to different assets and property. If the testator has recently purchased new possessions prior to his or her execution of a will, then impairment in short-term memory (the hallmark sign of early AD) can significantly impact his or her recall of these items. Testators also must be able to form working estimates of value for key pieces of property that reasonably approximate their true value; it is likely that executive function abilities play a role here.

Cognitive Functions Related to Knowing the Objects of One's Bounty. This legal element requires that the testator be cognizant of those individuals who represent his or her natural heirs, or other heirs who can place a reasonable claim on the estate (Marson et al., 2004). Historical and short-term episodic personal memory of these individuals and the nature of their relationships with the testator, would appear to be prominent cognitive abilities associated with this element. As dementias such as AD progress, testators may be increasingly unable to recall family members and acquaintances, leading ultimately to failure to recognize these individuals in photographs or even when present in person.

Cognitive Functions Related to a Plan for Distribution of Assets. This final legal element of TC requires that the testator be able to express a basic plan for distributing his or her assets to intended heirs (Marson et al., 2004). Insofar as this element integrates the first three elements in a supraordinate fashion, the proposed cognitive basis for this element arguably represents an integration of the cognitive abilities underlying the other three elements. Accordingly, higher-order executive function abilities are implied, because the testator must demonstrate a projective understanding of how future dispositions of specific property to specific heirs will occur.

The preliminary cognitive psychological model of TC proposed above represents a first step toward model building in this area. Such a model would require empirical verification in an older adult sample through use of a relevant TC instrument and neuropsychological test measures.

In summary, research in TC is in its infancy. Considerable work must be done in areas of theory and model building, instrument development and validation, clinical education, and targeted empirical studies. Such work will be of vital importance to the baby boomers and succeeding generations of the 21st century. The successful resolution of legal disputes concerning inheritance and property disposition among our elderly population will be a sentinel forensic issue over the next several decades, as our society continues to age and to grapple with the overwhelming reality of widespread dementing illnesses. Neuropsychological assessment can make crucial contributions to this process through informed and sophisticated understanding and assessment of capacity functioning and loss.

Driving

Background

In this final section we describe driving capacity, a fourth civil competency of importance to older adults in our society. We review the research on the impact of AD and related dementias on driving performance and examine neuropsychological studies of driving capacity in AD. We note the absence of conceptual models of driving capacity in aging adults and provide some indications for further work in this area. Finally, we offer basic recommendations regarding the assessment of driving competence in individuals with AD and discuss implications for public policy.

Driving is an advanced IADL that, like FC, is integral to the independence of community-dwelling older adults. Driving is a distinct capacity insofar as it comprises a set of overlearned and automatic motor, visuospatial, and procedural skills with simultaneous, intermittent demands on controlled processing abilities, including higher-order attention, judgment, and decision-making skills. As discussed below, it is probably the least verbally mediated of the four specific capacities presented here, and accordingly, it may be the least amenable to neuropsychological modeling.

The capacity of older adults to drive is a clinical and public policy issue of substantial and growing importance. Older adults represent the fastest growing segment of the driving population (Duchek, Hunt, Ball, Buckles, & Morris, 1997). In the United States the number of older drivers is projected to increase from 13 million in 1994 to 30 million by 2020 (Eberhard, 1994). Research suggests that older adults, particularly those over the age of 85, are at higher risk of automobile accidents than any other age group (Dubinsky, Stein, & Lyons, 2000). This finding is particularly concerning because increased risk associated with driving persists even in light of self-limiting behavior typical among older adult drivers, such as driving fewer miles and avoiding driving at night or in bad weather (Dubinsky et al., 2000; Fitten, 2003; Lundberg et al., 1997). Elderly drivers over the age of 65 are one to three times more likely to be injured in a motor vehicle accident than drivers between the ages of 25 and 64 years, and they have more fatal crashes per mile driven than any other age group except teenage males (Fitten, 2003; Grabowski, Campbell, & Morrisey, 2004; Levy, Wernick, & Howard, 1995; Lundberg et al., 1997; Lyman, Ferguson, Braver, & Williams, 2002). Furthermore, nearly one-third of all deaths occurring at intersections involve older adults, and 50% of these elders died while attempting left turns (Fitten, 2003).

Studies of Driving Capacity in Patients with AD

Medical conditions that compromise driving can occur at any age, but they are more likely to occur with advancing age (Dobbs, Carr, & Morris, 2002). In particular, AD and related dementias represent a direct challenge to driving capacity. Individuals with AD typically demonstrate progressive deficits in memory, executive functioning, visuospatial ability, and judgment that over time severely impair their ability to operate a motor vehicle (Adler, Rottunda, Bauer, & Kuskowski, 2000; Dubinsky et al., 2000). Studies of driving in AD have examined issues such as the prevalence of automobile accidents or "near-accidents" relative to other groups of drivers, causes of and factors contributing to automobile accidents, and the reliability and validity of neuropsychological tests or simulator performance in predicting driving aptitude (Drachman, Swearer, & group, 1993; Fitten et al., 1995; Hunt et al., 1997; Rizzo, Reinach, McGehee, & Dawson, 1997).

Patients with AD as a group drive more poorly and have a higher crash risk than their normal older peers (Ball, 2003; Dubinsky et al., 2000; Friedland et al., 1988; Lundberg et al., 1997). Dubinsky et al. (2000) conducted a systematic review of the literature to develop practice parameters for neurologists specific to driving and AD. Individuals with AD were found to demonstrate significantly poorer driving performance than controls for both on-the-road and simulator assessments as well as higher error rates on a simple traffic sign recognition task. Only one study failed to find increased risk of motor vehicle accidents and violations among individuals with AD relative to cognitively intact older drivers (Trobe, Waller, Cook-Flannagan, Teshima, & Bieliauskas, 1996). Friedland and colleagues (1988) found that a sample of AD drivers was 4.7 times more likely than the control group to have had at least one crash in the past 5 years, and these accidents were associated with errors related to maneuvering intersections, obeying traffic lights, and making lane changes. Moreover, individuals with AD are more likely than cognitively intact older drivers to experience disorientation in familiar as well as unfamiliar areas and a decrease in both comprehension of traffic signs and general driving performance relative to other groups of drivers (Carr, LaBarge, Dunnigan, & Storandt, 1998; Dubinsky et al., 2000; Rizzo et al., 1997). Increased risk in the AD group persists even though patients with AD reported driving less at night, on freeways, and in unfamiliar places (Adler et al., 2000). In fact, research has shown that individuals with AD report driving one-fourth as many kilometers as age-matched controls (Dubinsky et al., 2000; Trobe et al., 1996).

Some studies suggest that drivers in the *early stages of AD* have no more crashes than matched controls or drivers of all ages (Drachman et al., 1993; Trobe et al., 1996). Trobe and colleagues (1996) compared Michigan's driving records from 1986 to 1993 for 143 individuals with AD and 715 controls matched for age, sex, and county of residence. Crash rates were nearly identical between the two groups, with 77 to 78% of subjects in both groups having no crashes, 17 to 20% having one crash, and 3 to 5% having more than one crash. Several limitations of this study which may have resulted in equivalent crash and violation rates for AD drivers and controls include (1) the absence of cognitive status testing for control subjects who were presumed to be not demented, thereby potentially inflating cognitive deficits in the control group; (2) failure to include minor collisions that may not be reported to the police; and (3) confounding of reduced driving exposure among subjects with AD relative to controls.

As is true with other higher functional abilities such as FC (Wadley et al., 2003), patients with AD as a group appear to demonstrate anosognosia and denial with respect to their driving deficits. Research has found that AD drivers are no more likely than cognitively intact older adults to have discussed or made plans for driving cessation (Adler et al., 2000; Hebert, Martin-Cook, Svetlik, & Weiner, 2002). In fact, Adler and colleagues (Adler et al., 2000; Adler, Rottunda, & Kuskowski, 1999) found that 59 to 63% of AD drivers in each sample (n = 54 and 75) felt that their memory problems would not cause them to stop driving. Furthermore, 43% of collaterals (i.e., spouse or other individuals familiar with the subject's driving habits) believed that subjects with AD would be able to continue driving throughout the disease course (Adler et al., 1999). Additional research has shown that individuals with AD continue to drive after onset and diagnosis of dementia (Hebert et al., 2002; Lundberg et al., 1997). Thus the lack of awareness of impaired abilities among older drivers with dementia and their family members raise clear issues for public policymakers as they seek to protect both individual rights and public safety.

Neuropsychological Models of Driving Capacity in AD

A number of studies has examined the utility of neuropsychological test performance in predicting performance or at-risk behaviors in older adult drivers. Overall the results of these studies have been mixed.

Some studies have found reasonably high correlations between neuropsychological test performance and driving competency (Duchek et al., 1997; Lundberg et al., 1997). Measures of visual search and selective attention, visuospatial perception and construction, and executive function have been found to be highly correlated with driving status (i.e., drivers vs. nondrivers) and performance (Daigneault, Joly, & Frigon, 2002; Duchek et al., 1997; Ott et al., 2003; Rizzo, McGehee, Dawson, & Anderson, 2001; Rizzo et al., 1997). Rizzo and colleagues (1997) examined the effect of AD on driver collision avoidance using a driving simulator and found that performance on the Rey–Osterrieth Complex Figure Test (copy trial), WAIS-R Block Design, and TMT Part B were highly correlated with driving performance in drivers with AD. However, only the Rey–Osterrieth Complex Figure Test emerged as a significant predictor of driving performance. In a study comparing drivers with very mild (n = 12) and mild AD (n = 13) and healthy elderly controls (n = 13), Hunt, Morris, Edwards, and Wilson (1993) found that measures of general cognition (Short Blessed Test and Clinical Dementia Rating Scale), verbal and visual memory (Wechsler Memory Scale/WMS Logical Memory and Benton Visual Retention Test), visuoperceptual ability (Benton Visual Retention Test Copy), visual scanning and information processing (TMT Part A and WAIS Digit Symbol Coding), and language (Boston Naming Test) were significantly correlated with driving outcome. Daigneault and colleagues (2002) found that older adult male drivers with a history of motor vehicle accidents (MVAs) demonstrated poorer executive function as measured by the Color Trails Test, Wisconsin Card Sorting Test, Stroop Color–Word Test, and the Tower of London test than those with no history of MVAs. Although subject groups differed significantly in terms of performance speed, the number of errors and perseverative responses emerged as the best predictors of at-risk driving.

Whereas visual acuity has been found to be only weakly related to crash involvement, visual information processing and higher-order attentional skills as measured by the Useful Field of View (UFOV) play a critical role in driving performance errors and MVAs among older adult drivers (Ball, 2003; Rizzo et al., 2001; Rizzo et al., 1997). The UFOV is a computerized assessment comprised of three subtests designed to assess speed of visual information processing, divided attention, and selective attention. Loss of visual field as assessed by the UFOV has been found to be relevant to improper backing up or stopping and loss of control, as well as failure to merge, yield right of way, and notice other drivers at intersections (Rizzo et al., 1997). Research has shown that drivers with AD have greater loss in useful field of vision than older adult controls (Ball, 2003; Rizzo et al., 1997). The UFOV has been found to predict vehicle crashes better than neuropsychological test scores (Ball, 2003; Rizzo et al., 1997).

Several studies have found that neuropsychological tests do not help in identifying at-risk drivers or predicting future adverse driving events (Friedland et al., 1988; O'Neill et al., 1992; Trobe et al., 1996). For instance, Trobe and colleagues (1996) found that AD drivers with one or more MVAs following diagnosis did not differ significantly from AD drivers with no MVAs in terms of neuropsychological test performance. However, only five out of the 46 dementia patients had experienced an MVA, and the small sample sizes may have contributed to lack of significant findings. One study found that individuals with AD having greater crash rates demonstrate better performance on measures of memory (WMS-R Memory Quotient) as well as verbal and nonverbal intelligence (WAIS-R VIQ and PIQ) (Trobe et al., 1996). It is possible that these individuals lack awareness of their neurocognitive deficits and consider themselves competent to drive, thereby failing to self-impose limits on their driving and increasing their risk of crashes and violations (Trobe et al., 1996).

In summary, although neuropsychological test performance correlates with driving performance, the utility of these instruments in predicting driving competency of individual patients remains questionable (Dobbs et al., 2002; Friedland et al., 1988; Lundberg et al., 1997; O'Neill et al., 1992). As noted, some studies have found little or no difference in neuropsychological performance among those individuals who are at higher risk for MVA versus those who are not (Friedland et al., 1988). Furthermore, neuropsychological tests have not correlated sufficiently with the outcome of driving tests or future crash involvement to be considered reliable and valid predictors of driving competency for individuals with AD. As noted above, driving as a capacity probably involves nonverbal, procedural, judgment, and operational skills that are not easily measured by traditional neuropsychological assessment measures (Rizzo et al., 1997).

Need for Conceptual Models of Driving Capacity

Research on driving has focused on identifying cognitive risk factors of poor driving performance and developing clinical guidelines and tips for assessing driving ability (Dubinsky et al., 2000; Lundberg et al., 1997). Unfortunately, the results of these studies have not yet translated into unifying conceptual cognitive or neuropsychological models of driving. Given the importance of driving to everyday functioning and its direct impact on public safety, there is considerable need for sound, scientifically based models of driving capacity that can advance clinical practice and scientific research in this area.

Directions for future research here would include identifying the constituent components of driving capacity. The existing neuropsychological research is instructive here. Visuospatial skills, attention, judgment, and memory have been found to decline with disease progression, and these cognitive skills are directly relevant to driving safety. As described by Lundberg and colleagues (1997):

> Visuospatial skills are needed for a multitude of tasks such as appropriate positioning of the vehicle, estimating distances, and interpreting a traffic situation and predicting its evolution. Selective, divided and sustained attention are necessary to detect potential hazards, to deal with competing stimuli at intersections, and to maintain optimal vigilance during long trips. Judgment merits special consideration in this context, because it applies not only to the driving task but also to the awareness of deficits, making compensatory behavior possible. (p. 32)

In conjunction with declines in visuospatial abilities, memory deficits may pose difficulties for drivers in retaining information after glancing in the rearview mirror or getting lost, both of which can lead to driving errors and violations (Lundberg et al., 1997).

Thus a proposed working model of driving capacity would, at a minimum, include procedural motor skills (e.g., reaction times), visuospatial skills, attentional abilities such as those measured by the UFOV, semantic knowledge of signs and the rules of the road, and decision-making skills such as risk estimation and judgment abilities, particularly those called upon in novel situations. However, it is likely that not all of the variables of interest will be linked to traditional neuropsychological variables. The task ahead is to develop and test a truly comprehensive operational model in samples of cognitively normal and abnormal older drivers and determine how well it accounts for impairment and crash risk.

Summary

Overall, research supports the finding that the neurocognitive decline associated with AD results in impaired driving performance over time. Increased crash rate, significant impairment in driving ability, and significant deficits in visual processing have been associated with drivers who have AD, and these impairments may be evident even in the early stages of the disease process (Dubinsky et al., 2000; Duchek et al., 1997). However, significantly, the negative impact of dementia on driving performance is poorly understood by patients and their caregivers. As such, many individuals with AD continue driving for many months following diagnosis, thereby posing challenges to public safety as the disease course progresses (Adler et al., 2000; Hebert et al., 2002). Matters are further complicated in that some patients with mild AD retain good driving skills, suggesting that basic skills involved in driving are automatized and reflective of procedural knowledge, which is relatively spared in early AD (Duchek et al., 1997; Lundberg et al., 1997; Trobe et al., 1996). Although data on crash rates during the first few years after symptom onset and diagnosis of AD do not suggest a significant problem, the precise point in time at which risk becomes unacceptable remains to be determined (Lundberg et al., 1997). Unfortunately, tests of mental status, neuropsychological measures, and rating scales of functional performance administered within a clinical setting are limited in their ability to predict driving performance (Johansson & Lundberg, 1997; Trobe et al., 1996). As with other capacities, *direct assessment* of driving capacity, via simulator or on-the-road testing, remains the gold standard. However, although driving simulators are valid measures of driving aptitude, they are more costly, less accessible, and more difficult to administer than mental status tests, neuropsychological assessments, or state road tests (Dubinsky et al., 2000; Odenheimer, 1993).

The issue of driving capacity among older adults will become increasingly prominent over the next several decades, as our aging society struggles to balance the individual rights of our older adult population with the demands of public safety. Current needs at the present time include conceptual models of driving capacity, better assessment tools to identify individuals at high risk for crashes and violations, and the creation of alternatives to driving which are both appropriate and acceptable to high-risk older drivers (Adler et al., 2000).

CHAPTER SUMMARY

The assessment of everyday functioning in older adults is an integral part of gerontology and geriatric medicine. It is thus surprising that, until recently, evaluation of functional status has been a largely neglected aspect of geriatric neuropsychological assessment. For reasons of history and training, our field has focused primarily on cognitive and personality changes in normal and abnormal aging, with less attention paid to functional outcomes and the interrelationships of cognitive and functional change. The present chapter reflects how the field's emphasis is beginning to change and broaden in this regard. We have provided a conceptual overview of ADLs and IADLs, described two prevailing assessment approaches of self-informant report and direct assessment, and summarized literature linking cognitive and functional change in aging and dementia. In the second half of the chapter we focused in detail on four specific functional capacities that geriatric neuropsychologists frequently encounter (medical decision-making capacity, FC, testamentary capacity, and driving), describing applicable conceptual models, assessment instruments, and empirical studies.

The increasing interest of neuropsychology in functional change and capacity assessment is encouraging from both clinical and research standpoints. Neuropsychology as a discipline is perhaps uniquely positioned to explore the relationships between the aging brain, cognition, and everyday functioning. Utilizing functional brain imaging techniques, its own cognitive testing armamentarium, and increasingly sophisticated functional assessment methods, neuropsychology can elucidate the linkages between brain diseases/lesions, associated neurocognitive and neuropsychiatric changes, and the changes in everyday functioning and adaptation they occasion. This knowledge, in turn, can be translated into useful clinical knowledge to guide issues of diagnosis, placement, and intervention in community settings. In our view, the exploration and understanding of this continuum of brain–cognition–function represents one of the exciting scientific challenges for geriatric neuropsychology in the 21st century.

ACKNOWLEDGMENTS

Supported in part by an Alzheimer's Disease Research Center grant (NIH, NIA 1P50 AG16582) (Lindy Harrell, Principal Investigator) from the National Institute on Aging; a grant from the National Institute of Mental Health (NIH, NIMH 1 R01 MH55427); and the Alzheimer's Disease Cooperative Study (NIH, NIA AG 10483-12) (Leon Thal, Principal Investigator).

REFERENCES

Adler, G., Rottunda, S., Bauer, M., & Kuskowski, M. (2000). The older driver with parkinson's disease. *Journal of Gerontological Social Work, 34*(2), 39–49.

Adler, G., Rottunda, S., & Kuskowski, M. (1999). Dementia and driving: Perceptions and changing habits. *Clinical Gerontologist, 20*(2), 23–34.

Albert, M. (1997). Preclinical predictors of Alzheimer's disease. *Brain and Cognition, 35,* 284–303.

Albert, S. M., Michaels, K., Padilla, M., Pelton, G., Bell, K., Marder, K., et al. (1999). Functional significance of mild cognitive impairment in elderly patients without a dementia diagnosis. *American Journal of Geriatric Psychiatry, 7,* 213–220.

American Psychiatric Association. (1994). *Diagnostic and statistical manual of mental disorders* (4th ed.). Washington, DC: Author.

Angel, R. J., & Frisco, M. L. (2001). Self-assessments of health and functional capacity among older adults. *Journal of Mental Health and Aging, 7*(1), 119–135.

Appelbaum, P., & Grisso, T. (1988). Assessing patients' capacities to consent to treatment. *New England Journal of Medicine, 319,* 1635–1638.

Appelbaum, P., & Gutheil, T. (1991). *Clinical handbook of psychiatry and the law* (2nd ed.). Baltimore, MD: Williams & Wilkins.

Ball, K. (2003). Driving competence: It's not a matter of age. *Journal of the American Geriatric Society, 51,* 1499–1501.

Barberger-Gateau, P., Fabrigoule, C., Helmer, C., Rouch, I., & Dartigues, J. F. (1999). Functional impairment in instrumental activities of daily living: An early clinical sign of dementia. *Journal of the American Geriatrics Society, 47,* 456–462.

Becker, R. E., & LeBlang, T. R. (n.d.). *Assessing testamentary capacity in patients with Alzheimer's disease.* Unpublished manuscript.

Bell-McGinty, S., Podell, K., Franzen, M., Baird, A., & Williams, J. (2002). Standard measures of executive functions in predicting instrumental activities of daily living in older adults. *International Journal of Geriatric Psychiatry, 17,* 828–834.

Black, H. C. (1968). *Black's Law Dictionary* (4th ed.). St. Paul, MN: West.

Burns, T., Mortimer, J. A., & Merchak, P. (1994). Cognitive performance test: A new approach to functional assessment in Alzheimer's disease. *Journal of Geriatric Psychiatry and Neurology, 6,* 46–54.

Cahn-Weiner, D. A., Malloy, P. F., Boyle, P. A., Marran, M. E., & Salloway, S. (2000). Prediction of functional status from neuropsychological tests in community-dwelling elderly individuals. *Clinical Neuropsychologist, 14*(2), 187–195.

California Probate Code. Section 6100.5.

Carr, D., LaBarge, E., Dunnigan, K., & Storandt, M. (1998). Differentiating drivers with dementia of the Alzheimer type from healthy older persons with a traffic sign naming test. *Journal of Gerontology: Medical Sciences, 53*(2), M135–M139.

Chelune, G. J., & Moehle, K. A. (1986). Neuropsychological assessment and everyday functioning. In D. Welding & A. M. Horton, Jr. (Eds.), *The neuropsychology handbook: Behavioral and clinical perspectives* (pp. 489–525). New York: Springer.

Chen, S., Sultzer, D., Hinkin, C., Mahler, M. E., & Cummings, J. (1998). Executive dysfunction in Alzheimer's disease: Association with neuropsychiatric symptoms and functional impairment. *Journal of Neuropsychiatry and Clinical Neurosciences, 10,* 426–432.

Cohen-Mansfield, J., Werner, P., & Reisberg, B. (1995). Temporal order of cognitive and functional loss in a nursing home population. *Journal of the American Geriatrics Society, 43*(9), 974–978.

Cummings, J. (1993). Frontal–subcortical circuits and human behavior. *Archives of Neurology, 50,* 873–880.

Daigneault, G., Joly, P., & Frigon, J. (2002). Executive function in the evaluation of accident risk in older drivers. *Journal of Clinical and Experimental Neuropsychology, 24*(2), 221–238.

Daly, E., Zaitchik, D., Copeland, M., Schmahmann, J., Gunther, J., & Albert, M. (2000). Predicting conversion to Alzheimer disease using standardized clinical information. *Archives of Neurology*, *57*, 675–680.

DeBettignies, B. H., Mahurin, R. K., Roderick, K., & Pirozzolo, F. J. (1993). Functional status in Alzheimer's disease and multi-infarct dementia: A comparison of patient performance and caregiver report. *Clinical Gerontologist*, *12*(4), 31–49.

Demers, L., Oremus, M., Perrault, A., Champoux, N., & Wolfson, C. (2000). Review of outcome measurement instruments in Alzheimer's disease drug trials: Psychometric properties of functional and quality of life scales. *Journal of Geriatric Psychiatry and Neurology*, *13*, 170–180.

Diehl, M., Willis, S. L., & Schaie, K. W. (1995). Everyday problem solving in older adults: Observational assessment and cognitive correlates. *Psychology and Aging*, *10*, 478–491.

Dobbs, B. M., Carr, D. B., & Morris, J. C. (2002). Evaluation and management of the driver with dementia. *The Neurologist*, *8*, 61–70.

Drachman, D., Swearer, J., & group, C. S. (1993). Driving and Alzheimer's disease: The risk of crashes. *Neurology*, *43*, 2448–2456.

Dubinsky, R. M., Stein, A. C., & Lyons, K. (2000). Practice parameter: Risk of driving and Alzheimer's disease (an evidence-based review): Report of the quality standards subcommittee of the American Academy of Neurology. *Neurology*, *54*(12), 2205–2211.

Duchek, J., Hunt, L., Ball, K., Buckles, V., & Morris, C. M. (1997). The role of selective attention in driving and dementia of the Alzheimer's type. *Alzheimer Disease and Associated Disorders*, *11*(Suppl. 1), 48–56.

Earnst, K., Wadley, V., Aldridge, T., Steenwyk, A., Hammond, A., Harrell, L., et al. (2001). Loss of financial capacity in Alzheimer's disease: The role of working memory. *Aging, Neuropsychology, and Cognition*, *8*, 109–119.

Eberhard, J. (1994, May). *Mobility and safety: The mature driver's challenge*. Paper presented at the 14th International Technical Conference on the Enhanced Safety of Vehicles, Munich, Germany.

Fisk, J., & Warr, P. (1996). Age and working memory: The role of perceptual speed, the central executive, and the phonological loop. *Psychology and Aging*, *11*(2), 316–323.

Fitten, L. J. (1999). Frontal lobe dysfunction and patient decision making about treatment and participation in research. In B. L. Miller & J. L. Cummings (Eds.), *The human frontal lobes: Functions and disorders* (pp. 277–287). New York: Guilford Press.

Fitten, L. J. (2003). Driver screening for older adults. *Archives of Internal Medicine*, *163*(18), 2129–2131.

Fitten, L. J., Perryman, K. M., Wilkinson, C. J., Little, R. J., Burns, M. M., Panchana, N., et al. (1995). Alzheimer and vascular dementias and driving: A prospective road and laboratory study. *Journal of the American Medical Association*, *273*(17), 1360–1365.

Folstein, M., Folstein, S., & McHugh, P. (1975). Mini-Mental State: A practical guide for grading the cognitive state of the patient for the physician. *Journal of Psychiatry Research*, *12*, 189–198.

Fowles, D. (1991). *A profile of older Americans*. Washington, DC: American Association of Retired Persons.

Friedland, R., Koss, E., Kumar, A., Gaine, S., Metzler, D., Haxby, J., et al. (1988). Motor vehicle crashes in dementia of the Alzheimer's type. *Annals of Neurology*, *24*, 782–786.

Frolik, L. A. (2001). The strange interplay of testamentary capacity and doctrine of undue influence: Are we protecting older testators or overriding individual preferences? *International Journal of Law and Psychiatry*, *2–3*, 253–266.

Galasko, D., Bennett, D., Sano, M., Ernesto, C., Thomas, R., Grandman, M., et al. (1997). An inventory to assess activities of daily living for clinical trials in Alzheimer's disease. *Alzheimer Disease and Associated Disorders*, *11*(Suppl. 2), S33–S39.

Goode, K. T., Haley, W. E., Roth, D. L., & Ford, G. R. (1998). Predicting longitudinal change in caregiver physical and mental health: A stress process model. *Health Psychology*, *17*(2), 190–198.

Grabowski, D., Campbell, C., & Morrisey, M. (2004). Elderly licensure laws and motor vehicle fatalities. *Journal of the American Medical Association*, *291*(23), 2840–2846.

Greiffenstein, M. F. (1996). The neuropsychological autopsy. *Michigan Bar Journal*, (May), 424–425.

Griffith, H. R., Belue, K., Sicola, A., Krzywanski, S., Zamrini, E., Harrell, L. E., et al. (2003). Impaired financial abilities in mild cognitive impairment: A direct assessment approach. *Neurology, 60*(3), 449–457.

Grigsby, J., Kaye, K., Baxter, J., Shetterly, S. M., & Hamman, R. F. (1998). Executive cognitive abilities and functional status among community-dwelling older persons in the San Luis Valley health and aging study. *Journal of the American Geriatrics Society, 46,* 590–596.

Grisso, T. (1986). *Evaluating competencies: Forensic assessments and instruments* (Vol. 7). New York: Plenum Press.

Grisso, T. (2003). *Evaluating competencies: Forensic assessments and instruments* (Vol. 16, 2nd ed.). New York: Kluwer Academic/Plenum Publishers.

Grisso, T., & Appelbaum, P. (1995). The MacArthur treatment competence study: III. Abilities of patients to consent to psychiatric and medical treatments. *Law and Human Behavior, 19,* 149–174.

Grisso, T., Appelbaum, P., Mulvey, E., & Fletcher, K. (1995). The MacArthur treatment competence study: II. Measures of abilities related to competence to consent to treatment. *Law and Human Behavior, 19,* 127–148.

Groth-Marnat, G. (2000). Introduction to neuropsychological assessment. In G. Groth-Marnat (Ed.), *Neuropsychological assessment in clinical practice: A guide to test interpretation and integration* (pp. 3–25). New York: Wiley.

Haley, W. E., Roth, D. L., Coleton, M. I., Ford, G. R., West, C. A. C., Collins, R. P., et al. (1996). Appraisal, coping, and social support as mediators of well-being in black and white family caregivers of patients with Alzheimer's disease. *Journal of Consulting and Clinical Psychology, 64,* 121–129.

Heaton, R. K., & Pendleton, M. G. (1981). Use of neuropsychological tests to predict adult patients' everyday functioning. *Journal of Consulting and Clinical Psychology, 49*(6), 807–821.

Hebert, K., Martin-Cook, K., Svetlik, D., & Weiner, M. F. (2002). Caregiver decision-making and driving: What we say versus what we do. *Clinical Gerontologist, 26*(1–2), 17–29.

Houts, M. (1985). Alzheimer's disease and testamentary capacity. *Trauma, 26*(6), 1–29.

Hunt, L., Morris, C. M., Edwards, D., & Wilson, B. (1993). Driving performance in persons with mild senile dementia of the Alzheimer type. *Journal of the American Geriatrics Society, 41,* 747–753.

Hunt, L., Murphy, C., Carr, D., Duchek, J., Buckles, V., & Morris, J. (1997). Reliability of the Washington University road test: A performance-based assessment for drivers with dementia of the Alzheimer type. *Archives of Neurology, 54,* 707–712.

In re Estate of Raney. (1990). 247 kan 359, 799 p2d 986.

Ippen, C. G., Olin, J. T., & Schneider, L. S. (1999). Can caregivers independently rate cognitive and behavioral symptoms in Alzheimer's disease patients? A longitudinal analysis. *American Journal of Geriatric Psychiatry, 7,* 321–330.

Janofsky, J., McCarthy, R., & Folstein, M. (1992). The Hopkins competency assessment test: A brief method for evaluating patients' capacity to give informed consent. *Hospital and Community Psychiatry, 43,* 132–136.

Johansson, K., & Lundberg, C. (1997). The 1994 international consensus conference on dementia and driving: A brief report. *Alzheimer Disease and Associated Disorders, 11*(Suppl. 1), 62–69.

Jorm, A. (1986). Controlled and automatic information processing in senile dementia: A review. *Psychological Medicine, 16,* 77–88.

Kane, R., & Kane, R. (1981). *Assessing the elderly: A practical guide to measurement.* Lexington, MA: Lexington.

Kapp, M. (1992). *Geriatrics and the law: Patient rights and professional responsibilities.* New York: Springer.

Katz, M., Downs, T., Cash, H., & Gratz, R. (1970). Progress in the development of the index of ADL. *Gerontologist, 10,* 20–30.

Katz, S., & Akpom, C. A. (1976). A measure of primary sociobiological functions. *International Journal of Health Services, 6,* 493–507.

Kluger, A., & Ferris, S. (1991). Scales for the assessment of Alzheimer's disease. *Psychiatric Clinics of North America, 14*(2), 309–326.

Lawton, M. P. (1990). Aging and performance of home tasks. *Human Factors, 32*(5), 527–536.

Lawton, M. P., & Brody, E. (1969). Assessment of older people: Self-maintaining and instrumental activities of daily living. *Gerontologist, 9*, 179–185.

Lawton, M. P. (1982). Competence, environmental press, and adaptation of older people. In M. P. Lawton, P. Windley, & I. Byerts (Eds.), *Aging and the environment: Theoretical approaches* (pp. 33–59). New York: Springer.

Leckey, G. S., & Beatty, W. W. (2002). Predicting functional performance by patients with Alzheimer's disease using the problems in everyday living (PEDL) test: A preliminary study. *Journal of the International Neuropsychological Society, 8*, 48–57.

Lemsky, C. (2000). Neuropsychological assessment and treatment planning. In G. Groth-Marnat (Ed.), *Neuropsychological assessment in clinical practice: A guide to test interpretation and integration* (pp. 535–574). New York: Wiley.

Levy, D., Wernick, J., & Howard, K. (1995). Relationship between driver's license renewal policies and fatal car crashes involving drivers 70 years or older. *Journal of the American Medical Association, 274*, 1026–1030.

Lezak, M. (1995). *Neuropsychological assessment* (3rd ed.). New York: Oxford University Press.

Lichtenberg, P. A., & Nanna, M. (1994). The role of cognition in predicting activities of daily living and ambulation functioning in the oldest old rehabilitation patients. *Rehabilitation Psychology, 39*(5), 251–262.

Loewenstein, D. A., Arguelles, S., Bravo, M., Freeman, R. Q., Arguelles, T., Acevedo, A., et al. (2001). Caregivers' judgments of the functional abilities of the Alzheimer's disease patient: A comparison of proxy reports and objective measures. *Journal of Gerontology: Psychological Sciences, 56B*(2), P78–P84.

Loewenstein, D. A., & Mogosky, B. J. (1999). The functional assessment of the older adult patient. In P. A. Lichtenberg (Ed.), *Handbook of assessment in clinical gerontology* (pp. 529–554). New York: Wiley.

Loewenstein, D. A., Rupert, M., Berkowitz-Zimmer, N., Guterman, A., Morgan, R., & Hayden, S. (1992). Neuropsychological test performance and prediction of functional capacities in dementia. *Behavior, Health, and Aging, 2*(3), 149–158.

Lundberg, C., Johansson, K., Ball, K., Bjerre, B., Blomqvist, C., Braekhus, A., et al. (1997). Dementia and driving: An attempt at consensus. *Alzheimer Disease and Associated Disorders, 11*(1), 28–37.

Lyman, S., Ferguson, S., Braver, E., & Williams, A. (2002). Older driver involvement in police reported crashes and fatal crashes: Trends and projections. *Injury Prevention, 8*, 116–120.

Malloy, P. F., & Richardson, E. D. (1994). Assessment of frontal lobe functions. *Journal of Neuropsychiatry and Clinical Neurosciences, 6*, 399–410.

Marsiske, M., & Willis, S. L. (1995). Dimensionality of everyday problem solving in older adults. *Psychology and Aging, 10*(2), 269–283.

Marson, D. C. (1997). *Symposium: Loss of financial capacity in older adults with dementia.* Paper presented at the Annual Conference of the Gerontological Society of America, Cincinnati, OH.

Marson, D. C. (2001a). Loss of competency in Alzheimer's disease: Conceptual and psychometric approaches. *International Journal of Law and Psychiatry, 8*, 109–119.

Marson, D. C. (2001b). Loss of financial capacity in dementia: Conceptual and empirical approaches. *Aging, Neuropsychology and Cognition, 8*, 164–181.

Marson, D. C. (2002). *Assessment of civil competencies in the elderly: Theory, research, and clinical case studies.* Paper presented at the 22nd annual conference of the National Academy of Neuropsychology, Miami, FL.

Marson, D. C. (2002, Spring). Competency assessment and research in an aging society. *Generations*, 99–103.

Marson, D. C., & Briggs, S. D. (2001). Assessing competency in Alzheimer's disease: Treatment consent capacity and financial capacity. In S. Gauthier & J. Cummings (Eds.), *Alzheimer's disease and related disorders annual 2001* (pp. 1–28). London: Dunitz.

Marson, D. C., Chatterjee, A., Ingram, K. K., & Harrell, L. E. (1996). Toward a neurologic model of competency: Cognitive predictors of capacity to consent in Alzheimer's disease using three different legal standards. *Neurology, 46,* 666–672.

Marson, D. C., Cody, H. A., Ingram, K. K., & Harrell, L. E. (1995). Neuropsychologic predictors of competency in Alzheimer's disease using a rational reasons legal standard. *Archives of Neurology, 52,* 955–959.

Marson, D. C., Dymek, M., & Geyer, J. (2000). Ethical and legal issues of clinical care and research. In C. Clark & Trojanowski (Eds.), *Neurodegenerative dementias* (pp. 425–435). New York: McGraw-Hill.

Marson, D. C., Earnst, K., Jamil, F., Bartolucci, A., & Harrell, L. (2000). Consistency of physicians' legal standard and personal judgments of competency in patients with Alzheimer's disease. *Journal of the American Geriatrics Society, 48,* 911–918.

Marson, D. C., & Harrell, L. (1999). Executive dysfunction and loss of capacity to consent to medical treatment in patients with Alzheimer's disease. *Seminars in Clinical Neuropsychiatry, 4*(1), 41–49.

Marson, D. C., & Hebert, K. (2005). Assessing civil competencies in older adults with dementia: Consent capacity, financial capacity, and testamentary capacity. In G. Larrabee (Ed.), *Forensic neuropsychology* (pp. 334–377). New York: Oxford University Press.

Marson, D. C., Huthwaite, J., & Hebert, T. (2004). Testamentary capacity and undue influence in the elderly: A jurisprudent therapy perspective. *Law and Psychology Review, 28,* 71–96.

Marson, D. C., & Ingram, K. (1996). Competency to consent to treatment: A growing field of research. *Journal of Ethics, Law and Aging, 2,* 59–63.

Marson, D. C., Ingram, K. K., Cody, H. A., & Harrell, L. E. (1995). Assessing the competency of patients with Alzheimer's disease under different legal standards. *Archives of Neurology, 52,* 949–954.

Marson, D. C., Sawrie, S., Snyder, S., McInturff, B., Stalvey, T., Boothe, A., et al. (2000). Assessing financial capacity in patients with Alzheimer's disease: A conceptual model and prototype instrument. *Archives of Neurology, 57,* 877–884.

Marson, D. C., Schmitt, F., Ingram, K. K., & Harrell, L. E. (1994). Determining the competency of Alzheimer's patients to consent to treatment and research. *Alzheimer's Disease and Associated Disorders, 8*(Suppl. 4), 5–18.

Marson, D. C., & Zebley, L. (2001). The other side of the retirement years: Cognitive decline, dementia, and loss of financial capacity. *Journal of Retirement Planning, 4*(1), 30–39.

Matarazzo, J. D. (1972). *Wechsler's measurement and appraisal of adult intelligence* (5th ed.). Baltimore, MD: Williams & Wilkins.

Mayeux, R., Stern, Y., & Spanton, S. (1985). Heterogeneity in dementia of the Alzheimer type: Evidence of subgroups. *Neurology, 35,* 453–461.

McKhann, G., Drachman, D., Folstein, M., Katzman, R., Price, D., & Stadlan, E. (1984). Clinical diagnosis of Alzheimer's disease: Report of the NINCDS–ADRDA work group under the auspices of the Department of Health and Human Services task force on Alzheimer's disease. *Neurology, 34,* 939–944.

Morris, J. C. (2002). Challenging assumptions about Alzheimer's disease: Mild cognitive impairment and the cholinergic hypothesis. *Annals of Neurology, 51*(2), 143–144.

Mortimer, J. A., Ebbitt, B., Jun, S. P., & Finch, M. D. (1992). Predictors of cognitive and functional progression in patients with probable Alzheimer's disease. *Neurology, 42,* 1689–1696.

Moye, J. (1996). Theoretical frameworks for competency in cognitively impaired elderly adults. *Journal of Aging Studies, 10,* 27–42.

Nadler, J. D., Richardson, E. D., Malloy, P. F., Marran, M. E., & Hostetler-Brinson, M. E. (1993). The ability of the Dementia Rating Scale to predict everyday functioning. *Archives of Clinical Neuropsychology, 8,* 449–460.

Nerenberg, L. (1996). *Financial abuse of the elderly.* Washington, DC: National Center on Elder Abuse.

Norton, L. E., Malloy, P. F., & Salloway, S. (2001). The impact of behavioral symptoms on activities of daily living in patients with dementia. *American Journal of Geriatric Psychiatry, 9*(1), 41–48.

Odenheimer, G. L. (1993). Dementia and the older driver. *Clinical Geriatric Medicine, 9*(2), 349–364.

Olver, J. H., Ponsford, J. L., & Curran, C. A. (1996). Outcome following traumatic brain injury: A comparison between 2 and 5 years after injury. *Brain Injury, 10*(11), 841–848.

O'Neill, D., Neubauer, K., Boyle, M., Gerrard, J., Surmon, D., & Wilcock, G. (1992). Dementia and driving. *Journal of the Royal Society of Medicine, 85,* 199–201.

Ott, B. R., Heindel, W., Whelihan, W., Caron, Piatt, A. L., & DiCarlo, M. (2003). Maze test performance and reported driving ability in early dementia. *Journal of the American Geriatrics Society, 16,* 151–155.

Overman, W., & Stoudemire, A. (1988). Guidelines for legal and financial counseling of Alzheimer's disease patients and their families. *American Journal of Psychiatry, 145,* 1495–1500.

Patterson, M. B., Mack, J. L., Neundorfer, M. M., Martin, R. J., Smyth, K. A., & Whitehouse, P. J. (1992). Assessment of functional ability in Alzheimer disease: A review and a preliminary report on the Cleveland scale for activities of daily living. *Alzheimer Disease and Associated Disorders, 6*(3), 145–163.

Perr, I. (1981). Wills, testamentary capacity, and undue influence. *Bulletin of the American Association of Psychiatry and Law, 9,* 15–22.

Perry, R. J., & Hodges, J. R. (2000). Relationship between functional and neuropsychological performance in early Alzheimer's disease. *Alzheimer Disease and Associated Disorders, 14*(1), 1–10.

Petersen, R., Smith, G., Waring, S., Ivnik, R., Tangalos, E., & Kokmen, E. (1999). Mild cognitive impairment. *Archives of Neurology, 56,* 303–308.

Reisberg, B., Ferris, S., Armand, R., DeLeon, M. J., Schenck, M., Buttinger, C., et al. (1984). Functional staging of dementia of the Alzheimer's type. *Annals of the New York Academy of Sciences, 435,* 418–483.

Reisberg, B., Ferris, S., & Franssen, E. (1985). An ordinal functional assessment tool for Alzheimer's type dementia. *Hospital and Community Psychiatry, 36,* 593–595.

Ritchie, K., Artero, S., & Touchon, J. (2001). Classification criteria for mild cognitive impairment: A population based validation study. *Neurology, 56,* 37–42.

Rizzo, M., McGehee, D., Dawson, J., & Anderson, S. (2001). Simulated car crashes at intersections in drivers with Alzheimer disease. *Alzheimer Disease and Associated Disorders, 15*(1), 10–20.

Rizzo, M., Reinach, S., McGehee, D., & Dawson, J. (1997). Simulated car crashes and crash predictors in drivers with Alzheimer disease. *Archives of Neurology, 54*(5), 545–551.

Roth, L., Meisel, A., & Lidz, C. (1977). Tests of competency to consent to treatment. *American Journal of Psychiatry, 134,* 279–284.

Royall, D. R. (2003, April). Personal communication.

Royall, D. R., Cordes, J. A. N., & Polk, M. (1998). CLOX: An executive clock drawing task. *Journal of Neurology, Neurosurgery, and Psychiatry, 64*(5), 588–594.

Royall, D. R., Chiodo, L., & Polk, M. (2000). Correlates of disability among elderly retirees with "subclinical" cognitive impairment. *Journal of Gerontology: Medical Sciences, 55A*(9), M541–M546.

Royall, D. R., Cordes, J., & Polk, M. (1997). Executive control and the comprehension of medical information by elderly retirees. *Experimental Aging Research, 23,* 301–313.

Rubenstein, L. Z., Schairer, C., Wieland, G. D., & Kane, R. (1984). Systematic biases in functional status assessment of elderly adults: Effects of different data sources. *Journal of Gerontology, 39*(6), 686–691.

Sager, M. A., Dunham, N. C., Schwantes, A., Mecum, L., Halverson, K., & Harlowe, D. (1992). Measurement of activities of daily living in hospitalized elderly: A comparison of self-report and performance-based methods. *Journal of the American Geriatrics Society, 40,* 457–462.

Salthouse, T., & Miles, J. (2002). Aging and time-sharing aspects of executive control. *Memory and Cognition, 30*(4), 572–582.

Sbordone, R. J. (2000). *The executive functions of the brain.* New York: Wiley.

Schaie, K. W. (1996). *Intellectual development in adulthood: The Seattle longitudinal study.* New York: Cambridge University Press.

Sohlberg, M. M., & Mateer, C. A. (1989). Current perspectives in cognitive rehabilitation. In *Introduction to cognitive rehabilitation: Theory and practice* (pp. 3–17). New York: Guilford Press.

Spar, J. E., & Garb, A. (1992). Assessing competency to make a will. *American Journal of Psychiatry, 149,* 169–174.

Spar, J. E., Hankin, M., & Stodden, A. B. (1995). Assessing mental capacity and susceptibility to undue influence. *Behavioral Sciences and the Law, 13,* 391–403.

Spector, W., Katz, S., Murphy, J., & Fulton, J. (1978). The hierarchical relationship between activities of daily living and instrumental activities of daily living. *Journal of Chronic Diseases, 40,* 481–489.

Stern, Y., Hesdorffer, D., Sano, M., & Mayeux, R. (1990). Measurement and prediction of functional capacity in Alzheimer's disease. *Neurology, 40,* 8–14.

Tabert, M. H., Albert, S. M., Borukhova-Milov, L., Camacho, Y., Pelton, G., Liu, X., et al. (2002). Functional deficits in patients with mild cognitive impairment: Prediction of AD. *Neurology, 58,* 758–764.

Tepper, A., & Elwork, A. (1984). Competency to consent to treatment as a psychological construct. *Law and Human Behavior, 8,* 205–223.

Teri, L. (1997). Behavior and caregiver burden: Behavioral problems in patients with Alzheimer disease and its association with caregiver distress. *Alzheimer Disease and Associated Disorders, 11,* S35–S38.

Teunisse, S. (1995). Activities of daily living scales in dementia: Their development and future. In R. Levy & R. Howard (Eds.), *Developments in dementia and functional disorders in the elderly* (pp. 85–95). Philadelphia: Wrightson Biomedical.

Touchon, J., & Ritchie, K. (1999). Prodromal cognitive disorder in Alzheimer's disease. *International Journal of Geriatric Psychiatry, 14,* 556–563.

Trobe, J. D., Waller, P. F., Cook-Flannagan, C. A., Teshima, S. M., & Bieliauskas, L. A. (1996). Crashes and violations among drivers with Alzheimer disease. *Archives of Neurology, 53*(5), 411–416.

Vitaliano, P., Breen, A., Albert, M., Russo, J., & Prinz, P. (1984). Memory, attention, and functional status in community-residing Alzheimer type dementia patients and optimally healthy aged individuals. *Journal of Gerontology, 39*(1), 58–64.

Wadley, V. G., Harrell, L., & Marson, D. C. (2003). Self- and informant report of financial abilities in patients with Alzheimer's disease: Reliable and valid? *Journal of the American Geriatrics Society, 51,* 1621–1626.

Walsh, A. C., Brown, B. B., Kaye, K., & Grigsby, J. (1997). *Mental capacity: Legal and medical aspects of assessment and treatment* (2nd ed.). Deerfield, IL: Clark, Boardman, & Callaghan.

Walton, V. (2002, February 2). Con man sentenced to 20 years. *Birmingham News,* pp. 11A–12A.

West, R. L. (1996). An application of prefrontal cortex function theory to cognitive aging. *Psychological Bulletin, 120*(2), 272–292.

Wiener, J. M., Hanley, R. J., Clark, R., & Van Nostrand, J. F. (1990). Measuring the activities of daily living: Comparisons across national surveys. *Journal of Gerontology: Social Sciences, 45*(6), S229–S237.

Wild, K. V., & Cotrell, V. (2003). Identifying driving impairment in Alzheimer's disease: A comparison of self and observer reports versus driving evaluation. *Alzheimer Disease and Associated Disorders, 17*(1), 27–34.

Willis, S. L. (1996). Everyday cognitive competence in elderly persons: Conceptual issues and empirical findings. *Gerontologist, 36,* 595–601.

Willis, S. L., Allen-Burge, R., Dolan, M. M., Bertrand, R. M., Yesavage, J., & Taylor, J. L. (1998). Everyday problem solving among individuals with Alzheimer's disease. *Gerontologist, 38*(5), 569–577.

Willis, S. L., Jay, G. M., Diehl, M., & Marsiske, M. (1992). Longitudinal change and prediction of everyday task competence in the elderly. *Research on Aging, 14*(1), 68–91.

Wolinsky, F., Callahan, C., Fitzgerald, J., & Johnson, R. (1993). Changes in functional status and the risks of subsequent nursing home placement and death. *Journal of Gerontology: Social Sciences, 48*, S93–S101.

Wolinsky, F., & Johnson, R. (1991). The use of health services by older adults. *Journal of Gerontology: Social Sciences, 46*, 345–357.

Wolinsky, F., & Tierney, W. (1998). Self-rated health and adverse health outcomes: An exploration and refinement of the trajectory hypothesis. *Journal of Gerontology B: Psychological and Social Sciences, 53*(6), S336–S340.

"Woman out $5,300 in two cons." (1996, March 3). *Birmingham News.*

World Health Organization. (1980). *International classification of impairment, disabilities, and handicaps.* Geneva: World Health Organization.

Zimmerman, S. I., & Magaziner, J. (1994). Methodological issues in measuring the functional status of cognitively impaired nursing home residents: Use of proxies and performance-based measures. *Alzheimer Disease and Associated Disorders, 8*(Suppl. 1), S281–S290.

8

Cultural Issues

JENNIFER J. MANLY

During the next few decades, there will be significant changes in the ethnic and racial landscape among the elderly in the United States. These changes suggest that ethnic minority populations will bear an increased share of the economic and social burden associated with diseases that predominantly affect the elderly, such as Alzheimer's disease (AD) and other progressive dementias. The U.S. Census Bureau estimates that the proportion of elders who are white and non-Hispanic will decline from 87% (in 1990) to 67% in 2050. By 2010, the population of Hispanic elders is expected to double from that in 1990 and will be 11 times greater by 2050. Of the 80.1 million elderly projected for 2050, 8.4 million (10.4%) will be black, as compared to 8% of elders in 1990.

The growth in diversity of elders in the United States presents a unique opportunity for neuropsychologists to study the role of race, culture, and ethnicity in recognition, diagnosis, and treatment of age-related cognitive impairment and dementia. Scientists who believe that genetic risk factors differ by race hope that comparison of different ethnic/racial groups residing in the same environment may help to uncover genetic factors responsible for AD. At the same time, cross-cultural dementia research may provide an opportunity to identify different prevalence rates of AD among elderly within the same ethnic group (Osuntokun et al., 1992). For example, a comparative examination of Koreans living in Korea versus those living in Russia and Scandinavia will likely reveal genetically similar people who have been exposed to dramatically different environmental and cultural forces. This research could enhance the search for risk factors because these environmental and cultural forces may affect risk for dementia. Although both approaches are potentially fruitful, cross-cultural research on dementia must contend with the fact that assessments of both cognitive impairment and daily functioning are susceptible to culturally dependent definitions and are quantified by measures that are sensitive to cultural and educational backgrounds.

For illustrative purposes, two case examples are presented below that will be familiar to clinicians practicing in a memory disorders clinic that serves ethnically diverse patients and their families. These vignettes are provided as examples of the dilemmas that neuropsychologists face when evaluating patients from ethnic minorities.

Patient 1 is an 83-year-old retired factory worker with 6 years of schooling. Her husband passed away 3 years ago, and she now lives alone. Her oldest daughter, who visits infrequently but keeps in touch by phone, has arranged for an evaluation after noticing that she had to repeat conversations on several occasions during the last few months. The patient denies any decline in her ability to carry out day-to-day activities, including finances, shopping, navigating around the city and her neighborhood, and keeping up with friends. Patient 1 reports that although she thinks her memory is not as good as it used to be, she does not think that it is interfering with her daily functioning. Born and raised in Cuba, she identifies herself as Hispanic. She attended a one-room rural school in Cuba and worked on a farm on the days she did not attend school. She immigrated to New York City in her late 20s. Although she speaks English "pretty well," she is much more comfortable speaking Spanish, which she uses in her home and with her family and friends. Her score on a translated Folstein Mini-Mental State Examination, which was administered by a bilingual graduate student, was 23/30. She stated the incorrect date (but correctly reported the day of the week, month, year, and season), remembered two of three words after the delay, could not spell *world* backward, made an error on the phrase repetition, omitted a word and misspelled a word on her sentence, and failed the intersecting pentagons copy.

Patient 2 is a 67-year-old lawyer with 19 years of schooling. He is married and lives with his wife. He presents with complaints of memory difficulty over the past year. He states that he is relying more on his wife and secretary to keep track of his appointments, and that he cannot be relied on to remember a short list of groceries in the store. He stated that he has also noticed difficulty learning how to operate a new spreadsheet program on his computer. He reports no problems taking care of other daily activities. His wife and son corroborate that he has had increasing forgetfulness for appointments, but both suggest that he may be a bit depressed since deciding to reduce his busy work schedule and move toward full retirement. Patient 2 identifies himself as African American. He received his elementary and high school education in the integrated public schools of Brooklyn, New York. After attending the City College of New York, he worked in his father's construction business for a few years, then enrolled in the University of Minnesota Law School. He was a senior partner in a thriving practice in New York City for several decades. He is now semiretired, does mostly consulting, and sits on several boards for nonprofit organizations. His score on the Folstein Mini-Mental State Exam was 29/30; he could not recall one of the three words after a delay.

Although Patient 1's daily functioning is not impaired, it is concerning that her daughter has noticed a change in her memory over time. The cognitive screening test reveals a low score, but this performance may be within normal expectations given her age and educational and occupational background. Scores on more sensitive neuropsychological tests will probably also be relatively low, possibly in the impaired range in relation to published norms. Similar to most neuropsychologists in the United States, this neuropsychologist is not likely to speak Spanish and is most comfortable assessing English-speaking patients with English-language tests (Echemendia, Harris, Congett, Diaz, & Puente, 1997). Should the patient be tested in English? If not, the clinician will struggle to find a Spanish language battery that is normed for Caribbean Hispanic elders (rather than Mexican American elders) and also corrected for years of education, which is clearly a factor in this case. The clinician may not have access to a fully trained psychometrist who is able to administer the battery in Spanish.

Patient 2 also presents a dilemma, but for different reasons. He has cognitive complaints that may be related to mood, as suggested by his family, or could be early signs of a degenerative process. Heaton, Miller, and colleagues (Heaton, Miller, Taylor, & Grant, 2004) have recently published norms for African Americans, but it is unclear why these would provide a more appropriate comparison for this patient than norms established for well-educated European Americans, since Patient 2 was educated in mostly European American schools and worked alongside mostly European Americans throughout his career. The screening test suggests that sensitive tests of cognitive ability will be needed to detect a cognitive deficit (if there is one), and that the clinician's expectations for performance will have to be adjusted, given this individual's educational and occupational background.

Practical solutions for these common dilemmas are conspicuously inaccessible, despite the growth of the field of neuropsychology in clinical settings and research domains. In the absence of a substantial scientific body of literature that provides clear guidelines, this chapter presents a discussion of cultural and educational factors that should be considered systematically when assessing cognitive function among elders from ethnic minorities. In fact, I argue that acculturation, quality of education, literacy, and racial socialization are more meaningful and useful background variables to help adjust expectations for neuropsychological test scores and improve specificity of cognitive tests, regardless of race/ethnicity (Table 8.1). The chapter begins with a review of what we know about the rates of AD and dementia within African Americans, Hispanics, Asian/Pacific Islanders, and Native American living in the United States. I then explore the recognition of cognitive impairment in individuals from these populations, including issues of cultural bias in neuropsychological measurement of cognitive functioning and differences in presentation of cognitively impaired elders across ethnic and cultural groups. Within this discussion, I

TABLE 8.1. Background Factors That Influence Neuropsychological Test Performance

I. Culture
   A. Language
      1. Bilingualism
      2. Orthography–phonology consistency
      3. Articulatory time
   B. Acculturation
      1. Years in the United States
      2. Level of exposure to mainstream culture

II. Education
   A. Years of school
   B. Quality of education
      1. Segregation level
      2. Teacher–student ratio
      3. Per-pupil expenditures
      4. Length of school year
   C. Literacy level

III. Racial socialization
   A. Stereotype threat
   B. Perceived racism

use examples from my own work to highlight the issues and make recommendations for future research.

RATES OF AD AND DEMENTIA ACROSS ETHNIC GROUPS

Most U.S.-based studies have focused on comparing rates of dementia or AD among African Americans and Hispanics to rates among European Americans. These studies found higher rates of cognitive impairment, dementia, and AD among ethnic minorities than among European Americans (Prineas et al., 1995). For example, large longitudinal community studies in Northern Manhattan in New York City (Tang et al., 2001) and Indianapolis (Hendrie et al., 1995; Hendrie et al., 2001) reported higher rates of prevalent and incident dementia and AD among African Americans as compared to European Americans, but the Duke Established Populations for Epidemiological Studies of the Elderly (EPESE) project found no differences in frequency of dementia between African Americans and European Americans (Fillenbaum et al., 1998). These studies used National Institute of Neurological and Communicative Disorders and Stroke–Alzheimer's Disease and Related Disorders Associations (NINCDS–ADRDA) criteria, full neurological examinations, and administered extensive neuropsychological batteries; the differences in rates occurred even after correcting for differences in years of education. In addition, the rate of dementia on admission to nursing homes is higher among African American residents than among European American residents (Weintraub et al., 2000); however, findings from studies of long-term outcomes for African American elders with dementia are not consistent. Mortality associated with dementia was found to be higher among African Americans than non-Hispanic European Americans, especially among African American males (Lanska, 1998). However, there were no statistically significant differences in survival from time of entry into the CERAD study of European American and African Americans, after accounting for the effects of age, gender, and severity of dementia (Heyman, Peterson, Fillenbaum, & Pieper, 1996).

The role of immigration and changes in environmental risk factors was examined in several epidemiological studies of elders with Japanese ancestry. The age-standardized prevalence of dementia (using DSM-III criteria) among elderly Japanese American men living in Hawaii (White et al., 1996) was higher than Japanese men living in Japan, which was similar to European populations. The authors suggested that environmental or cultural exposures associated with migration from Japan to Hawaii influenced the development of AD in these Japanese Americans. Similar results were reported in a study of 1,985 Japanese American participants in the Kame project in King County, Washington (Graves et al., 1996). A cross-sectional study of dementia prevalence using the Alzheimer's Disease Diagnostic and Treatment Centers in California found that, as compared to European Americans, Asian Americans had a greater proportion of vascular dementia and lower proportion of AD (Yeo, Gallagher-Thompson, & Lieberman, 1996), similar to studies of Asians in Asia.

It appears that Native Americans have a lower rate of AD than European Americans, but equivalent rates of overall cognitive impairment or dementia. Hendrie et al. (1993) examined 192 Cree living on two reserves in Manitoba, Canada, ages 65 and over, and an age-stratified sample of 241 English-speaking European Canadians living in Winnipeg. Using the Community Screening Interview for Dementia (CSI-D) to screen for cognitive impairment, the authors found a significant difference between the age-adjusted prevalence of AD among the Cree Indians (0.5%) as compared to the European Canadians (3.5%), despite the two groups having an equivalent age-adjusted prevalence of dementia (4.2% in each population).

An interesting study of Cherokee Indians living in northeastern Oklahoma (Rosenberg et al., 1996) used NINCDS–ADRDA criteria to identify 26 people, with AD, ages 65 years and older, and then assessed an equal number of normal controls. The investigators found that as the genetic degree of Cherokee ancestry increased, the frequency of AD decreased. That is, independent of apoE4 allele status, elders with more than 50% genetic Cherokee ancestry were less likely to be in the AD group than the control group. Genetic degree of ancestry for each participant was calculated using genealogical records provided by the Cherokee Nation Tribal Registration Department. A limitation of this study is its case-control design; however, this study represents a more advanced method of examining the relationship of race/ethnicity to disease because the degree of ethnic ancestry was assessed (albeit not though formal genetic analysis), as opposed to classifying individuals into racial groups based on self-report or investigator observation.

Autopsy Confirmation of AD Pathology

Although the exact etiology cannot be definitively determined before an autopsy, there are research criteria for AD and vascular dementia that have been shown to predict the specific pathological determination upon autopsy with up to 90% accuracy. However, the supporting research has involved European American subjects almost exclusively. The research studies cited above showing ethnic differences in rates of AD and dementia use clinical criteria only; they would be greatly enhanced by studies in which autopsies were performed to obtain brain tissue for neuropathological investigation of individuals who were evaluated during life. However, African Americans and other ethnic minorities are less likely to consent to autopsy (Bonner, Darkwa, & Gorelick, 2000; Fillenbaum et al., 1996; Harrell, Callaway, & Powers, 1993). Therefore, there are few published studies comparing the rates of neuropathologically defined AD among different ethnic groups in the United States. The few studies with ethnically diverse samples have found either no racial differences in frequency of AD pathology among those autopsied (Miller, Hicks, D'Amato, & Landis, 1984), or that AD lesions were more prevalent among European Americans than among African Americans (de la Monte, Hutchins, & Moore, 1989). Small sample size is a problem for each of these studies, and because there is a much lower rate of consent for autopsy among African Americans, there may be a selection bias.

One study avoided selection bias by performing a survey of all autopsies on individuals ages 40–70 in the Maryland Chief Medical Examiner's office for an 8-year time period (Sandberg, Stewart, Smialek, & Troncoso, 2001). All died of "non-natural" causes, mostly accidents and homicides. The researchers assessed the prevalence of senile plaques (SPs) and neurofibrillary tangles (NFTs) in three brain areas: the hippocampus, entorhinal cortex, and inferior temporal cortex. In their sample of 138 individuals, 42% were African American and 61% were younger than age 65. NFTs were more common after age 54 and were found mostly in the hippocampus and entorhinal cortex. SPs were less frequent overall but were found mostly in people 75 years and older in the entorhinal cortex and inferior temporal cortex. Prevalence of neuritic plaques was consistently lower in African Americans than in European Americans. Although the authors confirmed that prevalence of mixed SPs and NFTs was strongly correlated with age, there was no evidence that these pathological changes had any differences in frequency by race.

Imaging Evidence

Brain imaging studies that use both structural and functional methods might provide an alternative line of evidence concerning AD pathology, which could support the epidemiological findings of ethnic discrepancies in the disease. However, there are very few studies of structural or functional brain imaging using diverse groups of elders. Studies of African American elders with clinical diagnoses of AD have shown that magnetic resonance imaging (MRI) measurements of hippocampal volume (Sencakova et al., 2001) and qualitative computed tomography (CT) and MRI findings (Charletta, Gorelick, Dollear, Freels, & Harris, 1995) were similar to those reported in other imaging studies of primarily European American patients. One study using MRI and single-photon emission computed tomography (SPECT) showed no major ethnic differences in degree of white matter hyperintensities, ventricle-to-brain ratio, and uptake among 3,301 nondemented community-dwelling elders without a history of stroke or transient ischemic attack (Longstreth et al., 2000). Other research has found a higher prevalence of white matter lesions among nondemented African American elders—a predictable finding, given that cardiovascular risk factors (e.g., hypertension, diabetes) are more common among African Americans (Liao et al., 1997; Lesser et al., 1996).

INTRUMENTATION ISSUES IN DETECTION OF DEMENTIA ACROSS CULTURES

Ethnic Differences and Cognitive Testing

One possible explanation for higher rates of AD and dementia among African Americans and Hispanics is that the neuropsychological tests used to assess cognitive function have not been properly validated for use among ethnic minorities in the United States. Lack of such validation may account for the fact that, based on neuropsychological test performance, ethnic minorities are judged to be cognitively impaired more often than non-Hispanic European American persons. This section reviews studies within and outside the United States that have compared the cognitive test performance of different ethnic groups and (2) describes constructs that might facilitate more sophisticated investigations of ethnic differences in the future.

Use of the standard cutoff of 23 on the Mini-Mental State Examination (MMSE) leads to overdiagnosis of dementia among African Americans, even after controlling for years of education (Bohnstedt, Fox, & Kohatsu, 1994). Racial, ethnic, and cultural differences have been found on MMSE performance and other screening measures before (Mast, Fitzgerald, Steinberg, MacNeill, & Lichtenberg, 2001; Unverzagt, Hall, Torke, & Rediger, 1996) and after adjusting for education (Escobar et al., 1986; Fillenbaum, Hughes, Heyman, George, & Blazer, 1988; Kuller et al., 1998; Salmon et al., 1989; Teresi, Albert, Holmes, & Mayeux, 1999; Welsh et al., 1995).

Difficulties in interpreting cognitive scores among ethnic minority elders are not limited to brief screening instruments; several studies have indicated that ethnic or cultural factors have a substantial effect on neuropsychological batteries (Adams, Boake, & Crain, 1982; Overall & Levin, 1978). Even when ethnic groups are matched on socioeconomic variables, discrepancies in neuropsychological test performance have remained (Jacobs et al., 1997; Kaufman, McLean, & Reynolds, 1988; Manly et al., 1998b; Reynolds, Chastain, Kaufman, & McLean, 1987). Roberts and Hamsher found that neurologically intact European Americans obtained significantly higher scores on a measure of visual naming ability than did neurologically intact African Americans, even after correcting for education level (Roberts & Hamsher, 1984). Several other studies also reported ethnic differences in performance on tests of visual confrontation naming (Carlson, Brandt, Carson, & Kawas, 1998; Ross, Lichtenberg, & Christensen, 1995; Welsh et al., 1995).

Ethnicity-related differences have been reported on measures of nonverbal abilities as well (Bernard, 1989; Brown et al., 1991; Campbell et al., 1996; Heverly, Isaac, & Hynd, 1986; Miller, Bing, Selnes, Wesch, & Becker, 1993). Jacobs et al. (1997) found that Spanish-speaking elders scored significantly lower than age- and education-matched English-speaking elders on a measure of nonverbal abstraction (i.e., the Identities and Oddities subtest from Mattis's Dementia Rating Scale); multiple choice matching and recognition formats of the Benton Visual Retention Test; and measures of category fluency and comprehension. In another study, healthy Spanish-speaking Mexicans and Mexican Americans who lived near a U.S.–Mexico border (*n* = 200) were compared with residents of Madrid, Spain (*n* = 218). After accounting for education, borderland residents obtained significantly lower scores on measures of recognition discriminability for stories and figures, learned fewer details from a story over five trials, and made more perseverative responses on the Wisconsin Card Sorting Task (Artiola i Fortuny, Heaton, & Hermosillo, 1998). There were some interactions between years of education and place of birth, suggesting that among those with high levels of education, borderland and Spanish participants performed similarly on several measures.

Several studies have reported significant differences in performance on neuropsychological test batteries designed to detect dementia among African American and European American elders, despite correcting for years of education, age, occupational attainment, and history of medical conditions such as hypertension and diabetes (Fillenbaum, Heyman, Huber, Ganguli, & Unverzagt, 2001; Manly et al., 1998b; Unverzagt et al., 1996). In contrast, a number of studies has failed to find discrepancies in test performance between racial, ethnic, or cultural groups after participants were matched on years of education (Carlson et al., 1998; Ford, Haley, Thrower, West, & Harrell, 1996), after statistically adjusting for education (Loewenstein, Ardila, Rosselli, & Hayden, 1992; Marcopulos, McLain, & Giuliano, 1997; Mungas, Marshall, Weldon, Haan, & Reed, 1996), or after cut-scores were adjusted for those with low education (Murden, McRae, Kaner, & Bucknam, 1991). However, the statistical power to detect a significant difference in some of these studies was severely limited by small sample sizes of non-white participants. For example, there were no significant ethnic differences among a small number of blacks (*n* = 11) and whites (*n* = 32) with AD on measures of naming, picture vocabulary, verbal abstraction, verbal list learning, and pragmatic language use after controlling for MMSE score and years of education (Ripich, Carpenter, & Ziol, 1997). Another study found that among 18 black and 114 white participants who met NINCDS–ADRDA criteria for AD, there were no significant differences by race on decline in MMSE score over an average 2.5-year period, whereas left-handedness, more years of education, and family history of dementia were associated with more rapid decline (Rasmusson, Carson, Brookmeyer, Kawas, & Brandt, 1996).

Taken together, most previous studies of ethnic group differences in performance on the MMSE and neuropsychological tests have shown that discrepancies between scores of different ethnic groups persist, despite equating groups on other demographics such as age, education, gender, and socioeconomic background. These discrepancies cause attenuated specificity of verbal and nonverbal neuropsychological tests, such that cognitively normal ethnic minorities are more likely than whites to be misdiagnosed as impaired (Ford-Booker et al., 1993; Klusman, Moulton, Hornbostle, Picano, & Beattie, 1991; Stern et al., 1992; Manly et al., 1998b; Welsh et al., 1995). These findings indicate that not all tasks are functionally equivalent (Helms, 1992; Ratcliff et al., 1998). In other words, although performance on a cognitive test may not reflect the same underlying construct across all racial and ethnic groups, many neuropsychologists assume that test scores provide valid indicators of ability regardless of cultural background (Nell, 2000). Although establishing separate test norms for ethnic minorities may help with mis-diagnosis (Miller, Heaton, Kirson, & Grant, 1997), there is variability of educational and cultural experiences within ethnicity that may decrease the accuracy of these norms. Sep-arate norms do not address the variability related to culture, race, and education that un-derlies ethnic group differences on cognitive test performance. It is therefore possible that separate ethnic group norms will create more problems than they solve, lead to increased misunderstanding of racial and ethnic group differences, and become unwieldy to the ev-eryday practitioner. Instead, direct measurement of more meaningful and predictive vari-ables that underlie test performance across cultural groups may serve to increase accuracy of cognitive assessment and the validity of all instruments used to diagnose dementia. In the following sections I review the relationship of cognitive test performance to some of the variables that differ within and between racial and ethnic groups.

Acculturation

Most previous research on ethnicity has classified participants on the basis of physical appearance or self-identified racial/ethnic classification, rather than measuring the cul-tural variables that accompany ethnic group membership. However, as suggested by Helms (1992), specification of the experiential, attitudinal, or behavioral variables that distinguish those belonging to different ethnic groups and that also vary among indi-viduals within an ethnic group, may allow investigators to understand better the under-lying reasons for the relationship between ethnic background and cognitive test perfor-mance.

Level of acculturation is one way in which social scientists have operationalized within-group cultural variability. *Acculturation* is defined as the level at which an individ-ual participates in the values, language, and practices of his or her own ethnic community versus those of the dominant culture (Landrine & Klonoff, 1996; Padilla, 1980). Previous studies have identified ideologies, beliefs, expectations, and attitudes as important com-ponents of acculturation, as well as cognitive and behavioral characteristics such as lan-guage and customs (Berry, 1976; Moyerman & Forman, 1992; Negy & Woods, 1992; Padilla, 1980).

Few studies have examined the relationship of cognitive test performance to within-group ethnic or cultural factors independent of those associated with socioeconomic status. Arnold et al. (Arnold, Montgomery, Castaneda, & Longoria, 1994) found a rela-tionship between Hispanic acculturation and performance on selected tests of the Halstead–Reitan Neuropsycholgical Battery among college students. Artiola et al. (1998) reported that among Mexican and Mexican American residents of a U.S. border region, percentage of life in which individuals lived in the United States was significantly and negatively related to number of words generated on a Spanish oral fluency measure, espe-cially among those with fewer than 8 years of education. In addition, those who spent a larger percentage of their life in the United States made more perseverative errors on the

Wisconsin Card Sorting Test, and bilingualism accounted for a significant amount of variance in performance on a Spanish verbal learning test.

Three studies have explored the relationship of African American acculturation (as measured by the African American Acculturation Scale (Landrine & Klonoff, 1994, 1995) to cognitive test performance. Manly, Miller, et al. (1998) found that among neurologically intact African Americans between the ages of 20 and 65, those who were less acculturated (more traditional) obtained lower scores on measures of general information and naming than more acculturated African Americans. Among elderly residents of northern Manhattan (Manly et al., 1998a), acculturation accounted for a significant amount of variance in several neuropsychological measures assessing verbal and nonverbal abilities, after accounting for age, education, and gender. Among elderly African Americans living in Jacksonville, Florida, acculturation accounted for a significant amount of variance in Verbal IQ (as measured by the Wechsler Adult Intelligence Scale), Boston Naming Test, and delayed recall of stories from the Wechsler Memory Scale—Revised (Lucas, 1998).

Taken together, investigations of acculturation level suggest that there are cultural differences within elders of the same ethnicity that relate to neuropsychological measures of verbal and nonverbal skills, and that accounting for acculturation may improve the accuracy of certain neuropsychological tests. Although previous research has focused on ethnic minority elders in the United States, it is likely that within-group cultural differences are also significant factors in the test performance of American elders who identify themselves as white or Caucasian, as well as ethnic groups outside the United States.

Years of Education, Quality of Education, and Literacy

Extreme differences in educational level are often found between ethnic minorities and European Americans. Illiteracy rates in the United States are highest among people ages 65 and over, but are especially elevated among elders from ethnic minorities (Kirsch, Jungeblut, Jenkins, & Kolstad, 1993). Cross-cultural researchers are therefore challenged to find measures that are sensitive to cognitive impairment across these broad educational backgrounds (Ratcliff et al., 1998). Although it is common for investigators to use covariance, matching procedures, or education-corrected norms in order to "equate" ethnic groups on years of education before interpreting neuropsychological test performance, as discussed above, these techniques ignore ethnic discrepancies in quality of education. Therefore, disparate school experiences could explain why many ethnic minorities obtain lower scores on cognitive measures, even after controlling for years of education. Table 8.2 provides examples of expenditures in selected states for African American and European American schools.

Therefore, even if an investigator "adjusts" for years of school, we cannot assume that the effect of educational experience has been removed from an analysis of ethnic and racial group differences in cognitive test performance. Along with several other authors (Kaufman, Cooper, & McGee, 1997; Loewenstein, Arguelles, Arguelles, & Linn-Fuentes, 1994; Whitfield & Baker-Thomas, 1999), I argue that due to the disparities in quality of education, matching on quantity of formal education does not necessarily mean that the quality of education received by each racial group is comparable. The variable "years of education" systematically differs between African Americans and European Americans (Margo, 1985, 1990; Smith, 1984; Smith & Welch, 1977; Welch, 1973, 1966) and is also related to cognitive test performance. If this variable is not commensurate between racial

TABLE 8.2. Per-Pupil Expenditures by State in 1935

State	Black	White	Ratio
Alabama	17.50	53.18	.33
Florida	17.71	39.80	.45
Maryland	80.63	102.84	.78
Mississippi	13.36	58.61	.23
North Carolina	32.92	51.43	.64
South Carolina	18.62	67.74	.28
Virginia	33.05	63.81	.52
New York		110.97	
Pennsylvania		75.74	

Note. Data from Blose and Caliver (1938).

groups, residual confounding will occur and spurious racial differences will be interpreted, despite matching groups on years of education.

Presence of poor literacy skills among elders is also a particularly relevant issue for neuropsychologists attempting to accurately detect dementia using cognitive measures. Reading level is a very powerful predictor of cognitive test performance, independent of years of education, age, or ethnicity (Ardila, Rosselli, & Rosas, 1989; Lecours et al., 1987; Manly et al., 1999; Matute, Leal, Zaraboso, Robles, & Cedillo, 1997; Reis, Guerreiro, & Castro-Caldas, 1994; Rosselli, Ardila, & Rosas, 1990; Scribner & Cole, 1981; Weiss, Reed, Kligman, & Abayd, 1995). Table 8.3 presents results from one study that suggest that performance on many verbal and nonverbal cognitive measures is more dependent on literacy or reading skills than years of education.

Our group recently reported a study that sought to determine if discrepancies in quality of education could explain differences in cognitive test scores between African American and European American elders matched on years of education (Manly, Jacobs, Touradji, Small, & Stern, 2002). A comprehensive neuropsychological battery was administered to a sample of nondemented African American and non-Hispanic European American participants in an epidemiological study of normal aging and dementia in the Northern Manhattan community. The Reading Recognition subtest from the Wide Range Achievement Test—Version 3 (WRAT-3) was used as an estimate of quality of education. African American elders obtained significantly lower scores than European Americans on measures of word-list learning and memory, figure memory, abstract reasoning, fluency, and visuospatial skill, even though the groups were matched on years of education. However, after adjusting the cognitive test scores for WRAT-3 performance, the overall effect of race was greatly reduced, and racial differences on all tests (except category fluency and a drawing measure) became nonsignificant. Reading score also attenuated the effect of race after accounting for an estimate of test-wiseness. *Test-wiseness* is defined as the ability to use the format and characteristics of a test to achieve a high score (Scruggs & Lifson, 1985), and the use of deduction and item cues to answer questions (Borrello & Thompson, 1985). This finding suggests that "years of education" is an inadequate measure of the educational experience among multicultural elders, and that adjusting for quality of education may improve the specificity of certain neuropsychological measures across racial groups.

These findings suggest that the full extent of discrepancies in educational experience between African Americans and European Americans is not captured by a simple "high-

TABLE 8.3. Proportion of Variance (R^2) in Neuropsychological Test Scores Accounted for by Demographics, Acculturation, and Reading Level

Test	Sex	Age	Years of education	Acculturation	WRAT-3 reading
Learning/memory					
SRT total recall	.001	.119	.166	.025	.189
SRT delayed recall	.001	.070	.091	.011[a]	.105
BVRT recognition memory	.004	.059	.156	.029	.211
Orientation					
MMSE Orientation	.004	.012[a]	.020	.002[a]	.033
Abstract reasoning					
WAIS-R Similarities Raw	.005	.062	.319	.060	.386
DRS Identities and Oddities	.005	.045	.077	.003[a]	.088
Language					
Boston Naming	.002	.025	.148	.048	.316
Letter fluency	.002	.046	.216	.030	.401
Category fluency	.000	.070	.184	.028	.184
BDAE repetition	.004	.010[b]	.057	.028	.095
BDAE Comprehension	.003	.012[a]	.096	.017	.137
Visuospatial ability					
Rosen Drawing	.001	.036	.071	.039	.116
BVRT matching	.001	.058	.139	.038	.156

Note. R^2 is the proportion of variance in the neuropsychological test score that is accounted for by the independent variable in a simple linear regression. All values shown had a p value less than .01 except that none of the R^2 values for the effect of sex was significant below the .01 level; and those values followed by [a] did not reach significance. SRT, Selective Reminding Test; BVRT, Benton Visual Retention Test; MMSE, Mini-Mental Status Examination; WAIS-R, Wechsler Adult Intelligence Scale—Revised; DRS, Dementia Rating Scale; BDAE, Boston Diagnostic Aphasia Examination. From Manly, Byrd, Touradji, and Stern (2004). Copyright 2004 by. Reprinted by permission.

est grade attained" variable, and thus residual confounding may explain findings of "persistent" race effects after matching groups on years of education. Nevertheless, despite the clear improvement in specificity that is provided by adjusting cognitive test scores for differences in educational experience across ethnic groups, some researchers caution against controlling for educational variables in studies of dementia, because low education may itself be a risk factor for disease.

The relationship of educational experience to performance on neuropsychological tests among normal elders across ethnic groups is a clear and consistent finding. However, because education has been found to be a risk factor for diagnosis of dementia (Kawas & Katzman, 1999), there is remaining controversy about whether norms that correct for years of school will reduce the sensitivity of cognitive tests. A higher prevalence of AD and dementia among elders with low levels of education has been found in Brazil (Caramelli et al., 1997), China (Hill et al., 1993; Zhang et al., 1990), Finland (Sulkava et al., 1985), France (Dartigues et al., 1991), Italy (Bonaiuto et al., 1990; Prencipe et al., 1996), Israel (Bowirrat, Treves, Friedland, & Korczyn, 2001; Korczyn, Kahana, & Galper, 1991), the Netherlands (Ott et al., 1995), Sweden (Fratiglioni et al.,

1991; Gatz et al., 2001), and the United States (Callahan et al., 1996; Gurland et al., 1995; Mortel, Meyer, Herod, & Thornby, 1995). Higher incidence of dementia has been demonstrated in several studies (Evans et al., 1993; Letenneur, Commenges, Dartigues, & Barberger-Gateau, 1994; Stern et al., 1994; White et al., 1994). Cognitive decline appears to be faster (Stern, Albert, Tang, & Tsai, 1999; Teri, McCurry, Edland, Kukull, & Larson, 1995; Unverzagt, Hui, Farlow, Hall, & Hendrie, 1998) and associated with increased risk of mortality (Stern, Tang, Denaro, & Mayeux, 1995) among highly educated minorities with AD, which suggests that the level of brain pathology is greater by the time well-educated individuals show the signs of dementia.

The studies reviewed in the previous section focus on the relationship of schooling and literacy to dementia or AD, specifically. But there is also evidence for a role of education in age-related cognitive decline. Several studies of normal aging have reported more rapid cognitive and functional decline among individuals with lower educational attainment (Albert et al., 1995; Butler, Ashford, & Snowdon, 1996; Chodosh, Reuben, Albert, & Seeman, 2002; Christensen et al., 1997; Farmer, Kittner, Rae, Bartko, & Regier, 1995; Finley, Ardila, & Roselli, 1991; Snowdon, Ostwald, & Kane, 1989). These studies suggest that the same education-related factors that delay the onset of dementia also allow individuals to cope more effectively with changes encountered in normal aging.

Cognitive reserve has been suggested as the mechanism for the link between low education and higher risk of dementia and cognitive decline observed in these studies (Mortimer, 1988; Satz et al., 1993; Stern, 2002). Reserve, or the brain's ability to tolerate the effects of dementia pathology, may result from native ability or from the effects of lifetime experience. Years of education may serve as a proxy for reserve, whether it results from ability or experience. In passive models of reserve (Stern, 2002), education would be a proxy for the brain's capacity (synaptic density or complexity) to tolerate either gradual or sudden insult. In active models, years of education would be an indicator of the brain's ability to compensate for pathology through more efficient use of existing cognitive networks or recruitment of alternate networks.

This paradox serves to illuminate the difficulty in comparing cultural groups with disparate backgrounds. However, there are cases in which the relationship between education and risk for cognitive impairment or dementia is weakened or absent. Two large international studies of incident dementia found that illiteracy or low levels of education did not increase the risk of AD among elders in India (Chandra et al., 2001) and West Africa (Hall et al., 1998; Hendrie, 2001). In fact, these studies had the lowest prevalence and incidence rates of dementia observed to date, despite the fact that a large proportion of the populations lacked formal schooling or literacy training. Reserve is measured by proxy variables (e.g., years of education, occupational level, or IQ measures), but there are a number of ways in which cultural, racial, and economic factors may affect the predictive power of these proxies. First, it is possible that race- and income-based limits on educational opportunity weaken the relationship between years of education and native ability, leading to underestimates of the relationship between education and cognitive decline. Minorities with strong intellectual abilities may not achieve high levels of academic or occupational status because their opportunities are limited by societal forces (e.g., racism, poverty) unrelated to their native intellect or drive to succeed. Although such individuals may be powerful or influential in their community, their abilities may not be reflected in years of schooling or traditional indicators of occupational status. Alternatively, rather than a reflection of innate ability, years of education could be an indicator of lifetime experiences that change the brain during childhood or adult life and thus create a reserve against disease pathology. However, use of years of education to represent a direct effect of experience on the brain or cognition is also problematic when employed among ethnic minorities and immigrants, due to the increased discordance between years of education and quality of education among these groups.

It is possible that literacy could be a more sensitive proxy for reserve than years of education because it more accurately reflects the quality of the educational experience provided to elders from ethnic minorities. In addition, literacy could be a more accurate reflection of native ability because it does not assume that all individuals get the same amount of learning from a certain grade level; the fact that some excel more than others or seek learning outside of school would be reflected in measurements of literacy.

I and my colleagues designed a study to explore the relationship of literacy level to change in memory ability over time among an ethnically diverse sample of English-speaking nondemented elders (Manly, Touradji, Tang, & Stern, 2003). Specifically, we wanted to determine if literacy was a stronger predictor of memory decline (and thus a more sensitive indicator of reserve) than years of education or racial/ethnic classification, although each of these variables was expected to influence baseline scores. We focused our analyses on immediate and delayed recall measures from a verbal word-list learning task, because these measures are sensitive to age-related memory decline and the earliest signs of AD. Among 136 participants, we found that elders with both high and low levels of literacy declined in immediate and delayed memory over time; however, the decline was more rapid among low-literacy elders (see Figure 8.1). This finding suggests that high literacy skills do not provide complete preservation of memory skills but rather a slowing of age-related decline. All participants had normal overall cognition and were functioning normally in daily activities; thus the decline in memory scores was not associated with the onset of a dementia disorder. There were no interactions between time and either years of education or ethnicity, suggesting that in this diverse population of normal elders, literacy was the most sensitive predictor of memory decline. Unlike many prior studies that examined the relationship of education to dementia or normal aging, we did not find that low education (less than 12 years) was a risk factor for cognitive decline. This finding may be

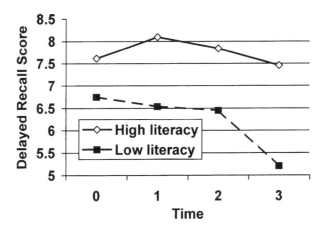

FIGURE 8.1. Change in Selective Reminding Test delayed recall score over time. From Manly, Touradji, Tang, and Stern (2003). Copyright 2003 by Taylor & Francis Publishers. Reprinted by permission.

related to the fact that we required that participants remain nondemented at each visit; future research that allows for significant decline in function and cognition after the baseline visit may more closely mirror the findings of previous studies.

Racial Socialization

Level of comfort and confidence during the testing session may also vary among participants from ethnic minorities. The concept of stereotype threat has been described as a factor that may attenuate the performance of participants from racial minorities on cognitive tests. *Stereotype threat* refers to the experience of diverting attention from the task at hand to the concern that one's performance will confirm a negative stereotype about one's group. Steele and his colleagues (Steele, 1997; Steele & Aronson, 1995) demonstrated that when a test consisting of difficult verbal Graduate Record Examination (GRE) items was described as measuring intellectual ability, black undergraduates at Stanford University performed worse than SAT-score-matched white undergraduates. However, when the same test was described as a "laboratory problem-solving task" or a "challenging test" that was unrelated to intellectual ability, the scores of black students matched those of white students. Researchers have also reported that when gender differences in math ability were invoked, stereotype threat undermined performance of women on math tests (Spencer, Steele, & Quinn, 1999) and white males (when comparisons to Asians were invoked; Aronson et al., 1999). The role of stereotype threat in neuropsychological test performance of blacks and Hispanics has not been investigated to date. In addition, it is likely that the salience of negative stereotypes differs among racial minorities and therefore that stereotype threat will likely affect some test takers more than others. Investigation of the experiential, social, and cultural variables that affect vulnerability to stereotype threat should be examined.

Linguistic Issues

Translation of English-Language Tests

Clinicians and researchers sometimes erroneously assume that instruments are equivalent across populations as long as the test is administered in the native language of the individual. However, literal translation may not produce items with comparable word frequency and/or salience in each culture, resulting in different difficulty levels (Loewenstein et al., 1994; Sano et al., 1997; Teng, 1996). In addition, idiosyncrasies of different languages may introduce problems in equating certain tests. For example, when asked to name as many animals as possible in a minute, Hispanics produce fewer exemplars than do Vietnamese. This discrepancy can be explained by the fact that most animal names in Spanish are multisyllabic, whereas most animal names in Vietnamese are monosyllabic (Kempler, Teng, Dick, Taussig, & Davis, 1998).

Translators of cognitive measures must use extreme caution and proper methods to adapt measures into another language. Artiola i Fortuny and Mullaney describe several examples of Spanish versions of tests that include syntactic, lexical, and spelling errors (Artiola i Fortuny & Mullaney, 1997). These authors also suggest that investigators consult only those who possess native fluency and in-depth knowledge of the culture before attempting to translate a measure. The accuracy of translated and adapted instruments should be checked following established guidelines (Artiola i Fortuny & Mullaney, 1997;

Brislin, 1970, 1980; Loewenstein et al., 1994; van de Vijver & Hambleton, 1996). Researchers and clinicians must also develop standards to determine in which language bilingual individuals should be assessed (Ponton et al., 1996).

Translation of measures is not simply a linguistic issue; measures must be culturally equivalent as well. That is, it must be determined whether the use of a particular test format to assess the cognitive skill of interest is equally valid within every culture in which the test will be administered (Teng, 1996; Teng et al., 1994).

Norms

Investigators must be aware that the published norms for tests administered in English are not necessarily valid when the tests are administered in another language. Further, they should not assume that test norms can be applied to distinct populations simply because they share a language. For example, there is evidence that several instruments developed in Spanish-speaking countries may not be functionally or linguistically equivalent when used among Spanish speakers in the United States (Artiola i Fortuny et al., 1998). Similarly, tests and norms developed among a particular group of immigrants to the United States (e.g., Cuban Americans) may not be valid among other groups in the United States who share a language (e.g., Dominicans or Puerto-Ricans; Loewenstein et al., 1994).

Use of Interpreters

Misinterpretation is a serious threat to the reliability and validity of testing. Family members are often used as translators, even though they are not likely to be objective. And even translators who are reasonably fluent in both languages may not be familiar with many of the terms used in neuropsychological testing (Ardila, Rosselli, & Puente, 1994; LaCalle, 1987). Increasing the linguistic diversity of testers and improving the availability of objective translators are thus worthwhile goals for investigators; when these accuracy measures are not feasible, the possibility of misinterpretation must be taken into consideration when interpreting results.

CONCLUSIONS

Issues

Racial and ethnic diversity is increasing among people ages 65 years and older in the United States. The share of the economic and social burden associated with AD and other dementias borne by African Americans will increase accordingly. Neuropsychologists are fundamentally unprepared for this growth in cultural, racial, and linguistic diversity, because neuropsychological tests have poor specificity among minority populations and cannot reliably differentiate subtle impairment associated with the early stages of dementia from the effects of normal aging. Misdiagnosis of dementia is thus more likely among cognitively normal ethnic minorities as compared to non-Hispanic whites.

The most prevalent attempt to address these issues has been to develop separate norms by race. Although this is a reasonable first step toward reducing misdiagnosis among culturally and linguistically different groups, separate norms have many disadvantages. The use of these norms depends on racial classifications that change over time and on geographical region, and is invalid for the growing number of individuals who self-identifies within multiple categories. Racial norms also lump together people who vary enormously in linguistic, geographic, economic, and educational experiences and level of exposure to European American culture.

A growing number or researchers has taken another approach to improving the specificity and utility of cognitive tests among elders from ethnic minorities. This work has identified aspects of cultural and educational experience that could be explicitly measured, related these variables to test performance both cross-sectionally and longitudinally, and included cultural experience, literacy, English fluency, and quality of education. Regardless of ethnicity, these factors may explain significant variance in test scores and thus should guide adjustment of expectations of performance before interpreting scores, just as age, years of education, and gender are now routinely taken into account. This work promises to expand our knowledge about the role of culture in affecting cognition and the aging brain.

Recommendations

Before administration of cognitive tests begins, a valid assessment of elders from ethnic minorities depends on the ability of neuropsychologists, psychometrists, and translators to reflect true understanding of cultural variations in interaction style and allow for sufficient time for thorough explanations of procedures and expanded inquiry regarding functional status. Even if these procedures and knowledge are in place, interpretation of neuropsychological test scores remains difficult, especially in cases of MCI or "questionable dementia," due to the poor specificity of our measures when used with individuals from minorities. Considering the relative lack of published research on this topic, any practical recommendations must be cautious and preliminary. Based on the work reviewed in this chapter, I advise the following:

- Do not assume to know an elder's race/ethnicity, because this is a self-identified classification. Ask patients/participants to self-identify their ethnicity, as well as to choose race and ethnicity in a manner consistent with the U.S. Census.
- Evaluate cultural experience by asking about the neighborhood characteristics of where patients/participants grew up and where they currently live.
- Evaluate educational experience by inquiring not only about highest grade achieved, but also obtain details about where primary, secondary, and post-secondary schooling took place, the segregation level of the school, whether it was a one-room school or had a low student–teacher ratio, and whether it was a rural or suburban/urban school.
- Become familiar with the number of years of compulsory education in the area where the elder was educated. For example, in Mexico, the length of compulsory education was raised from 6 to 9 years in 1992, but this requirement is enforced differentially throughout the country.
- Assess reading level using the WRAT-3 for English speakers and the Word Accentuation Test (Del Ser, Gonzalez-Montalvo, Martinez-Espinosa, Delgado-Villapalos, & Bermejo, 1997) for Spanish speakers.
- Among bilinguals or multilinguals, assess proficiency in each language.
- If you are using measures translated into another language, use published measures with large normative samples of individuals who are culturally similar to the patient/participant. For example, published norms for Mexican elders living in

Mexico may not be appropriate for an elderly second-generation Mexican American.

- Testing of non-English and non-native English speakers presents an ethical challenge for many English-speaking clinicians (Harris & Cullum, 2002). Although there are many complex considerations regarding this issue, it is clear that neuropsychologists should not use an interpreter (trained or untrained) to simply translate items and administer them to the patient/participant.
- Cautiously use the best available norms from the appropriate population.

Future Research Directions

The clear course for researchers is to measure and validate variables for which race/ethnicity serves as a proxy and determine the relationship of these variables with cognitive function. Some of these variables, such as quality of education, appear to have reliable and clinically significant relationships to test score across ethnic groups. However, it is possible that other variables will have a minimal effect on cognitive test performance or will be more meaningful in one cultural group but not others. Nevertheless, future studies can be designed to further our knowledge of the influence of cultural variables on test performance, as well as risk for cognitive decline over time, if they successfully address the following issues:

- Recruitment of large numbers of nondemented ethnic minority elders into longitudinal research studies is a difficult task, with which neuropsychologists have had spotty success, at best. Nevertheless, responsible and comprehensive examination of the relationships discussed in this chapter is impossible without achieving this goal.
- Research on the effect of region of birth and current residence on cognitive function among ethnic minorities is badly needed but will require large multisite cohorts. This is true not only of elders born in the United States, but also for immigrant groups. For example, it is of practical and theoretical interest to characterize any differences that may exist among Spanish speakers by nationality.
- Although biological and genetic factors may play a role in ethnic differences in cognitive test performance, these variables must be measured rather than assumed. Furthermore, the critical period during which chronic diseases such as diabetes and hypertension have an effect on cognitive function in aging and risk for dementia may occur in midlife; therefore, studies of the relationship of cardiovascular disease and cognitive aging must be longitudinal and enroll ethnically diverse people in their fourth and fifth decades of life.
- Finally, the role of race and racism on neuropsychological test performance of elders from ethnic minorities should not be ignored or underestimated. The operationalization of racism for the purposes of research on cognitive function among elders is an area that is ripe for exploration.

REFERENCES

Adams, R. L., Boake, C., & Crain, C. (1982). Bias in a neuropsychological test classification related to age, education and ethnicity. *Journal of Consulting and Clinical Psychology, 50*, 143–145.

Albert, M. S., Jones, K., Savage, C. R., Berkman, L., Seeman, T., Blazer, D., et al. (1995). Predictors of cognitive change in older persons: MacArthur studies of successful aging. *Psychology and Aging, 10,* 578–589.

Ardila, A., Rosselli, M., & Puente, A. E. (1994). *Neuropsychological evaluation of the Spanish speaker.* New York: Plenum Press.

Ardila, A., Rosselli, M., & Rosas, P. (1989). Neuropsychological assessment in illiterates: Visuo-spatial and memory abilities. *Brain and Cognition, 11,* 147–166.

Arnold, B. R., Montgomery, G. T., Castaneda, I., & Longoria, R. (1994). Acculturation and performance of Hispanics on selected Halstead–Reitan neuropsychological tests. *Assessment, 1,* 239–248.

Aronson, J., Lustina, M. J., Good, C., Keough, K., Steele, C. M., & Brown, J. (1999). When White men can't do math: Necessary and sufficient factors in stereotype threat. *Journal of Experimental and Social Psychology, 35,* 29–46.

Artiola i Fortuny, L., Heaton, R. K., & Hermosillo, D. (1998). Neuropsychological comparisons of Spanish-speaking participants from the U.S.–Mexico border region versus Spain. *Journal of the International Neuropsychological Society, 4,* 363–379.

Artiola i Fortuny, L., & Mullaney, H. (1997). Neuropsychology with Spanish speakers: Language use and proficiency issues for test development. *Journal of Clinical and Experimental Neuropsychology, 19,* 615–622.

Bernard, L. (1989). Halstead–Reitan neuropsychological test performance of black, Hispanic, and white young adult males from poor academic backgrounds. *Archives of Clinical Neuropsychology, 4,* 267–274.

Berry, J. W. (1976). *Human ecology and cognitive style.* New York: Sage-Halstead.

Blose, D., & Caliver, A. (1938). *Statistics of the Education of Negroes, 1933–34 and 1935–36. United States Office of Education, Bulletin No. 13.* Washington, DC: United States Government Printing Office.

Bohnstedt, M., Fox, P. J., & Kohatsu, N. D. (1994). Correlates of Mini-Mental Status Examination scores among elderly demented patients: The influence of race–ethnicity. *Journal of Clinical Epidemiology, 47,* 1381–1387.

Bonaiuto, S., Rocca, W. A., Lippi, A., Luciani, P., Turtu, F., Cavarzeran, F., et al. (1990). Impact of education and occupation on prevalence of Alzheimer's disease (AD) and multi-infarct dementia (MID) in Appignano, Macerata Province, Italy. *Neurology, 40*(Suppl. 1), 346.

Bonner, G. J., Darkwa, O. K., & Gorelick, P. B. (2000). Autopsy recruitment program for African Americans. *Alzheimer's Disease and Associated Disorders, 14,* 202–208.

Borrello, G. M., & Thompson, B. (1985). Correlates of selected test-wiseness skills. *Journal of Experimental Education, 53,* 124–128.

Bowirrat, A., Treves, T., Friedland, R. P., & Korczyn, A. D. (2001). Prevalence of Alzheimer's type dementia in an elderly Arab population. *European Journal of Epidemiology, 8,* 119–123.

Brislin, R. W. (1970). Back-translation for cross-cultural research. *Journal of Cross-Cultural Psychology, 1,* 185–216.

Brislin, R. W. (1980). Translation and content-analysis of oral and written material. In H. C. Triandis & J. W. Berry (Eds.), *Handbook of cross-cultural psychology, Vol. 2: Methodology* (pp. 389–444). Boston: Allyn & Bacon.

Brown, A., Campbell, A., Wood, D., Hastings, A., Lewis-Jack, O., Dennis, G., et al. (1991). Neuropsychological studies of blacks with cerebrovascular disorders: A preliminary investigation. *Journal of the National Medical Association, 83,* 217–229.

Butler, S. M., Ashford, J. W., & Snowdon, D. A. (1996). Age, education, and changes in the Mini-Mental State Exam scores of older women: Findings from the Nun Study. *Journal of the American Geriatrics Society, 44,* 675–681.

Callahan, C. M., Hall, K. S., Hui, S. L., Musick, B. S., Unverzagt, F. W., & Hendrie, H. C. (1996). Relationship of age, education, and occupation with dementia among a community-based sample of African Americans. *Archives of Neurology, 53,* 134–140.

Campbell, A., Rorie, K., Dennis, G., Wood, D., Combs, S., Hearn, L., et al. (1996). Neuropsychological assessment of African Americans: Conceptual and methodological considerations. In

R. Jones (Ed.), *Handbook of tests and measurement for black populations* (Vol. 2, pp. 75–84). Berkeley, CA: Cobb & Henry.

Caramelli, P., Poissant, A., Gauthier, S., Bellavance, A., Gauvreau, D., Lecours, A. R., et al. (1997). Educational level and neuropsychological heterogeneity in dementia of the Alzheimer type. *Alzheimer Disease and Associated Disorders, 11,* 9–15.

Carlson, M. C., Brandt, J., Carson, K. A., & Kawas, C. H. (1998). Lack of relation between race and cognitive test performance in Alzheimer's disease. *Neurology, 50,* 1499–1501.

Chandra, V., Pandav, R., Dodge, H. H., Johnston, J. M., Belle, S. H., DeKosky, S. T., et al. (2001). Incidence of Alzheimer's disease in a rural community in India: The Indo–U.S. study. *Neurology, 57,* 985–989.

Charletta, D., Gorelick, P. B., Dollear, T. J., Freels, S., & Harris, Y. (1995). CT and MRI findings among African-Americans with Alzheimer's disease, vascular dementia, and stroke without dementia. *Neurology, 45,* 1456–1461.

Chodosh, J., Reuben, D. B., Albert, M. S., & Seeman, T. E. (2002). Predicting cognitive impairment in high-functioning community-dwelling older persons: MacArthur Studies of Successful Aging. *Journal of the American Geriatrics Society, 50,* 1051–1060.

Christensen, H., Korten, A. E., Jorm, A. F., Henderson, A. S., Jacomb, P. A., Rodgers, B., et al. (1997). Education and decline in cognitive performance: Compensatory but not protective. *International Journal of Geriatric Psychiatry, 12,* 323–330.

Dartigues, J. F., Gagnon, M., Michel, P., Letenneur, L., Commenges, D., Barberger-Gateau, P., et al. (1991). Le programme de recherche paquid sur l'epidemiologie de la demence methodes et resultats initiaux [The Paquid research program on the epidemiology of dementia: Methods and initial results]. *Revue Neurologique (Paris), 147,* 225–230.

de la Monte, S. M., Hutchins, G. M., & Moore, G. W. (1989). Racial differences in the etiology of dementia and frequency of Alzheimer lesions in the brain. *Journal of the National Medical Association, 81,* 644–652.

Del Ser, T., Gonzalez-Montalvo, J.-I., Martinez-Espinosa, S., Delgado-Villapalos, C., & Bermejo, F. (1997). Estimation of premorbid intelligence in Spanish people with the Word Accentuation Test and its application to the diagnosis of dementia. *Brain and Cognition, 33,* 343–356.

Echemendia, R. J., Harris, J. G., Congett, S. M., Diaz, M. L., & Puente, A. E. (1997). Neuropsychological training and practices with Hispanics: A national survey. *Clinical Neuropsychologist, 11,* 229–243.

Escobar, J. I., Burnam, A., Karno, M., Forsythe, A., Landsverk, J., & Golding, J. M. (1986). Use of the Mini-Mental State Examination (MMSE) in a community population of mixed ethnicity: Cultural and linguistic artifacts. *Journal of Nervous and Mental Disease, 174,* 607–614.

Evans, D. A., Beckett, L. A., Albert, M. S., Hebert, L. E., Scherr, P. A., Funkenstein, H. H., et al. (1993). Level of education and change in cognitive function in a community population of older persons. *Annals of Epidemiology, 3,* 71–77.

Farmer, M. E., Kittner, S. J., Rae, D. S., Bartko, J. J., & Regier, D. A. (1995). Education and change in cognitive function: The epidemiologic catchment area study. *Annals of Epidemiology, 5,* 1–7.

Fillenbaum, G. G., Heyman, A., Huber, M. S., Ganguli, M., & Unverzagt, F. W. (2001). Performance of elderly African American and white community residents on the CERAD neuropsychological battery. *Journal of the International Neuropsychological Society, 7,* 502–509.

Fillenbaum, G. G., Heyman, A., Huber, M. S., Woodbury, M. A., Leiss, J., Schmader, K. E., et al. (1998). The prevalence and 3-year incidence of dementia in older black and white community residents. *Journal of Clinical Epidemiology, 51,* 587–595.

Fillenbaum, G. G., Huber, M. S., Beekly, D., Henderson, V. W., Mortimer, J., Morris, J. C., et al. (1996). The Consortium to Establish a Registry for Alzheimer's Disease (CERAD): Part XIII. Obtaining autopsy in Alzheimer's disease. *Neurology, 46,* 142–145.

Fillenbaum, G. G., Hughes, D. C., Heyman, A., George, L. K., & Blazer, D. G. (1988). Relationship of health and demographic characteristics to Mini-Mental State Examination score among community residents. *Psychological Medicine, 18,* 719–726.

Finley, G. E., Ardila, A., & Roselli, M. (1991). Envejecimento cognitivo en adultos colombianos analfabetos: ¿Una altseasion de patron clasico de envejecimento? [Cognitive aging in illiterate Colombian adults: A reversal of the classical aging pattern?] *Revista Interamericana de Psicologia*, 25, 103–105.

Ford, G. R., Haley, W. E., Thrower, S. L., West, C. A. C., & Harrell, L. E. (1996). Utility of Mini-Mental State Exam scores in predicting functional impairment among White and African American dementia patients. *Journals of Gerontology: Biological Sciences & Medical Sciences*, 51, 185–188.

Ford-Booker, P., Campbell, A., Combs, S., Lewis, S., Ocampo, C., Brown, A., et al. (1993). The predictive accuracy of neuropsychological tests in a normal population of African Americans. *Journal of Clinical and Experimental Neuropsychology*, 15, 64.

Fratiglioni, L., Grut, M., Forsell, Y., Viitanen, M., Grafstrom, M., Holmen, K., et al. (1991). Prevalence of Alzheimer's disease and other dementias in an elderly urban population: Relationship with age, sex and education. *Neurology*, 41, 1886–1892.

Gatz, M., Svedberg, P., Pederson, N. L., Mortimer, J. A., Berg, S., & Johansson, B. (2001). Education and the risk of Alzheimer's disease: Findings from the study of dementia in Swedish twins. *Journals of Gerontology*, 56B, 292–300.

Graves, A. B., Larson, E. B., Edland, S. D., Bowen, J. D., McCormick, W. C., McCurry, S. M., et al. (1996). Prevalence of dementia and its subtypes in the Japanese American population of King County, Washington state: The Kame Project. *American Journal of Epidemiology*, 144, 760–771.

Gurland, B. J., Wilder, D., Cross, P., Lantigua, R., Teresi, J. A., Barret, V., et al. (1995). Relative rates of dementia by multiple case definitions, over two prevalence periods, in three cultural groups. *American Journal of Geriatric Psychiatry*, 3, 6–20.

Hall, K. S., Gureje, O., Gao, S., Ogunniyi, A., Hui, S. L., Baiyewu, O., et al. (1998). Risk factors and Alzheimer's disease: A comparative study of two communities. *Australian and New Zealand Journal of Psychiatry*, 32, 698–706.

Harrell, L. E., Callaway, R., & Powers, R. (1993). Autopsy in dementing illness: Who participates? *Alzheimer's Disease and Associated Disorders*, 7, 80–87.

Harris, J. G., & Cullum, C. M. (2002). Ethical decision making with individuals of diverse ethnic, cultural, and linguistic backgrounds. In S. Bush & M. Drexler (Eds.), *Ethical issues in clinical neuropsychology* (pp. 223–241). Lisse, The Netherlands: Swets & Zeitlinger.

Heaton, R. K., Miller, S. W., Taylor, M. J., & Grant, I. (2004). *Revised comprehensive norms for an expanded Halstead–Reitan Battery: Demographically adjusted neuropsychological norms for African American and Caucasian adults*. Lutz, FL: Psychological Assessment Resources.

Helms, J. E. (1992). Why is there no study of cultural equivalence in standardized cognitive ability testing? *American Psychologist*, 47, 1083–1101.

Hendrie, H. C. (2001). Exploration of environmental and genetic risk factors for Alzheimer's disease: The value of cross cultural studies. *Current Directions in Psychological Science*, 10, 98–101.

Hendrie, H. C., Hall, K. S., Pillay, N., Rodgers, D., Prince, C., Norton, J., et al. (1993). Alzheimer's disease is rare in Cree. *International Psychogeriatrics*, 5, 5–14.

Hendrie, H. C., Ogunniyi, A., Hall, K. S., Baiyewu, O., Unverzagt, F. W., Gureje, O., et al. (2001). Incidence of dementia and Alzheimer disease in 2 communities: Yoruba residing in Ibadan, Nigeria, and African Americans residing in Indianapolis, Indiana. *Journal of the American Medical Association*, 285, 739–747.

Hendrie, H. C., Osuntokun, B. O., Hall, K. S., Ogunniyi, A. O., Hui, S. L., Unverzagt, F. W., et al. (1995). Prevalence of Alzheimer's disease and dementia in two communities: Nigerian Africans and African Americans. *American Journal of Psychiatry*, 152, 1485–1492.

Heverly, L. L., Isaac, W., & Hynd, G. W. (1986). Neurodevelopmental and racial differences in tactile–visual (cross-modal) discrimination in normal black and white children. *Archives of Clinical Neuropsychology*, 1, 139–145.

Heyman, A., Peterson, B., Fillenbaum, G., & Pieper, C. (1996). The Consortium to Establish a Registry for Alzheimer's Disease (CERAD): Part XIV. Demographic and clinical predictors of survival in patients with Alzheimer's disease. *Neurology*, 46, 656–660.

Hill, L. R., Klauber, M. R., Salmon, D. P., Yu, E. S. H., Liu, W. T., Zhang, M., et al. (1993). Functional status, education, and the diagnosis of dementia in the Shanghai survey. *Neurology*, *43*, 138–145.

Jacobs, D. M., Sano, M., Albert, S., Schofield, P., Dooneief, G., & Stern, Y. (1997). Cross-cultural neuropsychological assessment: A comparison of randomly selected, demographically matched cohorts of English- and Spanish-speaking older adults. *Journal of Clinical and Experimental Neuropsychology*, *19*, 331–339.

Kaufman, A. S., McLean, J. E., & Reynolds, C. R. (1988). Sex, race, residence, region, and education differences on the 11 WAIS-R subtests. *Journal of Clinical Psychology*, *44*, 231–248.

Kaufman, J. S., Cooper, R. S., & McGee, D. L. (1997). Socioeconomic status and health in blacks and whites: The problem of residual confounding and the resilience of race. *Epidemiology*, *8*, 621–628.

Kawas, C. H., & Katzman, R. (1999). Epidemiology of dementia and Alzheimer's disease. In R. D. Terry, R. Katzman, S. S. Sisodia, & K. L. Bick (Eds.), *Alzheimer's disease* (pp. 95–116). Philadelphia: Lippincott, Williams & Wilkins.

Kempler, D., Teng, E. L., Dick, M., Taussig, I. M., & Davis, D. S. (1998). The effects of age, education, and ethnicity on verbal fluency. *Journal of the International Neuropsychological Society*, *4*, 531–538.

Kirsch, I. S., Jungeblut, A., Jenkins, L., & Kolstad, A. (1993). *Adult literacy in America: The National Adult Literacy Survey*. National Center for Education Statistics, U.S. Department of Education. Washington, DC: U.S. Government Printing Office.

Klusman, L. E., Moulton, J. M., Hornbostle, L. K., Picano, J. J., & Beattie, M. T. (1991). Neuropsychological abnormalities in asymptomatic HIV seropositive military personnel. *Journal of Neuropsychological and Clinical Neurosciences*, *3*, 422–428.

Korczyn, A. D., Kahana, E., & Galper, Y. (1991). Epidemiology of dementia in Ashkelon, Israel. *Neuroepidemiology*, *10*, 100.

Kuller, L. H., Shemanski, L., Manolio, T., Haan, M., Fried, L., Bryan, N., et al. (1998). Relationship between apoE, MRI findings, and cognitive function in the Cardiovascular Health Study. *Stroke*, *29*, 388–398.

LaCalle, J. J. (1987). Forensic psychological evaluations through an interpreter: Legal and ethical issues. *American Journal of Forensic Psychology*, *5*, 29–43.

Landrine, H., & Klonoff, E. A. (1994). The African American Acculturation Scale: Development, reliability, and validity. *Journal of Black Psychology*, *20*, 104–127.

Landrine, H., & Klonoff, E. A. (1995). The African American Acculturation Scale II: Cross-validation and short form. *Journal of Black Psychology*, *21*, 124–152.

Landrine, H., & Klonoff, E. A. (1996). *African American acculturation: Deconstructing race and reviving culture*. Thousand Oaks, CA: Sage.

Lanska, D. J. (1998). Dementia mortality in the United States: Results of the 1986 National Mortality Followback Survey. *Neurology*, *50*, 362–367.

Lecours, A. R., Mehler, J., Parente, M. A., Caldeira, A., Cary, L., Castro, M. J., et al. (1987). Illiteracy and brain damage: 1. Aphasia testing in culturally contrasted populations (control subjects). *Neuropsychologia*, *25*, 231–245.

Lesser, I. M., Smith, M. W., Wohl, M., Mena, R. N., Mehringer, C. M., & Lin, K. M. (1996). Brain imaging, antidepressants, and ethnicity: Preliminary observations. *Psychopharmacology Bulletin*, *32*, 235–242.

Letenneur, L., Commenges, D., Dartigues, J. F., & Barberger-Gateau, P. (1994). Incidence of dementia and Alzheimer's disease in elderly community residents of south-western France. *International Journal of Epidemiology*, *23*, 1256–1261.

Liao, D., Cooper, L., Cai, J., Toole, J., Bryan, N., Burke, G., et al. (1997). The prevalence and severity of white matter lesions, their relationship with age, ethnicity, gender, and cardiovascular disease risk factors: The ARIC Study. *Neuroepidemiology*, *16*, 149–162.

Loewenstein, D. A., Ardila, A., Rosselli, M., & Hayden, S. (1992). A comparative analysis of functional status among Spanish- and English-speaking patients with dementia. *Journals of Gerontology*, *47*, 389–394.

Loewenstein, D. A., Arguelles, T., Arguelles, S., & Linn-Fuentes, P. (1994). Potential cultural bias in the neuropsychological assessment of the older adult. *Journal of Clinical and Experimental Neuropsychology, 16,* 623–629.

Longstreth, W. T., Jr., Arnold, A. M., Manolio, T. A., Burke, G. L., Bryan, N., Jungreis, C. A., et al. (2000). Clinical correlates of ventricular and sulcal size on cranial magnetic resonance imaging of 3,301 elderly people. The Cardiovascular Health Study, Collaborative Research Group. *Neuroepidemiology, 19,* 30–42.

Lucas, J. A. (1998). Acculturation and neuropsychological test performance in elderly African Americans. *Journal of the International Neuropsychological Society, 4,* 77.

Manly, J. J., Byrd, D., Touradji, P., & Stern, Y. (2004). Acculturation, reading level, and neuropsychological test performance among African American elders. *Applied Neuropsychology, 11,* 37–46.

Manly, J. J., Jacobs, D. M., Sano, M., Bell, K., Merchant, C. A., Small, S. A., et al. (1999). Effect of literacy on neuropsychological test performance in nondemented, education-matched elders. *Journal of the International Neuropsychological Society, 5,* 191–202.

Manly, J. J., Jacobs, D. M., Sano, M., Bell, K., Merchant, C. A., Small, S. A., et al. (1998a). African American acculturation and neuropsychological test performance among nondemented community elders. *Journal of the International Neuropsychological Society, 4,* 77.

Manly, J. J., Jacobs, D. M., Sano, M., Bell, K., Merchant, C. A., Small, S. A., et al. (1998b). Cognitive test performance among nondemented elderly African Americans and whites. *Neurology, 50,* 1238–1245.

Manly, J. J., Jacobs, D. M., Touradji, P., Small, S. A., & Stern, Y. (2002). Reading level attenuates differences in neuropsychological test performance between African American and White elders. *Journal of the International Neuropsychological Society, 8,* 341–348.

Manly, J. J., Miller, S. W., Heaton, R. K., Byrd, D., Reilly, J., Velasquez, R. J., et al. (1998). The effect of African-American acculturation on neuropsychological test performance in normal and HIV positive individuals. *Journal of the International Neuropsychological Society, 4,* 291–302.

Manly, J. J., Touradji, P., Tang, M.-X., & Stern, Y. (2003). Literacy and memory decline among ethnically diverse elders. *Journal of Clinical and Experimental Neuropsychology, 5,* 680–690.

Marcopulos, B. A., McLain, C. A., & Giuliano, A. J. (1997). Cognitive impairment or inadequate norms: A study of healthy, rural, older adults with limited education. *Clinical Neuropsychologist, 11,* 111–131.

Margo, R. A. (1985). *Disenfranchisement, school finance, and the economics of segregated schools in the United States South, 1880–1910.* New York: Garland.

Margo, R. A. (1990). *Race and schooling in the South, 1880–1950: An economic history.* Chicago: University of Chicago Press.

Mast, B. T., Fitzgerald, J., Steinberg, J., MacNeill, S. E., & Lichtenberg, P. A. (2001). Effective screening for Alzheimer's disease among older African Americans. *Clinical Neuropsychologist, 15,* 196–202.

Matute, E., Leal, F., Zaraboso, A., Robles, A., & Cedillo, C. (1997). Influence of literacy level on stick constructions in non-brain-damaged subjects. *Journal of the International Neuropsychological Society, 3,* 32.

Miller, E. N., Bing, E. G., Selnes, O. A., Wesch, J., & Becker, J. T. (1993). The effects of sociodemographic factors on reaction time and speed of information processing. *Journal of Clinical and Experimental Neuropsychology, 15,* 66.

Miller, F. D., Hicks, S. P., D'Amato, C. J., & Landis, J. R. (1984). A descriptive study of neuritic plaques and neurofibrillary tangles in an autopsy population. *American Journal of Epidemiology, 120,* 331–341.

Miller, S. W., Heaton, R. K., Kirson, D., & Grant, I. (1997). Neuropsychological (NP) assessment of African Americans. *Journal of the International Neuropsychological Society, 3,* 49.

Mortel, K. F., Meyer, J. S., Herod, B., & Thornby, J. (1995). Education and occupation as risk factors for dementia of the Alzheimer and ischemic vascular types. *Dementia, 6,* 55–62.

Mortimer, J. A. (1988). Do psychosocial risk factors contribute to Alzheimer's disease? In A. S. Henderson & J. H. Henderson (Eds.), *Etiology of dementia of Alzheimer's type* (pp. 39–52). Chichester, UK: Wiley.

Moyerman, D. R., & Forman, B. D. (1992). Acculturation and adjustment: A meta-analytic study. *Hispanic Journal of Behavioral Sciences, 14,* 163–200.

Mungas, D., Marshall, S. C., Weldon, M., Haan, M., & Reed, B. R. (1996). Age and education correction of Mini-Mental State Examination for English- and Spanish-speaking elderly. *Neurology, 46,* 700–706.

Murden, R. A., McRae, T. D., Kaner, S., & Bucknam, M. E. (1991). Mini-Mental State Exam scores vary with education in blacks and whites. *Journal of the American Geriatrics Society, 39,* 149–155.

Negy, C., & Woods, D. J. (1992). The importance of acculturation in understanding research with Hispanic-Americans. *Hispanic Journal of Behavioral Sciences, 14,* 224–247.

Nell, V. (2000). *Cross cultural neuropsychological assessment: Theory and practice.* Mahwah, NJ: Erlbaum.

Osuntokun, B. O., Hendrie, H. C., Ogunniyi, A. O., Hall, K. S., Lekwauwa, U. G., Brittain, H. M., et al. (1992). Cross-cultural studies in Alzheimer's disease. *Ethnicity and Disease, 2,* 352–357.

Ott, A., Breteler, M. M., van Harskamp, F., Claus, J. J., van der Cammen, T. J., Grobbee, D. E., et al. (1995). Prevalence of Alzheimer's disease and vascular dementia: Association with education. The Rotterdam study [see comments]. *British Medical Journal, 310,* 970–973.

Overall, J. E., & Levin, H. S. (1978). Correcting for cultural factors in evaluating intellectual deficit on the WAIS. *Journal of Clinical Psychology, 34,* 910–915.

Padilla, A. M. (1980). *Acculturation: Theory, models, and some new findings.* Boulder, CO: Westview Press.

Ponton, M. O., Satz, P., Herrera, L., Ortiz, F., Urrutia, C. P., Young, R., et al. (1996). Normative data stratified by age and education for the Neuropsychological Screening Battery for Hispanics (NeSBHIS): Initial report. *Journal of the International Neuropsychological Society, 2,* 96–104.

Prencipe, M., Casini, A. R., Ferretti, C., Lattanzio, M. T., Fiorelli, M., & Culasso, F. (1996). Prevalence of dementia in an elderly rural population: Effects of age, sex, and education. *Journal of Neurology, Neurosurgery, and Psychiatry, 60,* 628–633.

Prineas, R. J., Demirovic, J., Bean, J. A., Duara, R., Gomez-Marin, O., Loewenstein, D. A., et al. (1995). Assessing the prevalence of Alzheimer's disease in three ethnic groups. South Florida Program on Aging and Health. *Journal of the Florida Medical Association, 82,* 805–810.

Rasmusson, D. X., Carson, K. A., Brookmeyer, R., Kawas, C., & Brandt, J. (1996). Predicting rate of cognitive decline in probable Alzheimer's disease. *Brain and Cognition, 31,* 133–147.

Ratcliff, G., Ganguli, M., Chandra, V., Sharma, S., Belle, S., Seaberg, E., et al. (1998). Effects of literacy and education on measures of word fluency. *Brain and Language, 61,* 115–122.

Reis, A., Guerreiro, M., & Castro-Caldas, A. (1994). Influence of educational level of non brain-damaged subjects on visual naming capacities. *Journal of Clinical and Experimental Neuropsychology, 16,* 939–942.

Reynolds, C. R., Chastain, R. L., Kaufman, A. S., & McLean, J. E. (1987). Demographic characteristics and IQ among adults: Analysis of the WAIS-R standardization sample as a function of the stratification variables. *Journal of School Psychology, 23,* 323–342.

Ripich, D. N., Carpenter, B., & Ziol, E. (1997). Comparison of African-American and white persons with Alzheimer's disease on language measures. *Neurology, 48,* 781–783.

Roberts, R. J., & Hamsher, K. D. (1984). Effects of minority status on facial recognition and naming performance. *Journal of Clinical Psychology, 40,* 539–545.

Rosenberg, R. N., Richter, R. W., Risser, R. C., Taubman, K., Prado-Farmer, I., Ebalo, E., et al. (1996). Genetic factors for the development of Alzheimer disease in the Cherokee Indian. *Archives of Neurology, 53,* 997–1000.

Ross, T. P., Lichtenberg, P. A., & Christensen, B. K. (1995). Normative data on the Boston Naming Test for elderly adults in a demographically diverse medical sample. *Clinical Neuropsychologist, 9,* 321–325.

Rosselli, M., Ardila, A., & Rosas, P. (1990). Neuropsychological assessment in illiterates: II. Language and praxic abilities. *Brain and Cognition, 12*, 281–296.

Salmon, D. P., Riekkinen, P. J., Katzman, R., Zhang, M. Y., Jin, H., & Yu, E. (1989). Cross-cultural studies of dementia: A comparison of Mini-Mental State Examination performance in Finland and China. *Archives of Neurology, 46*, 769–772.

Sandberg, G., Stewart, W., Smialek, J., & Troncoso, J. C. (2001). The prevalence of the neuropathological lesions of Alzheimer's disease is independent of race and gender. *Neurobiology of Aging, 22*, 169–175.

Sano, M., Mackell, J. A., Ponton, M., Ferreira, P., Wilson, J., Pawluczyk, S., et al. (1997). The Spanish Instrument Protocol: Design and implementation of a study to evaluate treatment efficacy instruments for Spanish-speaking patients with Alzheimer's disease. The Alzheimer's Disease Cooperative Study. *Alzheimer's Disease and Associated Disorders, 11*(Suppl. 2), 57–64.

Satz, P., Morgenstern, H., Miller, E. N., Selnes, O. A., McArthur, J. C., Cohen, B. A., et al. (1993). Low education as a possible risk factor for cognitive abnormalities in HIV-1: Findings from the Multicenter AIDS Cohort Study (MACS). *Journal of Acquired Immune Deficiency Syndromes, 6*, 503–511.

Scribner, S., & Cole, M. (1981). *The psychology of literacy.* Cambridge, MA: Harvard University Press.

Scruggs, T. E., & Lifson, S. A. (1985). Current conceptions of test-wiseness: Myths and realities. *School Psychology Review, 14*, 339–350.

Sencakova, D., Graff-Radford, N. R., Willis, F. B., Lucas, J. A., Parfitt, F., Cha, R. H., et al. (2001). Hippocampal atrophy correlates with clinical features of Alzheimer disease in African Americans. *Archives of Neurology, 58*, 1593–1597.

Smith, J. P. (1984). Race and human capital. *American Economic Review, 4*, 685–698.

Smith, J. P., & Welch, F. (1977). Black–white male wage ratios: 1960–1970. *American Economic Review, 67*, 323–328.

Snowdon, D. A., Ostwald, S. K., & Kane, R. L. (1989). Education, survival and independence in elderly Catholic sisters, 1936–1988. *American Journal of Epidemiology, 130*, 999–1012.

Spencer, S. J., Steele, C. M., & Quinn, D. M. (1999). Stereotype threat and women's math performance. *Journal of Experimental and Social Psychology, 35*, 4–28.

Steele, C. M. (1997). A threat in the air: How stereotypes shape intellectual identity and performance. *American Psychologist, 52*, 613–629.

Steele, C. M., & Aronson, J. (1995). Stereotype threat and the intellectual test performance of African Americans. *Journal of Personality and Social Psychology, 69*, 797–811.

Stern, Y. (2002). What is cognitive reserve? Theory and research application of the reserve concept. *Journal of the International Neuropsychological Society, 8*, 448–460.

Stern, Y., Albert, S., Tang, M.-X., & Tsai, W.-Y. (1999). Rate of memory decline in AD is related to education and occupation: Cognitive reserve? *Neurology, 53*, 1942–1947.

Stern, Y., Andrews, H., Pittman, J., Sano, M., Tatemichi, T., Lantigua, R., et al. (1992). Diagnosis of dementia in a heterogeneous population: Development of a neuropsychological paradigm-based diagnosis of dementia and quantified correction for the effects of education. *Archives of Neurology, 49*, 453–460.

Stern, Y., Gurland, B., Tatemichi, T. K., Tang, M. X., Wilder, D., & Mayeux, R. (1994). Influence of education and occupation on the incidence of Alzheimer's disease. *Journal of the American Medical Association, 271*, 1004–1010.

Stern, Y., Tang, M. X., Denaro, J., & Mayeux, R. (1995). Increased risk of mortality in Alzheimer's disease patients with more advanced educational and occupational attainment. *Annals of Neurology, 37*, 590–595.

Sulkava, R., Wikstrom, J., Aromaa, A., Raitasalo, R., Lahtinen, V., Lahtela, K., et al. (1985). Prevalence of severe dementia in Finland. *Neurology, 35*, 1025–1029.

Tang, M. X., Cross, P., Andrews, H., Jacobs, D. M., Small, S., Bell, K., et al. (2001). Incidence of AD in

African-Americans, Caribbean Hispanics, and Caucasians in northern Manhattan. *Neurology*, 56, 49–56.

Teng, E. L. (1996). Cross-cultural testing and the Cognitive Abilities Screening Instrument. In G. Yeo & D. Gallagher-Thompson (Eds.), *Ethnicity and the dementias* (pp. 77–85). Washington, DC: Taylor & Francis.

Teng, E. L., Hasegawa, K., Homma, A., Imai, Y., Larson, E., Graves, A., et al. (1994). The Cognitive Abilities Screening Instrument (CASI): A practical test for cross-cultural epidemiological studies of dementia. *International Psychogeriatrics*, 6, 45–58.

Teresi, J. A., Albert, S. M., Holmes, D., & Mayeux, R. (1999). Use of latent class analyses for the estimation of prevalence of cognitive impairment and signs of stroke and Parkinson's disease among African-American elderly of central Harlem: Results of the Harlem Aging Project. *Neuro-epidemiology*, 18, 309–321.

Teri, L., McCurry, S. M., Edland, S. D., Kukull, W. A., & Larson, E. B. (1995). Cognitive decline in Alzheimer's disease: A longitudinal investigation of risk factors for accelerated decline. *Journals of Gerontology: Biological Sciences and Medical Sciences*, 50A, M49–M55.

Unverzagt, F. W., Hall, K. S., Torke, A. M., & Rediger, J. D. (1996). Effects of age, education and gender on CERAD neuropsychological test performance in an African American sample. *Clinical Neuropsychologist*, 10, 180–190.

Unverzagt, F. W., Hui, S. L., Farlow, M. R., Hall, K. S., & Hendrie, H. C. (1998). Cognitive decline and education in mild dementia. *Neurology*, 50, 181–185.

van de Vijver, F., & Hambleton, R. K. (1996). Translating tests: Some practical guidelines. *European Psychologist*, 1, 89–99.

Weintraub, D., Raskin, A., Ruskin, P. E., Gruber-Baldini, A. L., Zimmerman, S. I., Hebel, J. R., et al. (2000). Racial differences in the prevalence of dementia among patients admitted to nursing homes. *Psychiatric Services*, 51, 1259–1264.

Weiss, B. D., Reed, R., Kligman, E. W., & Abyad, A. (1995). Literacy and performance on the Mini-Mental State Examination. *Journal of the American Geriatrics Society*, 43, 807–810.

Welch, F. (1966). Measurement of the quality of education. *American Economic Review*, 56, 379–392.

Welch, F. (1973). Black–white differences in returns to schooling. *American Economic Review*, 63, 893–907.

Welsh, K. A., Fillenbaum, G., Wilkinson, W., Heyman, A., Mohs, R. C., Stern, Y., et al. (1995). Neuropsychological test performance in African-American and white patients with Alzheimer's disease. *Neurology*, 45, 2207–2211.

White, L., Katzman, R., Losonczy, K., Salive, M., Wallace, R., Berkman, L., et al. (1994). Association of education with incidence of cognitive impairment in three established populations for epidemiological studies of the elderly. *Journal of Clinical Epidemiology*, 47, 363–374.

White, L., Petrovitch, H., Ross, G. W., Masaki, K. H., Abbott, R. D., Teng, E. L., et al. (1996). Prevalence of dementia in older Japanese-American men in Hawaii: The Honolulu–Asia Aging Study. *Journal of the American Medical Association*, 276, 955–960.

Whitfield, K. E., & Baker-Thomas, T. (1999). Individual differences in aging minorities. *International Journal of Aging and Human Development*, 48, 73–79.

Yeo, G., Gallagher-Thompson, D., & Lieberman, M. (1996). Variations in demetia characteristics by ethnic category. In G. Yeo & D. Gallagher-Thompson (Eds.), *Ethnicity and the dementias* (pp. 21–30). Washington DC: Taylor & Francis.

Zhang, M., Katzman, R., Salmon, D., Jin, H., Cai, G., Wang, Z., et al. (1990). The prevalence of dementia and Alzheimer's disease in Shanghai, China: Impact of age, gender and education. *Annals of Neurology*, 27, 428–437.

9

Feedback

JOANNE GREEN

This chapter describes a critical phase in neuropsychological evaluation: the provision of feedback concerning the findings and implications of the testing. Guidelines of the American Psychological Association assert that individuals taking tests have a right to receive prompt and comprehensible feedback describing their test results (American Psychological Association, 1998), and part of the psychologist's responsibility is to ensure that such feedback is provided. Conducting a successful feedback session requires considerable expertise and skill, combining understanding of neuropsychological assessment with clinical skills derived from psychotherapeutic techniques. The quality of this feedback and the manner in which it is provided can be critical in determining the extent to which the outcomes of the assessment phase are translated into effective treatment plans.

The chapter begins by describing objectives and purposes for providing feedback, then describes common stages in the feedback process and offers guidelines for transversing these stages. Finally, therapeutic issues important to the feedback process are discussed.

PURPOSES FOR PROVIDING FEEDBACK

Providing feedback concerning the outcomes of a neuropsychological evaluation is often challenging, particularly when the patient is an older adult. The usual complexities of interacting with a patient are complicated by the special issues that face older adults, possibly including the onset of a devastating illness, the loss of independence, and the involvement of other family members in their care. While dealing with these issues, a number of important goals must be accomplished, usually in a limited amount of time.

Specific objectives of the feedback follow:

1. To specify the patient's neuropsychological strengths and weaknesses.
2. To explain how these strengths and weaknesses contribute to the memory, cognitive, personality, and other behavioral changes that have been observed.

223

3. To describe possible explanations for the changes, particularly in terms of neuro-logical, medical, psychiatric, or other disorders that might be contributing to the changes.

4. To identify any follow-up evaluations necessary for better identifying underlying disorders.

5. To discuss treatments likely to be effective for these disorders.

6. To determine whether treatments such as cognitive training or therapeutic support are needed to contribute to the patient's health, independence, safety, and comfort.

7. To identify those psychological issues affecting both the patient and involved family members or friends that may emerge from, or be exacerbated by, the patient's illness, and to begin planning interventions for addressing these.

Accomplishing these objectives requires not only understanding of neuropsychological assessment but also application of therapeutic skills that facilitate the patient and family's ability to process the information being presented during the session. A successful feedback session is dynamic, interactive, and often emotionally charged, particularly in the case of older patients who may feel threatened by anticipated changes in their lifestyle or level of independence. The neuropsychologist may find it necessary to manage not only the emotional responses of the patient and others, but also his or her own reactions to the issues facing them.

Despite these challenges, the extent to which feedback is provided to the patient and the quality of that feedback are critical in determining the usefulness of the overall evaluation. A successful feedback session can motivate both the patient and involved family members and friends to develop a new, more productive perspective for managing the difficulties they have been facing. After being presented with possible reasons for behavioral changes as well as treatment alternatives, the patient and family frequently feel empowered to develop more productive strategies for managing what was previously a distressing and confusing situation. The feedback session can also be critical in helping the patient feel better about him- or herself. Patients experiencing change in memory and cognition are vulnerable to negative self-concepts, such as feeling "stupid," "crazy," or "lazy." Naming and explaining the patient's experiences during the feedback session can have major therapeutic benefits in helping the patient to reorganize his or her self-concept (Finn & Tonsager, 1992). The session can help reframe a negative self-concept by clarifying that behavioral and mood changes are related to a definable and treatable disorder, not to undesirable personality traits.

STAGES IN PROVIDING FEEDBACK

Deciding How to Provide Feedback

During the clinical interview at the beginning of the assessment, alternative approaches to providing feedback are discussed with the patient. One issue of particular importance with older patients is specifying who will receive feedback. To avoid compromising principles of confidentiality, it is usually advisable for the neuropsychologist to suggest that both the patient and members of his or her support system be informed of the test findings. This permission is particularly important in the case of patients who are suspected of having significant neuropsychological dysfunction and who do not have a legal guardian. In most cases, patients will agree to sign a consent form allowing their test results to be shared with specified family members, friends, or professionals involved in their care.

Ideally, the neuropsychologist provides the feedback during a follow-up session occurring several weeks after the assessment report has been completed. Because the neuropsychologist fully understands the assessment, this approach increases the likelihood that the findings and their implications are presented in a comprehensible framework, and that follow-up services and treatment alternatives are pursued.

Ideally, both the patient and significant persons in his or her support system attend the feedback session, which typically includes family members and perhaps close friends or companions. The presence of involved family members or friends is particularly important for patients with significant neuropsychological dysfunction who may have difficulty remembering the content of the session. It is advisable that the feedback session include all individuals who are significantly involved in supporting the patient. If the major members of the patient's support system are present, then the neuropsychologist can help resolve any differences of opinion, address individual questions, and facilitate the interaction between patient and his or her support system. From a practical point of view, meeting simultaneously with the patient and his or her support system may avoid the need for additional meetings and phone conversations with individuals who did not attend the feedback session.

In reality, however, in-person feedback sessions with the neuropsychologist sometimes do not occur, or occur in only a highly abbreviated fashion. There are several reasons for this unfortunate reality. A major factor is the current health care environment, which does not necessarily support the provision of feedback by the psychologist who performed the assessment. Managed health care and other organizations often either do not allow reimbursement for feedback sessions or provide very limited reimbursement, encouraging the psychologist to perform only brief sessions that may not allow sufficient time for the outcomes of the assessment to be fully explained and processed.

In addition, some professionals and consumers of neuropsychological services incorrectly view neuropsychological assessment as a "procedure" similar to a medical procedure such as a blood test or an electroencephalogram. This perception implies that the findings consist of test scores that can be interpreted simply as "normal" or "abnormal" and grossly oversimplifies the outcomes of the evaluation and their potential implications for helping the patient. One aspect of the psychologist's responsibility during the feedback session is to educate others concerning the richness of both qualitative and quantitative data gathered during the evaluation and their relevance to a multitude of issues that may affect the patient.

Direct feedback from the neuropsychologist may be impractical if the patient is in frail health, lives at some distance from the psychologist's office, cannot afford additional costs, or wants to minimize appointments because he or she has to depend on a working adult child or friend for transportation. In these cases, several alternatives are common and practical. One possibility is that feedback be provided by another professional (most typically, an internist, neurologist, or psychiatrist) who is experienced with neurobehavioral disorders and is involved with the patient's ongoing care and treatment. Feedback by another professional can be highly effective when that professional is committed to the continued care of the patient and when the neuropsychological evaluation is presented within the context of other diagnostic tests (e.g., blood or other laboratory tests, brain imaging). An advantage to this approach is that the physician is able to prescribe any other necessary medical treatments.

If the patient chooses to receive feedback from another professional, it is particularly important that the neuropsychologist clearly communicate the neuropsychological findings. Ideally, that clinician should have a copy of the final report. The neuropsychologist may also want to speak directly with the clinician to stress issues that may affect the feedback session, such as the patient's or family's awareness of the patient's deficits, and psychological issues (e.g., defensiveness, a history of difficult family dynamics) that may affect the involved individuals' abilities to pursue treatment recommendations. If feedback is provided by another professional, the patient can be encouraged to contact the neuropsychologist later if he or she would like additional information concerning the neuropsychological findings.

To avoid additional appointments or costs, patients often request telephone feedback. This is generally a less desirable alternative because it limits the interaction between the patient and the neuropsychologist and reduces the opportunity for the neuropsychologist to monitor patient and family reactions, possibly decreasing the likelihood that recommended outcomes of the evaluation will be pursued. In some cases, however, telephone feedback may be the only practical alternative. In these cases, it is recommended that feedback be provided during a scheduled conference call that includes both the patient and an involved family member or friend. This format is particularly important for patients experiencing significant neuropsychological dysfunction. Both the time and the duration of the conference call can be established in advance, similar to formalizing these variables for an in-person feedback session. To the extent that this is possible, recommended practices for conducting in-person feedback sessions can be followed. Because the facial and bodily reactions cannot be observed, it is important to query those involved frequently by asking questions such as, "How does what we've just discussed seem to you?" "To make sure that we're communicating, can you summarize what I've just tried to explain?" "How are you feeling right now?"

It is not uncommon for patients or family members to request that they be mailed a copy of the report. Although they are legally entitled to the report, this practice may not be in the patient's best interests for a number of reasons. Patients are vulnerable to adverse emotional reactions if they misinterpret the technical language of the report or the test findings. Without the encouragement of the neuropsychologist, they may be less motivated to pursue follow-up evaluations and the treatment recommendations described in the report.

In most cases, patients can be persuaded that it is best for them to receive feedback from a person qualified to interpret the report. However, if they insist on receiving written findings of the evaluation, then it is often acceptable to prepare a letter summarizing the results and recommendations of the evaluation, rather than sending the full evaluation report. The neuropsychologist can talk with the patient briefly by phone after the letter has been received to answer any questions that may have arisen.

Preparing the Assessment Report

The assessment report is the basis for feedback to the patient. It becomes part of the patient's medical records and may be reviewed by a variety of professionals helping the patient, including physicians, therapists, and possibly attorneys. Thus it is critical that the report be clear, well organized, readable, and relevant to the referral question and the issues facing the patient. Because the report may be read by the patient or his or her family members, it is important to use nonjudgmental and constructive language, particularly in descriptions of the patient's behavior and the neuropsychologist's overall impression of him or her.

The evaluation report is organized in sections that have been described elsewhere (Green, 2000). These sections generally include the following:

1. The *referral* and *background information* section summarizes the major purposes for the evaluation; the symptoms of concern; relevant medical history, particularly concerning conditions that might be related to the symptoms (e.g., uncontrolled hypertension, previous history of stroke); the patient's educational and occupational history; and the patient's current support system.

2. The *behavioral observations* section describes the patient's behavior during the clinical interview and test administration, including descriptions of his or her awareness of cognitive change, level of effort during testing, emotional tone and range, ability to understand instructions and generate verbal responses, and ability to establish and maintain task sets.

3. The *tests administered* section lists the tests administered during the assessment.

4. The section on *test results* reports the quantitative findings from each test, organized by neuropsychological domains, such as general intellectual function, attention, executive functions, motor behavior, language, visuospatial and visuoconstructive abilities, memory, and affect/personality.

5. The section on *impressions and recommendations* forms an important basis for the feedback session, both in terms of content and organization. This section restates the purpose of the evaluation, followed by a summary of findings relevant to accomplishing that purpose. This includes a summary of the patient's neuropsychological profile, outlining neuropsychological strengths and weaknesses in specific domains as well in specific abilities with a domain. Conclusions relevant to the referral question are indicated. Diagnostic issues are addressed, and recommendations for follow-up evaluations and treatments are suggested. An opinion regarding the adequacy of the patient's current level of support and the need for additional support can be offered. The impression of the patient's competence for performing important functions such as cooking, driving, and managing finances might be suggested.

Focusing the Feedback Session

During the neuropsychological evaluation, a wealth of data concerning the patient's neuropsychological, emotional, and everyday functioning has been gathered and analyzed. Although this information is summarized in the neuropsychological assessment report, it is usually more than can be discussed and understood during the feedback session. Therefore, the neuropsychologist must make some decisions concerning which information will be presented when the patient and family return for feedback.

One important guideline for making this choice is to begin the feedback session by asking the patient and family to summarize, once again, what they hoped to learn from the evaluation, particularly the kind of help they are seeking. Addressing their issues and questions during the session will help ensure that the feedback is useful and directed toward helping the patient and family make future plans. In addition to helping the neuropsychologist determine which feedback will be provided, this initial questioning draws the patient/family into the session and encourages a more interactive process.

It is also important to present any information that might affect the patient's safety, general health, or ability to continue at his or her present level of independence. For example, if the patient is still driving but the test findings indicate that he or she has significant deficits in attention or visuospatial abilities, then it is important that these findings be discussed. If the patient has exhibited evidence of poor judgment, then his or her ability to make financial decisions may be questionable. If the patient has a complex medication regimen but also has impaired memory, then his or her ability to manage this medication regimen is probably poor, and plans for organizing the medications might be discussed.

Describing Neuropsychological Strengths and Weaknesses and Reasons for Change

A major purpose of most neuropsychological evaluations is to quantify the nature of strengths and weaknesses in attention, executive function, language abilities, visuospatial abilities, and memory. During the feedback session, the neuropsychologist clarifies the relative integrity of different neuropsychological domains, mentioning not only relative weaknesses but also relative strengths. It is sometimes a good idea to describe how the conclusions were reached in general terms by comparing the patient's actual test performance to normative data and to expectations concerning his or her characteristic level of functioning. Although some individuals will not totally understand this information, description of the principles adds credibility to the findings and extends patient and family understanding of the neuropsychologist's expertise.

It is a good idea to begin on a positive note by describing the patient's strengths before discussing weaknesses. The relationship of these strengths and weaknesses to the patient's behavioral changes is described. For example, if the family has been confused about why the patient repeats questions or manages his or her medication regimen unreliably, these behaviors may be explained if the patient has significant memory dysfunction. The irresponsible use of money and other unwise behaviors may be explained in terms of a deficit in executive function. It is common for families to become concerned when the patient exhibits decreased activity, such as a lack of interest in previously enjoyable hobbies. It is often important to clarify to what extent this change might reflect a deficit in executive function (e.g., inability to initiate behavior) or the onset of depression.

When describing dysfunction within a neuropsychological domain, it may be important to clarify the nature and severity of the dysfunction, particularly if this information has practical implications for improving the patient's functioning and comfort level. It is usually not sufficient to simply say that "memory" or "visuospatial function" is "impaired." Additional description often has implications for understanding the patient's behavior and for possible compensatory aides. For example, elucidation of the difference between long- and short-term memory can help explain why the patient can remember distant personal history but not recent conversations or the current date. It is often important to explain whether memory dysfunction primarily reflects a deficit in the initial acquisition of new information in memory, in the ability to retain (store) acquired information for longer time intervals, or in the finding (retrieval) of information that is stored in memory. In the first and last cases, characteristic of "subcortical disorders" such as Parkinson's disease, the use of structure, cuing, and repetition at the time of memory acquisition may facilitate both initial registration and retrieval. In the second case, more typical of "cortical" disorders such as Alzheimer's disease (AD), these aides may have less benefit.

When a storage deficit is prominent, description of the severity of this deficit may be helpful. The functioning of patients with a milder storage deficit may be improved if they can remember to record important information in a single small notebook that they carry with them at all times in the same location, for example, in a pant pocket or a handbag. These aides may be less effective for patients with a more severe storage deficit; they may want to ask for help from family members in remembering important information such as when to pay bills or take medications.

Most patient/families also want to gain some idea about the likely cause of the behavioral change. The psychologist can provide some feedback concerning the possible diagnoses, the relative certainty of the different alternatives, and additional information that would be useful in finalizing the diagnosis. For example, when family members are told that the patient's memory dysfunction may reflect AD, they may want to know how this disease is definitively diagnosed and that additional memory decline, in the absence of other illness, increases the likelihood that the patient has the disease. The patient/family may request reading materials or support services related to the disease. The neuropsychologist should be prepared to provide these resources.

In many cases, however, it is advisable that neuropsychologists take a conservative and cautious approach when discussing diagnostic and prognostic issues (Gass & Brown, 1992), particularly when medical or neurological disorders may be involved. It is important not to overstate the conclusiveness of the findings and to indicate clearly that these findings only suggest possible disorders or conditions that may contribute to cognitive dysfunction but do not provide a definitive diagnosis. It is often appropriate for the neuropsychologist to advise the family to seek consultation with a neurologist, psychiatrist, or other physician. These clinicians are often well qualified to make informed and more definitive statements about diagnostic and prognostic issues because of their expertise in interpreting a variety of other tests, including the findings of brain imaging, electroencephalography, and blood tests.

Discussing Treatment Alternatives, Patient Care, and Follow-Up Services

After the nature of and possible reasons for, neuropsychological change have been discussed, the implications of the findings for patient care, follow-up evaluations, and treatment alternatives are addressed. One important issue is the implication of the neuropsychological findings for the quality of the patient's everyday functioning and for his or her competence to continue assuming positions of responsibility. It is important to recognize that the neuropsychological test findings have limited value for directly predicting the quality of everyday functioning (Dunn, Searight, Grisso, Margolis, & Gibbons 1990; Heaton & Pendleton, 1981); other instruments have been specifically designed to assess both activities of daily living and instrumental activities of daily living (see Marson & Hebert, Chapter 7, this volume; Fillenbaum & Smyer, 1981; Katz, Ford, Moskowitz, Jackson, & Jaffee, 1963; Lawton, 1971; Lawton, Moss, Fulcomer, & Kleban 1982; Loewenstein et al., 1981). However, if the patient has significant neuropsychological dysfunction, the neuropsychologist can begin a discussion about the patient's competence for assuming specific responsibilities. These responsibilities may include driving a car, managing financial assets, controlling a firearm, following a medication regimen, maintaining adequate nutrition and personal hygiene, caring for grandchildren, and using a stove. Errors in handling such responsibilities may have grave implications not only for the comfort and health of the patient, but also for the safety of others.

Because they care about the patient and want to plan for his or her future well-being, it is not uncommon for family members to suggest relieving the patient of all responsibilities. This is often an overreaction, except in the case of a patient who has been determined to have severe and global dementia. The neuropsychologist may play an important role in helping the patient and family determine how a balance can be maintained between allowing the patient to remain independent as long as possible and preventing him or her from endangering self or others.

In most cases, the patient's competence to handle each responsibility should be considered separately, with the exception of patients who are determined to be severely and globally demented. Most patients are able to continue to handle some responsibilities but are better relieved of others. The neuropsychological test findings may help the neuropsychologist infer the types of responsibilities in which errors are likely and those which the patient can continue to perform adequately. For example, a patient with an amnestic syndrome is likely to have difficulty performing responsibilities dependent upon consideration of new information, such as the management of investments. However, this patient may still be competent to handle responsibilities dependent upon overlearned skills, such as driving on limited and familiar routes. Consideration of the patient's recent functioning may be helpful. A history of previous mistakes within a specific area of responsibility is often predictive that future errors are likely to occur, particularly for patients diagnosed with dementia. So, for example, if an amnestic patient has already caused minor automobile accidents or has become lost while driving, it is probably unwise for him or her to continue driving (see Marson & Hebert, Chapter 7, this volume).

In some cases, a formal competency evaluation may be necessary, particularly if there is disagreement between the patient and his or her family concerning his or her competence. Competency evaluations are often needed to evaluate continued ability to manage financial and legal affairs or to drive. Issues related to the evaluation of competence, including the need to determine the type of competence to be assessed, the nature of state regulations, and the use of evaluation instruments specific to different aspects of competence have been described elsewhere (Grisso, 1994; Marson & Hebert, Chapter 7, this volume).

Decisions concerning the continued competence to drive are often particularly complex and emotional. Patients who can no longer drive may also become unable to independently perform important activities such as grocery shopping, attending doctor's appointments, and participating in social activities. These changes may represent a major blow to patients' self-esteem and sense of efficacy. On the other hand, unsafe use of a car can easily cause serious injury or even death.

Although older individuals with cognitive dysfunction or dementia are at increased risk for driving poorly and having accidents (Friedland et al., 1988; Hunt et al., 1997; Lucas-Blaustein, Filipp, Dungan, & Tune, 1988), a diagnosis of dementia does not necessarily imply that the patient should stop all driving. Some patients with very mild or mild dementia can continue to drive safely (Kapust & Weintraub, 1992; Hunt, Morris, Edwards, & Wilson, 1993; Hunt et al., 1997; Trobe, Waller, Cook-Flannagan, Teshima, & Bieliauskas, 1996), particularly if they reduce the extent of their driving and confine themselves to familiar, low-traffic routes. However, as cognitive dysfunction or dementia severity increases, the patient is at increased risk for poor driving performance and accidents (Hunt et al., 1993; Hunt et al., 1997; Stutts, Stewart, & Martell, 1998; Tuokko, Hadjistavropoulos, Miller, Horton, & Beattie, 1995). An international consensus conference has recommended that patients with moderate to severe dementia not be allowed to drive (Johansson & Lundberg, 1997).

Variables that may be useful in evaluating the patient's driving safety include the recent driving history, certain neuropsychological findings, and the presence of a movement disorder (Logsdon, Teri, & Larson, 1992). A recent history of driving accidents or near-accidents, episodes of getting lost while driving, or poor judgment may be predictive of unsafe driving in the future. Patients with deficits in attention (particularly visual attention), in visuospatial and visuoconstructive abilities, or in mental speed are at increased risk for accidents (Fox, Bowden, Bashford, & Smith, 1997; Logsdon et al., 1992; Hunt et al., 1993; Lundberg, Hakamies-Blomqvist, Almkvist, & Johansson, 1998; Owsley, Ball, Sloane, Roenker, & Bruni, 1991; Parasuraman & Nestor, 1991, 1993). Patients with movement disorders such as Huntington's or Parkinson's disease are also more likely to drive poorly (Heikkila, Turkka, Korpelainen, Kallanranta, & Summala, 1998; Rebok, Bylsma, Keyl, Brandt, & Folstein, 1995). In some cases, the administration of a formal driving test, available in some medical centers, may be useful in clarifying the patient's continued ability to drive. Even when it is determined that it is likely to be safe for the patient to continue to drive, it is important that his or her driving be monitored carefully and that reassessment occur on a regular basis, particularly if there is evidence of increased cognitive dysfunction.

Another major decision that may be addressed during the feedback session involves the patient's continued ability to remain in his or her current living environment. The patient's response to considering a change is sometimes surprising. On the one hand, some patients who have been living in their own home may already be feeling overwhelmed by this responsibility. They may be relieved by the prospect of moving into an environment that provides more support, such as a retirement community, assisted living facility, or personal care home. However, some patients find it emotionally traumatic to consider moving into an unfamiliar setting. For some, this possibility heightens their awareness that they are approaching the last phase of their life and is perceived as involving difficult choices between many treasured possessions and abandoning rooms filled with happy memories to live in a smaller, unfamiliar space. The anticipation of learning the spatial organization and routines of a new environment may cause considerable anxiety for a patient with even mild dementia. The manner in which the patient has reacted to change in the past may be predictive of how well he or she will adjust to a new living environment. Individuals who have always been flexible and made friends easily are more likely to adapt well to future change.

If it is determined that the patient needs additional support and structure but would prefer not to move, approaches to strengthening his or her support system can be considered. If the support system consists of several individuals, they may benefit from counseling to help determine how different responsibilities will be distributed. For example, if the patient is no longer able to drive, a schedule for taking him or her to the grocery store or providing groceries can be devised. Other social services, such as senior day care or services that provide food (e.g., Meals on Wheels), can also be discussed, and a referral to a social worker familiar with the community's social service resources may be helpful. Ways of restructuring the patient's environment to help maintain his or her independence can be considered. For example, a patient may be able to continue following even a complex medication regimen if someone else organizes the medications and places them in labeled pill boxes that clearly indicate what should be taken and when. A patient may be able to keep better track of his or her own appointments and social engagements if someone else records these on a large calendar displayed in a prominent location, for example, on the refrigerator door. A patient who has caused fires while cooking may be able to continue cooking if he or she can remember to always use a loud timer or to rely on the microwave oven. Alternately, as noted, community resources for providing meals can be considered. For patients requiring considerable care at home, health insurance coverage can be considered. For example, some insurance plans provide in-home nursing care to assist with activities such as dressing and bathing.

In some cases, the patient is advised to seek further medical evaluations, and the neuropsychologist can provide advice on questions that might be addressed. Although the neuropsychologist is not qualified to provide medical treatments, he or she can play an important role in educating the family about what treatments are available. Because most neuropsychologists currently do not have prescriptions privileges, the psychologist must stress that he or she is only providing general information and that it is important for the patient to discuss these issues in greater detail with a physician.

For example, if vascular disease may be playing a role in the patient's cognitive dysfunction and the patient has not undergone brain imaging, then the patient/family might be encouraged to ask their physician whether such a procedure might be helpful. If the patient has not been eating adequately, then the patient/family might be advised to ask the physician whether blood tests have indicated that the patient has a vitamin B_{12} or other nutritional deficiency. For patients likely to have AD, the availability of medications (e.g., donepezil, galantamine, rivastigmine, vitamin E therapy) can be discussed in general terms. For patients likely to be depressed, discussing possible treatments can be a critical first step in determining whether the patient follows through in seeking treatment. Many patients are reluctant to seek treatment for depression, or even admit that they are depressed. If the patient is able to begin discussion of possible treatments with a psychologist that he or she has learned to trust, this rapport increases the likelihood that the patient will follow through on the treatment recommendations.

The neuropsychologist can also provide advice about psychological treatment programs that may be helpful, such as cognitive training or behavior management. Although the neuropsychologist may be specialized in assessment, he or she should be prepared to discuss treatment programs available in his or her region; the more knowledgeable the neuropsychologist is about the goals and advantages of specific programs, the greater the likelihood that further treatment will be pursued. For example, for patients having relatively mild or focal deficits, without generalized neuropsychological dysfunction, cognitive training may help develop relatively preserved abilities. A behavior management program may be helpful in encouraging agitated or aggressive patients to reduce the frequency of these behaviors. These approaches are described in greater detail in Part II of this book.

THERAPEUTIC ISSUES IN PROVIDING FEEDBACK

Therapy Skills Important in Neuropsychological Feedback

The neuropsychologist's clinical skills in interacting with patients and their support system are critical to the success of the feedback session. It is important that the session be interactive, such that all participants feel comfortable asking questions, voicing their concerns, and responding to the neuropsychologist's comments. Maintaining rapport with the patient as well as developing rapport with others attending the session are fundamental. As during the clinical interview and testing, it is important to maintain an alliance with the patient. However, the neuropsychologist's rapport with members of patients' support systems becomes especially critical for patients determined to have significant dementia. For each patient's best interests to be served, the patient and members of the support system must trust and have confidence in the neuropsychologist.

Careful listening and checking ensure that the information is being understood and accepted. In many cases, the language of neuropsychological reports will not be well understood by nonprofessionals. The neuropsychologist should be alert to verbal and nonverbal signs indicating that the feedback is being understood, and may even want to check this understanding by asking questions such as, "To make sure that I've communicated these results clearly to you, would you like to summarize your understanding of what's been described?"

It is important to be sensitive to the kind and amount of information the patient and family are ready to hear and to their reaction to this information. If they have been queried at the beginning of the feedback session concerning their purposes for seeking evaluation and their questions, then their answers can often provide excellent guidance about the kind of feedback that will be most helpful to them. For example, in many cases, they may be prepared to hear circumscribed information, such as a description of the neuropsychological weaknesses that may help explain unusual behaviors, but are not prepared to hear details of how a dementing illness is likely to progress over time, such that the patient ultimately becomes both mentally and physically incompetent. When the diagnosis is AD, some families prefer to obtain detailed information about the effectiveness (or limited effectiveness) of current medication treatments, whereas others prefer to know only that these treatments may help the patient. It is critical that the feedback not be presented in a manner that leaves the family and patient feeling hopeless, overwhelmed, and powerless.

As Knight has discussed, the success of the feedback session may be affected by the psychologist's personal characteristics and concerns (Knight, 1994, 1996). Some neuropsychologists find it difficult to provide feedback because of concerns that they are perceived as the bearer of bad news. Furthermore, although the evaluation may determine that a significant decline has occurred, the neuropsychologist may anticipate that the family expected to receive a more definitive diagnosis for these changes than can, in fact, be provided. The inability to provide a definitive diagnosis may make some neuropsychologists vulnerable to feeling less competent. Such feelings may make it more difficult to plan and lead an effective feedback session.

The neuropsychologist's success in leading a feedback session may also be affected by his or her personal reactions to the patient's condition. Delivery of feedback to a patient may heighten the neuropsychologist's concerns about what the future holds for someone he or she personally cares about, such as an aging parent or other relative. For older neuropsychologists, the feedback session may exacerbate personal issues about age-related changes in physical and psychological abilities and their own need for support in the future.

Neuropsychologists who have such reactions may become aware of their own unconstructive emotional response during the feedback session and may find it necessary to expend considerable internal resources trying to manage their personal feelings. It then becomes more difficult to maintain the professional perspective necessary to attend to the patient and family's reactions and needs. Therefore, it is important for neuropsychologists to be aware of their personal feelings and reactions throughout the evaluation process and to seek any necessary supervision or counseling.

Addressing Interpersonal and Family System Issues

Although neuropsychological evaluation focuses on the evaluation and treatment of an individual patient, family system and interpersonal issues often emerge during the feedback session. The patient usually functions as a member of an interpersonal system that may include a spouse, adult children, close friends, or a companion. The qualities of the interactions between the persons attending the feedback session, as well as the historical roles of each, may be important factors in determining the dynamics and outcome of the session. Knight provides an excellent discussion of how family system issues may impact the feedback session (Knight, 1994, 1996).

Decline in the neuropsychological functioning of an elder member of the family may have implications for the roles and responsibilities of each member of the family system. If an elderly parent who develops dementia has played a major role in nurturing and counseling the rest of the family, perceptions of his or her decreased ability to perform this role may cause a shift in the roles of other family members. Those who have been emotionally dependent upon the patient may experience a psychological crisis and require treatment themselves. In some cases, the family overreacts to the patient's illness and begins to make sudden, drastic changes in family roles, when this may not yet be necessary or appropriate. During the feedback session, it is important that the psychologist reinforce the family's perception of the patient as a family member with an illness, who can still assume important roles and responsibilities within the family.

If the patient needs support and structure, the process of deciding how these will be provided may highlight the nature of interactions between other family members. Discussion of how these responsibilities will be handled may revive longstanding or unspoken conflicts. Alliances and tensions between sibling pairs may be exacerbated. When necessary, family counseling may be suggested.

In many cases, the major responsibility for supporting the patient appears to fall on a single individual, often a spouse or an adult daughter. The patient's primary caregiver may become depressed or overwhelmed when confronted with knowledge of the patient's illness, and the psychologist may offer to meet with the caregiver separately to discuss his or her needs. Brief self-report instruments such as the Zarit Burden Inventory (Zarit, Reever, & Back-Peterson, 1980; Zarit, Tood, & Zarit, 1986) or the Brief Symptom Inventory (Derogatis & Spencer, 1982) may be helpful in assessing the nature and severity of caregiver distress. In their concern for caring for a family member, some caregivers neglect their own well-being, failing to maintain adequate levels of sleep, nutrition, and social activity. They may fail to appreciate that they may be better able to offer support for a longer period of time if they also continue caring for themselves.

A primary caregiver may benefit from an opportunity to talk frankly about his or her feelings concerning the patient's illness, to discuss better approaches for coping with these feelings, and to consider additional sources of support for the patient. If the primary caregiver is a spouse, the extent to which adult children can provide some support can be discussed. It is sometimes the case that the patient's spouse has not revealed the need for additional support to adult children because of the fear of burdening them, when, in fact, the children are very willing to provide some help. Some caregivers benefit from support groups that allow them to share their emotional responses with other caregivers and to work together to develop strategies for dealing with common issues and problems. It should be noted, however, that support groups are not necessarily helpful to all caregivers. For caregivers of patients with mild to moderate cognitive dysfunction, support group discussions of the problems associated with more severe disease may be depressing rather than supportive.

In summary, providing feedback on neuropsychological evaluation is an important and complex phase of helping older patients. Successful feedback requires that the neuropsychologist apply a variety of skills and knowledge, including expertise in principles of assessment, more general therapeutic skills important for interacting with patients and their families, and information about resources available to facilitate the patient's care in the future. If the feedback is accepted and understood, this can be an important transition to effective treatment for the patient in the future.

REFERENCES

American Psychological Association. (1998). *Rights and responsibilities of test takers: Guidelines and expectations*. Washington, DC: Author.

Derogatis, L., & Spencer, P. (1982). *Administration and procedures: Brief symptom checklist*. Baltimore: Johns Hopkins University Press.

Dunn, E., Searight, H., Grisso, T., Margolis, R., & Gibbons, J. (1990). The relation of the Halstead–Reitan Neuropsychological Battery to functional daily living skills in geriatric patients. *Archives of Clinical Neuropsychology*, 5, 103–117.

Fillenbaum, G., & Smyer, M. (1981). The development, validity, and reliability of the OARS Multidimensional Functional Assessment Questionnaire. *Journal of Gerontology*, 36, 428–434.

Finn, S., & Tonsager, M. (1992). Therapeutic effects of providing MMPI-2 test feedback to college students awaiting therapy. *Psychological Assessment*, 4, 278–287.

Fox, G., Bowden, S., Bashford, G., & Smith, D. (1997). Alzheimer's disease and driving: Prediction and assessment of driving performance. *Journal of the American Geriatrics*, 45, 949–953.

Friedland, R., Koss, E., Kumar, A., Gaine, S., Metzler, D., Haxby, J., et al. (1988). Motor vehicle crashes in dementia of the Alzheimer type. *Annals of Neurology*, 24, 782–786.

Gass, C., & Brown, M. (1992). Neuropsychological test feedback to patients with brain dysfunction. *Psychological Assessment*, 4, 272–277.

Green, J. (2000). *Neuropsychological evaluation of the older adult: A clinician's guidebook*. San Diego, CA: Academic Press.

Grisso, T. (1994). Clinical assessments for legal competence of older adults. In M. Storandt & G. VandenBos (Eds.), *Neuropsychological assessment of dementia and depression in older adults: A clinician's guide* (pp. 119–140). Washington, DC: American Psychological Association.

Heaton, R., & Pendleton, M. (1981). Use of neuropsychological tests to predict adult patients' everyday functioning. *Journal of Consulting and Clinical Psychology*, 49, 807–821.

Heikkila, V., Turkka, J., Korpelainen, J., Kallanranta, T., & Summala, H. (1998). Decreased driving ability in people with Parkinson's disease. *Journal of Neurology, Neurosurgery, and Psychiatry*, 64, 325–330.

Hunt, L., Morris, J., Edwards, D., & Wilson, B. (1993). Driving performance in persons with senile dementia of the Alzheimer type. *Journal of the American Geriatrics Society*, 41, 747–752.

Hunt, L., Murphy, C., Carr, D., Duchek, J., Buckles, V., & Morris, J. (1997). Reliability of the Washington University Road Test: A performance-based assessment for drivers with dementia of the Alzheimer type. *Archives of Neurology*, 54, 707–712.

Johansson, K., & Lundberg, C. (1997). The 1994 International Consensus Conference on dementia and driving: A brief report. *Alzheimer's Disease and Related Disorders*, 11(Suppl. 1), 62–69.

Kapust, L., & Weintraub, S. (1992). To drive or not to drive: Preliminary results from road testing of patients with dementia. *Journal of Geriatric Psychiatry and Neurology*, 5, 210–216.

Katz, S., Ford, A., Moskowitz, R., Jackson, B., & Jaffee, M. (1963). Studies of illness in the aged: The

Index of ADL, a standardized measure of biological and psychosocial function. *Journal of the American Medical Association, 185,* 94–99.

Knight, B. (1994). Providing clinical interpretations to older clients and their families. In M. Storandt & G. VandenBos (Eds.), *Neuropsychological assessment of dementia and depression in older adults: A clinician's guide* (pp. 141–154). Washington, DC: American Psychological Association.

Knight, B. (1996). *Psychotherapy with older adults* (2nd ed.). Thousand Oaks, CA: Sage.

Lawton, M. (1971). The functional assessment of elderly people. *Journal of the American Geriatrics Society, 19,* 465–481.

Lawton, M., Moss, M., Fulcomer, M., & Kleban, M. (1982). A research and service oriented multi-level assessment instrument. *Journal of Gerontology, 37,* 91–99.

Loewenstein, D., Amigo, E., Duara, R., Guterman, A., Hurwitz, D., Berkowitz, N., et al. (1981). A new scale for the assessment of functional status in Alzheimer's disease and related disorders. *Journal of Gerontology: Psychological Sciences, 44,* 114–121.

Logsdon, R., Teri, L., & Larson, E. (1992). Driving and Alzheimer's disease. *Journal of General Internal Medicine, 7,* 583–588.

Lucas-Blaustein, M., Filipp, L., Dungan, C., & Tune, L. (1988). Driving in patients with dementia. *Journal of the American Geriatric Society, 36,* 1087–1091.

Lundberg, C., Hakamies-Blomqvist, L., Almkvist, O., & Johansson, K. (1998). Impairments of some cognitive functions are common in crash-involved older drivers. *Accident Analysis and Prevention, 30,* 371–377.

Owsley, C., Ball, K., Sloane, M., Roenker, D., & Bruni, J. (1991). Visual/cognitive correlates of vehicle accidents in older drivers. *Psychology and Aging, 6,* 403–415.

Parasuraman, R., & Nestor, P. (1991). Attention and driving skills in aging and Alzheimer's disease. *Human Factors, 33,* 539–557.

Parasuraman, R., & Nestor, P. (1993). Attention and driving: Assessment in elderly individuals with dementia. *Clinics in Geriatric Medicine, 9,* 377–387.

Rebok, G., Bylsma, F., Keyl, P., Brandt, J., & Folstein, S. (1995). Automobile driving in Huntington's disease. *Movement Disorders, 10,* 778–787.

Stutts, J., Stewart, J., & Martell, C. (1998). Cognitive test performance and crash risk in an older driver population. *Accident Analysis and Prevention, 30,* 337–346.

Trobe, J., Waller, P., Cook-Flannagan, C., Teshima, S., & Bieliauskas, L. (1996). Crashes and violations among drivers with Alzheimer's disease. *Archives of Neurology, 53,* 411–416.

Tuokko, H., Hadjistavropoulos, T., Miller, J., Horton, A., & Beattie, B. (1995). *The clock drawing test: Administration and scoring manual.* Toronto, Ontario, Canada: Multi-Health Systems.

Zarit, S., Reever, K., & Back-Peterson, J. (1980). Relatives of the impaired elderly: Correlates of feeling of burden. *The Gerontologist, 20,* 649–655.

Zarit, S., Tood, P., & Zarit, J. (1986). Subjective burden of husbands and wives as caregivers. *The Gerontologist, 26,* 260–266.

PART II

GERIATRIC NEUROPSYCHOLOGICAL INTERVENTION

In contrast to the focus on assessment in the first part of this volume, Part II focuses on intervention, beginning with a model outlined in Chapter 10 to assist the process of evaluation, case conceptualization, and treatment planning. As with our assessment model, this intervention model is not presented as definitive or static, but rather as a dynamic beginning effort to redress the current gap of literature in this area. Section A outlines specific cognitive training interventions; Section B then presents approaches most appropriately classified as psychotherapeutic interventions.

We use the word *intervention*, in contrast to *rehabilitation*, because our elderly patients with significant cognitive compromise or dementia cannot be expected to make the magnitude and nature of gains seen with younger populations who experience a marked recovery of function after acute injury. The exception here is with elders suffering from recent stroke, who often do show remarkable gains. It is with elders who are well beyond acute recovery or who are in the early stages of a degenerative condition that intervention focuses upon compensation and coping in the manner that we address here. Indeed, there are also those who will not benefit from treatment, and ethical practice requires us to be forthcoming regarding these limits. However, we systematically consider each case, because successful identification of targets and treatments to reduce excess disability can often be found, even in the context of irreversible or progressive cognitive decline.

The chapters that follow clearly reveal that intervention can lead to improved management of memory deficits, functional status, and mood. As an extension of these gains, quality of life and health care outcomes may also improve. Indeed, over the past decade it has been exciting to watch as reports emerge detailing how treatment leads to less depression even among dementia patients, that systematic training can result in reliable calendar use among patients with Alzheimer's disease, that targeted training skills can lead to functional gains. Our own work has shown that training leads to better perceived memory functioning, with adequate insight. Some of these studies are reviewed in the chapters that follow.

The focus of Part II is unique to this text and is worth some emphasis in the introduction. We hope to underscore the important emerging truth: A neuropsychologist is not simply a diagnostician, as may have been true in the past. The neuropsychologist is also a therapist ideally trained to provide effective neurocognitive interventions to enhance individual patient outcomes through increased coping capacities in relation to losses. The intervention approach itself often involves systematic application of a specific technique, program, or therapy, as outlined in the chapters that follow. These interventions are informed by a clear understanding of the neurocognitive deficits present in each individual case, which allows delineation of target behaviors and facilitates the appropriate design of methodology with which to teach compensation. It is not the biological disease process that is the target of intervention. Indeed, test scores on our traditional measures often do not capture the gains. Additionally, the goal of intervention is rarely to fix or ameliorate a problem. Rather, it is the practical functional and emotional outcomes that are addressed through compensatory, training, and psychotherapeutic techniques.

It is our observation that many neuropsychologists do not feel that they have the skills necessary to do this kind of work. Perhaps others in related fields also underestimate their abilities in this arena. Some may attribute reluctance to practice in this area to lack of experience with intervention in this particular population—and indeed, those without adequate exposure will need to ensure appropriate training as they begin their work. However, our experience suggests that reluctance to practice is fueled by more basic concerns, such as a sense of inadequacy and powerlessness. This perspective often stems from lack of exposure to work that nets favorable outcomes, coupled with therapeutic nihilism—the belief that this particular population cannot benefit from intervention. With the promising outcomes that are reviewed in these sections, it becomes clear that the heretofore pervasive bias against treatment in this population was indeed premature and without merit. However, this evidence does little to empower the individual clinician with a sense of command and capacity. We would like to challenge this disempowerment and ask each clinician to carefully consider relevant skills he or she indeed possesses. What neuropsychologist is without training in behavioral principles and therapy? What clinician does not understand loss and grief? And we are inspired to challenge even further: Are not neuropsychologists in a uniquely qualified position to engage in this work, given that their expertise spans both the behavioral correlates to neuroanatomical compromise *and* the therapeutic arena? It is our belief, and perhaps bias, that many clinical neuropsychologists and related professionals are indeed qualified and quite skilled in intervention and that application of their intervention abilities awaits only their awareness and enthusiasm.

Cognitive Training and Compensatory Techniques

The chapters in Section A focus on specialized cognitive training and compensatory techniques.

Chapter 10 leads this section with a discussion of the intervention model. This model outlines the process of evaluation, case conceptualization, and treatment planning in a preliminary manner. Accordingly, cognitive training and compensatory techniques are considered as well as psychotherapeutic interventions, as discussed in Section B.

The remaining chapters in Section A focus on specialized cognitive training and compensatory techniques. As noted in this text, the primary targets of intervention tend to be either cognitive (e.g., memory, language) or functional in nature, but often involve a combination. As can be easily observed, many different techniques or combinations of techniques can address the same problem. Often, it is desirable to address behavior with a multimethod approach, because different patients have different strengths and preferences and are thus differentially able to use some techniques but not others. Indeed, patients should be informed about what is and is not known about each approach, and forewarned that multiple approaches may be needed to determine the best method for them. The reader is referred to the intervention model for consideration of factors that may affect intervention target and technique selection.

Chapter 11 describes a very specific program of cognitive and functional interventions. Importantly, this work emphasizes the need to target functional skills, which could improve qualify of life and possibly even delay disability. This chapter also presents follow-up data for what might be considered one of the most rigorous examples of intervention outcomes research.

Chapter 12 describes another approach: the increasingly applied and researched technique of spaced retrieval. This chapter outlines the strategy and provides examples of successful application of the method and efficacy data. There is also a discussion of issues relevant to the dissemination of the intervention, which applies to any effort to broadly deliver these relatively new approaches to the clinical care arena.

Chapter 13 provides a description of methods that employ multiple techniques. This multimethod approach is not only common in practice but is often clinically desirable.

Although this approach may lead to challenges in terms of researching effective components, it represents the first step in demonstrating clinical efficacy, and it is anticipated that additional study of program components will follow. The reader is encouraged to consider the many individual techniques that can be applied. Many are modified associative techniques that originated in traditional rehabilitation settings.

Chapter 14 addresses approaches for dealing with language deficits that are often applied with elders who have suffered stroke or have progressive aphasias. This work focuses on an area of functioning, language, that is often untreated in post-acute geriatric populations. Language impairments post obvious implications for social autonomy and function and are often quite distressing to patients when they occur. The neuropsychologist can assist by teaching strategies that compensate for acquired deficits; he or she is also in a position to provide comprehensive psychological care, incorporating targeted behavioral and adaptive coping strategies, a point highlighted later in the book.

Chapter 15 discusses the use of external auxiliary aids to facilitate function. The importance of establishing strong external methods of compensation for an impaired and possibly progressively declining cognitive function cannot be sufficiently underscored. The topics discussed here complement the other chapters dealing with specific psychological or behavioral compensatory strategies.

An Integrated Model for Geriatric Neuropsychological Intervention

DEBORAH K. ATTIX

The notion that dementia and other cognitive disorders is not treatable is a myth. The landscape of geriatric neuropsychological care services is unquestionably evolving, with treatment being a rapidly growing area of practice complementing traditional assessment. Reports demonstrating clinical efficacy of various intervention techniques are emerging and systematically dissolving previous biases against intervention with patients who have dementia. This promising work encourages the clinician to move beyond diagnosis in order to maximize functioning, coping, and quality of life, even in the context of debilitating dementia conditions (Koltai & Branch, 1998, 1999; Zarit & Zarit, 1998).

The neuropsychological interventions discussed in this text involve patient populations with progressive conditions or dementias that are stable, with any expected neuro-anatomical recovery already complete. Therefore, it is not the underlying neuropathology that is targeted for modification, but rather coping, adjustment, and the use of compensatory strategies and residual abilities (Koltai & Branch, 1998, 1999; Sohlberg & Mateer, 1989c).

In the chapters that follow, common intervention techniques are presented along with the associated research and anecdotal evidence supporting their utility. It seems obvious that these clinical approaches are best applied within an informed framework. It is well known among those working in any rehabilitation or intervention capacity that maximal benefit is contingent upon the development and execution of a carefully considered treatment plan. This chapter outlines one model that can be used to facilitate such planning. It is an approach used to conceptualize geriatric neuropsychological intervention services, built upon the clinical and research efforts within this emerging field. In this model data acquired or reviewed during the intervention evaluation are utilized to formulate the treatment plan.

INTERVENTION PLANNING: IDENTIFICATION OF
INTERVENTION TARGETS AND STRATEGY SELECTION

The initial intervention evaluation is the primary source of clinical data from which the treatment plan evolves, as variables relevant to the identification of treatment *targets* and *methods* are examined. Maximal benefit from neuropsychological intervention is achieved with careful, thorough planning. In this section variables relevant to the identification of treatment goals and methods, and the process of matching these in relation to the characteristics of each patient are described. The intervention evaluation is the context in which these variables are reviewed, which facilitates creation of the treatment plan. These variables include:

- Goals
- Motivation
- Neuropsychological evaluation
- Insight
- Affective status
- Unique patient and environmental factors
- Current compensatory methods and activities

These variables should be systematically reviewed and incorporated into the treatment plan. This step of the intervention process identifies the most feasible treatment targets and approaches by integrating neuropsychological data and identified intrapsychic or interpersonal concerns with a theoretical understanding of the neuroanatomical correlates of behavior and the appropriate psychotherapeutic approaches (Pramuka & McCue, 2000; Sohlberg & Mateer, 1989a).

Goals

Intervention planning begins with elucidation of the major complaints driving the need for treatment, because these give rise to treatment goals. Whereas some patients and families enter the treatment process with well-defined goals, others look to the provider for assistance in identifying targets. Regardless of the degree of goal identification that the patient and family bring to the initial meeting, the end point is to identify valued outcomes that are also amenable to treatment. The questions directly relevant to this factor include:

- What are the functional complaints of the patient? That is, what would he or she like to change?
- What are the patient's functional deficits from the perspective of the family? That is, what would they like to change?
- From the patient's perspective, what cognitive deficits are associated with the functional deficits?
- From the family's perspective, what cognitive deficits are associated with the patient's functional deficits?
- Does the patient report any affective distress?
- What is the patient's affective status from the perspective of the family?
- Is the affective distress in response to cognitive and functional failures (see below)?
- Is the affective distress of sufficient magnitude to contribute to the cognitive and functional deficits (see below)?

- Is there any discrepancy between patient and family reports of functional, cognitive, or affective status? If so, what accounts for the divergence?
- What cognitive and affective deficits are likely related to the functional complaints, given the neuropsychological data (see below)?
- Is there any discrepancy between patient and family reports? What would be expected, given the neuropsychological data (see below)? If there is a discrepancy, what accounts for it?

Typically, patients referred for intervention are beyond the acute stages of injury. In these instances few skill gains would be expected through natural history of recovery, and some patients may even be expected to decline over time. Therefore, goals should be structured within the context of an explicit understanding that cognitive deficits will be managed and compensated for rather than cured or "rehabilitated."

Although the patient and family will readily identify areas of functional disability, the clinician needs to understand the antecedents to such difficulties in order to best intervene. This understanding includes identifying sources of "functional dysfunction" from the perspective of both the patient and family members (Pramuka & McCue, 2000). For instance, is the patient not doing things listed on the "to-do list" because he or she forgets to check the list (memory disorder), does not follow the structure of the list (executive dysfunction), or lacks interest (apathetic depressive disorder)? Even if the target of intervention is the same, the strategy would vary considerably depending on the source of the problem.

To this end, the clinician should identify the presence of any cognitive dysfunction and affective distress that may be contributing to functional deficits. In addition, it is useful to know both patient and informant perspectives on the patient's cognitive and affective status. When patient and informant reports diverge, it is helpful to identify the source of discrepancy, because this information can also be helpful in planning (e.g., the patient may have anosognosia which can influence outcome or it may reflect caregiver burden). In addition, other sources of information, such as the neuropsychological evaluation, should be utilized to enhance the identification and quantification of cognitive and affective dysfunction.

Motivation

The patient's motivation to *actively* participate in the therapeutic process should be considered (Koltai & Branch, 1999). The state of being motivated involves feeling compelled, usually from a need or desire, to act. The questions directly relevant to this factor include:

- Is the patient sufficiently motivated to actively participate in treatment? Specifically, is he or she willing to attend sessions? Is he or she willing to participate in practice assignments that require effortful processing?
- If there is a lack of motivation, is it due to central nervous system dysfunction, resulting in poor initiation/apathy or emotional distress? Are personality factors operating, or is there another reason for poor motivation?

It is erroneous to assume that a patient will be inclined to expend the necessary effort to learn and practice new techniques or to use compensatory strategies just because he or she agrees that improving function is desirable. Similar to understanding the source of functional disability when establishing goals, it is useful to identify the source of diminished or absent motivation that may be a barrier to treatment. *Central nervous system*

(CNS) dysfunction, particularly that involving frontal systems, can result in apathy and impaired initiation of behavior that can be mistaken as a lack of motivation. *Depression* can also significantly impair interest and energy levels. Finally, *personality* factors may preclude adequate motivation to participate in treatment.

Because inadequate participation in the treatment process will likely preclude gains, less-than-optimal levels of motivation should be addressed prior to the initiation of the treatment plan. Of course, attention to personality and affective factors that influence motivation may result in a change that would allow for adequate participation. In contrast, CNS dysfunction that results in an inability to actively participate, despite the desire to do so, must be treated quite differently. In such instances the treatment plan would have to utilize approaches requiring minimal-to-no patient effort (e.g., spaced retrieval, behavioral conditioning). Thus lack of motivation does not completely preclude the possibility of benefit but, instead, significantly modifies the treatment approach.

Neuropsychological Evaluation

One of the most valuable sources of information for intervention planning is the neuropsychological evaluation, because it provides standardized, objective data to assist in both goal identification and strategy selection. The questions directly relevant to this factor include:

- What is the patient's general level of cognitive functioning?
- What diagnosis is supported by the data? What does this diagnosis suggest about the likely neuroanatomical structures and systems currently affected? What does it suggest about the likely cognitive deficits, behavioral changes, and emotional reactions of the patient? What does it suggest about likely progression and the neurobehavioral changes that will evolve over time?
- What type of and how severe a memory disorder is present? Is it characterized primarily by inadequate storage or poor retrieval?
- What types of executive deficits are present? Are the following processes affected: initiation, working memory, speed of processing, cognitive flexibility, sequential processing?
- Is there a processing advantage by modality (e.g., verbal over nonverbal)?
- Are expressive or receptive language skills affected? Visuospatial skills?
- What does the neuropsychological data suggest in terms of modification of technique? Are specific techniques unlikely to be acquired or utilized effectively? What modifications to techniques might prove beneficial, given the patients' cognitive presentation?
- Considering the data, are the identified goals realistic?
- Given the constellation of findings, which techniques might result in the greatest gains relevant to the identified goals?

General Level of Cognitive Functioning

General information about the stage of cognitive compromise—that is, mild, moderate, severe, profound—will set the tone for further exploration of the possibilities and limits of intervention. If an individual exhibits a moderate dementia, for instance, it is likely that both memory and executive deficits are present, whereas someone with a mild level of cognitive dysfunction may be suffering from an isolated memory deficit. Although hypotheses about intervention can be drawn from general stage information, more precise types of data should guide the inclusion or exclusion of specific types of techniques in the intervention plan.

Diagnosis

The importance of the diagnosis is two-fold. First, knowledge of the diagnosis allows for investigation of hypotheses related to the cognitive, emotional, and behavioral sequelae that typically attend various illnesses (Koltai & Branch, 1999). This appreciation of the neurobehavioral sequelae that characterize the presentation and course of neurological illnesses and syndromes guides the intervention process. For example, a patient in the early-to-middle stages of Alzheimer's disease (AD) will likely exhibit memory deficits (with constricted acquisition and rapid forgetting), executive compromises, and mild word-finding problems. A reactive depression and some mild changes in insight may also be present, because these deficits are common in early AD (Koltai & Welsh-Bohmer, 2000). In contrast, a patient with a history of a progressive language disorder (e.g., primary progressive aphasia) will likely demonstrate a moderate-to-severe aphasia syndrome, and depending on the stage of the illness, may demonstrate other cognitive deficits related to the compromise of frontal systems. Insight is likely to be spared in the early-to-middle stages of this illness. The intervention goals for these two patients would be very different, as would the patients' abilities to capitalize on strategies with varying levels of complexity.

Second, knowledge of the diagnosis allows the clinician to incorporate prognosis and likely patterns of future cognitive, affective, and behavioral changes into the intervention plan (Koltai & Branch, 1999). In both logical and ethical practice, strategies should be selected that would serve the patient well in the future.

Neuropsychological Profile

The clinician uses the obtained neuropsychological data to generate or revise hypotheses about cognitive strengths and weaknesses to further refine the treatment approach. The constellation of findings from testing allows for specific planning. Because the concerns of the patient and family often reflect the deficits observed on testing, these data allow for anticipation of the types of complaints and goals the patient and family may bring to the session. Ideally, the clinician is versed in how neuropsychological test performance relates to everyday functional capacities (e.g., driving, medication management, financial decision making; Pramuka & McCue, 2000). However, when complaints diverge significantly from test findings, the source of the discrepancy should be identified.

The neuropsychological profile not only contributes to appropriate goal selection but also includes and excludes the use of specific techniques. In the most obvious sense, strategies should be selected that allow the patient to use relative strengths to compensate for relative weaknesses. Beyond this principle, the potential influence of each compromised neurocognitive domain on each technique being considered should be reviewed. For instance, the clinician will want to determine the nature of the memory deficit: Is it characterized primarily by a storage or retrieval deficit? Obviously, techniques aimed at effortful processing, which increase the chance of storage, would be appropriate for the former (e.g., association techniques: story method, visual association methods), whereas search strategies would be most relevant for the latter. The clinician will also want to consider if there is a verbal over nonverbal processing advantage, or if there are any isolated but significant deficits that should be considered. If there is executive compromise, the clinician will want to understand in what way it may impact the initiation and implementation of various approaches. Feedback involving a review of results often benefits the patient and family and better prepares them for an intervention program that will be more relevant and feasible, given the data (see Green, Chapter 9, this volume).

Technique Modification

Specific cognitive deficits preclude the use of certain strategies. For instance, the method of loci, a mnemonic frequently used with normal elders that involves visually associating target items along a fixed visual route, has been found to be too complex for many cognitively impaired patients (Yesavage, Sheikh, Friedman, & Tanke, 1990; Hill, Yesavage, Sheikh, et al., 1989). Many times, however, specific approaches remain feasible, but only if they are adequately modified (Koltai & Branch, 1999). For instance, a very effective strategy to improve face–name pair learning and the length of retention duration with elders (Hill, Evankovich, Sheikh, & Yesavage, 1987; Wilson, 1987; Yesavage et al., 1990) is likely to have more benefit if modified when used with patients who have early dementia. The strategy typically involves first identifying a distinctive facial feature, then creating a visual association image with the name (e.g., *turtle* for the name "Tuttle"), and finally connecting the visual association image with a prominent facial feature. However, many dementia patients have difficulty executing the specific steps of this technique (Hill et al., 1987). An effective modification involves repetition of the name, creation of a visual association image based on the name, and visualization of the person with this image (e.g., a visualization of Mr. Tuttle interacting with the turtle).

In some instances only minor modifications will be necessary. For instance, the level of executive dysfunction may suggest that training in the use of a calendar is best approached in a series of simple, concrete steps, such as first mastering information extraction before the patient attempts to make systematic entries. Strategy modification may involve choosing one alternative over another based on ability, simplifying or eliminating more complex steps that are not essential to improve performance, or altering the timing of the introduction of strategy sections, as needed.

A critical element of intervention planning evolves during the intervention evaluation through consideration of goals in light of the neuropsychological data. Each goal should be considered in light of the test results. Specifically, the feasibility of targeting each goal should be considered and then, given the profile, the best strategy for targeting each should be identified.

Insight

Anosognosia, or the lack of awareness of deficits, is an indispensable patient variable to consider during the intervention evaluation. Although neuroanatomical theories have, for the most part, replaced motivational theories of "denial" in the dementia population (McGlynn & Schacter, 1989), motivated denial remains a potential psychodynamic construct that can influence intervention outcome and should be considered during the evaluation. More often than not, however, the patient with dementia suffers from an organically based inability to appraise accurately his or her skills. The questions directly relevant to this factor include:

- Is the patient aware of his or her cognitive deficits? Specifically, are both the presence and magnitude of deficit appreciated?
- Does the level of insight reflect other deficits in judgment or reasoning?
- Does the level of insight affect the patient's goals or motivation?

Among patients with dementia, severity of disease is more predictive of anosognosia than dementia duration or diagnosis (Anderson & Tranel, 1989; McDaniel, Edland,

Heyman, & CERAD clinical investigators, 1995; Migliorelli et al., 1995b; Sevush & Leve, 1993; Starkstein et al., 1997). Neuroimaging studies implicate the integrity of frontal-lobe structures in anosognosia (Reed, Jagust, & Coulter, 1993; Starkstein et al., 1995). Clinical observations also associate frontal dysfunction with lack of insight into diminished abilities or inappropriate behavior (e.g., Neary, 1990; see McGlynn & Schacter, 1989; Stuss, 1991). The ability of densely amnesic patients to assess their abilities accurately also suggests that "poor memory for memory failures" does not account for anosognosia (McGlynn & Schacter, 1989). Interestingly, AD subjects with poor insight into their own abilities retain the ability to predict their relatives' performance accurately, suggesting a monitoring defect restricted to the self (McGlynn & Kaszniak, 1991; McGlynn & Schacter, 1989). Alternatively, patients may be impaired in updating knowledge about the self as well as others, but because the informants have not changed, predictions about them remain more accurate (McGlynn & Kaszniak, 1991).

Additional evidence for the potential modifying effect of anosognosia on treatment outcome became apparent to investigators at our center in a preliminary investigation of a memory and coping program implemented with patients who had mild-to-moderate dementia and who were experiencing difficulty adjusting to their cognitive losses (Koltai, Welsh-Bohmer, & Schmechel, 2001). All participants with insight reported less memory failures after treatment. In contrast, subjects without insight or in the control group reported changes in memory failures with similar frequency. The difference between gains among those with and without insight was statistically significant ($p = .029$), suggesting that insight may well be an important variable that moderates actual treatment gain and/ or the perception of gain. In contrast, according to informants, there was a perceived benefit among the treatment group relative to controls, independent of insight status, which approached significance ($p = .065$). Clare, Wilson, Carter, Roth, and Hodges (2004) replicated these findings in a recent prospective study.

These investigations highlight the need for research to further delineate the influences of anosognosia and other potential outcome-modifying variables, such as baseline cognition and affective status. Further study to clarify the degree of *perceived* versus *actual* gain by insight status is needed and could have profound effects on selection of potential candidates for treatment. If anosognosia truly hinders treatment gain, as suggested by the perception of participants in this study, such services may be inappropriate for this subgroup. However, the greater gain perceived by treatment subject informants relative to control group informants, regardless of insight status, suggests that perhaps participants do benefit from treatment, although those with anosognosia may not be able to appreciate such gain, just as they do not appreciate the magnitude of deficits prior to treatment. Unawareness of deficit or its functional consequences logically does not promote the use of compensation (Crossen, 2000). If this is indeed the case, ethical practice would require a clear delineation of expected versus perceived gains within this context.

It is reasonable to hypothesize that the benefit of intervention among anosognostic patients may be hindered by decreased motivation resulting from a lack of appreciation for the need for effortful processing. There may also be a decreased ability to acquire intervention techniques due to the executive dysfunction frequently associated with this condition.

Because poor insight can significantly influence treatment outcome, the patient's degree of awareness should be considered carefully during the intervention evaluation. To the extent that is possible, the clinician should determine the degree of retained insight. An effort to differentiate between observations "echoed" by the patient from those that reflect a true appreciation of the presence and magnitude of deficits should be made.

Finally, this information can be considered in the context of the patient's ability to accurately judge and reason, and how these abilities (or their absence) may also affect motivation and goals.

Affective Status

No intervention evaluation is complete without a thorough assessment of the patient's affective status. Evaluation ideally involves structured interviews or questionnaires and observations of behavior. Patient interviews should be supplemented by informant reports, but with awareness of how caregivers' distress can affect their perceptions of their loved ones. Careful consideration of affective status is essential because it is both a target of treatment and a potential modifier of outcome. The questions directly relevant to this factor include:

- What is the patient's affective status from the perspective of the patient, family, and from the data?
- What is the magnitude of emotional distress?
- What characterizes the emotional distress (e.g., depressive symptoms, anxiety symptoms, irritability)?
- How does the emotional distress affect the patient's functioning?
- Does the patient have an affective disorder that warrants treatment?
- Is the emotional distress in response to cognitive demands and cognitive failures, or independent of them? Can the onset of emotional distress be tied to any clear event?
- Is there any history of an affective disorder?

Chapter 5 reviews cognitive dysfunction related to depression in detail. Because emotional distress can affect function and aggregate in a manner that undermines treatment progress, depression and its effects on behavior warrant some discussion here.

Depression and other emotional disorders can be considered sources of "excess disability," or *treatable* factors that can account for greater than warranted functional incapacity (Brody, Kleban, Lawton, & Silverman, 1971) and should be identified and targeted through intervention. Estimates of the prevalence of depression among elderly persons with dementia underscore the need for directed attention to this domain of functioning. One study of dementia patients found that 27% had minor depression and 25% had major depression (Ballard, Bannister, Solis, Oyebode, & Wilcock, 1996). Another study focusing on affective disorders among patients with AD revealed that 28% had dysthymia and another 23% met criteria for major depression (Migliorelli et al., 1995a). These prevalence figures far exceed those of depressed elderly patients without dementia (Myers, 1984). Not surprisingly, dysthymia typically starts after the onset of AD and is more prevalent in the early stages, whereas major depression typically has an earlier onset and similar prevalence across stages (Migliorelli et al., 1995a). Obviously some variance exists across typical affective symptoms encountered by disease severity and diagnosis. However, it is clear that emotional distress occurs frequently across dementia subtypes and at various times, and is thus a pivotal variable to consider during evaluation for intervention.

Another feature of depression beyond the obvious impact of emotional distress on quality of life is its potential to affect cognition. This cognitive effect can be observed in cases of "pseudodementia," the dementia syndrome of depression (Alexopoulos, Meyers,

Young, Mattis, & Kakuma, 1993, Barry & Muskowitz, 1988; Clarfield, 1988; Emery & Oxman, 1992; Nussbaum, 1994) in which cognitive sequelae are related to depression rather than a comorbid dementia. Also, some studies suggest additionally compromised cognition in cases of dementia when depression is comorbidly present. Further, although controversy exists as to the degree of discernible additional influence on cognition or functional status, some studies have found depression to contribute unique variance to cognitive performance among normal elders, patients with Parkinson's disease, and patients with AD (e.g., Lichtenberg, Ross, Millis, & Manning, 1995; Rovner, Broadhead, Spencer, Carson, & Folstein, 1989; Troster et al., 1995). Even among patients without marked affective disorders, reports of less efficient processing skills during periods of emotional distress are common.

Importantly, depression can also impair functional skills, both alone and in conjunction with cognitive impairment. Among behavior problems of patients with dementia in special care units, those related to emotional distress have been shown to be second only to problems related to memory impairment (Wagner, Teri, Orr-Rainey, 1995). Fitz and Teri (1994) remark that while both depression and cognitive status have been related to performance of basic activities of daily living (ADLS) and instrumental activities of daily living (IADLs) in patients with AD, the influence of depression on IADL performance may be contingent on the severity of cognitive dysfunction. In addition, the influence of depression on utilization of health care services has been well documented, even in the absence of dementia. Elderly depressed outpatients (1) are more likely to rate their health as fair or poor, (2) have more emergency room and outpatient visits, and (3) higher outpatient charges than nondepressed patients (Callahan, Hui, Nienaber, Musick, & Tierney, 1994). Koenig, Shelp, Goli, Cohen, and Blazer (1989) found significant health care utilization differences between older medically ill patients with and without major depression, with depressed patients having longer index inpatient stays, higher in-hospital mortality, and excess resource utilization after discharge.

Whereas the relationship between the domains of affect, cognition, and function awaits further clarification, it is evident that successful treatment of depression, even in the context of a neurodegenerative illness, may reduce cognitive and functional compromises and, in turn, affect health care utilization. The use of residual capacities and the need for formal care may also be impacted, given these interactive, multicausal domains (Koltai & Branch, 1998, 1999).

Finally, intervention efforts that targeting cognitive variables may be unsuccessful if attempted in the context of emotional distress. As noted above, emotional distress frequently leads to excess cognitive disability; many symptoms of affective disorders (e.g., apathy, anhedonia, irritability) tend to work against participation in cognitive techniques that require motivation and effort. Therefore, it is important to gain a thorough understanding of the emotional factors operating within the patient by differentiating emotional and personality changes that are a result of disease-based neurological changes from those that are reactive or premorbid, because treatment approaches differ as well (Crossen, 2000; Pramuka & McCue, 2000). Although there are rare exceptions, affective distress should always be targeted first in order to maximize the likelihood of benefit from other intervention efforts. Doing so will minimize or eliminate inefficiency introduced by the emotional distress and increase the patient's resources, which then can be applied during any cognitive-based intervention. In my experience, the only exception to this general approach occurs when patients refuse treatment of psychological distress and insist on focusing only on memory and processing skills. In such cases, the patient's refusal to consent to treatment of affective distress is, of course, honored, but with clear delineation of the limit to treatment progress in all areas, including the preferred treatment target. By honoring this decision, tension is minimized and an effective rapport is built that eventually allows for this area of functioning to be formally addressed.

In summary, it is apparent that appreciation of the patient's affective status is essential to consider both as a target of treatment and a potential modifier of outcome. Therefore, a thorough assessment of affective functioning should be incorporated into the intervention evaluation. In addition, it is important to understand not only the patient's overall affective status but also the antecedents and consequences of emotional distress for the patient. Finally, an understanding of the patient's history of depression can be useful in conceptualizing his or her current affective functioning, and may also provide historical data useful to the selection of treatment alternatives.

Unique Patient and Environmental Factors

One must be vigilant for factors unique to the patient or his or her situation that could influence the outcome of intervention. The questions directly relevant to this factor include:

- Are there unique factors about this patient that should be considered in the selection of treatment goals or methods?
- Who are the members of the household? How willing are they to be involved in treatment?
- Is the structure of the physical environment conducive to functioning? Is it conducive to the application of intervention techniques?

Although hard to anticipate at times, these factors are critical to identify and consider. For instance, if it becomes apparent that a patient has significant obsessive–compulsive tendencies, then caution must be exercised when teaching detailed structured techniques that risk being overused.

Likewise, there may be social or environmental factors operating that are likely to influence outcome. For instance, if the primary caregiver will not participate in treatment, the strategies will be limited to those that the patient can execute independently. Thus the patient's support and care system should be clearly identified, including the willingness of caregivers to be directly or indirectly involved in intervention efforts, and the patient's physical/environmental surroundings (Pramuka & McCue, 2000; Zarit & Zarit, 1998).

Current Compensatory Methods and Activities

The evaluation should consider what the patient is already doing to address cognitive and emotional dysfunction. Often, patients and families have initiated compensatory routines, many of which are quite effective (Pramuka & McCue, 2000). The questions directly relevant to this factor include:

- How does the patient and family presently keep track of important information? To what extent is this system working?
- Are there any other routine changes that have been made in an effort to compensate for the patient's cognitive losses?

- How does the patient spend his or her time? Is the patient sufficiently active?
- Do routines involve participation in rewarding and meaningful activities?

It is critical for the clinician to be aware of current efforts in order to avoid dismantling systems that are working or interfering with these by introducing competing routines. Sometimes only slight modifications to an established system will yield a markedly different outcome. For instance, the patient may require training in *when* to check an external aid such as an appointment calendar, because use is inconsistent but well enough established that abandonment of the aid would be illogical. Therefore, before the clinician dismantles current efforts, he or she should carefully consider each feature of the current compensatory scheme. Furthermore, careful review of such systems often provides insight into the capabilities of the patient to construct, initiate, and maintain compensatory strategies, either independently or with assistance.

Likewise, the clinician should be aware of the patient's activity level in order to make an informed assessment of whether alterations need to be made in this area. *Inactivity breeds depression.* Participation in rewarding, meaningful activities promotes emotional well-being.

CREATION OF THE TREATMENT PLAN

The information gathered during the intervention evaluation outlined above provides the essentials that contribute to the treatment plan. From this data a treatment plan evolves. Once the plan is established, it should be considered with the patient and family. The plan should specify the following:

- Targets of treatment, with rationale clarified, if needed
- Methods of treatment
- Estimated length of treatment
- Methods of outcome evaluation
- Ultimate goals of treatment

Once treatment goals have been formulated, any discrepancies between the patient/ his or her family and therapist perspectives should be directly reconciled. Such goal discrepancies arise frequently, both while treatment is planned and once it is initiated. Realism and education ideally guide discussion of goals and goal discrepancies. Treatment can proceed when the patient has provided consent, as appropriate.

Various models for intervention in geriatric dementia and neuropsychology have been described (e.g., Camp et al., 1993; Camp, 2001; Gross & Schutz, 1986; Lynch, personal communication, 2005; Zarit & Zarit, 1998). Whereas some of these focus on specific populations or techniques, others emphasize the identification of appropriate intervention approaches, given the patient's presentation. Examples of technique modifications for the geriatric dementia population can also be found, though sparingly. The following guide to using the information gathered during the intervention evaluation is not meant to be definitive, but rather to provide a general outline of how a clinician might proceed. Each clinician will capitalize on his or her background and expertise in creating a tailored approach to planning.

The information gathered during the evaluation provides the fundamental elements of the treatment plan, which will then be refined. One model for conducting this phase of the process is outlined in Figures 10.1 and 10.2. First, the clinician ascertains whether or not there is affective distress present that will interfere with cognitive management efforts. If so, the most effective means of treatment for this emotional distress should be identified. Guidelines for planning psychotherapeutic interventions are outlined in Figure 10.1. If no affective distress is present, planning can proceed to cognitive management, as outlined in Figure 10.2. Although intervention often encompasses treatment of cognitive, affective, and functional elements, we have found it useful to consider these domains independently during the planning phase.

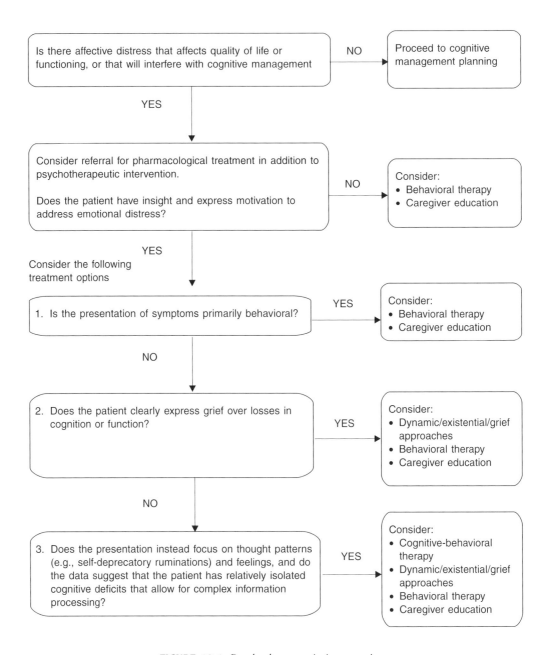

FIGURE 10.1. Psychotherapeutic interventions.

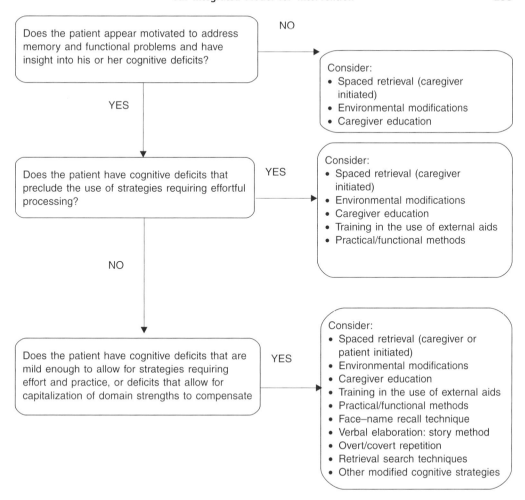

FIGURE 10.2. Cognitive management.

The chapters that follow outline many of these techniques, allowing for a more detailed appreciation of these methods. The examples of intervention approaches discussed here have all been shown to be effective in specific samples. It is such evidence-based efforts that will carry the intervention field forward to allow for beneficial, cost-effective, ethical services.

Once a carefully designed intervention plan has been initiated, the clinician will need to monitor treatment progress and should be prepared to make modifications to maintain optimal gains. The clinician should be cautioned not to rely solely or extensively on traditional objective tests of cognition, because many of these preclude the use of the techniques taught in intervention (Sohlberg & Mateer, 1989b). Neuropsychological measures should thus be supplemented with ratings of perceived gains that capture patient and family perceptions of treatment benefits and limitations. These are often well captured by measures of subjective well-being in the targeted area (e.g., everyday memory functioning) and measures of quality of life. In addition, it is ideal to include performance-based tasks that capture the targeted behavior and allow for strategy implementation, but these require psychometric validation to yield optimal data.

In the next section brief case examples outline the presentation and treatment plan of three patients. Patients with similar goals, levels of functioning, or diagnoses may require significantly different intervention approaches to maximize benefit while promoting an appropriate level of independence and autonomy. These examples are meant to be illustrative only.

CASE EXAMPLES

Case 1. Mrs. H, Mild Cognitive Impairment/Possible Early AD

Mrs. H was in her mid-60s when she was referred for intervention to develop compensatory and information-processing strategies to facilitate memory functioning and coping patterns.

Goals and Motivation

The patient was highly motivated to learn ways to minimize the impact of her memory disorder on her everyday functioning. Although she acknowledged mild anxiety and decreased self-confidence, she expressed a clear desire initially to focus on memory skills. She understood that intervention would not correct the memory disorder but that it could help her to manage the ensuing changes.

Neuropsychological Profile and Insight

Comprehensive neuropsychological evaluation revealed a marked verbal and nonverbal memory disorder, characterized by constricted learning and impaired recall. Performance improved on recognition memory testing, suggesting primarily a retrieval memory deficit at that time. In addition, the patient was mildly inefficient, although not impaired, on nonverbal timed sequencing tasks. The course of the illness was described as progressive, and no explanatory structural abnormality (e.g., vascular lesion) was revealed. The patient's presentation was consistent with the descriptive diagnosis of mild cognitive impairment, and longitudinal follow-up was anticipated to rule out the presence of a neurodegenerative illness. The patient was aware of her cognitive status and demonstrated insight into both the presence and magnitude of deficits.

Affective Status

As noted, mild emotional distress, characterized by anxiety and diminished confidence, was apparent during the initial evaluation. However, the patient expressed a desire to focus on the management of her memory difficulties and thus attention to these affective factors was initially deferred.

Unique Factors and Current Compensatory Methods and Activities

No consistent methods of addressing cognitive and functional deficits were being used, although the patient did keep inconsistent notes.

Intervention

The primary initial targets of intervention involved the patient's memory dysfunction. As treatment continued, her awareness of how cognitive and affective arenas influence one another increased, and she was more receptive to addressing her mood and coping style. Intervention thus evolved to address those aspects of functioning that the patient was able, willing, and motivated to address. Intervention focused on the following:

1. *Education.* Because the patient was high functioning and interested in understanding the nature of her memory disorder, intervention included an educational component addressing models of normal and abnormal memory functioning, as well as how passive versus active processing affects outcome.

2. *Learning and memory.* Although the patient's memory deficit was significant, her cognitive deficits did not impair her ability to initiate and practice complex techniques. Many different management and processing techniques were introduced, including spaced retrieval, the regular use of external aids, retrieval methods, verbal elaboration, repetition to facilitate concentration, conscious review of conversations, and a face–name recall technique.

3. *Affective functioning.* As the patient worked on various memory techniques, improving rapport and awareness of the influence of emotional factors on her processing led to a willingness to address this domain. Because the patient had minimal executive deficits and clearly articulated deprecatory thoughts, a cognitive-behavioral approach was chosen to address the patient's distress. Although not typically used in the geriatric dementia population, the cognitive-behavioral seemed suited to this patient, who spontaneously articulated judgments and perceptions. Little additional effort was needed to link her automatic thoughts with their negative emotional outcomes. The patient responded favorably to these efforts.

Case 2. Mr. C, Vasculitis

Mr. C was in his mid-50s and suffered marked neuropsychological deficits after having vasculitis, an inflammatory vascular disorder. He was referred for intervention approximately 1 year after the acute phase of the illness. Despite improvements, he had marked residual cognitive deficits.

Goals and Motivation

The patient was no longer able to work in his previous farming occupation, nor could he drive or participate in complex independent activities. However, in general, he was able to participate in basic ADLs, maintain religious and social activities, and play an active role in his family. He was motivated to improve his functioning, and his initial goals of addressing memory, confidence, and independence in specific skills were reasonable.

Neuropsychological Profile and Insight

The patient's functional deficits were driven by a dense amnesia, milder complex processing deficits, and mildly decreased awareness of both his deficits and his environment. Neuropsychological evaluation corroborated a profound memory deficit and milder executive compromises. Insight was clinically judged to be mildly compromised. Specifically, although the patient was aware of diminished skill levels, he did not always appreciate how these impairments manifested in everyday functioning, because he underestimated the magnitude of deficits and the frequency of memory failures.

Affective Status

Mr. C was concerned about his performance in many areas and exhibited diminished confidence, in response to which he was becoming increasingly withdrawn and demonstrating limited independence.

Current Compensatory Methods/Activities and Unique Factors

Interestingly, several compensatory methods and activities were in place, because the patient's wife realized early during the course of his recovery that cognitive stimulation and external aids were important. The patient recorded his activities and important information in a daily memory book that she had constructed for him, which, while detailed, was straightforward and effective. In addition, the patient participated in a number of "activities," or games/puzzles, to ensure cognitive "stimulation" in an effort to promote recovery. For the most part, the patient enjoyed these activities. No unique factors relevant to intervention were notable.

Intervention

The initial treatment targets included memory functioning, confidence and independence, with later work related to awareness.

1. *Memory functioning.* Intervention first targeted memory skills. The patient made significant gains using a combination of regular calendar use (which was systematically trained; see the following point), spaced retrieval, and retrieval search techniques.

2. *External aids and compensatory exercises.* Modification of established compensatory activities was appropriate during the course of intervention at two time points. First, education about our current understanding (and its limits) of the utility of cognitively stimulating activities was provided. This information gave the patient and his wife a context within which to choose how much to emphasize participation in games/puzzles in hopes of enhancing functioning through cognitive stimulation. They were discouraged from using in frustrating activities of any kind, given that these were more likely to undermine confidence than provide any tangible gains. They modified their regimen accordingly. Second, as the patient continued to improve, it became evident that the level of detail and structure involved in his memory book was not necessary the way it had been during the more acute stages of his illness. We therefore progressed this system toward the use of a regular appointment calendar. This was done by systematically collapsing the established categories of entry, to the point that entries could be made in a regular calendar in a few relevant domains (e.g., health-related tasks, social/recreational activities, appointments).

3. *Awareness.* The focus of intervention then evolved to identification of methods that would assist the patient in compensating for his reduced awareness. An example of a practical intervention in this area involved a disruptive functional issue: The patient could not track whether or not he had taken a shower each day, so he would have to rely on his wife to either cue him to do so or to inform him that he had taken one already when he asked (repeatedly, of course). This problem was resolved in the following simple manner: Spaced retrieval (see Camp, Chapter 12, this volume) was used to teach the patient to take a towel out of the drawer and put it on the bathroom counter first thing every morning before starting any other activity. With systematic repetition, this became an estab-

lished part of his routine. Later, when curious about whether or not he had showered, he needed only to look at the counter—if the towel was there, he had not yet showered; if it was not there, it had been used, indicating that he had showered. He no longer needed to (repeatedly) ask his wife for assistance with this aspect of self-care. This simple solution took 10 minutes of a session to introduce and review and approximately 10 morning spaced-retrieval sessions (with the patient being cued by his wife) to establish this pattern as an independent behavior.

4. *Emotional functioning.* Throughout treatment, the patient was encouraged to identify and participate in meaningful and rewarding projects (see Logsdon, McCurry, & Teri, Chapter 16, this volume) to address the overlapping areas of affect, confidence, and independence.

Case 3. Mrs. L, Disconnection Syndrome

Mrs. L suffered from a vascular disconnection syndrome in her early 60s that had left her with elements of aphasia. She was referred for intervention services with a specific functional complaint.

Goals and Motivation

The primary functional complaint of this patient and her husband was that she could no longer shop to prepare meals. She was completely capable of cooking—of planning and executing the process—with the exception of the shopping, which she had previously done daily for each evening meal. She was highly motivated to identify and participate in a solution.

Neuropsychological Profile and Insight

Specifically, she was anomic (could not name pictures or objects); she could not name specific objects when she was trying to express something that she desired. She therefore could not ask for specific items at the store. She also could not comprehend written language and therefore could not follow a shopping list. Insight was intact.

Affective Status

Although Mrs. L was frustrated by her language deficits, she remained relatively euthymic and free from excessive emotional distress.

Current Compensatory Methods/Activities and Unique Factors

There was no compensatory strategy in place and no relevant unique factors.

Intervention

Treatment targeted the patient's specific functional complaint. Because Mrs. L could not comprehend written language, she could not effectively use a prepared shopping list. She likewise could not tell anyone what ingredients she needed due to her anomia, so even her husband could be of little assistance. And although she could visually recognize (but not name) the desired items, canvassing an entire store (e.g., "Do I need this? Do I need this? Do I need this?") would be unwieldy. This problem was targeted and resolved in the following simple manner: A pocket-sized picture photo album displaying the most common grocery items Mrs. L used was constructed. Prior to shopping, she would mark the items she wanted with stickies and then take the album with her as her shopping list. In contrast to written words, she could visually recognize pictures, and could thus match the picture with the store item for purchase.

SUMMARY

This chapter outlined a model to guide intervention planning for individuals with dementia and other geriatric cognitive disorders. It reviewed fundamental aspects of treatment planning based on the best current approaches reported in the research literature. Those working in intervention anticipate and welcome continued efforts in this arena, so that treatment approaches and planning methods become more refined as new research helps to further define this promising area of practice. The chapters that follow highlight efficacious and promising outcomes in specific areas of clinical intervention. Rigorously defined research needs to continue to ensure that these services remain available in the context of evidence-based practice.

The vignettes presented in this chapter illustrate intervention planning and the yield of practical functional interventions at the individual level. The reader is encouraged to consider the meaning of these simple practical gains in terms of patient well-being, autonomy, and quality of life. Regardless of the targets and techniques employed, this work indeed reflects how people try to find and use the degrees of freedom they have within the constraints of their illness.

So what, then, is intervention? One answer is that *it is the work that occurs at the intersection of biology and existentialism*. It is here that people try to find, and move themselves within, the context of their experience. Although treatment progress sometimes centers on simple, practical solutions to specific complaints, it is more common that patients are debilitated and depressed by their functional deficits, and in these cases intervention encompasses much more. In these cases *intervention often involves a restructuring of the patient's responsibilities, expectations, and sense of self, largely to yield a transformation in role identity that is adaptive in the behavioral context of the illness.*

Many patients emphasize the favorable impact of intervention on quality of life, functional outcomes, and sense of well-being, dignity, and purpose. The potential reduction of costs and disability should also not be overlooked. The chapters that follow illustrate these outcomes. At present, there are few treatment options for our rapidly aging population of elders with cognitive compromise. Until prevention and cure of geriatric cognitive disorders becomes a reality, it remains our obligation to continue devoting effort to both clinical and research-based intervention. We enthusiastically look ahead as this promising area continues to be defined.

REFERENCES

Alexopoulos, G., Meyers, B., Young R., Mattis, S., & Kakuma, T. (1993). The course of geriatric depression with reversible dementia: A controlled study. *American Journal of Psychiatry, 150,* 1693–1699.

Anderson, S., & Tranel, D. (1989). Awareness of disease states following cerebral infarction, dementia, and head trauma: Standardized assessment. *Clinical Neuropsychologist, 3,* 327–339.

Ballard, C., Bannister, C., Solis, M., Oyebode, F., & Wilcock, G. (1996). The prevalence, associations and symptoms of depression amongst dementia sufferers. *Journal of Affective Disorders, 36,* 135–144.

Barry, P., & Moskowitz, M. (1988). The diagnosis of reversible dementia in the elderly: A critical review. *Archives of Internal Medicine, 148,* 1914–1918.

Brody, E., Kleban, M., Lawton, M. P., & Silverman, H. (1971). Excess disabilities of mentally impaired aged: Impact of individualized treatment. *Gerontologist, 11*(2), 124–133.

Callahan, C., Hui, S., Nienaber, N., Musick, B., & Tierney, W. (1994). Longitudinal study of depression and health services use among elderly primary care patients. *Journal of the American Geriatrics Society, 42,* 833–838.

Camp, C. (2001). From efficacy to effectiveness to diffusion: Making the transitions in dementia intervention research. *Neuropsychological Rehabilitation, 11*(3–4), 495–517.

Camp, C., Foss, J., Stevens, A., Reichard, C., McKitrick, L., & O'Hanlon, A. (1993). Memory training in normal and demented elderly populations: The E-I-E-I-O model. *Experimental Aging Research, 19*(3), 277–290.

Clare, L., Wilson, B., Carter, G., Roth, I., & Hodges, J (2004). Awareness in early-stage Alzheimer's disease: Relationship to outcome of cognitive rehabilitation. *Journal of Clinical and Experimental Neuropsychology, 26,* 215–226.

Clarfield, A. (1988). The reversible dementias: Do they reverse? *Annals of Internal Medicine, 109,* 476–486.

Crossen, B. (2000). Application of neuropsychological assessment results. In R. Vanderploeg (Ed.), *Clinician's guide to neuropsychological assessment* (pp. 195–244). Mahwah, NJ: Erlbaum.

Emery, V., & Oxman, T. (1992). Update on the dementia spectrum of depression. *American Journal of Psychiatry, 149,* 305–317.

Fitz, A., & Teri, L. (1994). Depression, cognition, and functional ability in patients with Alzheimer's disease. *Journal of the American Geriatrics Society, 42,* 186–191.

Gross, Y., & Schutz, L. (1986) Intervention models in clinical neuropsychology. In B. Uzzell & Y. Gross (Eds.), *Clinical neuropsychology of intervention.* Boston: Martinus Nijhoff.

Hill, R., Evankovich, K., Sheikh, J., & Yesavage, J. (1987). Imagery mnemonic training in a patient with primary degenerative dementia. *Psychology and Aging, 2,* 204–205.

Hill, R., Yesavage, J., Sheikh, J., & Friedman, L. (1989). Mental status as a predictor of response to memory training in older adults. *Educational Gerontology, 15,* 633–639.

Koenig, H., Shelp, F., Goli, V., Cohen, H., & Blazer D. (1989). Survival and health care utilization in elderly medical inpatients with major depression. *Journal of the American Geriatrics Society, 37,* 599–606.

Koltai, D. C., & Branch, L. G. (1998). Consideration of intervention alternatives to optimize independent functioning in the elderly. *Journal of Clinical Geropsychology, 4,* 333–349.

Koltai, D. C., & Branch, L. G. (1999). Cognitive and affective interventions to maximize abilities and adjustment in dementia. *Annals of Psychiatry: Basic and Clinical Neurosciences, 7,* 241–255.

Koltai, D. C., & Welsh-Bohmer, K. A. (2000). Geriatric neuropsychological assessment. In R. Vanderploeg (Ed.), *Clinician's Guide to Neuropsychological Assessment* (2nd ed., pp. 383–415). Mahwah, NJ: Erlbaum.

Koltai, D. C., Welsh-Bohmer, K. A., & Schmechel, D. E. (2001). Influence of anosognosia on treatment outcome among dementia patients. *Neuropsychological Rehabilitation, 11,* 455–475.

Lichtenberg, P., Ross, T., Millis, S., & Manning, C. (1995). The relationship between depression and cognition in older adults: A cross-validation study. *Journal of Gerontology, 50,* P25–P32.

McDaniel, K., Edland, S., Heyman, A., & CERAD clinical investigators (1995). Relationship between level of insight and severity of dementia in Alzheimer disease. *Alzheimer Disease and Associated Disorders, 9,* 101–104.

McGlynn, S., & Kaszniak, A. (1991). When metacognition fails: Impaired awareness of deficit in Alzheimer's disease. *Journal of Cognitive Neuroscience, 3,* 183–189.

McGlynn, S., & Schacter, D. (1989). Unawareness of deficits in neuropsychological syndromes. *Journal of Clinical and Experimental Neuropsychology, 11,* 143–205.

Migliorelli, R., Teson, A., Sabe, L., Petracchi, M., Leiguarda, R., & Starkstein, S. (1995a). Prevalence and correlates of dysthymia and major depression among patients with Alzheimer's disease. *American Journal of Psychiatry, 152,* 37–44.

Migliorelli, R., Teson, A., Sabe, L., Petracca, G., Petracchi, M., Leiguarda, R., et al. (1995b). Anosognosia in Alzheimer's disease: A study of associated factors. *Journal of Neuropsychiatry, 7,* 338–344.

Myers, J., Weissman, M., Tischler, G., Holzer, C., Leaf, P., Orvaschel, H., et al. (1984). Six-month prevalence of psychiatric disorders in three communities 1980 to 1982. *Archives of General Psychiatry, 41*(10), 959–967.

Neary, D. (1990). Dementia of frontal lobe type. *Journal of the American Geriatrics Society, 38,* 71–72.

Nussbaum, P. (1994). Pseudodementia: A slow death. *Neuropsychology Review, 4,* 71–90.

Pramuka, M., & McCue, M. (2000). Assessment to rehabilitation: Communicating across the gulf. In R. Vanderploeg (Ed.), *Clinician's guide to neuropsychological assessment* (pp. 337–355). Mahwah, NJ: Erlbaum.

Reed, B., Jagust, W., & Coulter, L. (1993). Anosognosia in Alzheimer's disease: Relationships to depression, cognitive function, and cerebral perfusion. *Journal of Clinical and Experimental Neuropsychology, 15,* 231–244.

Rovner, B., Broadhead, J., Spencer, M., Carson, K., & Folstein, M. (1989). Depression and Alzheimer's disease. *American Journal of Psychiatry, 146,* 350–353.

Sevush, S., & Leve, N. (1993). Denial of memory deficit in Alzheimer's disease. *American Journal of Psychiatry, 150,* 748–751.

Sohlberg, M. M., & Mateer, C. A. (1989a). A process-specific approach to cognitive rehabilitation. In M. M. Sohlberg & C. A. Mateer (Eds.), *Introduction to cognitive rehabilitation: Theory and practice* (pp.18–36). New York: Guilford Press.

Sohlberg, M. M., & Mateer, C. A. (1989b). A three-pronged approach to memory rehabilitation. In M. M. Sohlberg & C. A. Mateer (Eds.), *Introduction to cognitive rehabilitation: Theory and practice* (pp. 136–175). New York: Guilford Press.

Sohlberg, M. M., & Mateer, C. A. (1989c). Applications of cognitive rehabilitation in special populations. In M. M. Sohlberg & C. A. Mateer (Eds.), *Introduction to cognitive rehabilitation: Theory and practice* (pp. 382–406). New York: Guilford Press.

Starkstein, S., Chemerinski, E., Sabe, L., Kuzis, G., Petracca, G., Teson, A., et al. (1997). Prospective longitudinal study of depression and anosognosia in Alzheimer's disease. *British Journal of Psychiatry, 171,* 47–52.

Starkstein, S., Vazquez, S., Migliorelli, R., Teson, A., Sabe, L., & Leiguarda, R. (1995). A single-photon emission computed tomographic study of anosognosia in Alzheimer's disease. *Archives of Neurology, 52,* 415–420.

Stuss, D. (1991). Disturbance of self-awareness after frontal system damage. In G. Prigatano & D. Schacter (Eds.), *Awareness of deficit after brain injury* (pp. 63–83). New York: Oxford University Press.

Troster, A., Paolo, A., Lyons, K., Glatt, S., Hubble, J., & Koller, W. (1995). The influence of depression on cognition in Parkinson's disease: A pattern of impairment distinguishable from Alzheimer's disease. *Neurology, 45,* 672–676.

Wagner, A., Teri, L., & Orr-Rainey, N. (1995). Behavior problems of residents with dementia in special care units. *Alzheimer Disease and Associated Disorders, 9,* 121–127.

Wilson, B. A. (1987). *Rehabilitation of memory.* New York: Guilford Press.

Yesavage, J., Sheikh, J., Friedman, L., & Tanke, E. (1990). Learning mnemonics: Roles of aging and subtle cognitive impairment. *Psychology and Aging, 5,* 133–137.

Zarit, S., & Zarit, J. (1998). Treatment of dementia. In S. Zarit & J. Zarit (Eds.), *Mental disorders in older adults: Fundamentals of assessment and treatment* (pp. 277–289). New York: Guilford Press.

Training of Cognitive and Functionally Relevant Skills in Mild Alzheimer's Disease

An Integrated Approach

DAVID LOEWENSTEIN
AMARILIS ACEVEDO

Cognitive rehabilitation has been employed as an effective means of improving memory and other cognitive functions in patients who have suffered traumatic brain injury or stroke (Prigatano, 1997; Salazar et al., 2000; Wilson, 1999). In the cognitively normal older adult, training in the use of several memory techniques, including imagery, organization, and the method of loci, has been accompanied by memory improvement (see Backman, 1996). However, most of these techniques, including organizational instructions (Diesfeldt, 1984), semantic orienting tasks (Corkin, 1982), as well as visual imagery and verbal mediation (Butters et al., 1983), have been shown to be relatively ineffective when used with individuals with Alzheimer's disease (AD). The lack of efficacy of these techniques in AD may be due to their reliance on episodic memory, which is vulnerable to early impairment in the disease process. Episodic memory greatly depends on brain structures (e.g., the hippocampus) that are compromised in patients with AD (see Braak & Braak, 1995; Eslinger & Damasio, 1986; Fox, Warrington, & Freebourough, 1996). In contrast, techniques such as spaced retrieval, dual cognitive support, and procedural motor learning, which do not seem to rely on episodic memory and the implicated brain structures, have been shown to improve cognition and/or function in patients with AD.

In this chapter we provide an overview of techniques that have demonstrated efficacy in enhancing cognitive and/or functional performance among patients diagnosed with AD. We then present data from a recently developed cognitive and functional rehabilitation paradigm that indicate efficacy in improving both cognitive and functional skills of patients with mild AD. Finally, the limitations of previous empirical research, the conceptual differentiation between cognitive and functional skills training, the importance of developing targeted interventions to address specific outcomes, and potential directions for future interventions are discussed.

BRIEF REVIEW OF THE LITERATURE

First described by Landauer and Bjork in 1978, the expanding rehearsal method or spaced retrieval technique (SRT) was one of the earliest interventions that had direct applicability to patients with AD. This approach, which is more fully described in Chapter 12, involves the incorporation of progressive increases in time intervals (in which other activities prevent rehearsal) between the presentation of the to-be-remembered information and its recall. In the event that a retrieval error occurs, the patient receives corrective feedback, and the interval between stimulus presentation and recall is decreased to the previous interval in which recall was correct. In contrast to other memory strategies such as visual imagery, which requires effortful and elaborative processing that most brain-impaired individuals are unable to achieve spontaneously, SRT seems to require little cognitive effort, to be effective when used with patients who have AD (Bird & Kinsella, 1996; Camp & Stevens, 1990; Clare, Wilson, Carter, Roth, & Hodges, 2002; Davis, Massman, & Doody, 2001), and to be spontaneously used by patients (Schacter, Rich, & Stampp, 1985). It has been postulated that SRT works via a priming mechanism (Camp, Bird, & Cherry, 2000) by engaging implicit rather than explicit memory processes, by tapping procedural systems, and by decreasing reliance on semantic or declarative memory systems (Eslinger & Damasio, 1986). This last component is important, because both procedural and implicit memory systems have been shown to remain relatively preserved in AD (Backman, 1992).

Dual cognitive support, the provision of extensive support at both the encoding and retrieval stages of learning and memory, has also been shown to facilitate memory in patients with AD (Backman, 1992). Support at encoding is sometimes achieved (1) by increasing item richness (Davis & Mumford, 1984), (2) by anchoring the to-be-remembered information to personal life material (De Vreese, Neri, Fioravanti, Belloi, & Zanetta, 2001), (3) by providing guidance to engage in self-generated semantic encoding (Lipinska, Backman, Mantyla, & Vitanen, 1994), (4) by activating event-relevant prior knowledge (Johnson & Smith, 1998), or (5) by utilizing to-be-remembered stimuli that allow a higher degree of organization (Herlitz & Vitanen, 1991). The use of material that is emotionally laden (Moayeri, Cahil, Jin, & Potkin, 2000) or that is encoded in a multimodal fashion (Lipinska & Backman, 1997) has also been found to result in better recall in patients with AD. Support at retrieval may be accomplished by providing appropriate recall cues that are compatible with the approach used during the encoding stage (Bird & Kinsella, 1996).

Activation of procedural memory and motor learning has also been shown to facilitate memory in patients with AD. Supportive evidence for the efficacy of procedural memory in improving memory in AD stems from the finding that in the mild to moderate stages of dementia, patients tend to recall their self-selected movements better than movements selected by the experimenter (Dick, Kean, & Sands, 1988). In addition, patients who have AD with varying severities of dementia recall command sentences better when they perform the requested action (e.g., lift a cup, put on a glove) than when they read but do not perform the command (Karlsson et al., 1989). Procedural motor learning in patients with AD has been shown on (1) mirror tracing tasks (Gabrieli, Corkin, Mickel,

& Growdon, 1993), (2) rotary pursuit motor tasks (Eslinger & Damasio, 1986), (3) finger maze tasks (Kuzis et al., 1999), and (4) in learning-to-dance tasks (Rosler et al., 2002). The effectiveness of procedural memory and motor learning in AD likely reflects the relative sparing of the basal ganglia and sensory motor cortex in patients in the early stages of the illness (Backman, 1999; Haxby, Grady, & Koss, 1990; Loewenstein, Barker, et al., 1989). These brain structures are involved in the selection, initiation, sequencing, and modulation of motor activity (Adams, Victor, & Ropper, 1997; Kandel, Schwartz, & Jessel, 2000).

In addition to the aforementioned techniques, individual (see Squires, Hunkin, & Parkin, 1997) and meta-analytic studies (see Kessels & de Haan, 2003) have shown the effectiveness of errorless learning (i.e., the reduction of errors during learning) in improving memory in amnestic patients. Errorless learning used alone or in combination with SRT has been shown to improve the ability of patients with AD to use memory resources to improve orientation to time (Clare et al., 2000) and to learn face–name associations (Clare et al., 2000; Clare et al., 2002; Clare, Wilson, Carter, & Hodges, 2003). (See Clare, Chapter 13, this volume, for a more in-depth discussion of errorless learning approaches.)

These studies demonstrate improvement in memory in patients with AD after the utilization of specific training techniques. Other studies have demonstrated functional improvement in this population following participation in functional training programs. Zanetti, Magni, Binetti, Bianchetti, and Trabucchi (1994) trained patients with mild AD during a 3-week program on basic activities of daily living (ADLs) and instrumental activities of daily living (IADLs; e.g., writing a check, preparing coffee). At the end of the program, patients were faster at completing not only the trained tasks but also untrained tasks, suggesting transfer of skill learning. On the other hand, performance on cognitive tasks for which subjects were not trained (i.e., memory) did not improve. Zanetti, Rozzini, Bianchetti, and Trabucchi (1997) also studied the time it took to perform 20 ADLs in a group of untreated cognitively normal older adults versus a group of patients with AD who participated in procedural memory training sessions for 3 weeks. Half of the patients with AD were trained on 10 of the ADL outcome measures, and the other half were trained on the alternate 10 ADL tasks. Results showed that not only were trained patients with AD from 3.6 to 1.9 standard deviations faster than normal older adults in the completion of the tasks, but that they improved in the untrained tasks as well, completing them faster than the control group at postintervention. Consistent with other studies, however, no change in performance was noted on neuropsychological measures tapping cognitive abilities for which the subjects were not trained.

In a more recent study, Lekeu, Wojtasik, Van der Linden, and Salmon (2002) successfully employed an errorless learning paradigm to teach patients with AD to use a mobile telephone. Farina and colleagues (2002) described an intensive 5-week program with 22 AD inpatients who participated in individual sessions, twice a day, 3 days a week. The investigators compared the efficacy of a procedural memory training intervention that was based on practicing ADLs (e.g., identifying currency, sending a letter) to a residual cognitive function intervention that was based on activities aimed to stimulate cognitive processes (e.g., looking for specific words in an array, recalling digits, naming pictures). Results indicated significant postintervention improvement in performance of patients in both groups on the Functional Living Skills Assessment, a measure that directly measures performance on everyday functional tasks. They also found a slight improvement in the procedural memory training group on two neuropsychological measures. Unfortunately, all gains tended to regress to pretraining levels at 3 months postintervention. These researchers suggested that training ADLs with a strong procedural memory component may be more effective than stimulating "residual" cognitive functions in patients with AD. More importantly, the above results suggest that functional training can generalize to untrained tasks and to real-world functioning in patients who have AD.

LIMITATIONS OF PREVIOUS RESEARCH

Although spaced retrieval, dual cognitive support, and activation of procedural and motor memory have been found to enhance memory in AD patients, these procedures have often been utilized in isolation. Over the last several years, our laboratory has been engaged in developing an integrated cognitive and functional training program specifically developed for patients with mild and very mild AD. The conceptual underpinnings of the paradigm that has been developed are as follows:

1. Memory and functional skills in mildly and very mildly impaired patients with AD can be improved by the integrated utilization of SRT, dual cognitive support, and procedural motor activation, all of which have been suggested to rely on brain processes and systems (i.e., implicit memory, basal ganglia) that are relatively preserved in mild AD.
2. Training should focus on the acquisition and maintenance of skills that are directly related to the patient's everyday life.

We have also developed a greater appreciation of the potential value of participation in booster training sessions, which are likely to extend the period during which cognitive and functional gains are maintained.

Many previous intervention studies have failed to address important issues such as the need to increase cognitive processing speed and enhance prospective memory (i.e., remembering to remember an intended action). This omission may be related to the fact that although prospective memory problems are a common complaint among cognitively normal and memory-impaired older adults, neuropsychologists rarely assess this important aspect of memory. Further, a number of cognitive rehabilitation interventions have not incorporated compensatory strategies (e.g., memory notebooks) or training of a family member or a friend who can assist the patient as a therapy extender when practicing learned skills at home and in the real-world environment.

To address these weaknesses in other intervention programs, our training program incorporates compensatory techniques such as a memory notebook and the training of a family member or friend who can integrate the in-office training to the patient's everyday environment. In addition, given that speed of cognitive processing has been postulated to underlie many component cognitive abilities in the elderly (Salthouse, 1996; Salthouse & Somberg, 1982), we have incorporated training of cognitive processing speed in our intervention program. Cognitive processing speed has been shown to be improved in cognitively normal older adults after their participation in a 5- to 6-week cognitive intervention program (see Ball et al., 2002). These investigators also demonstrated that individuals who participated in postintervention booster sessions were more likely to maintain these gains at 2 years postintervention, as compared to their peers who did not participate in the booster sessions. Unfortunately, this paradigm has not been well studied in AD.

DATA FROM OUR INTEGRATED COGNITIVE REHABILITATION PROGRAM

The cognitive rehabilitation (CR) intervention developed in our laboratory incorporates the techniques described above that have been shown to be effective in AD. For example, we utilized the SRT and dual cognitive support in face–name association training, which also incorporated the use of phonetic cues related to specific features of the to-be-remembered face (e.g., Smiling Sam). In addition, our intervention incorporated procedural and motor memory in the training of specific functional tasks, such as making change for a purchase, balancing a checkbook, and enhancing memory through the manipulation of objects in a way consistent with their use (e.g., use a hammer as though hammering; use a can opener as though opening a can). We also employed an orientation and memory notebook (Loewenstein & Acevedo, 2000a) for in-session exercises that would benefit from the use of anchoring information that was of relevance to the patient (e.g., birthday, anniversaries), as suggested by De Vreese and coworkers (2001).

The efficacy of our training program was recently demonstrated in a cognitive rehabilitation trial that was funded by the National Institutes of Health/National Institute on Aging. The study included 44 subjects with probable or possible AD, according to the criteria established by the National Institute of Neurological and Communicative Disorders and Stroke and the Alzheimer's Disease and Related Disorders Association (NINCDS–ADRDA; McKhann et al., 1984). Patients were diagnosed by an experienced neurologist after a thorough neurological and neurocognitive evaluation, blood laboratories, and brain magnetic resonance imaging (MRI). Subjects had been on a stable dose of an acetylcholinesterase inhibitor (AChEI) for at least 8 weeks. In this initial trial (see Loewenstein, Acevedo, Czaja, & Duara, 2004), we compared the effects of our CR intervention to that of a nonspecific mental stimulation (MS) intervention that consisted of participation in interesting, commercially available computer games (e.g., "hangman," word scramble) that were presented by the therapist. Results of the investigation indicated that subjects in the CR intervention evidenced improvements at both postintervention and 3-month follow-up in cognitive processing speed, face–name association, orientation, and functional skills such as making change for a purchase. As expected, there were no training effects on traditional neuropsychological measures of component abilities, such as memory, language, visuospatial skills and executive function, that were not directly targeted by the CR intervention.

We have now collected new data on additional cases, for a total of 57 subjects, who have completed their 3-month postintervention evaluation. Subjects were randomly assigned to the CR (n = 33, 42% females) or MS (n = 24, 50% females) intervention. The CR group had a mean age of 76.8 years (SD = 4.7), mean education of 12.1 years (SD = 4.3), and a mean score on the Mini-Mental State Examination (MMSE; Folstein, Folstein, & McHugh, 1975) of 23.5 (SD = 3.1). The MS group had a mean age of 74.8 years (SD = 6.8), mean education of 14.3 years (SD = 3.0), and mean MMSE score of 24.5 (SD = 4.1). Of the total sample, 36 patients (63.2%) were English speakers and 21 (36.8%) were Spanish speakers, with all components of the program (i.e., in-office sessions, at-home exercises, neuropsychological functional battery) conducted in patients' primary language. The neuropsychological functional battery, which consisted of tests that were related or unrelated to the CR training tasks, was administered at baseline, postintervention, and at 3 and 6 months postintervention.

To assess the potential impact of the training interventions, we used traditional cognitive measures (e.g., Continuous Performance Test, CPT, Conners, 2000; orientation subtest of the MMSE) as well as tests developed in our laboratories. The latter included the Procedural Object-Memory Evaluation (POME; Loewenstein et al., 2004), the Face–Name Association Test (FNAT; Acevedo & Loewenstein, 2001), the Balancing-A-Checkbook Task (Loewenstein & Acevedo, 2000b), and the Modified Making Change for a Purchase Test (Loewenstein & Acevedo, 2000b)—the latter two of which are revised versions of the corresponding subtests that are part of the Direct Assessment of Functional Status Scale (Loewenstein, Amigo, et al., 1989). The POME consists of 12 common objects (e.g., key, straw) that are placed in front of the subject, who is allowed to manipulate them during the 10-second item exposure time. The subject is asked to recall the items across three learning trials and after a 30-minute delay. The FNAT involves the presentation of 10 faces, each with a corresponding name, across three learning trials in which the faces are presented in a different order. Recall is assessed immediately after each trial, with corrective feedback provided if the subject was unable to recall the correct name. Recall is again assessed after a 30-minute delay. In the Modified Balancing the Checkbook Test, the subject is asked to calculate, by hand and with the aid of a calculator, the balance in a checking account after paying three utility bills (i.e., water, electricity, and telephone). The Modified Making Change for a Purchase Test consists of five trials in which the patient is asked to make change of different amounts from a $20 bill. All tests in the initial and outcome battery that were related to the CR consisted of items that were different from those used in the training sessions. The only exception was the inclusion in the CR training sessions of 5 of the 10 faces that comprise the FNAT.

A series of 2 × 3 group (CR or MS) by time (baseline, postintervention, 3-month follow-up) repeated-measures mixed-model analysis of variance (ANOVA) was conducted using the 57 subjects. Given that education was slightly higher in the MS group, education was entered as a covariate in all analyses. Table 11.1 depicts the different means associated with statistically significant group × time interactions. Relative to baseline, patients in the CR group achieved higher scores on the three-trial learning and delayed recall of the FNAT, on the Making Change for a Purchase Task, and on reaction time on the CPT, both at postintervention and the 3-month follow-up. The CR group demonstrated improved scores on the Orientation subtest of the MMSE at postintervention relative to baseline, but scores had returned to baseline at the 3-month follow-up. In contrast, performance of the MS group, which did not evidence improvement on orientation at postintervention, showed deterioration from baseline levels of performance at the 3-month follow-up. Except for higher scores on the three-trial learning score of the FNAT at postintervention and the 3-month follow-up, and a lower number of commission errors on the CPT at the 3-month follow-up, there were no differences between baseline and follow-up performance for the MS group. These results remained consistent when factors such as primary language (i.e., English vs. Spanish) and medication dosage were entered into the statistical models.

SIX-MONTH POSTINTERVENTION DATA COMPARED TO BASELINE DATA

Our previous data were limited to a 3-month postintervention follow-up. Here we present data on 51 of the 57 subjects who completed their 6-month postintervention evaluation. Twenty-seven of these subjects participated in the CR intervention (mean age = 76.86, SD = 4.3; 53% females) and 24 participated in the MS intervention (mean age = 74.61, SD = 6.9; 47% females). The interaction term in a series of 2 × 2 group (CR or

TABLE 11.1. Mean (Standard Deviation) of Cognitive Rehabilitation and Mental Stimulation Groups on Tasks Related to Cognitive Rehabilitation Training

Trained skills	Group	Baseline	Postintervention	3-month follow-up	Group × time interaction p value
FNAT three-trial learning	CR	7.46 (5.5)	14.79 (7.9)***	14.65 (8.8)***	.022
	MS	6.95 (5.3)	9.32 (7.4)*	10.43 (7.7)**	
FNAT delay recall	CR	2.52 (2.5)	5.36 (3.0)***	5.16 (3.4)***	< .001
	MS	3.45 (2.4)	3.73 (3.3)	3.52 (3.0)	
Orientation	CR	7.63 (1.8)	8.30 (1.4)*	7.84 (1.9)	.009
	MS	7.79 (2.2)	7.25 (2.1)	6.75 (2.5)**	
POME three-trial learning	CR	19.58 (6.2)	20.48 (7.3)	21.36 (7.2)	.254
	MS	20.17 (6.2)	20.13 (7.3)	20.21 (8.1)	
POME delay recall	CR	5.12 (3.5)	4.97 (3.4)	5.39 (3.8)	.681
	MS	5.33 (3.4)	5.58 (3.7)	5.38 (3.8)	
Making Change for a Purchase Task	CR	4.91 (3.2)	6.18 (3.3)*	5.81 (3.4)*	.023
	MS	5.08 (3.9)	4.00 (4.0)	4.92 (3.9)	
Balancing checkbook (by hand)	CR	2.25 (1.7)	2.03 (1.7)	1.97 (1.7)	.386
	MS	1.50 (1.5)	1.63 (1.6)	1.74 (1.5)	
Balancing checkbook (with calculator)	CR	2.66 (1.6)	3.28 (1.5)	3.25 (1.4)	.357
	MS	2.71 (1.8)	2.63 (1.6)	2.74 (1.7)	
CPT omission errors	CR	19.33 (24.0)	18.17 (31.1)	12.29 (40.2)	.828
	MS	19.50 (19.6)	18.30 (21.4)	17.70 (25.2)	
CPT commission errors	CR	13.29 (5.2)	16.37 (7.6)*	15.71 (7.9)	.014
	MS	10.38 (6.6)	8.38 (6.3)	7.60 (5.0)*	
CPT reaction time	CR	514.50 (153.5)	431.88 (66.2)**	472.44 (133.9)**	.005
	MS	519.97 (67.1)	506.40 (78.7)	504.51 (78.5)	

Note. Mean performance at follow-up and 3-month evaluations for a specific group with a statistically significant interaction term is significantly different from baseline. n = 33 for cognitive rehabilitation (CR) group; n = 24 for mental stimulation (MS) group. FNAT, Face–Name Association Test; POME, Procedural Object-Memory Evaluation; CPT, Continuous Performance Test. The bold items are statistically significant at $p < .05$.

* $p < .05$; ** $p < .01$; *** $p < .001$.

MS) by time (baseline vs. 6-month follow-up) repeated measures ANOVAs revealed that the CR group evidenced improvement relative to baseline at 6 months postintervention on the three-trial learning score, $F(1,49) = 6.06$; $p < .02$, and the delayed recall score $F(1,46) = 17.39$; $p < .001$, of the FNAT, as well as on reaction time on the CPT, $F(1,38) = 4.84$, $p < .02$. CR and MS groups did not differ on Orientation and the Making Change for a Purchase Task at the 6-month postintervention follow-up.

FURTHER DEVELOPMENT OF COGNITIVE AND FUNCTIONAL REHABILITATION PARADIGMS

Our previous work indicates that certain cognitive and functional skills can be trained in mildly impaired patients with AD on AChEIs and that these gains can generally be maintained from 3 to 6 months postintervention. Although successful, there were some limitations in our pilot study that we have attempted to address in our ongoing work. First, the

CR intervention consisted mostly of tasks that were cognitive in nature, and it only included direct training of a limited number of functional tasks (e.g., making change for a purchase). In addition, there was limited training to address prospective memory problems, an aspect of memory with considerable real-world relevance (see Loewenstein & Mogosky, 1999), and one that constitutes a frequent complaint among both cognitively intact and memory-impaired elderly patients. Because cognitive and functional training tasks were presented together, our previous study did not allow us to disentangle the independent effects of cognitive versus functional approaches as they related to the outcome measures. Disentangling their relative contributions is important because it has been postulated that reduced cognitive processing speed may result in impairment in other component cognitive processes and in functional skills in normal elderly adults (Salthouse, 1996; Salthouse & Somberg, 1982). Finally, another limitation of our previous research is the lack of postintervention maintenance sessions, which may have prolonged treatment gains over longer periods of time.

CONCEPTUAL DIFFERENCES BETWEEN COGNITIVE AND FUNCTIONAL TASKS

One of the more complex issues in developing cognitive intervention paradigms is the theoretical and conceptual delineation between what constitutes a cognitive task and what constitutes a functional task. Some cognitive scientists believe that functional performance and its measurement can be thought of as cognitive in nature, because a complex array of component cognitive abilities and their interactions underlie many functional skills. This belief has long been held by a number of professionals in the area of cognitive rehabilitation, which has traditionally attempted to train underlying cognitive abilities such as memory and attention in an effort to remediate real-world functional deficits resulting from traumatic brain injury or cerebrovascular events. However, the available literature in AD does not support the efficacy of training component cognitive abilities to improve cognitive outcomes; even the results of the large trial by Ball and collaborators (2002) with normal elders indicate that training and maintenance of specific cognitive skills do not result in changes in functional outcomes. Of course, more studies with further longitudinal follow-up are required.

In a previous analysis of the literature, we argued that a significant amount of variance in independent ADLs among mild to moderately impaired patients with AD is not explained by knowledge of neuropsychological test performance alone (see Loewenstein & Mogosky, 1999). Although our view is that functional capacity and performance on real-world functional tasks rely on specific cognitive abilities, the traditional view likely underestimates the complexity of the various factors that underlie relevant real-world function. In this regard, we believe that internal subject variables (e.g., motivation, fluctuations in alertness) as well as external environmental variables (e.g., task difficulty, contextual cues) are critical in the successful completion of functional tasks within the person's home environment. Thus task performance is affected by (1) cognitive abilities and other internal characteristics of the individual, (2) the nature of the specific task, and (3) environmental factors that interact with each other and may affect the relationship between these variables or their relative importance over time. For these reasons, the study of both mediator and moderator variables is likely to be critical to our understanding of these processes. Given that traditional least-square regression models may not be adequate to examine mediating variables and any changes in performance over time, the use of multilevel models that apply structural equation modeling (SEM) and latent growth curve approaches seems to be the appropriate way to proceed.

Until more complex conceptual models are developed that better elucidate the relationship among cognitive and functional variables, we have employed a useful set of heuristics to help distinguish between cognitively and functionally based training tasks for mildly impaired patients with AD. This set of heuristics has allowed us build different types of intervention models that lend themselves to empirical evaluation. We believe that cognitive rehabilitation intervention and functional enhancement interventions differ in three important ways: (1) their theoretical foundations, (2) their primary goals, and (3) their training techniques. The theoretical foundation of the cognitive rehabilitation intervention stems from clinical neuropsychology and cognitive neurosciences, whereas the functional enhancement intervention has its theoretical foundations in rehabilitation psychology and occupational therapy. The primary goal of the cognitive intervention is the remediation of cognitive deficits, such as impaired memory and slowed cognitive processing speed. In contrast, the primary goal of the functional enhancement intervention is to directly train targeted functional tasks that have traditionally been considered to be IADLs (e.g., making change for a purchase) and that have high correspondence to real-world situations. It is important to note that the functional enhancement paradigm acknowledges that component cognitive abilities such as cognitive processing speed may affect task performance. However, this intervention does *not* rely on the training of cognitive skills but rather on the training of actual functional tasks. The main techniques (i.e., spaced retrieval, dual cognitive support) used in the cognitive intervention and in our previous pilot trial have been associated with improvement in memory and other cognitive domains that are frequently affected in mild AD (see Loewenstein et al., 2004). Conversely, the primary technique used in the functional enhancement intervention (i.e., procedural motor learning) has been associated with improved performance on functional tasks. In summary, although they both have strong theoretical and empirical foundations, cognitive and functional enhancement interventions are based on different theoretical models, have different primary goals, and use different techniques to attain these goals.

DEVELOPMENT OF MORE FUNCTIONALLY RELEVANT OUTCOMES

Although patients with AD are able to learn targeted skills and maintain gains over time, further work is required to develop training tasks that have real-world counterparts and functional relevance. Some of these tasks could be related to medication adherence, basic money management, and learning to interface with existing technology (e.g., use of a cellular telephone, navigating of a telephone menu system to perform specific functions, such as refilling a prescription or reporting a power outage). Training patients on ways to improve prospective memory in the real world (e.g., remembering to make a medical appointment or to take medications) would also have high generalizability to real life. We have recently conducted pilot work that indicates that it is possible to train prospective memory in patients with mild AD by utilizing the Orientation and Memory Notebook, in which prospective memory training is enhanced by the provision of specific cues. Using this approach, patients have been taught to periodically check their notebooks for specific to-be-remembered assignments that were previously written by the patients in their notebooks. For example, a patient might be told to page the therapist the following day at 11:30 A.M. or to call our office at 3:00 P.M. on a different day. The use of memory note-books has been shown to decrease future remembering deficits in brain-injured individu-als (Mateer & Sohlberg, 1988). Improvement in prospective memory in patients with AD has also been accomplished by the utilization of SRT and errorless learning techniques (Kixmiller, 2002).

As mentioned above, Zanetti and coworkers (1994, 1997) found that trained pa-tients with AD performed trained and untrained ADLs at a faster speed than at baseline. In our laboratories, we have collected data on a different type of functional skill—the ability to learn to use a mock menu-driven automated telephone banking system. The sys-tem, developed by Dr. Sara Czaja and her colleagues at the University of Miami, requires patients to call a mock bank, where, by selecting the appropriate menus, they could ob-tain information such as the balance of mock savings, checking, and credit card accounts, transfer funds, and verify if a payment has been posted to one of the mock accounts (see Czaja, Sankaran, & Lee, 2002). This mock telephone banking system is similar to those routinely used by banking institutions. The reliability and validity of the tasks that can be performed using this system were tested on a group of 14 mildly impaired patients with AD (6 males and 8 females) with mean Mini-Mental State Examination (MMSE) score of 23.0 ($SD = 3.6$.) The mean age of this group was 79.9 ($SD = 6.9$), and the average level of educational attainment was 12.54 years ($SD = 3.6$). Test–retest reliability for the total number of items answered correctly on this telephone banking task was excellent ($r = .85$; $p < .001$). Test–retest reliabilities for specific aspects of the task were also high, especially for the savings account task, $r = .92$ ($p < .001$), the checking account task, $r = .77$ ($p < .01$), and the credit card task, $r = .65$ ($p < .02$). In a recent pilot study, we trained 13 mildly impaired patients with AD (7 males and 6 females) to use the system. The mean age of this group was 78.41 ($SD = 5.3$), the mean level of educational attainment was 13.12 ($SD = 3.5$), and the mean MMSE was 24.18 ($SD = 3.6$). Results using similar items included in the training sessions indicated improvement, as compared to baseline, in the patients' ability to use the system to obtain correct financial data related to the mock ac-counts ($df = 12$) = 2.9; $p < .02$. Post-hoc tests demonstrated a particular improvement in the number of correct responses on questions related to the checking account (12) = 2.3, $p < .04$, and in the time it took the patients to complete the task, $t(12) = -2.50$, $p < .04$. Faster rates of completion were also found in a similar task related to the savings ac-count, $t(12) = 2.31$, $p < .04$. (See Attix, Chapter 10, this volume, for a more detailed de-scription of targeted interventions for specific functional tasks.)

TARGETED INTERVENTIONS

As mentioned above, there is little evidence that merely training component cognitive skills such as memory, language, attention, or cognitive processing speed in patients with AD generalizes to performance in real-world tasks. Furthermore, the use of traditional nonspecific memory drills is of questionable value with patients who have AD. By train-ing skills that are directly related to important real-world tasks and that allow continued practice at home, the intervention becomes more meaningful to the patient and his or her family.

As already discussed, we believe that the effectiveness of cognitive and functional in-terventions would be extended by the administration of periodic booster sessions that would give patients the opportunity to practice the skills under the supervision of a trained professional. Maintaining treatment gains over an extended period of time could have a significant impact in the independence and quality of life of both the patient and the caregiver. Further, extending cognitive and functional independence in the patient with AD for even 6 months to 1 year would result in considerable cost-savings to many societies. Of course, these aspirational goals can only be attained with continued vigorous research to develop targeted interventions that would be optimally effective for patients with AD.

FUTURE DIRECTIONS

There is an emerging literature that demonstrates that mildly and perhaps even moderately impaired patients with AD can learn and maintain cognitive and/or functional gains over time. The extent to which moderately and more severely impaired patients with AD, and those with other neurodegenerative disorders, can benefit from integrative cognitive and functional rehabilitation approaches awaits further research. As newer pharmacological agents become increasingly effective, a larger window of opportunity may arise during which we would be able to work with patients on both cognitively and functionally relevant skills. As pharmacological, genetic, or other approaches are developed that can effectively halt the progression of AD and other dementias, there will continue to be a critical need to rehabilitate the cognitive and functional sequelae of the already damaged neural structures and systems that are essential to everyday life. These resultant deficits may best be addressed with targeted cognitive and functional rehabilitation interventions that will likely become more sophisticated as we further our understanding of the intervention process.

What only a decade ago seemed quite unlikely, cognitive and functional rehabilitation using specific techniques to bypass the episodic memory deficits associated with AD seems to hold a refreshing promise. This promise can only be realized through continued novel research on effective cognitive and functional approaches that have real life impact and that increase the quality of life of both the patient and the caregiver. We owe our patients and their families no less.

ACKNOWLEDGMENTS

This work was supported by the National Institute on Aging (Grant No. R01 AG018401-03) and by the Johnnie B. Byrd Sr. Alzheimer's Center and Research Institute, Tampa, Florida (David Loewenstein, principal investigator).

REFERENCES

Acevedo, A., & Loewenstein, D. (2001). *The Face–Name Association Test: Administration and scoring manual.* Unpublished manuscript, University of Miami School of Medicine, Miami, FL.

Adams, R. D., Victor, M., & Ropper, A. H. (1997). *Principles of neurology* (6th ed.). New York: McGraw-Hill.

Backman, L. (1992). Memory training and memory improvement in Alzheimer's disease: Rules and exception. *Acta Neurologica Scandinavica* (Suppl. 139), 84–89.

Backman, L. (1996). Utilizing compensatory task conditions for episodic memory in Alzheimer's disease. *Acta Neurologica Scandinavica* (Suppl. 165), 109–113.

Backman, L., Andersson, J. L. R., Nyberg, L., Winblad, B., Nordberg, A., & Almkvist, O. (1999). Brain regions associated with episodic retrieval in normal aging and Alzheimer's disease. *Neurology, 52*, 1861–1870.

Ball, K., Berch, D. B., Helmers, K. F., Jobe, J. B., Marisiske, M., Morris, J. N., et al. (2002). Effect of cognitive training interventions with older adults: A randomized controlled trail. *Journal of the American Medical Association, 288*, 2271–2281.

Bird, M., & Kinsella, G. (1996). Long-term cued recall of tasks in senile dementia. *Psychology and Aging, 11*, 45–56.

Braak, H., & Braak, E. (1995). Staging of Alzheimer's disease-related neurofibrillary changes. *Neurobiology of Aging, 16*, 271–278.

Butters, N., Albert, M. S., Sax, D. S., Miliotis, P., Nagode, J., & Sterste, A. (1983). The effect of verbal mediation on the pictorial memory of brain-damaged patients. *Neuropsychologia, 21*, 307–323.

Camp, C. J., Bird, M. J., & Cherry, K. E. (2000). Retrieval strategies as a rehabilitation aid for cognitive loss in pathological aging. In R. D. Hill, L. Backman, & A. S. Neely (Eds.), *Cognitive rehabilitation in old age* (pp. 224–248). New York: Oxford University Press.

Camp, C. J., & Stevens, A. B. (1990). Spaced-retrieval: A memory intervention for dementia of the Alzheimer's type (DAT). *Clinical Gerontologist, 10*, 58–60.

Clare, L., Wilson, B. A., Carter G., Breen, K., Gosses, A., & Hodges, J. R. (2000). Intervening with everyday memory problems in dementia of Alzheimer type: An errorless learning approach. *Journal of Clinical and Experimental Neuropsychology, 22*, 132–146.

Clare, L., Wilson, B. A., Carter G., & Hodges, J. R. (2003). Cognitive rehabilitation as a component of early intervention in Alzheimer's disease: A single case study. *Aging and Mental Health, 7*, 15–21.

Clare, L., Wilson, B. A., Carter G., Roth, I., & Hodges, J. R. (2002). Relearning face–name associations in early Alzheimer's disease. *Neuropsychology, 16*, 538–547.

Conners, C. K. (2000). *Continuous Performance Task*. Odessa, FL: Psychological Assessment Resources.

Corkin, S. (1982). Some relationships between global amnesias and the memory impairments in Alzheimer's disease. In S. Corkin, K. L. Davies, J. H. Growden, E. Usdin, & R. J. Wurtman (Eds.), *Alzheimer's disease: A report of progress*. New York: Springer.

Czaja, S. J., Sankaran, N., & Lee C. (2002). *Development and implementation of the Simulated Automated Telephone Menu System, Automated Teller Machine (ATM), and Messaging Voice Mail System for cognitively intact and memory impaired older adults*. Unpublished manuscript, University of Miami School of Medicine, Miami, FL.

Davis, P. E., & Mumford, S. J. (1984). Cued recall and the nature of the memory disorder in dementia. *British Journal of Psychiatry, 144*, 383–386.

Davis, R. N., Massman, P. J., & Doody, R. S. (2001). Cognitive intervention in Alzheimer's disease: A randomized placebo-controlled study. *Alzheimer Disease and Associated Disorders, 15*, 1–9.

De Vreese, L. P., Neri, M., Fioravanti, M., Belloi, L., & Zanetti, O. (2001). Memory rehabilitation in Alzheimer's disease: A review of progress. *International Journal of Geriatric Psychiatry, 16*, 794–809.

Dick, M. B., Kean, M. L., & Sands, D. (1988). The preselection effect on the recall facilitation of motor movements in Alzheimer-type dementia. *Journal of Gerontology, Psychological Sciences, 43*, P127–P135.

Diesfeldt, H. F. A. (1984). The importance of encoding instructions and retrieval cues in the assessment of memory in senile dementia. *Archives of Gerontology and Geriatrics, 3*, 51–57.

Eslinger, P. J., & Damasio, A. R. (1986). Preserved motor learning in Alzheimer's disease: Implications for anatomy and behavior. *Journal of Neuroscience, 6*, 3006–3009.

Farina, E., Fioravanti, R., Chiavari, L., Imbornone, E., Alberoni, M., Pomati, S., et al. (2002). Comparing two programs of cognitive training in Alzheimer's disease: A pilot study. *Acta Neurologica Scandinavica, 105*, 365–371.

Folstein M., Folstein S., & McHugh P. (1975). Mini-Mental State: A practical method for grading the cognitive state of patients for the physician. *Journal of Psychiatric Research, 12*, 189–198.

Fox, N. C., Warrington, E. K., & Freebourough, P. A. (1996). Presymptomatic hippocampal atrophy in Alzheimer's disease. *Brain, 119*, 2001–2007.

Gabrieli, J. D. E., Corkin, S., Mickel, S. F., & Growdon, J. H. (1993). Intact acquisition and long-term retention of mirror-tracing skill in Alzheimer's disease and global amnesia. *Behavioral Neuroscience, 107*, 899–910.

Haxby, J. V., Grady, C. L., & Koss, E. (1990). Longitudinal study of cerebral metabolic asymmetries and associated neuropsychological patterns in early dementia of the Alzheimer type. *Archives of Neurology, 47*, 753–760.

Herlitz, A., & Viitanen, M. (1991). Semantic organization and verbal episodic memory in patients with mild to moderate Alzheimer's disease. *Journal of Clinical and Experimental Neuropsychology, 13*, 559–574.

Kandel, E. R., Schwartz, J. H., & Jessel, T. M. (2000). *Principles of Neural Science* (4th ed.). New York: McGraw-Hill.

Johnson, D. L., & Smith, S. D. (1998). Effects of familiarity and temporal organization on memory for events schemas in aged and Alzheimer subjects: Implications for clinical management. *Alzheimer's Disease and Associated Disorders, 12*, 18–25.

Karlsson, T., Backman, L., Herlitz, A., Nilsson, L. G., Winblad, B., & Osterlind, P. O. (1989). Memory improvement at different stages of Alzheimer's disease. *Neuropsychologia, 27*, 737–742.

Kessels, R. P., & de Haan, E. H. (2003). Implicit learning in memory rehabilitation: A meta-analysis on errorless learning and vanishing cues methods. *Journal of Clinical and Experimental Neuropsychology, 25*, 805–814.

Kixmiller, J. S. (2002). Evaluation of prospective memory training for individuals with mild Alzheimer's disease. *Brain and Cognition, 49*, 237–241.

Kuzis, G., Sabe, L., Tiberti, C., Merello, M., Leiguarda, R., & Starkstein, S. E. (1999). Explicit and implicit learning in patients with Alzheimer's disease and Parkinson's disease with dementia. *Neuropsychiatry, Neuropsychology, and Behavioral Neurology, 12*, 265–269.

Landauer, T. K., & Bjork, R. A. (1978). Optimal rehearsal patterns and name learning. In M. Greenberg, P. Morris, & R. Sykes (Eds.), *Practical aspects of memory*. London: Academic Press.

Lekeu, F., Wojtasik, V., Van der Linden, M., & Salmon, E. (2002). Training early Alzheimer patients to use a mobile phone. *Acta Neurologica Belgica, 102*, 114–121.

Lipinska, B., & Backman, L. (1997). Encoding-retrieval interactions in mild Alzheimer's disease: The role of access to categorical information. *Brain and Cognition, 34*, 274–286.

Lipinska, B., Backman, L., Mantyla, T., & Vitanen, M. (1994). Effectiveness of self-generated cues in early Alzheimer's disease. *Journal of Clinical and Experimental Neuropsychology, 16*, 809–819.

Loewenstein, D. A., & Acevedo, A. (2000a). *Development and utilization of an orientation and memory notebook for cognitive rehabilitation of patients with mild Alzheimer's disease.* Unpublished manuscript, University of Miami School of Medicine, Miami, FL.

Loewenstein, D. A., & Acevedo, A. (2000b). *The Modified Making Change for a Purchase Test and the Modified Balancing the Checkbook Test.* Unpublished manuscript, University of Miami School of Medicine, Miami, FL.

Loewenstein, D. A., & Acevedo, A. (2001). *The Prospective Memory Test: Administration and scoring manual.* Unpublished manuscript, University of Miami School of Medicine, Miami, FL.

Loewenstein, D. A., Acevedo, A., Czaja, S., & Duara, R. (2004). Cognitive rehabilitation of mildly impaired Alzheimer's disease patients on cholinesterase inhibitors. *American Journal of Geriatric Psychiatry, 12*, 395–402.

Loewenstein, D. A., Amigo, E., Duara, R., Guterman, A., Hurwitz, D., Berkowitz, N., et al. (1989). A new scale for the assessment of functional status in Alzheimer's disease and related disorders. *Journal of Gerontology, 44*, 114–121.

Loewenstein, D. A., Barker W. W., Chang, J. Y., Apicella, A., Yoshii, R., Kothari, P., et al. (1989). Predominant left hemisphere dysfunction in dementia. *Archives of Neurology, 46*, 146–152.

Loewenstein, D. A., & Mogosky, B. (1999). Functional assessment in the older adult patient. In P. Lichtenberg (Ed.), *Handbook of assessment in clinical gerontology* (pp. 529–554). New York: Wiley.

Mateer, C. A., & Sohlberg, M. M. (1988). A paradigm shift in memory rehabilitation. In H. A. Whitaker (Ed.), *Neuropsychological studies of nonfocal brain damage: Dementia and trauma* (pp. 202–225). New York: Springer-Verlag.

McKhann, G., Drachman, D., Folstein, M., Katzman, R., Price, D., & Stadlan, E. M. (1984). Clinical diagnosis of Alzheimer's disease: Report of the NINCDS-ADRDA work group under the auspices of Department of Health and Human Services task force on Alzheimer's disease. *Neurology, 34*, 939–944.

Moayeri, S. E., Cahil, L., Jin, Y., & Potkin, S. G. (2000). Relative sparing of emotionally influenced memory in Alzheimer's disease. *Neuroreport, 11*, 653–655.

Prigatano, G. P. (1997). Learning from our successes and failures: Reflections and comments on "Cognitive rehabilitation: How it is and how it might be." *Journal of the International Neuropsychological Society, 3*, 497–499.

Rosler, A., Seifritz, E., Krauchi, K., Spoerl, D., Brokuslaus, I., Proserpi, S. M., et al. (2002). Skill learning in patients with moderate Alzheimer's disease: A prospective pilot-study of waltz-lessons. *International Journal of Geriatric Psychiatry, 17*, 1155–1156.

Salazar, A. M., Warden, D. L., Schwab, K., Spector, J., Braverman, S., Walter, J., et al. (2000). Cognitive rehabilitation for traumatic brain injury: A randomized trial. *Journal of the American Medical Association, 283*, 3075–3081.

Salthouse, T. A. (1996). The processing-speed theory of adult age differences in cognition. *Psychological Review, 103*, 403–428.

Salthouse, T. A., & Somberg, B. L. (1982). Isolating the age deficit in speeded performance. *Journal of Gerontology, 37*, 59–63.

Schacter, D. L., Rich, S. A., & Stampp, M. S. (1985). Remediation of memory disorders: Experimental evaluation of the spaced-retrieval technique. *Journal of Clinical and Experimental Neuropsychology, 7*, 79–96.

Squires, E. J., Hunkin, N. M., & Parkin, A. J. (1997). Errorless learning of novel associations in amnesia. *Neuropsychologia, 35*, 1103–1111.

Wilson, B. A. (1999). Memory rehabilitation in brain-injured people. In D. T. Stuss, G. Winocur, & I. H. Robertson (Eds.), *Cognitive neurorehabilitation* (pp. 333–346). Cambridge, UK: Cambridge University Press.

Wilson, R. S., Mendes de Leon, C. F., & Barnes, L. L. (2002). Participation in cognitively stimulating activities and incident risk of Alzheimer's disease. *Journal of the American Medical Association, 287*, 742–748.

Zanetti, O., Magni, E., Binetti, G., Bianchetti, A., & Trabucchi, M. (1994). Is procedural memory stimulation effective in Alzheimer's disease? *International Journal of Geriatric Psychiatry, 9*, 1006–1007.

Zanetti, O., Rozzini, M. E., Bianchetti, A., & Trabucchi, M. (1997). Procedural memory stimulation in Alzheimer's disease: Impact of a training programme. *Acta Neurologica Scandinavica, 95*, 152–157.

Spaced Retrieval

A Model for Dissemination of a Cognitive Intervention for Persons with Dementia

CAMERON J. CAMP

It is not enough to be right—we must also be effective.
—Unofficial motto of the Myers Research Institute

Recently I was presenting a workshop on cognitive interventions for dementia to a group of staff from nursing homes in the Midwest. One attendee had heard a previous presentation of mine on an intervention known as spaced retrieval. She related that she had tried the intervention at her facility with a resident who had dementia and who was a "low talker," to use a phrase made famous by a long-running TV sitcom. The resident usually spoke in an unintelligible whisper. Using this intervention, the attendee trained the resident to talk louder when she would prompt the resident with the question "How should you talk to me?" A few weeks later, the resident evidenced a sudden bout of agitation and was pacing up and down the halls, speaking aloud (softly) and grimacing. The resident ignored questions from staff seeking to discern the source of discomfort. Staff were deciding whether to attempt to administer an antianxiety drug orally or through injection when the staff member who had trained the resident intervened. The resident was asked "How should you talk to me?" and responded, "TALK LOUDER." The staff member then asked, "What's wrong?" and the resident shouted in response, "MY FEET HURT!" The resident's feet were then examined and treatment administered for an aching bunion.

Research in neuroscience and cognitive aging must inform and influence treatment of persons with dementia. A better understanding of the trajectories of different cognitive abilities over the course of dementia is critical to the continuing evolution of better care and enhanced quality of life for persons with dementing illnesses. Although cholinergic drugs work to reestablish neurotransmission in brain regions damaged by dementing illness, they cannot enable reorganization of the nervous system to compensate for deficits (Requena et al., 2004). This lacuna in treatment argues strongly for the use of cognitive training interventions in dementia, perhaps in conjunction with pharmacological interventions (Loewenstein, Acevedo, Czaja, & Duara, 2004; Requena et al., 2004). Findings from research must be translated into best-care practices and delivered by nonresearchers as part of job routines. Psychologists can play a vital role in making such transitions a reality.

This chapter focuses on a cognitive intervention for persons with dementia, initially researched and developed by psychologists, called spaced retrieval (SR). First, the spaced retrieval technique is described. Research associated with this intervention and possible mechanisms responsible for the effects produced are reviewed. A case study is then presented to illustrate the obstacles to adoption of interventions that exist in real-world settings, along with recommendations for overcoming such obstacles.

DESCRIPTION OF THE SR TECHNIQUE

SR refers to a technique in which clients practice the successful retrieval of information over successively longer time intervals. Camp, Bird, and Cherry (2000) have documented the evolution of SR from a lab-based research topic to a therapeutic intervention for persons with dementia. Here let us consider an example of how SR might be used to address a common problem seen in care settings for persons with dementia.

A long-term care resident often complains that her daughter "never comes to visit," though the daughter visits two or three times a week, and the resident regularly asks staff "When is my daughter coming back to see me?" The intervention in this case might involve two components. First, there is a need to create an external memory aid that can store information about past and future visits. This aid might consist of a "guest book" in the resident's room. When the daughter comes to visit, she signs the guest book at the end of the visit, briefly describes the content of their visit, and notes when she will be returning next. The external aid is a necessary, though not sufficient, aspect of the intervention, for the older woman must learn to access the guest book when her anxiety rises concerning her daughter's visits. This is where SR can be most useful—creating new associations that link an external aid with a strategy for its effective use. (See Bourgeois, Chapter 15, this volume, for additional illustrations of external aids for persons with dementia.)

To create such an association, the therapist shows the external aid to the resident, with a page or two filled out, describes its function and content, and asks the resident "What would you call this?" If the resident supplies a reasonable name for the aid, that name would be used as the correct response. If no name was suggested, the name "guest book" would be provided and the resident asked "Does that sound like a good name for this?" If so, that name would be used for the aid during SR training. To establish the link between the guest book and its role in reducing visitation-related anxiety, the therapist would ask "When is your daughter coming to visit you?" When the resident says "I don't know" or provides an erroneous response, the therapist says "You can find out about your daughter's visit in your guest book. Now, where can you find out about your daughter's visit?" The resident, upon this prompt for immediate recall, should answer something like "In my guest book."

The therapist would then provide the prompt at expanding intervals, such as after 30 seconds, then after 60 seconds, then 2 minutes, 4 minutes, 8 minutes, and 16 minutes. If the resident does not provide a correct response, the therapist says the correct response and then the prompt is given again to elicit immediate recall. Thus each trial ends with a success. Then the next recall trial is shortened to that of the last previous successful recall interval. For example, if recall was successful at 2 minutes but not over a 4-minute interval, the next recall interval would be set back to 2 minutes. If the person is successful at 2 minutes, the intervals would begin expanding again.

The SR intervention is usually provided in 15-minute segments, because such segments are often used as billing increments for provision of rehabilitation (Malone, Camp, & Rose, 2002). As a result, within a session the longest expansion interval reached is usually 16 minutes, though this time frame does not have to become an upper limit if circumstances allow additional expansion. It is our experience that once expansion intervals begin to exceed 10 minutes, long-term retention of information (i.e., retention across training sessions) becomes very probable. In some instances, even shorter retention intervals can be predictive of a transfer of information into long-term memory (Camp, Foss, Stevens, & O'Hanlon, 1996, p. 359).

At the next therapy session, usually 1–7 days later, the therapist begins the session by providing the prompt. If the client provides the appropriate response, no further training is given in that session. Appropriate retention at the start of two or three consecutive therapy sessions signals a transition to maintenance training for the targeted information. If the client does not remember the correct response at the start of a session after initial training, the correct response is provided, immediately followed by another prompt and immediate recall by the client. This allows the recall probe trial to end with a success. The next recall trial interval will be of a length equal to the longest successful recall interval achieved in the previous therapy session. Expansion or contraction of subsequent recall intervals will depend on whether the client provides correct or incorrect responses to recall probes.

Brush and Camp (1998a) along with Malone et al. (2002) provide detailed instructions on the application of SR as a therapeutic intervention. These instructions include topics such as implementing a quick screening procedure to document evidence that a client shows potential to benefit from SR; how to proceed if a client does not answer; how to proceed if the client does (or does not) provide the correct response at the start of latter sessions; how to ensure that learned strategies are actually performed; and how to avoid most common errors in applying SR. Staff from the Myers Research Institute provide training seminars in appropriate application of SR (for more information, visit our website at www.myersresearch.org).

ESTABLISHING SR GOALS

SR goals vary according to the needs of clients. At a functional level, the specific cause of dementia is not as relevant to designing a goal as determining the features that lead to failure and the abilities that remain, on which to base the intervention. Basic issues in designing goals include:

- Can the client read (and, if so, can the client follow written directions)?
- Can the client manipulate objects?
- Why is the client failing to achieve a goal or engaging in problematic behavior?
- Does the intervention require training the client to remember factual information, the use of a strategy, the use of an external aid, or some combination of these?

In general, goals for SR involve training clients to learn or remember specific facts (e.g., adult children's names); where they (i.e., the clients) live; their room number; or the use of a strategy, which often involves the use of external aids (e.g., checking the guest book when they want to know about visitations). Two case studies illustrating the use of SR within the context of the Attix intervention model for geriatric neuropsychological intervention (Chapter 10, this volume) are now presented.

CASE EXAMPLES

Case 1. Mr. J, Alzheimer's Disease—Moderate Level Dementia

Mr. J was referred for intervention because of repetitive questioning. He would repeatedly go to the nursing station on his special care unit for dementia, asking when the next meal would be served.

Goals and Motivation

The client was motivated to be able to find this information for himself. He did not like to admit to having memory impairment or to have to depend on others to answer questions. (For repetitive question asking, it is critical to determine whether the behavior is driven by information seeking or by other factors such as a need for attention, social contact, reassurance, etc. SR can be very useful when repetitive questioning is driven by information seeking, but not for other causes. See Camp and Nasser [2003] for a discussion of methods to determine underlying causes and resultant interventions for agitation in persons with dementia.)

Neuropsychological Profile and Insight

Mr. J had significant difficulties retaining new episodic information for periods longer than 90 seconds. Mobile, verbal, and intelligent, he was aware of having some memory difficulties but did not want to discuss them because to do was embarrassing to him.

Affective Status

Mild emotional distress characterized by anxiety and changes in confidence were noted; his inability to remember mealtimes seemed to trigger increases in anxiety.

Current Compensatory Methods and Activities

Staff tried to be patient with the resident and answer his question whenever he asked "When is the next meal going to be served?" However, this strategy became stressful when the frequency of the behavior was high and staff had other demands on their time.

Intervention

The therapist determined that the client could read and comprehend printed instructions, configured to accommodate changes in vision often seen in persons with dementia (e.g., large print size, sans serif font, thick letters, high contrast). A quick evaluation of this ability is generally part of our initial examination. The therapist also noted that the client always carried a wallet. The therapist wrote the times of meals on an index card (e.g., "Breakfast is at 7 o'clock, lunch is at 12 o'clock, dinner is at 5 o'clock") and asked the client to read the card aloud and then put the card in his wallet. The therapist then initiated an SR training session in which the recall probe was "How can you find out when meals are served?" The client was to respond verbally "I've got it in my wallet," and then physically take out the card and read it aloud.

Note how practicing both the verbalization of the strategy and the motoric execution of the strategy—use of an external aid—creates multiple routes to assist the client in implementing the use of the aid. After SR training, the client generally would say the strategy aloud and execute it when his anxiety about mealtimes rose. If he went to the nursing station and asked the question, nursing staff would respond with the recall probe used during therapy to help reinitiate the desired response. One month after initial mastery of SR training, Mr. J was still successfully implementing the technique.

Case 2. Ms. L, HIV-Associated Dementia

Ms. L was referred for intervention because of problems remembering to take her medications appropriately.

Goals and Motivation

The client wanted to take her medications appropriately and understood that it was important for her to do this so that she would not start to feel worse.

Neuropsychological Profile and Insight

Ms. L had significant short-term memory deficits, along with evidence of executive dysfunction. She had limited insight into her condition.

Affective Status

Ms. L generally showed no great concern regarding her difficulties with medication adherence, possibly due to lack of insight. However, social isolation was a primary concern of hers and cause for some distress.

Current Compensatory Methods and Activities

As is typically the case for persons being treated for HIV, the client had been given a pillbox to organize her medications. However, she was not using it appropriately, though she was not aware of this.

Intervention

As is always the case, the key to designing a successful intervention was to determine where and why the client was failing. Discovering this information usually involves a task breakdown/analysis approach. Ms. L, for example, sometimes forgot to put medications into slots in her pillbox or she put in incorrect amounts, or she did not remember to take the pills at the appropriate time.

The intervention involved creating a template with life-size pictures of the pills the client was to put into the pillbox for the next week. She was trained to put the template next to the pillbox, to cover all of the pictures on the template with their corresponding pills, and then to put the pills into the pillbox. This task was to be done each Sunday before dinner. SR was used to create the association of getting out the template, pills, and pillbox when setting the Sunday dinner table, and of taking her pills when she heard a signal from a digital timekeeper set by a staff member. The client liked the template because it "did not make me have to think about what pills I had to put where." Interestingly, successful use of the template and the signals led the client to admit that she had not been as good as she had previously believed at taking her medications appropriately.

A wide variety of goals can be developed for SR interventions. Examples include safety issues (e.g., remembering to use a walker; "putting nose over toes" before standing; safe transfer techniques), repetitive questioning, anxiety reduction, anger management (e.g., "What should you do when you are about to lose it?"—"Get away and cool off in my room"). Examples of different goals that have been used with SR are shown in Table 12.1. In addition, consider the following example.

A long-term care resident was repetitively going to the nursing station on his unit and asking about his wife and when she would be coming to see him. The man's wife had died about 2 years before. Staff generally attempted delaying tactics ("She'll be here soon") or redirection with him, because they did not want to confront him with the bare fact that his wife was dead. These approaches were becoming less and less effective, and the resident's agitation was escalating. The next step seemed to be selecting the appropriate pharmacological intervention and method of its administration.

At that point a therapist who was training in the use of SR intervened. Using SR, she created the following association for the resident: "What should you do when you want to know about your wife?"—"Pick up and read the card" (i.e., a card kept at the nursing station). The therapist had created a card that read "Where is my wife?" on one side and a series of answers to the question on the other side. During SR training, the resident was trained to pick up the card (which was facing up with the question "Where is my wife?" on that side), turn it over, and read the text on the back side of the card. On that side, the text read:

"My wife isn't here because she cannot find me."
This makes no sense. She would move heaven and earth to find me.

"My wife isn't here because she is ill."
This probably isn't true. She was healthy all of her life, and my children would let me know if she was too ill to see me.

"My wife isn't here because she doesn't want to see me."
This cannot be true. We were in love all of our lives.

"My wife isn't here because she is with God now."
She passed away and is waiting for me. I'll be with her again in heaven.

This man had a strong religious faith, which the therapist took into consideration. When he first read the text on the back of the card, he nodded silently after seeing each answer. On completing the last lines of the text, the resident looked at the therapist and said, "Yes, if God will have her." These answers satisfied him, and he learned to go to the nursing station and pick up the card and read it whenever he became anxious about the whereabouts of his wife.

One way of approaching goal setting is to ask yourself what therapy you would use if the client did not have an episodic memory deficit for new information. The key is to identify causes of failure to benefit from therapy along with remaining skills. To the extent that the inability to remember new information is the chief barrier to benefiting from therapy, SR can help circumvent such deficits. In other words, SR creates a type of cognitive prosthesis. Of course, this prosthesis generally requires that therapeutic interventions can be written down or presented in a pictorial or auditory format (e.g., using a tape recording), and that use of such external aids can indeed allow interventions to be executed by the client.

In addition to its use for a variety of goals, SR also has been shown to work across a variety of dementing conditions: Alzheimer's disease (Anderson, Arens, Johnsom, & Coppens, 2001; Arkin, 1991; Bird, Alexopoulos, & Adamowicz, 1995; Bourgeois et al., 2003; Brush & Camp, 1998b, 1998c; Camp et al., 1996; McKitrick, Camp, & Black, 1992); dementia related to Parkinson's disease (Hayden & Camp, 1995) and HIV (Lee & Camp, 2001; Neundorfer et al., 2004); and mixed dementia (Abrahams & Camp, 1993). Bourgeois et al. (2003) also demonstrated that SR can produce better learning and retention than cueing hierarchies (e.g., the use of phonemic and semantic cues to assist recall)

TABLE 12.1. Examples of SR Goals

Type of goal	Diagnosis	Source
Using a calendar to remember daily tasks	AD	Camp et al. (1996)
Remembering to redeem a coupon	AD	McKitrick, Camp, & Black (1992)
Object naming	AD with vascular dementia	Abrahams & Camp (1993)
Remembering to eat	HAD	Neundorfer et al. (2004)
Describing an item if patient cannot name it	CVA	Brush & Camp (1998b)
Remembering room number	Dementia	Brush & Camp (1998b)
Speaking into a voice amplifier when talking	CVA/dysarthria	Brush & Camp (1998b)
Taking a sip of liquid after eating a bite of food	Dementia/dysphagia	Brush & Camp (1998c)
Building face–name associations	AD	Clare et al. (2002); Loewenstein et al. (2004)
Using a notebook to find answers to questions	AD and vascular dementia	Bird & Kinsella (1996)
Addressing "paranoid delusions" and violent behavior	AD	Bird (2001)
Addressing obsessive toileting	Hypoxic brain damage	Bird (2001)
Facilitating anger management	Traumatic brain injury	M. Bourgeois (personal communication, March 2004)

Note. AD, Alzheimer's disease; HAD, HIV-associated dementia; CVA, cerebrovascular accident.

in persons with dementia. Why should this be the case? Possible mechanisms underlying SR that might be responsible for its effects are examined next. It should be noted that these mechanisms are not mutually exclusive, and some elements of each may be acting in concert during therapy sessions in which SR is used.

SR as Spacing Effect

One way of viewing SR is that it represents a variation of a general memory phenomenon known as the spacing effect. The term *spacing effect* refers to the finding that information is learned and retrieved more effectively when learning trials are distributed over time (i.e., distributed practice) compared to consecutive presentation of all learning trials (i.e., massed practice; Camp et al., 2000; Cermak, Verfaellie, Lanzoni, Mather, & Chase, 1996; Ebbinghaus, 1885/1964; Hillary et al., 2003). In the case of SR, the distributed practice of learning trials includes an expansion function, such that successive trials occur at ever-increasing intervals.

There are multiple explanations for why the spacing effect should produce better learning than massed practice (see Braun & Rubin, 1998; Cermak et al., 1996; Green, 1992; Hillary et al., 2003; Hintzman, 1974; Murdock, 2003). A discussion of this topic is beyond the scope of this chapter. However, a summary comment is possible. Hillary et al. (2003) noted that any explanation of the spacing effect (and hence of SR) "must accommodate the fact that the [spacing effect] is a natural phenomenon of the human memory system that does not, necessarily, require conscious effort, training, or additional mental operations by the individual" (pp. 50–51). It is interesting these researchers demonstrated that the spacing effect was present in a sample of adults with traumatic brain injury (TBI), who demonstrated impaired memory on a standardized neuropsychological test battery. Cermak et al. (1996) demonstrated spacing effects for both recognition and recall in amnesia patients, attributing at least some of the spacing effects in recall to automatic processes.

SR as Priming

Squire (1992, 1994) describes memory as primarily composed of two systems: declarative memory and nondeclarative memory (also called procedural memory). The declarative memory system is believed to involve conscious, effortful learning, such as remembering what you had for breakfast; what was said to you 5 minutes ago; where you parked your car; your address when you were in high school; or general information about the world (the capitals of France and Cambodia). The nondeclarative/procedural memory system is believed to involve relatively unconscious, automatic, and effortless learning. In Squire's model, this system has multiple components, one of which involves *priming*, a form of nondeclarative (or implicit) memory in which prior exposure to a stimulus exerts an effect on the later detection or identification of that stimulus. For example, semantic priming is the effect in which a response to items from a particular class of words (e.g., animals) is facilitated by the presentation of a different item from the same semantic class.

Squire (1992, 1994) and other researchers (e.g., Cermak, Talbot, Chandler, & Wolbarst, 1985; Haist, Musen, & Squire, 1991; Verfaellie & Cermak, 1994; Verfaellie, Cermak, Letourneau, & Zuffante, 1991; Weingartner et al., 1993) have demonstrated that persons with memory deficits can show priming effects in the absence of conscious recollection of practice episodes or of having encountered information previously that has now been learned (see Reichard, Camp, & Strub, 1995, for an example of this in persons with Alzheimer's disease). Camp and Foss (1997) have described SR as a form of "ecologically valid priming" and presented experimental evidence that SR seems to involve nondeclarative/procedural memory systems rather than declarative memory systems (see also Cherry, Simmons, & Camp, 1999; Cherry & Simmons-D'Gerolamo, 1999, 2005).

SR as Conditioning

Bjork (1988) referred to SR as shaping applied to memory. From this perspective, SR uses *operant conditioning* techniques to enable persons with short-term memory deficits to achieve closer and closer approximations to the desired goal of putting information into long-term memory. Successful recall serves as an intrinsic reinforcer—perhaps especially so for persons with memory deficits. Thus, once a goal has been established that is meaningful to the client with dementia, successful SR recall trials are often highly motivating. Evoking motivation addresses a key component of the model of geriatric neuropsychological intervention described by Attix (Chapter 10, this volume). To the extent that clients are aware of memory deficits, SR also interfaces with the *insight* component of Attix's intervention model, in that the successful recall performance in SR contrasts with recall failures under ordinary circumstances in these persons.

An optional way of viewing SR is as a *classical conditioning* paradigm. Certainly, strong associations are created between a prompt and the recall of the target behavior after multiple pairings. In a case study reported elsewhere (Stevens, O'Hanlon, & Camp, 1993), a man with dementia initially had difficulty learning to say the response "Look at my calendar" when prompted with the questions "How do you know what to do today?" The study describes how the target response was changed from saying the answer to turning a card over and reading the answer that had been written on the other side (see the discussion to follow on SR as errorless learning). A fading cues approach was then used, to the point that the man was able to effectively learn and execute the strategy of looking at his calendar and following its directions regarding daily chores or appointments to keep. What was not reported was that initially the participant confided to a research assistant that he "didn't care for" the lead trainer in the study. This occurred at a time when the participant was experiencing initial failures in our training. However, after the training began to involve the use of SR in conjunction with an external cue and motor response (i.e., turning the card over and reading the answer), the participant confided that he "really liked" the lead trainer. At the conclusion of the study, the participant asked if the lead trainer would like to accompany him and his family on their yearly vacation. The *goals* and *motivation* components of the Attix intervention model are impacted by classical conditioning in SR. The above example also illustrates that SR can be effective in the absence of significant *insight*.

This phenomenon is often observed by our rehabilitation staff at Menorah Park, where clients may not remember sessions they have had with their therapist but will make positive comments to the therapist, such as saying "I like you—I think you make me smarter or something." Whether classical conditioning is the primary mechanism underlying SR or a secondary feature of the clinical process remains to be discovered. In either case the ability to elicit positive associations between clients and their therapists/therapy sessions is a potent adjunct to the use of SR for persons with dementia, and seems to contribute to its success.

SR as Errorless Learning

Errorless learning involves attempts to reduce or eliminate the production of errors during learning trials. This method was first described in the operant conditioning literature, in which Terrace (1963) used this approach to teach discrimination learning to pigeons. Barbara Wilson and her colleagues (Baddeley, 1992; Clare et al., 2000; Wilson, Baddeley, Evans, & Sheil, 1994; Wilson & Evans, 1996) have discussed the need to use errorless learning when designing training programs for persons with memory impairment. The idea behind this line of work is that trial-and-error learning is less effective for persons with memory impairment, including persons with dementia, than learning paradigms that prevent error. These researchers assume that the automatic nature of procedural/ nondeclarative (implicit) memory makes it particularly vulnerable to interference when errors occur in learning, especially in persons with impaired declarative (explicit) memory, because they lack conscious access to recent training trails. This lack of access makes it difficult for persons with memory impairment (such as persons with dementia) to use past episodes to evaluate and correct current erroneous responses.

Not all researchers agree that errorless learning is solely dependent on nondeclarative/procedural memory (e.g., Hunkin, Squires, Parkin, & Tidy, 1998; see Anderson et al., 2001, for an additional discussion of this topic). Fillingham, Hogsdon, Sage, and Ralph (2003) offer a model based on Hebbian learning and feedback modulation that can accommodate errorless learning processes in both normal and memory-impaired populations. They also make a distinction in the errorless learning literature between training that involves *error elimination* versus *error reduction*, in which errors are reduced but not completely eliminated during training. It should be noted that in rehabilitative contexts, where tasks are made gradually harder for clients, error reduction may be a more realistic goal.

DISSEMINATION OF SR

The biggest barrier to the dissemination of nonpharmacological interventions for persons with dementia is *therapeutic nihilism*—the belief that a person or a population cannot benefit from intervention (see Clark, 1995). In its extreme form, this nihilism assumes that anyone who attempts to intervene is dishonest and/or naïve and therefore are not to be trusted, assisted, or believed. As a case in point, until 2002, provision of rehabilitation services to persons with dementia was severely constricted, especially in the area of cognitive disabilities. The reasoning behind this stance was that persons with AD and related dementing conditions could not remember what was trained in therapy and thus could not benefit from it—a clear case of therapeutic nihilism.

However, due to pressure from two forces—consumer groups such as the national Alzheimer's Association and a growing body of research indicating that learning could take place in persons with dementia—this policy was revoked (CMS-Pub. 60AB, dated 9/25/01). Note that the policy revocation occurred in the fall of 2001 but was not publicized until the spring of 2002. Resistance to change is inherent in health delivery systems (see Berwick, 2003). However, in essence, a new market for services has been opened. Persons with dementia represent a growing public health concern, so this change in policy is quite timely.

Therapeutic nihilism exists at many levels of health care systems: in the physician who refuses to refer a client for therapy; in the reimbursing agency that will not provide payment for therapy delivered; in the course curriculum of an academic department where treatment of persons with dementia is either scantily addressed within more generic course content, or missing entirely; in the family members who tell a clinician that their older relative will not be able to benefit from a psychosocial intervention; in the staff members who say that their clients or residents have no capacity to improve. In essence, therapeutic nihilism is an example of learned helplessness at a systemic level. The chapters in this volume provide examples of a wide variety of efficacious nonpharmacological interventions for problems associated with dementia (see also Camp, Cohen-Mansfield, & Capezuti, 2002), with SR being one weapon in this arsenal. Indeed, other researchers are now embedding SR within multicomponent interventions for persons with dementia (Clare et al., 2000; Clare, Wilson, Carter, Roth, & Hodges, 2002; Koltai, Welsh-Bohmer, & Schmechel, 2001; Loewenstein et al., 2004). But therapeutic nihilism is a ubiquitous impediment to the implementation of any intervention. How, therefore, can this insidious obstacle be overcome?

SR as a Case Study

Fillingham et al. (2003) noted that a challenge to the use of errorless learning paradigms for persons with memory impairment (and, by extension, to any intervention initially focused on demonstrations of efficacy) is to do so in a cost-effective manner within the constraints of standard clinical practice. Many errorless learning paradigms involve protocols that are time intensive. This approach conflicts with a managed care environment that demands quick, quantifiable improvement. This requirement addresses a necessary but not sufficient condition for dissemination—an intervention must be shown to be effective within real-world contexts.

With regard to SR, as described earlier, this intervention utilizes an error-reduction process in which clients are continually challenged to recall information at longer and longer intervals. The use of expanding schedules of recall trials makes SR a nonintensive approach. In addition, we have demonstrated (Brush & Camp, 1998a, 1998b, 1998c; Brush & Camp, 1999; Malone, Camp, & Rose, 2003) that it can be implemented as a reimbursable therapy procedure. But demonstration of the effectiveness, in addition to the efficacy, of nonpharmacological intervention does not remove most obstacles to dissemination of interventions for persons with dementia (see Camp, 2001, for a general review of transitions between efficacy, effectiveness, and dissemination involved in interventions for dementia).

The Need for Multilevel Intervention

Intervention for this population must occur on many levels. At the level of policy change, advocacy from organizations such as the American Psychological Association and the American Psychological Society must be combined with advocacy from consumer groups such as the Alzheimer's Association. In addition, data from research demonstrating that psychosocial interventions developed for persons with dementia are both an efficacious and cost-effective means of providing better care for these clients must be made available and their relevance demonstrated to policymakers. Again, the successful attempt to allow reimbursement for rehabilitation provided to persons with Alzheimer's disease serves as a useful template for this process.

At the level of physician referral sources, education regarding psychosocial intervention often lags far behind access to information provided by pharmaceutical companies. There is no sales force for psychosocial treatment options to compare with that marshaled by drug companies. As a result, therapists wishing to increase referrals from physicians must be entrepreneurial. For example, when we talked to physicians about what would persuade them to make referrals for psychosocial interventions, their responses were clear and straightforward:

- The efficacy of the intervention should be research- and evidence-based.
- There should be an indication that a screening process has been used or is available to indicate that the treatment is both called for and likely to produce positive results for a particular client.
- The prescription for the intervention should not be viewed as open-ended; there should be a clear criterion for whether the therapy is generating progress toward a legitimate goal, as well as a clear criterion for when to stop therapy as a result of lack of progress or goal attainment.
- There should be a clearly articulated system in place to ensure maintenance of treatment effects.

As a result of these discussions, SR training provided by staff of the Myers Research Institute includes provision of templates for letters to physicians addressing each of these issues. We also include pages of research references documenting the effectiveness of SR for these physicians to peruse. (References are provided in a format usually found in medical journals, such as *The Journal of the American Medical Association*.)

At the level of staff, family members, or others responsible for maintenance of effects produced by therapy, it is important that these individuals overcome a version of therapeutic nihilism that contains two "sub-beliefs," if you will. The first sub-belief is that the therapist cannot produce positive change in a client with dementia. There is only one way to address this contention—by demonstrating that the client is capable of improving. Demonstrating this improvement must be done under the gaze of persons who will then become responsible for maintaining the effects produced by the therapy. A report of progress made in an office may not (usually *will* not?) be believed, and often will not result in an effective maintenance program.

Consider the case of a nurse assistant on a special care unit for persons with dementia in a skilled nursing facility. A therapist takes a resident off unit and then returns, instructing the assistant to undertake additional activities for maintenance of an intervention never seen by him or her. The outcome of this process is as predictable as it is relatively unavoidable. As a result, we suggest that cognitive interventions be undertaken on the units where residents live, whenever possible. Client training in an office cannot be observed by persons who will be asked to maintain therapy outcomes. Additionally, for persons with dementia, generalization from an office environment to their living environments may be unrealistic.

The second sub-belief is that the therapist can produce successful outcomes, but not the caregiver. Again, this perspective can only be addressed by including the caregiver in a transitional training phase in which the caregiving will take place. Working with a client at the dinner table will make it easier to enlist and empower a nurse assistant in maintaining effects of cognitive interventions for eating or hydration. Persons charged with maintaining effects of SR therapy initially can be supervised and coached when SR is provided in real-world time frames and contexts. In addition, the therapist can discuss the benefits of SR maintenance and the negative consequences for both the client and the therapy maintainer, should maintenance not be attempted or continued over time.

For administrators, it is important to link interventions to four key factors. The first is the *mission statement* of a facility or organization. It must be made clear that provision of an intervention, and support for staff working to maintain the intervention, is clearly connected with the mission of an organization (Jitka Zgola, personal communication, November, 2003). Establishing this link makes it more difficult for midlevel managers, unit coordinators, or supervisors who have yet to overcome therapeutic nihilism to undermine interventions: To oppose the intervention is to oppose the mission of their organization.

The next three factors relate to what is known as the *health care triangle model* (Camp & Brush, 2003). These are three key areas of interest to administrators of facilities providing care for persons with dementia: *reimbursement*, *marketing*, and *surviving state inspections*. We start with the assumption that for an intervention to be effective in real long-term care facilities where dementia care is provided, any intervention must be demonstrated to positively impact at least one of these areas (preferably, all three). These are the areas paramount to chief executive officers, regardless of whether a facility is nonprofit or for profit. Interventions that do not positively address these areas are likely to disappear as soon as the psychologist responsible for introducing them leaves the building. It is therefore critical to point out that a good intervention can also mean good business, and that provision of a better quality of care makes a facility more competitive in the marketplace. Once a chief executive approves of an intervention, then work can begin to convince middle managers and line staff to implement and maintain it.

An example of this dissemination process can be illustrated by the working relationship that exists between Myers Research Institute (MRI) and HCR ManorCare, Inc. (ManorCare), a for-profit national company that owns skilled nursing facilities, assisted care facilities, and home health care agencies. After listening to a presentation on SR research for persons with dementia, executive staff of ManorCare expressed an interest in learning more about the intervention. Further contacts resulted in a demonstration project in which speech–language pathologists (SLPs) working for ManorCare in the greater Cleveland area were trained by staff from the MRI in the use of SR. After ManorCare conducted an internal study of the effects of this training on measures such as goals attained and increases in billable hours, which were confirmed independently by our own research (Malone et al., 2003), outcomes were so impressive that MRI was asked to begin training their therapists nationally. In addition, staff from MRI assisted in development of a corporate training model so that ManorCare's staff could begin to disseminate SR training within their company. To date, SLPs and other therapists from over 100 ManorCare facilities nationally have been trained in the application of SR. For executives and staff of ManorCare, use of SR is a win–win situation: It increases their billable hours (addressing the issue of reimbursement, the first component of the health care triangle model), and provides effective means of addressing a host of goals for their clients with dementia that could not be addressed as readily before SR was made available to their therapists.

With regard to marketing, ManorCare now advertises the availability of SR to their clients. Implementation of SR by their therapists is referred to as their "MemorEase Program." The ability to provide SR is seen as a marketing advantage for ManorCare, thus addressing the second component of the health care triangle model.

Finally, ManorCare executives view SR as a helpful means of facilitating improvement in quality indicators (QIs), addressing the third component of the health care triangle model. For example, an SLP working for ManorCare related an example to her trainers in which she used SR with a client living in a skilled nursing facility. This resident was not drinking water or fluids when these were placed in front of her. Nursing staff were resorting to the use of IVs to keep the resident hydrated and thereby avoid flagging the resident for the QI of dehydration. The therapists newly trained in SR used the technique to train the resident to drink water from her glass when given a verbal prompt. This training was carried out at the dinner table, during meals, and in the presence of nursing staff who were charged with administering the IVs to the resident. Given the choice between providing an IV or a verbal prompt for maintaining the effects of SR, nursing staff immediately saw the relevance of the therapist's intervention and enthusiastically adopted it. In addition, administrators at every level value inexpensive and effective means of providing good quality care that results in preventing residents from being flagged for QIs.

A final lesson we have learned through this experience is that executives in the business of delivering dementia care value research. We are continually asked by administrators and managers if the interventions we propose are supported by research and are evidence-based. The ability to respond that research on SR has been federally funded and has generated publications in academic journals is valued in the marketplace. Businesspersons want to know that research involving interventions such as SR have credibility in the scientific community. Good science is appreciated and seen as enhancing marketability of services delivered by this industry.

CONCLUSIONS

Researchers in neuroscience and cognitive aging as well as practicing clinical geropsychologists and neuropsychologists are making great strides in the development and delivery of efficacious and effective interventions for care of persons with dementia. By training and circumstance, psychologists in this area have focused on treatment of the individual client or on training staff within a specific facility. In this chapter, intervention at a systems level has been discussed. This perspective was taken in the hope that readers would view their efforts in a larger context, and perhaps that some would begin the work of attempting to carry forward interventions through the process of dissemination.

Berwick (2003) provides a fascinating overview of the diffusion of innovation (i.e., novel interventions) in health care systems. For those readers who have not rejected the implications of this chapter and who have continued reading to this point, Berwick's article is highly recommended. One component of Berwick's work (out of many) is a discussion of the five perceived attributes of an innovation that help determine speed of adoption and change.

The first (and most powerful) is the perceived *benefit* of the change. The intervention must be helpful, but it must also be viewed as low in risk. Unfamiliar change requires extra burdens of proof. That is why we consciously consider the health care triangle model when discussing SR, and why we assume that an intervention such as SR must be seen as providing benefit with low risk to therapists, clients, and the organization that employs the therapists.

The second attribute is *compatibility*. To diffuse quickly, an intervention must be seen as compatible with the values, history, and current needs of an organization and its staff. This is why we discuss the mission statement of a facility and organization when describing SR. Therapists need interventions that are effective, not time intensive, and that generate both billable hours and continuing referrals because of a good track record. When we provide training in SR to these persons, we address all of these issues.

For two reasons, the third attribute, *simplicity*, may be an especially difficult issue (and barrier) for researchers who wish to see their interventions disseminated. The first, as Berwick astutely notes, is that "individuals who develop an innovation often are not its best salespeople, because they are at least as invested in its complexity as its elegance. They tend to insist on absolute replication, not adaptation" (p. 1971). Simple interventions generally spread more quickly than complicated ones.

This point relates to the second reason: Interventions/innovations do not actually spread, they are "reinvented." Adopters will take complex interventions and simplify them during the implementation process. Adopters will also change interventions to suit their own needs. Berwick likens this process to the way children learn language. As he states, "In fact, children who only repeat what they hear are not good learners; they are autistic. Individuals in organizations are learners. They do not merely repeat what they hear, they change it" (p. 1971). Furthermore, for interventions to be disseminated widely, originators must not only accept this change process, they must encourage it. Readers can judge for themselves how well this principle might be tolerated by researchers.

The fourth attribute is *trialability*: Interventions must be tested on a small scale before widespread adoption takes place. At MRI, we are ideally suited for this process. As part of Menorah Park Center for Senior Living, we can first develop interventions such as SR "in-house." Next, we work with nearby facilities, as we did with ManorCare, to test the intervention on a small scale in new settings before attempting dissemination.

The final attribute is *observability*, which relates to the ease with which potential adopters and implementers can watch others try the change first. This is why we insist that therapists implementing SR must do so in the presence of caregivers who will be asked to maintain effects of therapy. This is also why we use video recordings extensively in our training. Adopters must see interventions being implemented, and this process must result in their belief that they too can utilize the intervention. Only then will the defense of therapeutic nihilism be overcome.

This chapter has not provided a "how to" description of SR. Such instructions already have been published, as described previously. Instead, this chapter has focused on the translation of SR into an effective intervention that can be widely disseminated. A description of the theoretical explanations underlying effects of SR was given. To date, no single explanation has emerged as definitive, and perhaps no such single explanation will ever emerge.

A description of the process of dissemination of interventions was then presented. At MRI we have focused our energies on the dissemination of SR, an intervention that can help persons with dementia. For whatever underlying reason, SR works (pragmatic validity, if you will). This process has served as a model for dissemination of other interventions for dementia, such as Montessori-based Dementia Programming. In response to this second dissemination process, ManorCare, and MRI were jointly awarded recognition for outstanding achievement in health care practice by the American Society of Aging in 2004. At MRI we take Berwick's (2003) final admonition for dissemination of innovation to heart—*lead by example*.

ACKNOWLEDGMENTS

Preparation of this manuscript was partially supported through Grant No. R21 MH069199 from the National Institute of Mental Health and Grant Nos. R01 AG17908 and R03 AG19016 from the National Institute on Aging to Cameron J. Camp. I wish to thank Jennifer Brush, Michelle Bourgeois, Megan Malone, Jaime Carr, Miriam Rose, Audrey Holland, and Blanche White for their comments in the development of spaced retrieval as an intervention that could be disseminated on a large scale. I especially thank the Rehabilitation Department (Rehab Plus) of Menorah Park Center for Senior Living and the residents and clients of Menorah Park, without whom this work would not have proceeded.

REFERENCES

Abrahams, J. P., & Camp, C. J. (1993). Maintenance and generalization of object naming training in anomia associated with degenerative dementia. *Clinical Gerontologist, 12,* 57–72.

Anderson, J., Arens, K., Johnson, R., & Coppens, P. (2001). Spaced retrieval vs. memory tape therapy in memory rehabilitation for dementia of the Alzheimer's type. *Clinical Gerontologist, 24*(1/2), 123–139.

Arkin, S. M. (1991). Memory training in early Alzheimer's disease: An optimistic look at the field. *American Journal of Alzheimer's and Related Disorders Care and Research, 6,* 17–25.

Baddeley, A. D. (1992). Implicit memory and errorless learning: A link between cognitive psychology and neuropsychological rehabilitation? In L. R. Squire & N. Butters (Eds.), *Neuropsychology of memory* (2nd ed., pp. 309–314). New York: Guilford Press.

Berwick, D. M. (2003). Disseminating innovations in health care. *Journal of the American Medical Association, 289*(15), 1969–1975.

Bird, M. (2001). Behavioural difficulties and cued recall of adaptive behaviour in dementia: Experimental and clinical evidence. *Neuropsychological Rehabilitation, 11,* 357–375.

Bird, M., Alexopoulos, P., & Adamowicz, J. (1995). Success and failure in five case studies: Use of cued recall to ameliorate behaviour problems in senile dementia. *International Journal of Geriatric Psychiatry, 10,* 305–311.

Bird, M., & Kinsella, G. (1996). Long-term cued recall of tasks in senile dementia. *Psychology and Aging, 11,* 45–56.

Bjork, R. A. (1988). Retrieval practice and the maintenance of knowledge. In M. M. Gruneberg, P. Morris, & R. Sykes (Eds.), *Practical aspect of memory* (Vol. 2, pp. 396-401). London: Academic Press.

Bourgeois, M. S., Camp, C. J., Rose, M., White, B., Malone, M., Carr, J., & Rovine, M. (2003). A comparison of training strategies to enhance use of external aids by persons with dementia. *Journal of Communication Disorders, 36,* 361–378.

Braun, K., & Rubin, D. C. (1998). The spacing effect depends on an encoding deficit, retrieval, and time in working memory: Evidence from once-presented words. *Memory, 6*(1), 37–65.

Brush, J. A., & Camp, C. J. (1998a). *A therapy technique for improving memory: Spaced retrieval.* Beachwood, OH: Menorah Park Center for Senior Living.

Brush, J. A., & Camp, C. J. (1998b). Using spaced retrieval as an intervention during speech–language therapy. *Clinical Gerontologist, 19,* 51–64.

Brush, J. A., & Camp, C. J. (1998c). Using spaced retrieval to treat dysphagia in a long-term care resident with dementia. *Clinical Gerontologist, 19*(2), 96–99.

Brush, J. A., & Camp, C. J. (1999). Effective interventions for persons with dementia: Using spaced retrieval and Montessori techniques. *Neurophysiology and Neurogenic Speech and Language Disorders, 9*(4), 27–32.

Camp, C. J. (2001). From efficacy to effectiveness to diffusion: Making the transitions in dementia intervention research. *Neuropsychological Rehabilitation, 11,* 495–517.

Camp, C. J., Bird, M. J., & Cherry, K. E. (2000). Retrieval strategies as a rehabilitation aid for cognitive loss in pathological aging. In R. D. Hill, L. Bäckman, & A. S. Neely (Eds.), *Cognitive rehabilitation in old age* (pp. 224–248). New York: Oxford University Press.

Camp, C. J., & Brush, J. A. (2003, January). *Managing residents with dementia utilizing the successful health care triangle model.* Symposium presented for Northern Speech Services, Austin, TX.

Camp, C. J., Cohen-Mansfield, J., & Capezuti, E. A. (2002). Use of nonpharmacologic interventions among nursing home residents with dementia. *Psychiatric Services, 53,* 1397–1401.

Camp, C. J., & Foss, J. W. (1997). Designing ecologically valid memory interventions for persons with dementia. In D. G. Payne & F. G. Conrad (Eds.), *Intersections in basic and applied memory research* (pp. 311–325). Mahwah, NJ: Erlbaum.

Camp, C. J., Foss, J. W., Stevens, A. B., & O'Hanlon, A. M. (1996). Improving prospective memory task performance in Alzheimer's disease. In M. A. Brandimonte, G. O. Einstein, & M. A. McDaniel (Eds.), *Prospective memory: Theory and applications* (pp. 351–367). Mahwah, NJ: Erlbaum.

Camp, C. J., & Nasser, E . H. (2003). Nonpharmacological aspects of agitation and behavioral disorders in dementia: Assessment, intervention, and challenges to providing care. In P. A. Lichtenberg, D. L. Murman, & A. M. Mellow (Eds.), *Handbook of dementia: Psychological, neurological, and psychiatric perspectives* (pp. 359–401). New York: Wiley.

Cermak, L. S., Talbot, N., Chandler, K., & Wolbarst, L. R. (1985). The perceptual priming phenomenon in amnesia. *Neuropsychologia, 21,* 615–622.

Cermak, L. S., Verfaellie, M., Lanzoni, S., Mather, M., & Chase, K. A. (1996). Effect of spaced repetitions on amnesia patients' recall and recognition performance. *Neuropsychology, 10,* 219–227.

Cherry, K. E., Simmons, S. S., & Camp, C. J. (1999). Spaced-retrieval enhances memory in older adults with probable Alzheimer's disease. *Journal of Clinical Geropsychology, 5,* 159–175.

Cherry, K. E., & Simmons-D'Gerolamo, S. S. (1999). Effects of a target object orientation task on recall in older adults with probable Alzheimer's disease. *Clinical Gerontologist, 20,* 39–63.

Cherry, K. E., & Simmons-D'Gerolamo, S. (2005). Long-term effectiveness of spaced-retrieval memory training for older adults with probable Alzheimer's Disease. *Experimental Aging Research, 31,* 1–29

Clare, L., Wilson, B. A., Carter, G., Breen, K., Gosses, A., & Hodges, J. R. (2000). Intervening with everyday memory problems in dementia of the Alzheimer's type: An errorless learning approach. *Journal of Clinical and Experimental Neuropsychology, 22*(1), 132–146.

Clare , L., Wilson, B. A., Carter, G., Roth, I., & Hodges, J. R. (2002). Relearning face–name associations in early Alzheimer's disease. *Neuropsychology, 16,* 538–547.

Clark, L. W. (1995). Interventions for persons with Alzheimer's disease: Strategies for maintaining and enhancing communicative success. *Topics in Language Disorders, 15,* 47–65.

Ebbinghaus, H. (1964). *Memory: A contribution to experimental psychology.* New York: Dover. (Original work published in 1885)

Fillingham, J. K., Hogsdon, C., Sage, K., & Ralph, M. A. L. (2003). The application of errorless learning to aphasic disorders: A review of theory and practice. *Neuropsychological Rehabilitation, 13,* 337–363.

Green, R. L. (1992). Repetition paradigms. In R. L. Green (Ed.), *Human memory: Paradigms and paradoxes* (pp. 132–152). Hillsdale, NJ: Erlbaum.

Haist, F., Musen, G., & Squire, L. R. (1991). Intact priming of words and nonwords in amnesia. *Psychobiology, 19,* 275–285.

Hayden, C. M., & Camp, C. J. (1995). Spaced-retrieval: A memory intervention for dementia in Parkinson's disease. *Clinical Gerontologist, 16*(3), 80–82.

Hillary, F. G., Schultheis, M. T., Challis, B. H., Millis, S. R., Carnevale, G. J., Galshi, T., et al. (2003). Spacing of repetitions improves learning and memory after moderate and severe TBI. *Journal of Clinical and Experimental Neuropsychology, 25,* 49–58.

Hintzman, D. L. (1974). Theoretical implications of the spacing effect. In R. L. Solso (Ed.), *Theories in cognitive psychology: The Loyola Symposium* (pp. 77–99). Potomac, MD: Erlbaum.

Hunkin, N. M., Squires, E. J., Parkin, A. J., & Tidy, J. A. (1998). Are the benefits of errorless learning dependent on implicit memory? *Neuropsychologia, 36*(1), 25–36.

Koltai, D. C., Welsh-Bohmer, K. A., & Schmechel, D. E. (2001). Influence of anosognosia on treatment outcome among dementia patients. *Neuropsychological Rehabilitation*, *11*, 455–475.

Lee, M. M., & Camp, C. J. (2001). Spaced-retrieval: A memory intervention for HIV+ older adults. *Clinical Gerontologist*, *22*(3/4), 131–135.

Loewenstein, D. A., Acevedo, A., Czaja, S. J., & Duara, R. (2004). Cognitive rehabilitation of mildly impaired Alzheimer disease patients on cholinesterase inhibitors. *American Journal of Geriatric Psychiatry*, *12*, 395–402.

Malone, M., Camp, C., & Rose, M. (2002). *The spaced-retrieval technique: A training seminar manual*. Beachwood, OH: Menorah Park Center for Senior Living.

Malone, M., Camp, C., & Rose, M. (2003). The spaced-retrieval technique: A "Train the Trainer" program for rehabilitation staff [Abstract]. *Gerontologist*, *43*(Special Issue 1), 135.

McKitrick, L. A., Camp, C. J., & Black, W. (1992). Prospective memory intervention in Alzheimer's disease. *Journals of Gerontology: Psychological Sciences*, *47*, P337–P343

Murdock, B. (2003). The mirror effect and the spacing effect. *Psychonomic Bulletin and Review*, *10*, 570–588.

Neundorfer, J. J., Camp, C. J., Lee, M. M., Skrajner, M. J., Malone, M. L., & Carr, J. R. (2004). Compensating for cognitive deficits in persons aged 50 and over with HIV/AIDS: A pilot study of a cognitive intervention. *Journal of HIV/AIDS and Social Services*, *3*, 79–97.

Reichard, C. C., Camp, C. J., & Strub, R. L. (1995). Effects of sudden insight on long-term sentence priming in Alzheimer's disease. *Journal of Clinical and Experimental Neuropsychology*, *17*, 325–334.

Requena, C., Lopez Ibor, M. I., Maestu, F., Campo, P., Lopez Ibor, J. J., & Ortiz, T. (2004). Effects of cholinergic drugs and cognitive training on dementia. *Dementia and Geriatric Cognitive Disorders*, *18*, 50–54.

Schacter, D. L., Rich, S. A., & Stampp, M. S. (1985). Remediation of memory disorders: Experimental evaluation of the spaced-retrieval technique. *Journal of Clinical and Experimental Neuropsychology*, *7*, 79–96.

Squire, L. R. (1992). Memory and the hippocampus: A synthesis from findings with rats, monkeys, and humans. *Psychological Review*, *99*, 195–231.

Squire, L. R. (1994). Declarative and nondeclarative memory: Multiple brain system supporting learning and memory. In D. L. Schacter & E. Tulving (Eds.), *Memory systems 1994* (pp. 203–232). Cambridge, MA: MIT Press.

Stevens, A. B., O'Hanlon, A. M., & Camp, C. J. (1993). Strategy training in Alzheimer's disease: A case study. *Clinical Gerontologist*, *13*, 106–109.

Terrace, H. S. (1963). Discrimination learning with and without "errors." *Journal of the Experimental Analysis of Behavior*, *6*, 1–27.

Verfaelli, M., & Cermak, L. S. (1994). Acquisition of generic memory in aphasia. *Cortex*, *30*, 293–303.

Verfaelli, M., Cermak, L. S., Letourneau, L., & Zuffante, P. (1991). Repetition effects in a lexical decision task: The role of episodic memory in the performance of alcoholic Korsakoff patients. *Neuropsychologia*, *29*, 641–657.

Weingartner, H., Eckardt, M., Grafman, J., Molchan, S., Putnam, K., Rawlings, R., & Sunderland, T. (1993). The effects of repetition on memory performance in cognitively impaired patients. *Neuropsychology*, *7*, 385–395.

Wilson, B. A., Baddeley, A., Evans, J., & Sheil, A. (1994). Errorless learning in the rehabilitation of memory impaired people. *Neuropsychological Rehabilitation*, *4*, 307–326.

Wilson, B. A., & Evans, J. (1996). Error-free learning in persons with memory impairments. *Journal of Head Trauma Rehabilitation*, *11*, 54–64.

Multitechnique Program Approaches

LINDA CLARE

Theoretical models from neuropsychology provide a strong rationale for the relevance of interventions directed at the cognitive difficulties experienced by people with dementia, especially in the earlier, mild to moderate stages. Understanding of the typical patterns of preserved and impaired cognitive functions found in different diagnostic subtypes of dementia allows interventions to be targeted accordingly, with the aim of either building on relatively preserved aspects or making the most of residual abilities in impaired domains (Clare, 2002, 2003). Evidence from experimental studies clearly shows that people with dementia (1) can alter their behaviour in response to changed environmental contingencies (Burgess, Wearden, Cox, & Rae, 1992), (2) can learn new skills (Salmon, Heindel, & Butters, 1992), and (3) can take in and recall new verbal information (Little, Volans, Hemsley, & Levy, 1986), given appropriate conditions and adequate support (Bäckman, 1992). There is, therefore, a strong foundation on which to base the application of cognition-focused interventions.

This chapter considers the extent to which we are currently able to make optimal use of these possibilities to provide clinically relevant interventions that improve well-being and quality of life for people with dementia and their family members or caregivers. In this respect, it is essential to begin with methods and techniques for which there is specific evidence of effectiveness. This is not, however, the sole consideration, and clinically relevant cognition-focused interventions are likely in practice to combine methods and techniques in order to achieve desired outcomes. Furthermore, there are strong arguments for adopting an integrative approach that addresses not just cognitive functioning but also affective and interpersonal domains in an holistic, person-centered manner (Kitwood, 1997), based on a biopsychosocial understanding of the impact of dementia. This view is consistent with a rehabilitation-oriented approach to optimizing functioning and well-being and reducing excess disability, thus helping to maintain engagement and social participation (World Health Organization, 1998).

TECHNIQUES OF COGNITION-FOCUSED THERAPY

An extensive literature delineates a number of specific cognition-focused methods that have been used effectively with people who have dementia, including, for example, spaced retrieval (Camp, 1989; Camp, Bird, & Cherry, 2000; see also Camp, Chapter 12, this volume), deep-level semantic processing (Bird & Luszcz, 1991, 1993), self-generation of cues (Lipinska, Bäckman, Mantyla, & Viitanen, 1994), visual and verbal elaboration and mnemonics (Hill, Evankovich, Sheikh, & Yesavage, 1987), and various forms of cueing (Thöne & Glisky, 1995). There is developing evidence to support the value of each of these techniques in addressing practical difficulties arising from impairments in memory and other aspects of cognition and thus improving well-being for the person with dementia and caregiver alike. For example, Clare et al. (2000) used a simple cueing technique to teach a woman with dementia to use a daily calendar as an alternative to repetitively questioning her husband. The participant, who was very aware of the difficulties caused by her need to ask questions repetitively, was happy to have an alternative strategy, the husband commented following this intervention that things were "100 per cent better," and both were subsequently able to work together to apply a similar problem-solving approach to other everyday situations.

COMBINING TECHNIQUES TO ADDRESS SPECIFIC REHABILITATION GOALS

Cognitive rehabilitation involves individually designed interventions aimed at addressing specific practical difficulties relevant to daily life, identified by the person with dementia and/or the family caregiver. Because of this focus on practical relevance, these interventions are likely to combine techniques in order to optimize the likelihood of a clinically effective outcome. When applying this approach to the rehabilitation of everyday memory difficulties, a central concern in early-stage dementia, interventions typically fall into one of two categories: either making the most of remaining aspects of memory or cognitive functioning, or developing the use of compensatory aids and strategies in order to reduce demands on memory.

This kind of approach is demonstrated in a study reporting a series of six single case studies in which goals for rehabilitation were identified by the person with Alzheimer's disease (AD) and his or her family member (Clare et al., 2000). The interventions involved either learning or relearning information, such as names of people in the person's social circle (four participants), or learning to use a memory aid as an alternative to repetitive questioning of the spouse, as described above (two participants). The aim was to ensure effective learning or behavior change by basing the interventions on the twin guiding principles of effortful processing and errorless learning. Individual interventions drew on techniques of known efficacy, such as mnemonics and elaboration, spaced retrieval or vanishing cues, as appropriate to the rehabilitation goal and the person's neuropsychological profile. For three of the four participants who learned personally relevant information, techniques were combined to produce a comprehensive approach to addressing the selected goal; the remaining case allowed a comparison of different techniques, demonstrating differential effectiveness (Clare & Wilson, 2004). Significant improvements on targeted goals were achieved for all four of these individuals, with good long-term maintenance over the following 6–9 months. Two of the cases, which focused on learning names, were also reported in more detail. For one individual, the intervention involved a combination of a mnemonic strategy with vanishing cues and expanding rehearsal (Clare, Wilson, Breen, & Hodges, 1999); for the other, a combination of mnemonics and rehearsal was used (Clare, Wilson, Carter, & Hodges, 2003). In one of these (Clare et al., 1999), a further evaluation over an additional 2-year follow-up period demonstrated very long-term maintenance of gains (Clare, Wilson, Carter, Hodges, & Adams, 2001). This successful approach to learning names of familiar people, using multiple techniques within an errorless learning paradigm, was subsequently replicated in a controlled group study (Clare, Wilson, Carter, Roth, & Hodges, 2002). Taking a similar approach, Bird (2001) has applied cognitive rehabilitation methods, again including specific techniques such as spaced retrieval and fading cues, to help ameliorate significant behavioral difficulties for people with mild to moderate dementia.

A recent comprehensive review (De Vreese, Neri, Fioravanti, Belloi, & Zanetti, 2001) concluded that there is sound evidence to support the effectiveness of this kind of individual approach to memory rehabilitation for people with early-stage dementia. However, a systematic review conducted for the Cochrane Collaboration[1] (Clare, Woods, Moniz-Cook, Orrell, & Spector, 2003), and further discussed in Clare and Woods (2004), found no randomized controlled trials (RCTs) of cognitive rehabilitation and commented that at present the evidence base is limited, although the indications are cautiously positive. Further, variability in response requires elucidation of the factors that may impact on outcome for a given individual. Despite these current limitations, this approach offers a promising way forward that can take into account the needs and context of each person and adapt the selection of goals and methods accordingly, with the potential for integration into a broader psychosocial intervention context.

COMBINING TECHNIQUES IN COGNITIVE TRAINING PROGRAMS

The individualized and goal-oriented cognitive rehabilitation approach can be contrasted with the hitherto more widely used cognitive training model. Cognitive training involves guided practice on a set of standardized tasks that aims to address several specific aspects of cognition, such as memory, language, attention, or executive function. Thus this kind of approach, by definition, is likely to incorporate multiple techniques and methods. Within the provision of standardized tasks, varying difficulty levels may be offered to permit a degree of adaptation to different degrees of severity of cognitive impairment. Although this focus on practice with standardized tasks forms the central element of cognitive training interventions, there is considerable variation in the approaches described, and cognitive training interventions take place in a variety of formats and with varying content. These include one-to-one training sessions with a therapist, individual computerized practice, and facilitation by family members. Some studies have sought to use cognitive training in conjunction with, or as a comparison for, pharmacological interventions.

A number of studies have evaluated the effects of individual cognitive training sessions that incorporated a range of techniques. Beck and colleagues (Beck, Heacock,

---

[1] The Cochrane Collaboration (www.cochrane.org) is an international not-for-profit organization, providing up-to-date information about the effects of health care. The Collaboration includes a specialist dementia group, the Cochrane Dementia and Cognitive Improvement Group (www.jr2.ox.ac.uk/cdcig). The Cochrane Library (www.thecochranelibrary.com) contains regularly updated evidence-based health care databases.

Mercer, Thatcher, & Sparkman, 1988) compared cognitive training involving exercises to improve attention, reading, concentration, and memory, given in 30-minute sessions three times per week for 6 weeks, with standard treatment for hospital or nursing home residents with mild/moderate AD or mixed dementia. No significant differences were found on cognitive tests following treatment. Davis and colleagues (Davis, Massman, & Doody, 2001) reported an RCT for people with AD in which cognitive training was compared to a "mock" placebo intervention. The cognitive training, given in weekly 60-minute sessions over 5 weeks, involved learning face–name associations and using spaced retrieval to rehearse personal information. The trained group improved significantly, compared to baseline, on recall of face–name associations and personal information, but neither group improved on standardized cognitive tests. The only between-group difference was that the trained group did better on one attentional task; there were no other differences in cognitive test scores, depression, or caregiver-rated quality of life. As would be expected, these studies indicate that cognitive training does not significantly improve performance on standardized measures of impairment. However, they do suggest that it is possible to demonstrate some training-specific improvements on target tasks; that is to say, there may be an effect at the level of disability or handicap, with the potential, given appropriate support, for some generalization to the context of everyday functioning.

An alternative approach to cognitive training, based on enhancement of relatively preserved aspects of memory (Zanetti et al., 2001), has evaluated the effectiveness of daily, hour-long procedural memory training sessions given 5 days per week over 3 weeks for day hospital attenders with mild/moderate AD, in comparison to a control group. This training focused on practice of 13 basic and instrumental activities of daily living (ADLs and IALs). Following intervention, the trained group performed the activities significantly faster than controls. However, it remains unclear to what extent this change had any clinical significance and whether gains generalized to the everyday setting. Farina and colleagues (Farina et al., 2002) compared a similar approach of training residual cognitive functions that focused on impaired elements of memory and involved exercises targeting attention, short-term memory, semantic memory, language, and visuospatial perception. Following intervention, both groups improved significantly on ratings of functional living skills, but there were no differences between groups on any other measure of ADL, memory and behavior problems, or quality of life. The only difference on measures of cognitive functioning was that the procedural memory group did significantly better on attentional matrices after training, but there were no differences in memory or verbal fluency, or in Mini-Mental State Examination (MMSE) scores. These findings were interpreted as showing that procedural memory training was more beneficial than training of residual cognitive functions.

Some studies have evaluated individual cognitive training delivered by computer. Schreiber and colleagues (Schreiber, Lutz, Schweitzer, Kalveram, & Jaencke, 1998; Schreiber, Schweizer, Lutz, Kalveram, & Jaencke, 1999) compared 2 weeks of daily half-hour computerized cognitive training sessions involving practice of immediate and delayed recall with social contact for people with mild/moderate dementia. In a pre–post comparison of cognitive test results, the training group improved significantly on a test assessing immediate recall of visual information only, whereas the control group showed no significant improvement. In a between-group comparison, the training group performed significantly better than the control on this test and on delayed route recall, but not on other cognitive tests. Heiss and colleagues (Heiss, Kessler, Mielke, Szelies, & Herholz, 1994) compared twice-weekly 60-minute computerized cognitive training sessions involving practice on memory, perceptual, and motor tasks with a social support placebo condition for people with mild/moderate AD. The intervention period was 26 weeks. No differences were found between the two groups. These studies, therefore, suggest that computerized cognitive training has few benefits for people with early-stage dementia.

A different approach to individual cognitive training is reflected in the development of a cognitive training program facilitated by family members in the home setting (Quayhagen, Quayhagen, Corbeil, Roth, & Rodgers, 1995; Quayhagen et al., 2000; Quayhagen & Quayhagen, 2001). This program involved 60 minutes per day of practice on ecologically valid tasks addressing memory, problem solving, and conversational fluency, facilitated by the family caregiver, and given over an 8- or 12-week period. When compared to placebo and wait-list control conditions with a group of people having mild to moderate AD (Quayhagen et al., 1995), there were significantly better outcomes for the cognitive training group on general and nonverbal memory and fluency, but not verbal memory or problem solving, and the cognitive training group remained stable on caregiver ratings of behavioral problems, whereas the other groups declined. When this program was further compared with three other forms of psychosocial intervention and a wait-list control (Quayhagen et al., 2000), the cognitive training group again performed significantly better on delayed memory, problem solving, and verbal fluency, and caregivers of cognitive training group participants were less depressed than caregivers in the other conditions.

COMBINING COGNITIVE TRAINING TECHNIQUES IN WORKING WITH GROUPS

Coming together in groups may present particular challenges for individuals who are experiencing cognitive difficulties, but it also provides opportunities to harness a wider range of resources and facilitate the expression of mutual support (Scott & Clare, 2003). Cognitive training has been applied in group formats in which the groups consist either of individuals with dementia or of these individuals plus their spouses or other family members. In this context, cognitive training principles are likely to be combined with other elements of intervention, including group discussion, and the group itself provides a forum for practice of newly introduced strategies and techniques, allowing a sense of ecological validity. A related, though distinct, form of intervention is that of general cognitive stimulation or reality orientation, which involves engagement in a range of group activities and discussions aimed at enhancing general cognitive and social functioning (Breuil et al., 1994; Spector, Orrell, Davies, & Woods, 1998). This approach has usually been applied with people who have more advanced dementia and therefore is not considered further here.

Group cognitive training can fit well into residential care provision. Bernhardt and colleagues (Bernhardt, Maurer, & Frölich, 2002) developed a group memory training program for residents with a diagnosis of mild/moderate dementia, involving hour-long sessions given twice weekly for 6 weeks. Following training, the intervention group performed significantly better than the control group on a short standardized cognitive test, and in a pre–post comparison, significant improvements were found in the memory and attention subcomponents. There were no significant differences between groups on the Brief Cognitive Rating Scale, but in a pre–post comparison the trained group members significantly improved their scores, whereas the control group members' scores declined.

Participants evaluated the program positively, although they did not consider that their memory functioning had improved as a result.

Most people with early-stage dementia continue to live at home with family members. Some group intervention formats have been extended to allow persons with dementia and their spouse or family member to participate together. Zarit and colleagues (Zarit, Zarit, & Reever, 1982) compared two forms of group memory training, attended by participant–caregiver dyads and involving a series of seven, twice-weekly, 90-minute sessions, and a wait-list control condition. The two forms of training were didactic training classes, involving training in forming visual mental images and making associations, and problem-solving classes, involving discussion of practical steps that could be taken to manage everyday problems. Following intervention, recall scores were better for the two training groups than for the control group, and it was noted additionally that participants in the didactic training condition showed within-session gains that were lost by posttesting. However, caregivers who attended either type of class were more depressed following intervention than control caregivers, although there were no differences in burden or reports of memory and behavior problems. This finding seems to have resulted in a widespread negative evaluation of cognitive training and its possible impact on caregivers (e.g., Small et al., 1997), although the few other cognitive training studies that have considered outcomes for caregivers report more positive, or at least neutral, findings. Another group memory program for people with dementia and their spouses or other family caregivers (Kesslak, Nackoul, & Sandman, 1997; Moore, Sandman, McGrady, & Kesslak, 2001; Sandman, 1993), involving a series of five weekly meetings, demonstrated significant improvements over baseline performance for participants with dementia on recall of names and effortful recall, and significant short-term benefits from a "significant event" technique in which couples were asked to undertake novel, enjoyable activities together. Participants with dementia improved significantly on one cognitive measure, Kendrick Digit Copy, and on depression scores, but not in ADL ratings. Caregivers did not report any differences in level of stress, nor did they rate participants' memory functioning differently.

Koltai and colleagues (Koltai, Welsh-Bohmer, & Schmechel, 2001) compared individual (an average of six sessions) and group memory training (five weekly 60-minute sessions) in a "memory and coping" program. This program incorporated several cognitive training techniques, including spaced retrieval, face–name recall, verbal elaboration, and practice on concentration tasks. These techniques were combined with the introduction of external memory aids and group discussion of coping strategies. Caregivers joined the last 10–15 minutes of sessions, when available. No differences were found between the individual and group modalities, or between these and a wait-list control condition, although sample sizes were small. An important contribution of this study was the demonstration, through a careful retrospective analysis, of the possible role that variations in awareness of memory difficulties might play in determining response to intervention. Participants who were rated as having greater awareness of their memory and cognitive difficulties showed improvements following intervention, whereas those who showed limited awareness did not. This association has now been demonstrated in a prospective study (Clare, Wilson, Carter, Roth, & Hodges, 2003), which showed that greater awareness of memory difficulties was associated with better learning outcomes. These findings highlight the need to target interventions appropriately for each individual, depending on a careful assessment of psychological and social factors as well as neuropsychological profiles. However, few studies have considered the factors that may influence outcome in the individual case, and this area requires further research.

Taken together, the multicomponent cognitive training studies reviewed here suggest that small gains can be observed in some domains of cognitive functioning in some cases, although the extent to which these result in clinically significant benefits remains unclear. One recent comprehensive review (Gatz et al., 1998) describes cognitive training procedures as "probably efficacious" in slowing decline in dementia. However, a systematic review of RCTs of cognitive training for people with early-stage dementia (Clare, Woods, Moniz-Cook, Orrell, & Spector, 2003) found no significant benefits of cognitive training in any domain, as measured by standardized cognitive tests. In addition to general difficulties with RCTs of psychosocial interventions, such as impossibility of blinding participants to condition, this review identified a number of methodological limitations that may impact the conclusions; many of these limitations apply equally to other studies of cognitive training that could not be included in the systematic review. Additionally, in any future developments, it will be important to seek to integrate cognition-focused approaches with interventions targeting other domains of functioning, and it is to this issue that discussion now turns.

COMBINING COGNITIVE TRAINING AND PHARMACOLOGICAL INTERVENTION

The realities of clinical practice dictate that psychosocial interventions are likely to be offered alongside other forms of intervention, especially pharmacological treatment. With the development of pharmacological treatments for people with early-stage dementia, it might be anticipated that cognition-focused interventions could potentiate drug effects (Newhouse, Potter, & Levin, 1997), and several studies have explored the combination of individual cognitive training and drug treatments. Brinkman and colleagues (1982) compared the effects of treatment with lecithin (a putative cognitive enhancer) plus memory training with placebo for people with mild/moderate AD in a double-blind crossover design. Lecithin treatment did not produce any beneficial effects on cognitive functioning, but memory training did produce significant improvements on a memory task compared to placebo therapy.

In addition to comparing computerized cognitive training (CT) and social support, as described above, Heiss and colleagues (1994), also considered the possible effects of combining CT and pharmacological treatment. Two further conditions explored the effect of adding either pyritinol (CT-P, 600 mg twice daily) or phosphatidylserine (CT-PS, 200 mg twice daily) to the CT. In a between-group comparison, the CT-PS group was significantly better than both CT and SS on orientation at 8 and 16 weeks, but at 26 weeks there were no significant differences on any cognitive measure. In a pre–post comparison, the CT-P group had significantly improved orientation at 8 weeks and verbal fluency at 16 weeks, and the CT-PS group had significantly improved orientation at 8 and 16 weeks and Corsi-Block-Tapping-Test at 26 weeks.

De Vreese and colleagues (1998, 2001; de Vreese & Neri, 1999) compared acetylcholinesterase-inhibiting medication (AChEI), a combination of this with CT (AChEI + CT), and placebo medication in an RCT with people who had a diagnosis of mild AD. Medication was given for 6 months. In the AChEI + CT condition, CT was introduced after 3 months on the drug and given for a 3-month period. The authors reported significantly better MMSE and ADL scores for the AChEI + CT group than for

AChEI alone or placebo, and significant improvements on the Alzheimer's Disease Assessment Scale—Cognitive subscale (ADAS-Cog) for both AChEI and AChEI + CT, which were more marked for the latter group.

Clare and colleagues (2002) were able to compare learning outcomes for participants who were, or were not, receiving AChEI medication at the same time as engaging in cognitive rehabilitation, and found no difference between the two groups.

The evidence on combining cognitive training with pharmacological treatments remains equivocal, although the recent work of De Vreese and colleagues provides encouraging results, with potential for direct applicability to current clinical practice. At present, therefore, the availability of some positive results suggests that further work in this area is warranted in the future.

COMBINING COGNITIVE TRAINING AND OTHER ELEMENTS IN BROADER PROGRAMS

Although changes in cognition are central to our understanding of dementia, they cannot be viewed in isolation. People with dementia, and their family members or caregivers, have a range of emotional, interpersonal, and practical needs. Although it is important to consider specific domains of functioning and evaluate the effectiveness of interventions that directly target those domains, it is clinically desirable to address the full spectrum of need in an integrated way. Therefore, some programs have sought to combine cognitive training methods with other elements in broad-based programs (see also Loewenstein & Acevedo, Chapter 11, this volume).

In an early approach to including cognitive training within a broader program (Brodaty & Gresham, 1989; Brodaty, Gresham, & Luscombe, 1997), a residential 10-day memory training program was provided either in conjunction with a caregivers' program or on a "respite" basis. Caregiver and patient outcomes were better in the caregivers' program group, suggesting that integration with other intervention elements is important. In keeping with this finding, the Memory Clinic in Basel, Switzerland, offers weekly, hour-long, group memory training sessions for people with early-stage dementia, as part of a "milieu therapy" that provides advice and counseling, social activities, exercise, holidays, caregiver support, and organization of practical help (Ermini-Fünfschilling & Meier, 1995; Meier, Ermini-Fünfschilling, & Zwick, 2000). Patients continue in the group for as long as needed, typically between 18 months and 3 years. In one study, patients receiving memory training improved significantly on mood and fluency, but not memory, whereas a comparison group who did not receive memory training declined. A second study reported that patients who received memory training remained stable on the MMSE and quality of life, whereas those in the control group declined. This study suggests that memory training is a useful element within this kind of milieu therapy.

Other studies have taken a more community-based approach, for example, an "elder rehab" program for people with mild to moderate Alzheimer's disease, comprising memory training, language activities, an exercise intervention, and partnered volunteering, as well as participation in other group events (Arkin, 2001). Both rehabilitation and control groups improved significantly in mood, and the rehabilitation group scored significantly better on MMSE and some project-specific measures of memory and language, although not on other standardized cognitive tests or measures of physical fitness. Werner (2000) describes a "memory club" that aimed to provide social and clinical support for older people with severe memory problems living in the community. The club met two or three times a week for 4 hours at a time. Sessions included practice on memory training exercises alongside other activities. In the context of an overall decrease in MMSE scores over the year, memory functioning was maintained, with significant improvements only in verbal fluency. However, there was no comparison group, the participants had memory difficulties for a range of reasons (61.3% had a dementia diagnosis), and MMSE scores varied widely (range 0–29), so it is difficult to draw specific conclusions from these findings.

Finally, one study explored the applicability of cognitive training as an element of physical rehabilitation in medical settings, with the aim of reducing excess disability resulting from a hospital stay (Guenther, Fuchs, Schett, Meise, & Rhomberg, 1991). This study used cognitive training as an element of rehabilitation in a medical setting for women who had organic memory impairment but were receiving rehabilitation for a physical condition. Individual 45-minute sessions were given daily over 9 days. Participants in the training group improved significantly on task-specific assessments, but the only difference on standardized measures of cognitive functioning was in object naming. Trained participants also performed better than controls on evaluations of social behavior, lethargy, and affective disturbance, though not cognitive impairment or somatic problems. These findings suggest potentially useful avenues, not only for reducing excess disability among people with early-stage dementia in medical settings, but also perhaps for helping to ensure that people with dementia receive equitable access to physical health care and rehabilitation.

CONCLUSIONS

I began this chapter by saying that neuropsychological and experimental studies provide a strong basis for developing effective cognition-focused interventions, and that specific techniques of proven efficacy are available. However, in order to develop clinically meaningful interventions that are geared to each individual's profile of strengths and difficulties, and that take account of the emotional and interpersonal context, a combination of methods and techniques is likely to be needed (see Attix, Chapter 10, this volume). This chapter has reviewed a range of studies that demonstrate that some progress has been made in this direction. See Table 13.1 for an overview of the studies discussed in this chapter.

Cognitive rehabilitation studies have shown that combining techniques can help achieve specific rehabilitation goals, but there is a need for more evidence from rigorously designed trials in order to support the further development and wider application of this approach. Cognitive training approaches draw on a range of techniques, exercises, and methods to address a number of domains of cognitive functioning, and these multimodal cognitive training interventions have been combined, in turn, with other specific forms of intervention and within broad-based psychosocial intervention programs. Evidence for the efficacy of cognitive training, as such, remains limited, however. This limitation may be due, in part, to methodological issues, but it is likely that it also reflects the difficulty of applying an essentially standardized approach to a very heterogeneous participant group, in the absence of a clear understanding of the factors that influence individual outcomes.

In future research on cognitive rehabilitation and cognitive training, it will be important to overcome the methodological limitations that are evident in many of the existing

TABLE 13.1. Overview of Multitechnique Studies Reviewed in This Chapter

Study	Type	Aims	Participants/Conditions	Interventions	Outcomes
Individual goal-oriented cognitive rehabilitation					
Clare et al. (1999, 2000, 2001, 2003); Clare & Wilson (2004)	Individual goal-oriented cognitive rehabilitation	Six single case studies	6 people with mild AD	Learning/relearning personally relevant information or face–name associations (4 participants); learning to use a memory aid (2 participants).	Significant improvement on target goals in 5 of the 6 participants. No changes on measures of cognition or mood, or caregiver ratings of mood/strain. Long-term follow-up of one participant showed benefits were maintained up to 3 years after the intervention.
Bird (2001)	Individual goal-oriented cognitive rehabilitation	Two case studies	2 people with mild/moderate dementia	Application of spaced retrieval and fading cues methods to address behavioral problems.	Successful outcome in both cases.
Cognitive training in individual sessions					
Beck et al. (1988)	Cognitive training in individual sessions	Assess effectiveness of cognitive skills remediation training compared with standard treatment	20 people with AD or mixed dementia resident in VA hospital or nursing home (method of assignment unclear).	1. Cognitive skills remediation training given individually in 30- to 40-minute sessions, three times a week for 6 weeks. 2. Standard treatment only.	No significant differences between groups on tests of attention, reading, remembering, or concentrating on detail.
Guenther et al. (1991)	Cognitive training in individual sessions	Evaluate efficacy of cognitive training as part of rehabilitation within medical setting	14 women with organic cognitive impairment, receiving rehabilitation for a physical health condition with organic condition supported by relative report of decline since admission	1. Cognitive training ($n = 7$) 2. Control ($n = 7$); general conversation with therapist	Training group improved performance on each component of training; controls showed no change. Training group improved compared to controls on some cognitive subtests but not others, and caregivers reported improvements in some behavioral domains for the training group.

Davis et al. (2001)	Cognitive training in individual sessions	RCT comparing cognitive training and placebo in crossover design	37 people with probable AD (16 male, 21 female)	1. Cognitive training (n = 19)—1-hour individual session weekly for 5 weeks, and home practice 2. Placebo (n = 18)—"mock" intervention	Cognitive training group improved on recall of face–name associations and personal information. No significant changes for either group in cognitive functioning, and no significant differences between groups on depression or quality-of-life scores.
Zanetti et al. (2001)	Cognitive training in individual sessions	Evaluate effectiveness of procedural memory training on 13 basic and instrumental activities of daily living (ADLs, IADLs).	18 day-hospital attenders with mild/moderate AD	1. Procedural memory training (n = 11)—1-hour session each day for 5 days per week for 3 weeks 2. Control (n = 7)—unspecified	Training group were significantly faster in completing ADLs than controls following intervention.
Farina et al. (2002)	Cognitive training in individual sessions	Compare two cognitive training programs	22 consecutive outpatients with mild/moderate AD sequentially allocated to one or other group	1. Procedural memory training (n = 11) 2. Training of residual cognitive functions (n = 11) Both groups had two 45-minute individual sessions per day for 3 days per week over 5 weeks.	Postintervention, both groups improved significantly on performance of functional living skills. The procedural training group was better than the comparison group on attentional matrices, but there were no differences on other cognitive tests or questionnaire measures. At 3-month follow-up both groups had returned to baseline levels of performance.
Clare et al. (2002)	Cognitive training in individual sessions	Group replication of Clare et al. (1999)	12 people with mild AD	Training in face–name associations using paradigm developed in 1999 paper.	Significant improvement from baseline to postintervention for recall of trained but not control items. No changes on measures of mood or general tests of cognition. Awareness assessed prior to intervention predicted outcome; higher levels of awareness were associated with better learning outcomes.

(continued)

TABLE 13.1. (continued)

Study	Type	Aims	Participants/Conditions	Interventions	Outcomes
			Computer-based cognitive training		
Schreiber et al. (1998, 1999)	Computer-based cognitive training in individual sessions	Evaluate effects of interactive computer-based memory training program	14 people with mild/moderate dementia, alternately assigned to treatment or control group; assessment blind to group allocation	1. Training (*n* = 7) 2. Control (*n* = 7); chat with a psychologist Ten 30-minute sessions, held on 5 days per week, over 2 weeks	Training group performed significantly better on two subtests (immediate visual recall and delayed recall of a route) compared to controls; this represented a significant improvement, compared to baseline, for immediate visual recall.
			Cognitive training in group sessions		
Zarit et al. (1982)	Cognitive training in groups	Compare two types of cognitive training and wait-list control	35 people with dementia and their family caregivers	1. Didactic training classes (*n* = 14) twice weekly for 90 minutes for 3.5 weeks 2. Problem-solving classes (*n* = 11) twice weekly for 90 minutes for 3.5 weeks Patients and caregivers attended together, with 6–8 people per group. 3. Wait-list control (*n* = 10)	Recall scores better for the two training groups than controls. No differences in recognition scores. Caregivers who attended the classes (in either condition) were significantly more depressed afterward.

Study	Intervention	Aim	Sample	Method	Results
Brodaty & Gresham (1989); Brodaty et al. (1997)	Cognitive training in groups	Reduce psychological distress and improve coping skills in caregivers of people with dementia	96 patient–caregiver pairs; patients had mild/moderate dementia	1. Caregivers' program (*n* = 33)—couples admitted together in cohorts up to 4. Caregivers had 10 days training in coping. Patients had memory training sessions. 2. Respite for caregivers (*n* = 31)—patients admitted alone and had memory training. 3. Wait-list control (*n* = 32) The 1997 paper reports an 8-year follow-up.	Caregivers receiving the caregivers' program had significantly better scores for general well-being after 12 months, and there was a significantly higher rate of survival at home for the people with dementia for whom they cared. The people with dementia otherwise showed no differences. At 8-year follow-up, patients whose caregivers had received the caregivers' program stayed at home significantly longer and tended to live longer.
Sandman (1993)	Cognitive training in groups	Evaluate 4-week memory group	11 people with mild/moderate AD and their spouses	Group of two to four dyads met for four weekly sessions.	People with dementia were able to learn and recall names of other participants by session 3 or 4. On remembering details from a TV program, learning with "extra effort" produced equivalent performance to that of spouses learning under normal conditions. People with dementia recalled more on planned "special event" days than noneventful days.
Kesslak et al. (1997)	Cognitive training in groups	Evaluate efficacy of a 4-week memory training program	11 people with mild/moderate dementia and their spouses, who acted as age-matched controls	Group of two to four dyads met for four weekly sessions.	People with dementia improved on task-specific measures of name recall, on a digit copying task, and on depression scores, and rated themselves as having improved (although caregivers disagreed). Caregivers also showed improvements on task-specific measures.

(continued)

TABLE 13.1. (*continued*)

Study	Type	Aims	Participants/Conditions	Interventions	Outcomes
Moore et al. (2001)	Cognitive training in groups	Evaluate efficacy of 5-week memory training program	25 people with mild/moderate dementia and their caregivers, who acted as age-matched controls	Group of two to four dyads met for five weekly sessions. Additional caregiver support provided.	People with dementia improved on task-specific measures of name recall, on a digit copying task, and on depression scores, and rated themselves as having improved (although caregivers disagreed). Caregivers also showed improvements on task-specific measures but no reduction in caregiver stress.
Bernhardt et al. (2002)	Cognitive training in groups	Evaluate efficacy of cognitive training program designed to generalize to daily life	26 people with dementia living in seniors homes	1. Cognitive training ($n = 13$)—two 1-hour sessions per week for 6 weeks; two groups each with six or seven members. 2. Control ($n = 13$)—weekly 1-hour conversation group	The cognitive training group performed significantly better than controls on the short cognitive test. Training group improved own performance on memory and attention, and were rated better on cognitive function than before intervention, but did not differ significantly from controls.
			Cognitive training comparing individual and group sessions		
Koltai et al. (2001)	Cognitive training in individual or group sessions	Evaluate effects of a memory and coping intervention; RCT	24 participants with mild/moderate dementia	1. Individual memory and coping program ($n = 8$)—individual sessions (mean of 6). 2. Group memory and coping program ($n = 8$)—five 1-hour weekly sessions in groups of 4 3. Wait-list control ($n = 8$)	No significant differences in depression and memory ratings or on cognitive tests; participants with higher levels of awareness reported fewer memory failures after treatment.

Quayhagen et al. (1995)	Cognitive training facilitated by family caregivers	RCT comparing cognitive training with placebo and wait-list control	79 people with mild/ moderate AD and their family caregivers (data available for 78)	1. Cognitive training ($n = 25$)—60 minutes/ day facilitated by caregiver. 2. Placebo ($n = 28$)— passive observation of cognitive training activities. 3. Wait-list control ($n = 25$) Duration: 12 weeks	Significantly better outcome for cognitive training group on general cognitive functioning and composite scores for general and nonverbal memory and problem solving. Significantly fewer behavioral problems reported for cognitive training group.
Quayhagen et al. (2000)	Cognitive training facilitated by caregivers	RCT comparing cognitive training with three other psychosocial interventions and wait-list control	103 people with mild/ moderate dementia (AD, VaD, Parkinson's) and their spouse caregivers	1. Cognitive training ($n = 21$), facilitated by spouse 2. Dyadic counseling ($n = 29$) 3. Dual supportive seminar groups ($n = 22$) 4. Early-stage day care ($n = 16$) 5. Wait-list control ($n = 15$) Duration 8 weeks	Cognitive training group significantly better on delayed memory, problem solving, and verbal fluency. Caregivers of participants in this group were less depressed.
Quayhagen & Quayhagen (2001)	Cognitive training facilitated by caregivers	Compare two studies using different forms of cognitive train ng intervention	Study 1—56 couples, in which one partner had mild to moderate dementia Study 2—30 couples, in which one partner had mild to moderate dementia	Each study had cognitive training, placebo (passive stimulation), and wait-list control groups. The two cognitive training conditions were: Study 1—12 weeks Study 2—8 weeks	Both cognitive training groups improved on immediate memory, delayed memory, verbal fluency, and problem solving, indicating that shortening the program did not affect outcome.

(continued)

307

TABLE 13.1. (*continued*)

Study	Type	Aims	Participants/Conditions	Interventions	Outcomes
		Cognitive training combined with pharmacological interventions			
Brinkman et al. (1982)	Cognitive training in individual sessions combined with drug treatment	Compare lecithin + memory training with placebo drug and therapy in double-blind crossover design	10 people with mild/ moderate AD	Lecithin + memory training condition: 35 mg/day of lecithin for 2 weeks. During last 5 days had daily 45- to 60-minute individual memory training sessions. Placebo condition: placebo medication for 2 weeks. During last 5 days had 45- to 60-minute individual unstructured conversation sessions.	Lecithin did not produce any beneficial effects on memory. Memory training produced significant improvements compared to placebo.
Heiss et al. (1994)	Computer-based cognitive training in individual sessions combined with drug treatment	Evaluate efficacy of computer-based cognitive training given alone and with two different drugs, compared with social support placebo	70 people with probable AD, mild/ moderate; MMSE score range 13–26	1. CT ($n = 18$)—1 hour twice a week of computer-based training 2. CT-P—CT plus pyritinol 600 mg twice daily ($n = 17$) 3. CT-PS—CT plus phosphatidylserine 200 mg twice daily ($n = 18$) 4. Social support placebo—1 hour weekly talking about past and present experiences and personal issues ($n = 17$) Intervention lasted 26 weeks.	No significant differences between groups in MMSE scores after 26 weeks. On cognitive tests there were no significant between-group differences. In pre–post comparison, the CT–PS group had improved visual span at 26 weeks.

| De Vreese et al. (1998, 1999, 2001); unpublished data provided by author | Individual cognitive training combined with drug treatment | Compare CT alone, AChEI alone, CT plus drug, and placebo (1998 paper). Design later amended (2001 paper) to drop the cognitive training alone condition | (2001 paper) 1. 27 people with mild AD (MMSE score range 20–26) | 1. AChEI alone (n = 9), 6 months
2. AChEI + CT in twice weekly individual 45-minute sessions. CT introduced after 3 months on drug and lasted 3 months
3. Placebo medication (n = 9), 6 months | AChEI + CT group significantly better on scores for general cognitive functioning and ratings of ADL performance. |

Cognitive training as part of a broader psychosocial intervention program

| Ermini-Fuenfschilling & Meier (1995) | Cognitive training in group sessions as part of broad-based program | Evaluate efficacy of memory training offered as component of "milieu therapy" | People with mild dementia (MMSE score at least 23)
Study 1—44 patients; treatment group n = 22; control n = 22
Study 2—53 patients; treatment group n = 17; control n = 36 | Memory training in weekly 1-hour sessions in groups of 8. People continue as long as needed in the group (AD patients typically 18 months; other patients 2–3 years). This is part of a wider program run by the Memory Clinic. Control group: no memory training, but receive all other aspects of program. | Study 1: Training group significantly improved in mood, verbal fluency, nonverbal fluency. No improvement in memory. Control group worsened on all aspects.
Study 2: Patients in training group were stable on MMSE scores and quality-of-life ratings, whereas control group worsened. Caregivers of patients in the training group improved on quality-of-life ratings. |

(continued)

TABLE 13.1. (continued)

Study	Type	Aims	Participants/Conditions	Interventions	Outcomes
Werner (2000)	Cognitive training in groups as part of broad-based program	Evaluate effectiveness of a "memory club" for people with cognitive impairment over a 1-year period	31 older persons, of whom 61.3 % had a dementia diagnosis	Meetings took place twice or three times a week for 4 hours each time	MMSE scores decreased significantly over the year. Memory functioning, in general, was maintained over the year.
Arkin (2001)	Cognitive training in individual sessions as part of broad-based program	Evaluate efficacy of rehabilitation program conducted by students under supervision	11 persons with mild/moderate AD	1. Rehabilitation group (n = 7)—range of activities with student partner. 2. Control group (n = 4)—unstructured time with student.	Rehabilitation group significantly better on MMSE scores, on project-specific biographical memory test, some aspects of language function, and physical ability, but not on other cognitive tests. Both groups showed significant improvements in mood.

Note. AchEI, acetylcholinesterase inhibitor; AD, Alzheimer's disease; ADLs, activities of daily living; CT, cognitive training; CT-P, cognitive training plus pyritinol; CT-PS, cognitive training plus phosphatidylserine; IADLs, instrumental activities of daily living; MMSE, Mini-Mental State Examination; RCT, randomized controlled trial; VA, Veterans Administration; VaD, vascular dementia.

studies. These include limited statistical power due to small sample sizes; insufficient duration and intensity of intervention; comparison with other active treatments rather than placebo; repetition of neuropsychological tests as outcome measures over short intervals, rendering the results liable to practice effects; and selection of outcome measures that reflect impairment rather than disability and therefore fail to capture some changes that do occur as a result of intervention (Clare, Woods, et al., 2003). Future well-designed trials should provide more reliable evidence. However, any further research in this area should seek to demonstrate an impact on disability, rather than impairment, and should attempt to produce benefits that are of significance for everyday functioning and quality of life. Attention must also be paid to an exploration of the factors that influence outcome at the individual level. Most importantly, it will be necessary to ensure that the implications of any findings are integrated into general clinical practice with people who have early-stage dementia.

In summary, future research will need to build on existing knowledge in this area in order to develop clinically relevant and personally meaningful interventions that take account of individual differences, and to evaluate outcome in terms of the impact on disability and the potential for improving quality of life for persons with dementia and their family members and supporters.

ACKNOWLEDGMENTS

This chapter draws on an earlier review article (Clare, 2003b).

REFERENCES

Arkin, S. (2001). Alzheimer rehabilitation by students: Interventions and outcomes. *Neuropsychological Rehabilitation, 11*, 273–317.

Bäckman, L. (1992). Memory training and memory improvement in Alzheimer's disease: Rules and exceptions. *Acta Neurologica Scandinavica, Supplement 139*, 84–89.

Beck, C., Heacock, P., Mercer, S., Thatcher, R., & Sparkman, C. (1988). The impact of cognitive skills remediation training on persons with Alzheimer's disease or mixed dementia. *Journal of Geriatric Psychiatry, 21*, 73–88.

Bernhardt, T., Maurer, K., & Frölich, L. (2002). Der Einfluss eines alltagsbezogenen kognitiven Trainings auf die Aufmerksamkeits- und Gedächtnisleistung von Personen mit Demenz [The effects of cognitive training based on everyday activities on the attention and memory performance of people with dementia]. *Zeitschrift für Gerontologie und Geriatrie, 35*, 32–38.

Bird, M. (2001). Behavioural difficulties and cued recall of adaptive behaviour in dementia: Experimental and clinical evidence. *Neuropsychological Rehabilitation, 11*, 357–375.

Bird, M., & Luszcz, M. (1991). Encoding specificity, depth of processing, and cued recall in Alzheimer's disease. *Journal of Clinical and Experimental Neuropsychology, 13*, 508–520.

Bird, M., & Luszcz, M. (1993). Enhancing memory performance in Alzheimer's disease: Acquisition assistance and cue effectiveness. *Journal of Clinical and Experimental Neuropsychology, 15*, 921–932.

Breuil, V., de Rotrou, J., Forette, F., Tortrat, D., Ganasia-Ganem, A., Frambourt, A., et al. (1994). Cognitive stimulation of patients with dementia: Preliminary results. *International Journal of Geriatric Psychiatry, 9*, 211–217.

Brinkman, S. D., Smith, R. C., Meyer, J. S., Vroulis, G., Shaw, T., Gordon, J. R., et al. (1982). Lecithin and memory training in suspected Alzheimer's disease. *Journals of Gerontology, 37*, 4–9.

Brodaty, H., & Gresham, M. (1989). Effect of a training programme to reduce stress in carers of patients with dementia. *British Medical Journal, 299,* 1375–1379.

Brodaty, H., Gresham, M., & Luscombe, G. (1997). The Prince Henry Hospital dementia caregivers' training programme. *International Journal of Geriatric Psychiatry, 12,* 183–192.

Burgess, I. S., Wearden, J. H., Cox, T., & Rae, M. (1992). Operant conditioning with subjects suffering from dementia. *Behavioural Psychotherapy, 20,* 219–237.

Camp, C. J. (1989). Facilitation of new learning in Alzheimer's disease. In G. Gilmore, P. Whitehouse, & M. Wykle (Eds.), *Memory and aging: Theory, research and practice* (pp. 212–225). New York: Springer.

Camp, C. J., Bird, M. J., & Cherry, K. E. (2000). Retrieval strategies as a rehabilitation aid for cognitive loss in pathological aging. In R. D. Hill, L. Backman, & A. S. Neely (Eds.), *Cognitive rehabilitation in old age* (pp. 224–248). Oxford, UK: Oxford University Press.

Clare, L. (2002). Assessment and intervention in Alzheimer's disease. In A. D. Baddeley, B. A. Wilson, & M. D. Kopelman (Eds.), *Handbook of memory disorders* (pp. 711–739). Chichester, UK: Wiley.

Clare, L. (2003a). Rehabilitation for people with dementia. In B. A. Wilson (Ed.), *Neuropsychological rehabilitation: Theory and practice* (pp. 197–215). London: Swets & Zeitlinger.

Clare, L. (2003b). Cognitive training and cognitive rehabilitation for people with early-stage dementia. *Reviews in Clinical Gerontology, 13,* 75–83.

Clare, L., & Wilson, B. A. (2004). Memory rehabilitation techniques for people with early-stage dementia. *Zeitschrift für gerontopsychologie und psychiatrie, 17,* 109–117.

Clare, L., Wilson, B. A., Breen, K., & Hodges, J. R. (1999). Errorless learning of face–name associations in early Alzheimer's disease. *Neurocase, 5,* 37–46.

Clare, L., Wilson, B. A., Carter, G., Gosses, A., Breen, K., & Hodges, J. R. (2000). Intervening with everyday memory problems in early Alzheimer's disease: An errorless learning approach. *Journal of Clinical and Experimental Neuropsychology, 22,* 132–146.

Clare, L., Wilson, B. A., Carter, G., & Hodges, J. R. (2003). Cognitive rehabilitation as a component of early intervention in dementia: A single case study. *Aging and Mental Health, 7,* 15–21.

Clare, L., Wilson, B. A., Carter, G., Hodges, J. R., & Adams, M. (2001). Long-term maintenance of treatment gains following a cognitive rehabilitation intervention in early dementia of Alzheimer type: A single case study. *Neuropsychological Rehabilitation, 11,* 477–494.

Clare, L., Wilson, B. A., Carter, G., Roth, I., & Hodges, J. R. (2002). Relearning of face–name associations in early-stage Alzheimer's disease. *Neuropsychology, 16,* 538–547.

Clare, L., Wilson, B. A., Carter, G., Roth, I., & Hodges, J. R. (2003). Awareness in early-stage Alzheimer's disease: Relationship to the outcome of cognitive rehabilitation. *Journal of Clinical and Experimental Neuropsychology, 26,* 215–226.

Clare, L., & Woods, R. T. (2004). Cognitive training and cognitive rehabilitation for people with early-stage Alzheimer's disease: A review. *Neuropsychological Rehabilitation, 14,* 385–401.

Clare, L., Woods, R. T., Moniz-Cook, E. D., Orrell, M., & Spector, A. (2003). Cognitive rehabilitation and cognitive training for early-stage Alzheimer's disease and vascular dementia (Cochrane Review). *Cochrane Library,* Issue 4. Chichester, UK: Wiley. Available www.thecochranelibrary.com.

Davis, R. N., Massman, P. J., & Doody, R. S. (2001). Cognitive intervention in Alzheimer disease: A randomized placebo-controlled study. *Alzheimer Disease and Associated Disorders, 15,* 1–9.

de Vreese, L. P., & Neri, M. (1999). Ecological impact of combined cognitive training programs (CTP) and drug treatment (ChE-I) in AD [Abstract]. *International Psychogeriatrics, 11*(Suppl.), S187.

de Vreese, L. P., Neri, M., Fioravanti, M., Belloi, L., & Zanetti, O. (2001). Memory rehabilitation in Alzheimer's disease: A review of progress. *International Journal of Geriatric Psychiatry, 16,* 794–809.

de Vreese, L. P., Verlato, C., Emiliani, S., Schioppa, S., Belloi, L., Salvioli, G., et al. (1998). Effect size of a three-month drug treatment in AD when combined with individual cognitive retraining: Preliminary results of a pilot study [Abstract]. *Neurobiology of Aging, 19*(4S), S213.

Ermini-Fünfschilling, D., & Meier, D. (1995). Gedaechtnistraining: Wichtiger Bestandteil der

Milieutherapie bei seniler Demenz [Memory training: Important component of milieu therapy in senile dementia]. *Zeitschrift für Gerontologie und Geriatrie, 28*, 190–194.

Farina, E., Fioravanti, R., Chiavari, L., Imbornone, E., Alberoni, M., Pomati, S., et al. (2002). Comparing two programs of cognitive training in Alzheimer's disease: A pilot study. *Acta Neurologica Scandinavica, 105*, 365–371.

Gatz, M., Fiske, A., Fox, L., Kaskie, B., Kasl-Godley, J. E., McCallum, T. J., et al. (1998). Empirically validated psychological treatments for older adults. *Journal of Mental Health and Aging, 4*(1), 9–45.

Guenther, V., Fuchs, D., Schett, P., Meise, U., & Rhomberg, H. P. (1991). *Kognitives Training bei organischem Psychosyndrom* [Cognitive training in organic psycho-syndrome]. *Deutsche Medizinische Wochenschrift, 116*, 846–851.

Heiss, W.-D., Kessler, J., Mielke, R., Szelies, B., & Herholz, K. (1994). Long-term effects of phosphatidylserine, pyritinol and cognitive training in Alzheimer's disease. *Dementia, 5*, 88–98.

Hill, R. D., Evankovich, K. D., Sheikh, J. I., & Yesavage, J. A. (1987). Imagery mnemonic training in a patient with primary degenerative dementia. *Psychology and Aging, 2*, 204–205.

Kesslak, J. P., Nackoul, K., & Sandman, C. A. (1997). Memory training for individuals with Alzheimer's disease improves name recall. *Behavioural Neurology, 10*, 137–142.

Kitwood, T. (1997). *Dementia reconsidered: The person comes first.* Buckingham, UK: Open University Press.

Koltai, D. C., Welsh-Bohmer, K. A., & Schmechel, D. E. (2001). Influence of anosognosia on treatment outcome among dementia patients. *Neuropsychological Rehabilitation, 11*, 455–475.

Lipinska, B., Bäckman, L., Mantyla, T., & Viitanen, M. (1994). Effectiveness of self-generated cues in early Alzheimer's disease. *Journal of Clinical and Experimental Neuropsychology, 16*, 809–819.

Little, A. G., Volans, P. J., Hemsley, D. R., & Levy, R. (1986). The retention of new information in senile dementia. *British Journal of Clinical Psychology, 25*, 71–72.

Meier, D., Ermini-Fünfschilling, D., & Zwick, V. (2000). Gedächtnistraining für Patienten mit beginnender Demenz [Memory training for people with early-stage dementia]. *Geriatrie Praxis, 3*, 48–51.

Moore, S., Sandman, C. A., McGrady, K., & Kesslak, J. P. (2001). Memory training improves cognitive ability in patients with dementia. *Neuropsychological Rehabilitation, 11*, 245–261.

Newhouse, P. A., Potter, A., & Levin, E. D. (1997). Nicotinic system involvement in Alzheimer's and Parkinson's diseases: Implications for therapeutics. *Drugs and Aging, 11*, 206–228.

Quayhagen, M. P., & Quayhagen, M. (2001). Testing of a cognitive stimulation intervention for dementia caregiving dyads. *Neuropsychological Rehabilitation, 11*, 319–332.

Quayhagen, M. P., Quayhagen, M., Corbeil, R. R., Hendrix, R. C., Jackson, J. E., et al. (2000). Coping with dementia: Evaluation of four nonpharmacologic interventions. *International Psychogeriatrics, 12*, 249–265.

Quayhagen, M. P., Quayhagen, M., Corbeil, R. R., Roth, P. A., & Rodgers, J. A. (1995). A dyadic remediation program for care recipients with dementia. *Nursing Research, 44*, 153–159.

Salmon, D. P., Heindel, W. C., & Butters, N. (1992). Semantic memory, priming and skill learning in Alzheimer's disease. In L. Backman (Ed.), *Memory functioning in dementia* (pp. 99–118). Amsterdam: Elsevier.

Sandman, C. A. (1993). Memory rehabilitation in Alzheimer's disease: Preliminary findings. *Clinical Gerontologist, 13*(4), 19–33.

Schreiber, M., Lutz, K., Schweitzer, A., Kalveram, K. T., & Jaencke, L. (1998). Development and evaluation of an interactive computer-based training as a rehabilitation tool for dementia. *Psychologische Beiträge, 40S*, 85–102.

Schreiber, M., Schweizer, A., Lutz, K., Kalveram, K. T., & Jaencke, L. (1999). Potential of an interactive computer-based training in the rehabilitation of dementia: An initial study. *Neuropsychological Rehabilitation, 9*, 155–167.

Scott, J., & Clare, L. (2003). Do people with dementia benefit from psychological interventions offered on a group basis? *Clinical Psychology and Psychotherapy, 10*, 186–196.

Small, G. W., Rabins, P. V., Barry, P. P., Buckholtz, N. S., DeKosky, S. T., Ferris, S. H., et al. (1997). Diagnosis and treatment of Alzheimer disease and related disorders: Consensus statement of the American Association for Geriatric Psychiatry, the Alzheimer's Association and the American Geriatrics Society. *Journal of the American Medical Association*, 278, 1363–1371.

Spector, A., Orrell, M., Davies, S., & Woods, R. T. (1998). *Reality orientation for dementia: A review of the evidence for its effectiveness* (Issue 4). Oxford, UK: Update Software.

Thöne, A. I. T., & Glisky, E. L. (1995). Learning of face–name associations in memory impaired patients: A comparison of different training procedures. *Journal of the International Neuropsychological Society*, 1, 29–38.

Werner, P. (2000). Assessing the effectiveness of a memory club for elderly persons suffering from mild cognitive deterioration. *Clinical Gerontologist*, 22, 3–14.

World Health Organization. (1998). *International classification of impairments, disabilities and handicaps* (2nd ed.). Geneva: World Health Organization.

Zanetti, O., Zanieri, G., de Giovanni, G., de Vreese, L. P., Pezzini, A., Metitieri, T., et al. (2001). Effectiveness of procedural memory stimulation in mild Alzheimer's disease patients: A controlled study. *Neuropsychological Rehabilitation*, 11, 263–272.

Zarit, S. H., Zarit, J. M., & Reever, K. E. (1982). Memory training for severe memory loss: Effects on senile dementia patients and their families. *Gerontologist*, 22, 373–377.

Language Interventions in Dementia

CYNTHIA K. THOMPSON
NANCY JOHNSON

Most of the literature in the area of language rehabilitation has focused almost exclusively on the treatment of aphasia due to stroke. Although the techniques described in this chapter are also applicable to specific language impairments that occur as a result of cerebrovascular accidents, we focus on the management of progressive language impairments in individuals with primary progressive aphasia (PPA), a form of dementia. Because this form of dementia is relatively rare, the first section of the chapter provides additional background information, including clinical presentation and diagnosis, neuroimaging and genetic findings, and neuropathological substrates associated with this clinical syndrome.

OVERVIEW OF PPA

PPA is a form of dementia defined by the insidious onset and progressive dissolution of language skills, despite the relative sparing of other cognitive domains, specifically memory, for at least 2 years. Language impairments are readily detected on formal neuropsychological measures, but patients with PPA may also score abnormally on tests of memory or attention and on standard dementia screening batteries, due to the dependence of these measures on verbal instructions and responses. Patients with PPA typically remain independent well into the middle and advanced stages of the disease, demonstrating sound judgment, preserved social skills, and intact ability to recall daily events (Mesulam, 2001). PPA can be differentiated from the clinical syndrome typical of Alzheimer's disease (AD) by the relative preservation of memory (especially nonverbal and episodic memory), and from frontotemporal dementia (FTD) by the relative sparing of frontal lobe functions and appropriateness of behavior.

Several related clinical syndromes have been described as subtypes of frontotemporal lobar degeneration (FTLD). Neary, Snowden, et al. (1998) have designated one subtype as "progressive nonfluent aphasia," which, in this nomenclature, is characterized by impairments in expressive language (e.g., effortful speech production; word-retrieval deficits) but relatively preserved comprehension. Another subtype, defined by a severe naming deficit and language comprehension and visual recognition deficits, but with intact fluency, has been termed "semantic dementia." According to our nomenclature, however, PPA encompasses all types of aphasia, both with and without comprehension deficits. The diagnosis of PPA is not made if visual recognition deficits are also present.

In order to distinguish PPA from other forms of degenerative diseases that also involve progressive aphasia, it is important to monitor the course of symptoms over time. When aphasia remains the only symptom for many years (at least 2 years, but 5 years on average), the diagnosis is consistent with PPA. Aphasia that occurs along with problems in strength and movement is referred to as cortical–basal ganglionic degeneration (CBGD; Mimura, Oda, et al., 2001). When aphasia occurs in conjunction with alterations in personality and behavior, the clinical syndrome is known as frontal lobe dementia. Aphasia can also occur in the context of significant memory loss, and in those cases, the symptoms would be consistent with a diagnosis of AD. In rare cases, individuals may present exclusively with problems in articulation, with preservation of underlying language functions; this condition is referred to as progressive dysarthria (Broussole, Bakchine, et al., 1996). In some cases, a condition may start as PPA and then develop into one of the other disorders described above.

The course of symptom progression in PPA has been investigated in a few individual case studies and in group studies with relatively small sample sizes (De Oliveira, Castro, & Bittencourt, 1989; Pachana, Boone, Miller, Cummings, & Berman, 1996; Sapin, Anderson, & Pulaski, 1989). Some cases have been described in which anomia remains the primary symptom for many years. In other cases, language dysfunction may progress to include comprehension deficits and agrammatism. Weintraub, Rubin, et al. (1990), for example, followed four patients with a nonfluent profile of PPA for a period of 3–5 years, using a battery of neuropsychological tests. All patients declined in naming, based on scores on the Boston Naming Test (Kaplan, Goodglass, et al., 1983). In addition, declines in auditory comprehension, repetition of words and sentences, oral reading, and word fluency were noted. Relative stability of memory, visuospatial skills, reasoning, comportment, and most activities of daily living (ADLs) was observed. Cognitive decline in nonlanguage areas, however, has been noted in some patients, often occurring after the initial 2 years, but the language deficit remains the most salient aspect of the clinical picture. The time course for the emergence of other symptoms is variable (Green, Morris, Sandson, McKeel, & Miller, 1990; Karbe, Kertesz, et al., 1993; Kempler, Metter, et al., 1990; Weintraub, Rubin, et al., 1990).

An important issue pertaining to the progression of symptoms concerns the language profile of the patient with PPA. Patients with aphasia resulting from stroke are often characterized as fluent versus nonfluent, based on patterns of spoken language and comprehension deficits. Fluent patients generally produce speech at normal to fast rates and show relatively normal phrase length, with often marked difficulty in auditory comprehension; in contrast, nonfluent patients show slow rates of speech with effortful production, reduced phrase length, and relatively spared auditory comprehension. The language disorder seen in PPA rarely fits neatly into these two categories (Mesulam, 1987). It has been suggested that patients with PPA who have early complaints of auditory comprehension difficulty and nonverbal semantic deficits and who fulfill criteria for a diagnosis of semantic dementia eventually exhibit fluent production patterns (Hodges & Patterson,

1996), whereas those with nonfluent aphasia exhibit preserved language comprehension in early stages. It has also been suggested that patients with a fluent deficit may evidence an earlier course of generalized cognitive involvement, as compared to patients showing a nonfluent profile (Snowden, Neary, et al., 1992). However, this observation has not been replicated, and in our own clinical experience, patients with nonfluent PPA may also develop additional comportmental and executive function deficits in later stages.

Further research is needed to clarify not only patterns of language deficits and decline, but also patterns of decline in nonlanguage domains. However, it is important to keep in mind that patients with PPA do not represent a homogeneous group. Indeed, in a review of published cases of patients with PPA, Westbury and Bub (1997) reported that word-finding and naming difficulty was prevalent in 41% of cases, 28% showed difficulty with language production; and 20% showed impairments in comprehension. Some patients also presented with difficulties in reading and writing. Symptoms vary across patients and within patients over time. Thus clinical management for these patients will also vary, to some degree, as we address below.

Multiple studies have demonstrated both structural and functional disruption in the language network in PPA. This network is almost always located in the left hemisphere and includes perisylvian parts of the inferior frontal and temporoparietal regions, respectively known as Broca's and Wernicke's areas, as well as surrounding regions of the frontal, parietal, and temporal cortices. Many patients with PPA display cortical atrophy (indicative of neuronal loss), electroencephalographic slowing, decreased blood flow (measured by single-photon emission computed tomography [SPECT]) and decreased glucose utilization (measured by positron emission tomography [PET]) in these regions of the brain (Catani, Piccirilli, et al., 2003; Chawluk, Mesulam, et al., 1986; Kempler, Metter, et al., 1990; Mesulam & Weintraub, 1992; Tyrrell, Warrington, et al., 1990). The clinical focality of PPA is thus matched by the anatomical selectivity of the underlying pathological process. This distribution of structural and functional deficits is distinctly different from what is seen in typical AD. Patients with nonfluent PPA and intact language comprehension tend to have metabolic dysfunction within anterior perisylvian language areas, including the left inferior frontal cortex, whereas fluent patients with comprehension deficits tend to have dysfunction that favors the middle, inferior, and polar parts of the temporal lobe (Abe et al., 1997; Mummery et al., 1999). Despite marked left-hemisphere dysfunction, the metabolic state of the contralateral right hemisphere can remain within the normal range, especially early in the disease (Chawluk et al., 1986).

Functional neuroimaging allows the identification of brain areas that become engaged in the performance of specific cognitive tasks. In one study of word processing, patients with PPA activated components of the language network to the same extent as age-matched controls. The one significant abnormality in the patients consisted of greater neuronal activation during the performance of the language tasks, but in areas outside of the traditional language network (Sonty, Mesulam, et al., 2003). The magnitude of this compensatory or deviant activation was correlated with the degree of impairment in a standardized naming test.

Recent research has begun to explore the molecular basis of PPA and other focal degenerations. Patients with PPA have apoE genotypes that are distinctly different from those of patients with AD (Mesulam, Johnson, et al., 1997) and also display an overrepresentation of the tau H1 haplotype (Sobrido, Abu-Khalil, et al., 2003). No differences have been found, to date, in either tau haplotype or genotype distribution on the basis of fluent and nonfluent clinical subtypes of PPA.

Neuropathological studies in PPA have revealed heterogeneous findings. Individual cases of PPA have shown an association with the neuropathology of AD (Benson & Zaias, 1991; Cummings et al., 1985; Galton, Patterson, et al., 2000; Green et al., 1990; Greene, Patterson, et al., 1996; Kempler, Metter, et al., 1990; Li, Iseki, et al., 2000), Pick's disease (Graff-Radford et al., 1990), Creutzfeldt–Jakob disease (Mandell et al., 1989), and "nonspecific focal atrophy" (also referred to as "dementia lacking distinctive histology" [DLDH]; Kertesz et al., 1994; Kirshner et al., 1987; Mesulam, 1982; Snowden et al., 1992). In a review of 16 autopsied published cases of PPA, Westbury and Bub (1997) found that approximately 20% of cases were associated with AD pathology, 15% were associated with Pick's disease, and the majority was described pathologically as DLDH. More recent advances in immunohistochemical subtyping of the frontotemporal dementias (FTDs) suggest the possibility that many cases previously diagnosed as DLDH would now be shown to have tau- or ubiquitin-positive inclusions characteristic of "FTD with motor neuron disease-like inclusions," "cortical–basal ganglionic degeneration," or other non-AD tauopathies (Lipton et al., 2001).

Because of the clinical heterogeneity in symptoms of language impairment, it has been hypothesized that there may be pathological subtypes of PPA. In a study of three patients with nonfluent aphasia, Turner et al. (1996) demonstrated that the neuropathological findings on autopsy were consistent with DLDH. The authors reviewed other autopsied cases of PPA and found that DLDH was associated significantly more often with nonfluent aphasia, whereas AD, Pick's disease, and Creutzfeldt–Jakob disease were associated most frequently with fluent forms of PPA. However, although this study demonstrates a possible relationship between aphasia type and neuropathological findings, both nonfluent (Turner et al., 1996) and fluent aphasia (Schwarz et al., 1998) have been associated with nonspecific focal atrophy at autopsy. Neuropathological data from a larger sample of clinically well-characterized patients is needed to clarify the relationship between neuropathological processes and clinical presentations.

LANGUAGE DEFICITS AND THE DECLINE OF LANGUAGE IN PPA

As noted above, the symptoms of PPA vary from individual to individual; however, word finding and naming difficulties are the most commonly reported deficits, at least in the early phases. As the disease progresses, other domains of language become affected. The specific language functions that become impaired may also differ from one patient to another. In an in-depth study of language decline in four patients with nonfluent-type PPA who experienced difficulty retrieving words in the early phases of PPA, we noted two patterns of language decline (Thompson et al., 1997). Using spontaneous language samples collected for up to 11 years post-onset of PPA symptoms, extensive analysis of lexical and morphosyntactic variables was undertaken, revealing that three of the patients experienced declines in grammatical aspects of production, showing language behavior similar to that of patients with agrammatic aphasia resulting from stroke. These patients showed increasing difficulty with morphology and syntax—verb endings and other affixes were deleted from words, small grammatical words such as prepositions were omitted, and sentences were ill-formed. For example, the words in sentences were not produced in proper order, and verbs were often missing. The fourth patient showed a very different pattern that was characterized by advancing naming difficulty. He had little difficulty with morphology or syntax; his main problem remained one of word retrieval, which affected primarily nouns. Although there are other patterns of language decline that may be seen in patients with PPA, our study highlights the fact that different patients present with different patterns of decline. Thus it is important that (1) the language abilities of patients with PPA be carefully examined before treatment is applied, (2) treatment be applied to aspects of language that are impaired, and (3) the patient's language abilities be followed as they decline, with treatment adjusted accordingly.

TREATMENT OF PPA

The primary goal of treatment for individuals with PPA is to improve their ability to communicate. In order to fully address how best to accomplish this goal, we make reference to the World Health Organization (WHO; 1980, 1997) model of disablement. According to this model, disablement is considered on three levels: the impairment (impairment level), the impact of the impairment on performance of activities (activity limitation or functional level), and the impact of the impairment on participation in life (participation restriction level). Although the WHO model was developed to conceptualize problems associated with any disease entity, it is particularly applicable to patients with PPA. These individuals clearly show language impairments, as described above; because of these impairments they often evidence difficulties carrying out ADLs that require language comprehension or use (e.g., talking on the telephone; reading train schedules), and their language deficits often limit or restrict their access to opportunities associated with full participation in society (e.g., carrying out family and work responsibilities; involvement in social activities). Like the language impairment itself, the impact of the impairment on activities and participation also varies across patients and is associated with many factors, including personality and motivation to improve communication.

Assessment of Language

Because the language deficit in patients with PPA differs from individual to individual and changes over time, it is important that a careful assessment of language be performed early after the onset of symptoms, as well as periodically as symptoms progress. Although a review of assessment tools for aphasia is beyond the scope of this chapter, we recommend using a full aphasia test battery such as the Boston Diagnostic Aphasia Examination (BDAE; Goodglass & Kaplan, 2001) or the Western Aphasia Battery (WAB; Kertesz, 1982), as well as tests designed to examine naming of both nouns and verbs. The Boston Naming Test (BNT; Kaplan et al., 2001) is recommended to test naming of nouns, and the Object and Action Naming Test (Druks & Masterson, 2000) or the Verb and Sentence Test (VAST; Bastiaanse, Edwards, & Rispens, 2002) may be used to examine the naming of verbs. We also note that the Northwestern Naming Battery (Thompson & Weintraub, 2004) will be available soon. It is designed to examine naming of nouns by semantic category and verbs based on their syntactic status. Tests designed to examine the source of naming failure, such as the Psycholinguistic Assessment of Language Skills (PALPA; Kay et al., 1992), are also recommended, as are tests designed to examine comprehension and production of sentences of varying syntactic difficulty (e.g., the VAST). Tests examining grammatical morphology and phonology also may be indicated for some patients; subtests of the PALPA and/or the BDAE may be utilized for this purpose. Narrative language analysis also helps to establish patterns of production deficits across language domains (e.g., semantic, syntactic, morphological, and phonological deficits patterns). In addition, functional assessment of communication is important, using tests such as the American Speech-Language-Hearing Association Functional Assessment of Communication Skills for Adults (ASHA FACS; Frattali, Thompson, Holland, Wohl, & Ferketic, 1995). Data derived from these tests should be used to guide treatment.

Approaches to Treatment

There are two basic approaches to treatment for PPA. One approach is to focus treatment directly on the language impairment—that is, on the language skills that show impairment on testing. The other approach is to focus on functional language ability (the WHO activities/limitation level). Augmentative/alternative communication (AAC) strategies or devices also are provided, in anticipation of future declines in language. We recommend that, at least in early stages of language decline, both impairment-based and functional treatment approaches be used. When the language intervention is focused on the impairment, functional language targets should be provided as much as possible, and opportunities to practice using language in functional contexts with communication partners should be included. AAC strategies also should be introduced early in treatment, with instruction about how to use them, so that patients can practice using them for functional communication. In later stages of language decline, impairment-based treatment may be discontinued as the focus shifts to functional communication using AAC strategies.

We emphasize the importance of impairment-level treatment for PPA, even though the degree to which such treatment will improve language function or retard its decline is largely unknown. Based on what is known about neural plasticity—that is, that the brain has the capacity to reorganize after injury, even in adulthood—we suggest that such treatment may result in recruitment of uncompromised neural tissue. For example, extra perisylvian areas in the left hemisphere and/or right hemisphere areas of the brain have been shown to be recruited to support language recovery in stroke patients with aphasia (Calvert et al., 2000; Heiss, Kessler, Thiel, Ghaemi, & Karbe, 1999; Thompson, 2000; Thulborn, Carpenter, & Just, 1999). It is thus reasonable to assume that unimpaired cortical tissue may be utilized by patients with PPA for language processing (Sonty, Mesulam, et al., 2003). In the following sections we highlight potential approaches for training patients who have impairments in naming, sentence comprehension, and production. We follow this with a discussion of some augmentative/alternative approaches to treatment. It is important to recognize that because PPA is caused by a degenerative brain disease, the goals of treatment are very different from traditional language intervention for aphasia due to stroke or head injury. As in other neurodegenerative diseases, the goals of treatment are to (1) *maintain* functional communication skills for as long as possible, and (2) *retard decline* of communication skills over time as the disease progresses.

Approaches to Training Naming

Because most patients with PPA evidence early word-finding or naming difficulty, treatment focused on enhancing access to words will likely be appropriate. Whether treatment is focused on nouns or verbs (or other word classes) will depend on the results of language testing. In addition, tests revealing the source of naming errors will help to guide treatment. For example, some patients may show difficulty naming and orally reading nouns but have no difficulty comprehending or repeating words or nonwords. Such a profile would indicate problems in accessing the phonological form of words; thus treatment aimed at improving phonological access would be indicated. Other patients may show reduced naming secondary to difficulty accessing the meaning representation of certain words. These patients often have difficulty both comprehending and producing words, and they show semantic deficits on subtests of the PALPA (Kay et al., 1992), such as, for example, Spoken Word to Picture Matching and Auditory Word Pair Judgment. Patients presenting with this profile might benefit from treatments focused on the semantic aspects of words.

Numerous researchers have undertaken studies aimed at examining the effects of treatment for naming deficits in patients with aphasia resulting from stroke. These treatments also may be used successfully with patients who have PPA. Many such treatments are focused on the source of impaired naming. For individuals with phonological access problems, cueing hierarchies have often been employed. For example, Thompson and Kearns (1981) used sentence completion cues, phonetic cues, and verbal modeling to train a patient with anomic aphasia to improve naming. Raymer, Thompson, Jacobs, and LeGrand (1993) used a similar approach with nonfluent aphasic patients who had naming deficits. They used a phonologically based cuing hierarchy, first presenting pictures of words to name (e.g., *cat*), then presenting a word rhyming with the target word (e.g., *hat*), next presenting the first phoneme of the word (e.g., /k/), and finally presenting the target word for the patient to repeat. This strategy improved both naming and oral reading of target words.

Treatments aimed at improving access to semantics also have been useful for aphasic patients. The most successful treatments are those that exploit what is known about normal language representation and processing. The mental lexicon is thought to be organized (at least, in part) by networks of items, based on features defining their semantic class. Drew and Thompson (1999) trained nonfluent aphasic patients who showed semantic deficits to name items within semantic categories by training them to (1) sort items by semantic class, (2) sort items by perceptual and functional features, (3) match written words to pictures and names to definitions, and (4) answer questions involving the semantic attributes of words. Boyle and colleagues have used a similar approach, known as semantic feature analysis (Boyle & Coelho, 1995). This approach involves training patients to name the semantic category of selected items, the use of the item, its action, physical properties, usual location, and something typically associated with it. Results of this treatment have indicated improved naming in case studies of patients with several types of aphasia.

Another semantic approach is one based on the typicality of items within semantic categories. Kiran and Thompson (2003) trained four fluent aphasic patients to name items within the categories of *birds* and *vegetables* by controlling the featured details of items. Some items within categories were typical (e.g., a *robin* is a typical bird that flies, has a beak, etc.), and some items were atypical (e.g., an *ostrich* is an atypical bird that does not fly but has some features that are similar to typical birds). Training aphasic patients to name atypical items resulted not only in improved production of the trained items, but also improvement on untrained items within category (e.g., training the naming of *ostrich* improved the naming of *robin*). Interestingly, however, training patients to name typical items improved naming of these items, but had no affect on naming atypical items. These findings suggest not only that naming can be improved with treatment, but that treatment of more complex items (e.g., those with features that are distant from the prototype) facilitates generalization to less complex items (typical items). Although seemingly counterintuitive, this finding is in keeping with Thompson et al.'s complexity account of treatment efficacy (CATE) for aphasia (Thompson, Shapiro, et al., 2003), suggesting that treatment beginning with more complex material will result in generalization to less complex material that is linguistically related. Training typical items repeatedly emphasized only a few features that were in common among items within categories; training atypical items highlighted the featural variation with categories.

Although there are few reports of the effects of naming treatment for patients with PPA in the literature, there is evidence that treatments focused on word-retrieval skills may prove useful. McNeil and colleagues (McNeil, Small, et al., 1995), for example, reported improved word-finding ability in their patient with PPA when treatment focused directly on word finding was provided. Interestingly, throughout the training period, their patient showed declines in aspects of language that were not treated, suggesting, albeit inconclusively, that treatment may retard the decline of language. Further research exploring the effects of naming treatment in patients with PPA is needed, particularly studies examining the effects of various treatment approaches that have been shown to be successful in stroke patients. In patients with PPA who have not completely lost their access to language, training more complex material prior to training less complex material may prove beneficial.

Approaches to Training Sentence Comprehension and Production Deficits

There are several approaches to training sentence comprehension and production in patients with aphasia resulting from stroke. These approaches vary from direct-production treatment focused on the surface form of sentences (e.g., syntax stimulation; Helm-Estabrooks & Ramsberger, 1986) to approaches that are based on theories of language disruption in aphasia (e.g., mapping therapy; Byng, 1988; Haendiges, Berndt, & Mitchum, 1996; Jones, 1986; Mitchum, Haendiges, & Berndt, 1995; Schwartz et al., 1994); and treatment of underlying forms (TUF; Thompson, 2001; Thompson, Ballard, & Shapiro, 1998; Thompson, Shapiro, Tait, Jacobs, & Schneider, 1996; Thompson et al., 1997; Thompson et al., 2003). Mapping therapy is based on models of normal sentence production (e.g., Bock & Levelt, 1994; Garret, 1975, 1980; Levelt, 1999) and focuses on the link between sentence meaning and sentence structure. The aim of treatment is to help patients understand the relation between the verb(s) and nouns in sentences, using both simple active and complex (e.g., passive) sentences and probe questions, such as "What is the verb?", "Who is doing the verb-ing?", and "Who or what is [he or she] verb-ing?"

TUF is similar to mapping therapy. However, the theoretical framework is slightly different. TUF is based on linguistic theory as well as what is known about normal language representation and processing. In addition, in TUF, both comprehension and production of sentences are trained; the focus is on complex rather than simple sentences; and, in addition to emphasizing the relation between the verb(s) and nouns in sentences, as occurs in mapping therapy, the linguistic operations required to derive complex from simple sentence structures are emphasized.

In general, all approaches used with stroke patients have shown that sentence deficits can be improved with treatment. In some cases, however, generalization to untrained structures may be limited, in particular, with direct-production approaches (Doyle,

Goldstein, & Bourgeois, 1987; Wambaugh & Thompson, 1989). Such treatments, focused on the surface form of structures, give little attention to the lexical and syntactic properties of constructions learned in treatment and those tested for generalization. In contrast, more successful generalization appears to occur when treatment considers important linguistic aspects of sentences. Then generalization occurs across structures that are linguistically related to one another. For example, using TUF for training complex sentences with object relative clauses—for example, "The man saw the child whom the doctor saved"—improves both comprehension and production of untrained sentences of this type. In addition, generalization is seen to untrained but linguistically related structures such as *wh-* questions (e.g., "Whom did the doctor save?"). We (Thompson et al., 2003) also have found better generalization from complex (e.g., object relatives) to simple sentences (e.g., *wh-* questions), than from simple to complex sentences, again across sentences that are linguistically related. For example, of 17 patients trained using TUF, 70% (seven of ten) showed generalization from complex to simple structures, whereas only 14% (one of seven patients) showed generalization from simple to complex structures.

Interestingly, the one patient who showed generalization from simple to complex sentences was a 62-year-old woman with PPA. At the time of treatment, she was 1-year postsymptom onset, and language testing showed a mild aphasia. Her aphasia quotient (AQ) on the Western Aphasia Battery was 93.6; she showed mild sentence comprehension deficits (i.e., she scored 92% correct comprehension of complex sentences and 100% correct of simple active sentences); naming was mildly impaired (i.e., she scored 98 on the Test of Adult/Adolescent Word Finding (TAWF; German, 1990); and she showed mild to moderate difficulty with sentence production (i.e., in narrative language samples she showed a reduced mean length of utterance (MLU; 6.06) as compared to normal (13.57); she produced more simple sentences (59%) than normal (45%) and a lower proportion of grammatical sentences (38%) than normal (88%).

Because of her difficulty with sentence comprehension and production, she was provided with 10 weeks of TUF focused on simple *wh-* questions (e.g., "Whom did the man follow every morning?"), which resulted in several interesting patterns of acquisition and generalization. First, training who-questions resulted in improved who-question comprehension and production. In addition, improved what-question comprehension and production was noted (e.g., "What did the horse follow every morning?"). Secondly, training *wh-* questions with both direct and indirect objects (e.g., "Whom did the man chase every morning?") resulted in improved production and comprehension of simpler *wh-* questions with only a direct object (e.g., "Whom did the woman follow?"). These two patterns were also noted in our patients with Broca's aphasia (focal lesions); that is, treatment resulted in improvement on structures that are linguistically related to one another (e.g., who- and what-questions), and improvement on structures that are simpler than those trained (e.g., from questions with three constituents to those with only two). In addition, improvement was noted in narrative language production, with an increase in production of grammatical sentences (57%). However, unlike our patients with aphasia resulting from stroke, treatment in the patient with PPA also improved more complex, linguistically related object-cleft sentence comprehension and production (e.g., "It was the woman whom the man chased"). This latter finding may have occurred because the patient's language network was only mildly impaired at the time of treatment; thus treatment likely enhanced access to normal (and still available) language comprehension and production routines.

Augmentative/Alternative Communication Strategies

AAC strategies also should be used. We suggest that, even in early stages of language de-cline, the patient (and family members) be trained in nonverbal communication strate-gies. For example, a gesture + verbal treatment strategy, in which patients are trained to produce gestures and words simultaneously, may be useful for improving word-retrieval skills. The gestures may, at first, serve to augment verbal communication. In later stages of decline when verbal language is no longer available, they may serve as an alternative communication system.

We (Schneider, Thompson, & Luring, 1996) used this strategy with one of our pa-tients who was 2½ years postdiagnosis of PPA. At the time, she had some difficulty re-trieving words, but she had greater difficulty putting words together in sentences and us-ing proper verb tense. We selected several verbs and nouns that could be combined to form sentences. Then we selected gestures to go with each of the words as well as gestures to denote grammatical morphemes for present, past, and future tense (the patient helped select the gestures that she wanted to use). Iconic gestures—that is, gestures that look much like the words that they depict—were used and were easily understood by others. The therapy involved training gestures for the nouns, verbs, and grammatical mor-phemes, followed by practice producing a variety of sentences by pairing spoken words with corresponding gestures. Results of treatment showed improved production of trained and untrained sentences, both on clinical testing and when she communicated with others outside of treatment. Interestingly, we noted that when she did not use the gestures, her ability to produce sentences was much poorer. Following treatment, the patient's language skills continued to decline; she was nearly nonverbal at 5 years postdiagnosis. However, she continued to use gestures as a primary means of communication.

Other nonverbal strategies that can be paired with verbal production include writing and drawing. Provided with pencil and paper, patients can often cue verbal language by writing the first letter of words, or they may draw pictures that depict the ideas that they wish to communicate. A treatment program developed by Morgan and Helm-Estabrooks (1987) called Back to the Drawing Board, involves training patients to draw pictures with increasing detail and speed to communicate. For example, patients are trained to draw static representations of objects or places, or to depict events by drawing sequences of pictures.

Patients also may be provided with communication devices, including communica-tion notebooks containing pictures, written words, or electronic voice output devices. Communication notebooks are personalized for individual patients, often organized by category (e.g., family members, including a family tree), food items, greetings, questions/ requests, emotional expressions) or by topics (e.g., words or phrases used in certain com-munication contexts or conversational situations, such as visiting the doctor or talking to grandchildren). Maps and calendars are also often included to help the patient communi-cate about places and time. Alphabet boards (or an alphabet page in the communication notebook) can be useful to help patients cue their communication with letters. (See Rog-ers et al., 2000, for an excellent discussion of communication notebook construction.) Importantly, the patient and his or her communication partner(s) should be consulted to determine the content and organization of communication notebooks and given training in how they can be used to facilitate successful communication. In addition, because patients' communication needs change as their language declines, the communication notebook will require periodic updating and adaptation (e.g., a switch from words to pic-tures; changes in communication topics and vocabulary).

There are several voice output devices available commercially, a review of which is beyond the scope of this chapter. Again, these should be personalized as much as possible and provided in early stages of language compromise, even if they are not used extensively until later in the course of language decline. In addition, training of communication partners is necessary to familiarize them with how the communication device can be used and to train them to provide prompts and assistance during communication attempts. Finally, electronic devices require modification over time and are sometimes discontinued as language deteriorates.

Regardless of which strategy is provided to patients, it is important to encourage their use of the strategy outside of the therapy environment. Murray (1998) reported the results of a case study with a patient with PPA in which drawing treatment was provided. Despite positive treatment effects in the clinic, the patient showed little use of drawing in other situations. This is a common problem when alternative communication strategies are used. Practicing functional use of the strategy during therapy and involving family members in treatment may help patients to use trained strategies more successfully in the natural environment.

In conclusion, the following guidelines are offered for intervention with patients who have PPA:

- A complete evaluation of speech, language, and other cognitive skills should be completed in early stages of PPA.
- Frequent follow-up evaluations are needed to determine patterns of language decline and corresponding treatment needs.
- Treatment should be provided in early stages, focused directly on aspects of language that are impaired; approaches used successfully with patients who have aphasia resulting from stroke may also be useful for patients with PPA.
- The focus of treatment should be adjusted as language abilities decline.
- AAC strategies should be introduced in early stages; patients shown these strategies in later stages of language decline may have difficulty learning to use them.
- Involvement of family members or other individuals with whom the patient communicates is important, not only to enhance awareness of successful communication strategies but also to practice using these strategies with the patient.
- As language declines, patients will rely more on AAC strategies; some strategies may be more useful than others, and some patients may use more than one.
- Treatment likely will not reverse the progression of the aphasia; however, it may retard the decline of language, and it will greatly enhance communication ability, diminish isolation, and give the patient a sense of control.

CASE EXAMPLE[1]

Relevant History

RP was referred for a comprehensive evaluation in the Northwestern Alzheimer's Disease Center PPA Program by his primary care physician. He reported an approximately 4-year history of progressive word-finding difficulties. These problems began following vascular

---

[1]Some details have been changed to maintain confidentiality.

surgery, but had worsened progressively since that time. His daughter stated that RP frequently appeared to have problems expressing his thoughts, may use the wrong word in conversation, and occasionally had difficulty understanding single words. For example, when asked by his daughter to get the margarine out of the refrigerator, he asked her what *margarine* was. He recently told his daughter he was going outside to "cut the sandwich," when he meant to say "cut the grass." RP remains relatively independent in all ADLs. He continues to drive and has had no accidents or tickets and has not gotten lost. He continues to manage his finances, including paying bills on time, balancing his checkbook, and making purchases. His daughter recently began to help him write out checks due to problems in writing. RP has always been very handy with home repairs and woodworking, and no decline in these skills has been noted. He continues to make household repairs without error, including recently rewiring a room in his daughter's basement. RP has withdrawn somewhat from social interactions outside of his immediate family. He reported it is becoming more difficult for him to follow conversations in a group setting and that he is hesitant to speak in public because he is embarrassed by his word-finding difficulties.

Demographic Information

RP is a 58-year-old, right-handed European American male with a bachelor's degree in education. He had worked as a high school geometry teacher but was forced to retire 6 months prior to the evaluation because of language difficulties. RP is widowed and lives alone, although his daughter and son-in-law live nearby.

Medical/Family History

RP's medical history was significant for hypertension, hypercholesterolemia, and arthritis. His medications included Toprol, simvistatin, and Celebrex. There is no reported family history of dementia or other neurological disorders in his parents, siblings, or children.

Evaluation Results

Neurological Evaluation

A brain magnetic resonance imaging (MRI) done 2 years ago was unremarkable. A PET scan done approximately 6 months prior showed marked decrease of metabolism in the temporal lobes bilaterally, but greater decrease on the left side. Additional areas of hypometabolism were noted in the parietal lobes bilaterally and the anterior frontal lobes. All laboratory investigations (homocysteine, thyroid-stimulating hormone, Vitamin B_{12}, complete blood count) and electroencephalogram were normal. Examination of cranial nerves and sensory motor function was normal, and there was no evidence of fasciculations.

Neuropsychological Evaluation

All nonverbal testing, including nonverbal reasoning, spatial and form perception, and attention were within normal limits for age and education. Memory scores were below normal for both verbal and nonverbal information, although by report, his memory in day-to-day activities was intact.

Speech and Language Evaluation

RP was tested with the Western Aphasia Battery (WAB; Kertesz, 1982), and the Boston Naming Test—Second Edition (BNT; Kaplan et al., 2001). A narrative retell, an oral–motor assessment, and hearing screening were also completed. The results of the evaluation were consistent with an anomic aphasia. Verbal output was fluent and appropriate, but word-finding difficulties were frequently observed. Circumlocution attempts and revisions were demonstrated with occasional hesitations and interjections. Confrontation naming impairments were present for both high- and low-frequency nouns. Naming was better for colors, body parts, and verbs compared to objects and shapes. Errors in naming were frequently phonemically or semantically related to the target. In attempting to generate the name, associated gestures were produced on some items. Tactile cues were not helpful, and phonemic cues were of limited benefit. Although the main difficulty was in oral expression, semantically related errors occurred occasionally on single-word auditory verification tasks, reading comprehension, and written expression tasks.

Treatment Recommendations

General Communication Aids

Initially, communicative gesture techniques were introduced. Handouts containing general communication strategies with individuals with PPA were provided to RP and his family. A communication card in the form of a business card containing emergency information and an explanation of PPA was provided (see Figure 14.1).

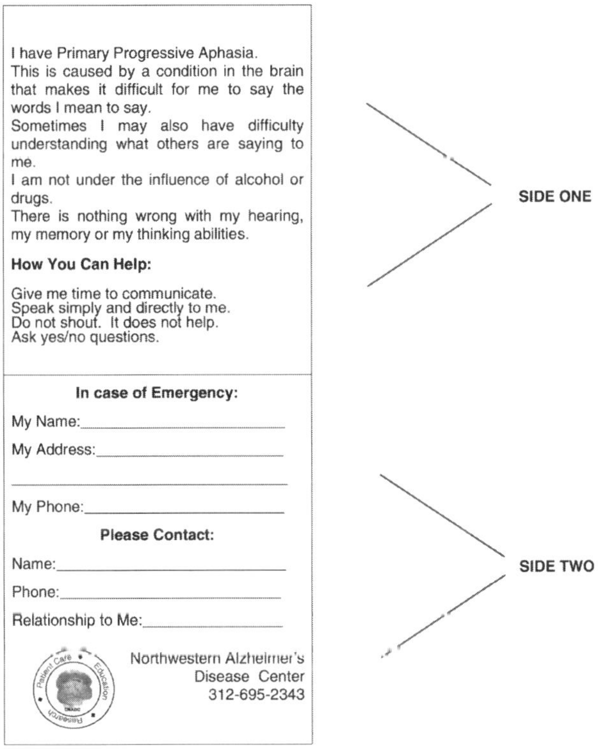

I have Primary Progressive Aphasia.
This is caused by a condition in the brain that makes it difficult for me to say the words I mean to say.
Sometimes I may also have difficulty understanding what others are saying to me.
I am not under the influence of alcohol or drugs.
There is nothing wrong with my hearing, my memory or my thinking abilities.

How You Can Help:

Give me time to communicate.
Speak simply and directly to me.
Do not shout. It does not help.
Ask yes/no questions.

SIDE ONE

In case of Emergency:

My Name:_____
My Address:_____
_____
My Phone:_____

Please Contact:

Name:_____
Phone:_____
Relationship to Me:_____

Northwestern Alzheimer's
Disease Center
312-695-2343

SIDE TWO

FIGURE 14.1. PPA Card.

Guidelines for Ongoing Treatment

Goals of language treatment were to develop strategies and techniques to maximize current communication as well as establish compensatory skills, given the potential for additional language decline. Suggested treatment activities included:

1. Self-cueing methods to facilitate lexical access:
    a. Gesture plus verbal techniques
    b. Associative and automatic phrases to cue closure techniques
    c. Generating verb phrase starters to cue nouns
2. Techniques to compensate for word finding difficulties:
    a. Semantic description
    b. Representational gesture
    c. Communicative drawing

TABLE 14.1. General Language Stimulation Activities

Listening

Retrieving specifically requested objects when assisting with a project
Listening to and following directions read aloud (games, cooking crafts)
Listening to and discussing a letter than has been read aloud
Listening for specific information such as weather reports and sports scores, while watching the news or listening to the radio
Listening for specific information on pre-recorded messages (movie times, store hours, etc).
Listening for specific songs on a CD or tape

Reading

Reading signs in the environment such as street names, restaurant names, gas stations, traffic signs, information signs, store hours, billboards
Looking through the newspaper for ads, coupons or logos
Sorting coupons
Sorting the mail
Reading cards
Reading mail
Alphabetizing
Reading daily appointments from a calendar or daily planner
Reading labels on household products
Reading advertisements in newspapers and magazines
Completing word search puzzles
Reading recipes
Looking up information in the newspaper (weather, horoscope, special events)
Reading newspaper articles
Reading stories aloud to children

Writing

Signing, writing, or copying name
Copying important names, addresses and phone numbers onto a reference sheet
Writing grocery lists, shopping lists, or "to-do" lists
Entering appointments and activities onto a calendar or daily planner
Labeling photographs
Writing captions for pictures in photo albums or scrapbooks
Writing the names of household objects
Copying a recipe from a book or magazine
Writing a summary of an event
Writing phone messages from the answering machine

3. Development and generalization of communication cards to facilitate receptive and expressive skills. Initial content may include situationally relevant terminology and categories, as well as specific names.

4. Semantic stimulation exercises, including semantic sort/resort tasks and alternate formulation activities.

5. Language stimulation program for home practice to facilitate generalization and carryover of skills addressed in treatment. Supplemental language stimulation exercises can also be completed individually. Table 14.1 includes list of general language stimulation activities related to daily living activities.

6. Computer-based language stimulation and functional communication activities (e.g., Web-based searches, e-mail, word games) may also be utilized.

REFERENCES

Abe, K., Ukita, H., et al. (1997). Imaging in primary progressive aphasia. *Neuroradiology, 39*(8), 556–559.

Bastiaanse, R., Edwards, S., & Rispens, J. (2002). *The verb and sentence test (VAST)*. Thurston, Suffolk, UK: Thames Valley Test Company.

Benson, D., & Zaias, B. (1991). Progressive aphasia: A case with postmortem correlation. *Neuropsychiatry, Neuropsychology, and Behavioral Neurology, 4*, 215–223.

Bock, K., & Levelt, W. (1994). Language production: Grammatical encoding. In M. A. Gernsbacher (Ed.), *Handbook of psycholinguistics* (pp. 945–984). San Diego: Academic Press.

Boyle, M., & Coehlo, C. A. (1995). Application of semantic feature analysis as a treatment for dysnomia. *American Journal of Speech–Language Pathology, 4*, 94–98.

Broussole, E., Bakchine, S., et al. (1996). Slowly progressive anarthria with late anterior opercular syndrome: A variant form of frontal cortical atrophy syndromes. *Journal of Neurological Sciences, 144*, 44–58.

Byng, S. (1988). Sentence processing deficits: Theory and therapy. Cognitive *Neuropsychology, 5*, 629–676.

Calvert, G., Brammer, M., Morris, R., Williams, S., King, N., & Matthews, P. (2000). Using fMRI to study recovery from acquired dysphasia. *Brain and Language, 71*, 391–399.

Catani, M., Piccirilli, M. et al. (2003). Axonal injury within language network in primary progressive aphasia. *Annals of Neurology, 53*(2), 242–247.

Chawluk, J. B., Mesulam, M. M. et al. (1986). Slowly progressive aphasia without generalized dementia: Studies with positron emission tomography. *Annals of Neurology, 19*(1), 68–74.

Cummings, J., Benson, F., et al. (1985). Aphasia in dementia of the Alzheimer type. *Neurology, 35*, 394–397.

De Oliveira, S. A., Castro M., J., & Bittencourt, P. R. (1989). Slowly progressive aphasia followed by Alzheimer's dementia: A case report. *Arquivos de Neuro-Psiquiatria, 47*, 72–75.

Doyle, P. J., Goldstein, H., & Bourgeois, M. (1987). Experimental analysis of syntax training in Broca's aphasia: A generalization and social validation study. *Journal of Speech and Hearing Disorders, 52*, 143–155.

Drew, R. L., & Thompson, C. K. (1999). Model based semantic treatment for naming deficits in aphasia. *Journal of Speech, Language, and Hearing Research, 42*, 972–990.

Druks, J., & Masterson, J. (2000). *An object and action naming test*. Hove, UK: Psychology Press.

Frattali, C., Thompson, C. K., Holland, A. L., Wohl, C. B., & Ferketic, M. M. (1995). *ASHA Functional Assessment of Communication Skills for Adults (FACS)*. Rockville, MD: American Speech–Language–Hearing Association.

Galton, C. J., Patterson, K., et al. (2000). Atypical and typical presentations of Alzheimer's disease: A clinical, neuropsychological, neuroimaging and pathological study of 13 cases. *Brain*, *123*(Pt. 3), 484–498.

Garret, M. F. (1975). The analysis of sentence production. In G. Bower (Ed.), *Psychology of learning and motivation* (Vol. 9, pp. 133–177). New York: Academic Press.

Garret, M. F. (1980). Levels of processing in sentence production. In B. Butterworth (Ed.), *Language production* (Vol. 1, pp. 177–220). New York: Academic Press.

German, D. J. (1990). *Test of Adult/Adolescent Word Finding*. Allen, TX: DLM.

Goodglass, H., & Kaplan, E. (2001). *Boston Diagnostic Aphasia Examination* (3rd ed.). Philadelphia: Lea & Febiger.

Graff-Radford, N. R., Damasio, A. R., et al. (1990). Progressive aphasia in a patient with Pick's disease: A neuropsychological, radiologic, and anatomic study. *Neurology*, *40*(4), 620–626.

Green, J., Morris, J. C., Sandson, J., McKeel, D. W., Jr., & Miller, J. W. (1990). Progressive aphasia: A precursor of global dementia? *Neurology*, *40*, 423–429.

Greene, J. D., Patterson, K., et al. (1996). Alzheimer disease and nonfluent progressive aphasia. *Archives of Neurology*, *53*(10), 1072–1078.

Haendiges, A. N., Berndt, R. S., & Mitchum, C. C. (1996). Assessing the elements contributing to a "mapping deficit": A targeted treatment study. *Brain and Language*, *52*, 276–302.

Heiss, W. D., Kessler, J., Thiel, A., Ghaemi, M., & Karbe, H. (1999). Differential capacity of left and right hemispheric areas for compensation of poststroke aphasia. *Annals of Neurology*, *45*, 430–438.

Helm-Estabrooks, N., & Ramsberger, G. (1986). Treatment of agrammatism in longterm Broca's aphasia. *British Journal of Disorders of Communication*, *21*, 39–45.

Hodges, J. R., & Patterson, K. (1996). Nonfluent progressive aphasia and semantic dementia: A comparative neuropsychological study. *Journal of the International Neuropsychological Society*, *2*(6), 511–524.

Jones, E. V. (1986). Building the foundations for sentence production in a non-fluent aphasic. *British Journal of Disorders of Communication*, *21*, 63–82.

Kaplan, E., Goodglass, H., et al. (1983). *The Boston Naming Test*. Philadelphia: Lea & Febiger.

Kaplan, E., Goodglass, H., et al. (2001). *The Boston Naming Test—Second Edition*. Philadelphia: Lea & Febiger.

Karbe, H., Kertesz, A., et al. (1993). Profiles of language impairment in primary progressive aphasia. *Archives of Neurology*, *50*(2), 193–201.

Kay, J., Lesser, R., & Culheart, M. (1992). *The psycholinguistic assessment of language processing in aphasia (PALPA)*. Hove, UK: Erlbaum.

Kempler, D., Metter, E. J., et al. (1990). Slowly progressive aphasia: Three cases with language, memory, CT and PET data. *Journal of Neurology, Neurosurgery, and Psychiatry*, *53*(11), 987–993.

Kertesz, A. (1982). *Western Aphasia Battery (WAB)*. San Antonio, TX: Psychological Corporation.

Kertesz, A., Hudson, L., et al. (1994). The pathology and nosology of primary progressive aphasia [see comments]. *Neurology*, *44*(11), 2065–2072.

Kiran, S., & Thompson, C. K. (2003). The role of semantic complexity in treatment of naming deficits: Training semantic categories in fluent aphasia by controlling exemplar typicality. *Journal of Speech, Language, and Hearing Research*, *46*, 773–787.

Kirshner, H. S., Tanridag, O., et al. (1987). Progressive aphasia without dementia: two cases with focal spongiform degeneration. *Annals of Neurology*, *22*(4), 527–532.

Levelt, W. (1999). Producing spoken language: A blueprint of the speaker. In C. M. Brown & P. Hagoort (Eds.), *The neurocognition of language* (pp. 83–122). New York: Oxford University Press.

Li, F., Iseki, E., et al. (2000). An autopsy case of Alzheimer's disease presenting with primary progressive aphasia: A clinicopathological and immunohistochemical study. *Neuropathology*, *20*, 239–245.

Lipton, A., White, C., III, et al. (2001). Frontal lobe dementia with ubiquitinated inclusions predominates in 40 cases of frontotemporal degeneration. *Journal of Neuropathology and Experimental Neurology*, *60*, 514.

Mandell, A. M., Alexander, M. P., et al. (1989). Creutzfeldt–Jakob disease presenting as isolated aphasia. *Neurology, 39*(1), 55–58.

McNeil, M. R., Small, S. L., Masterson, R. J., & Fossett, T. R. D. (1995). Behavioral and pharmacological treatment of lexical–semantic deficits in a single patient with primary progressive aphasia. *American Journal of Speech–Language Pathology, 4,* 76–87.

Mesulam, M. M. (1982). Slowly progressive aphasia without generalized dementia. *Annals of Neurology, 11*(6), 592–598.

Mesulam, M. M. (1987). Primary progressive aphasia—differentiation from Alzheimer's disease [Editorial]. *Annals of Neurology, 22*(4), 533–534.

Mesulam, M. M. (2001). Primary progressive aphasia. *Annals of Neurology, 49,* 425–432.

Mesulam, M. M., Johnson, N., et al. (1997). Apolipoprotein E genotypes in primary progressive aphasia. *Neurology, 49*(1), 51–55.

Mesulam, M. M., & Weintraub, S. (1992). Primary progressive aphasia: Sharpening the focus on a clinical syndrome. In F. Boller, F. Forette, Z. Khachaturian, M. Poncet, & Y. Christen (Eds.), *Heterogeneity of Alzheimer's Disease* (pp. 43–66). Berlin: Springer-Verlag.

Mimura, M., Oda, T. et al. (2004). Corticobasal degeneration presenting with nonfluent primary progressive aphasia: A clinicopathologic study. *Journal of Neurological Sciences, 183,* 19–26.

Mitchum, C. C., Haendiges, A. N., & Berndt, R. S. (1995). Treatment of thematic mapping in sentence comprehension: Implications for normal processing. *Cognitive Neuropsychology, 12,* 503–547.

Morgan, A., & Helm-Estabrooks, N. (1987). Back to the drawing board: A treatment for nonverbal aphasic patients. *Clinical Aphasiology, 16,* 34–39.

Mummery, C. J., Patterson, K., et al. (1999). Disrupted temporal lobe connections in semantic dementia. *Brain, 122*(Pt. 1), 61–73.

Murray, L. L. (1998). Longitudinal treatment of primary progressive aphasia: A case study. *Aphasiology, 12,* 651–672.

Neary, D., Snowden, J. S., et al. (1998). Frontotemporal lobar degeneration: a consensus on clinical diagnostic criteria. *Neurology, 51*(6), 1546–1554.

Pachana, N. A., Boone, K. B., Miller, B. L., Cummings, J. L., & Berman, N. (1996). Comparison of neuropsychological functioning in Alzheimer's disease and frontotemporal dementia. *Journal of the International Neuropsychological Society, 2,* 505–510.

Raymer, A. M., Thompson, C. K., Jacobs, B., & LeGrand, H. R. (1993). Phonological treatment of naming deficits in aphasia: Model-based generalization analysis. *Aphasiology, 7,* 27–53.

Rogers, M., King, J., et al. (2000). Proactive management of primary progressive aphasia. In D. Beukelman, K. Yorkston, & J. Reichle (Eds.), *Augmentative communication for adults with neurogenic and neuromuscular disabilities* (pp. 305–337). Baltimore, MD: Brookes.

Sapin, L. R., Anderson, F. H., & Pulaski, P. D. (1989). Progressive aphasia without dementia: Further documentation. *Annals of Neurology, 25,* 411–413.

Schneider, S. L., Thompson, C. K., & Luring, B. (1996). Effects of verbal plus gestural matrix training on sentence production in a patient with primary progressive aphasia. *Aphasiology, 10,* 297–316.

Schwartz, M. F., Saffran, E., Fink, R. B., Myers, J. L., & Martin, N. (1994). Mapping therapy: A treatment programme for agrammatism. *Aphasiology, 8,* 19–54.

Schwarz, M. F., De Bleser, R., et al. (1998). A case of primary progressive aphasia: A 14-year follow-up study with neuropathological findings. *Brain, 121*(Pt. 1), 115–126.

Snowden, J. S., Neary, D., et al. (1992). Progressive language disorder due to lobar atrophy. *Annals of Neurology, 31*(2), 174–183.

Sobrido, M., Abu-Khalil, A., et al. (2003). Tau polymorphisms and primary progressive aphasia: Further evidence for a broad role of the tau gene in neurodegeneration. *Neurology, 60*(5), 862–864.

Sonty, S., Mesulam, M., et al. (2003). Primary progressive aphasia: PPA and the language network. *Annals of Neurology, 53,* 35–49.

Thompson, C. K. (2000). The neurobiology of language recovery in aphasia. *Brain and Language, 71,* 245–248.

Thompson, C. K. (2001). Treatment of underlying forms: A linguistic specific approach for sentence production deficits in agrammatic aphasia. In R. Chapey (Ed.), *Language intervention strategies in adult aphasia* (4th ed., pp. 605–628). Baltimore: Williams & Wilkins.

Thompson, C. K., Ballard, K. J., et al. (1997). Patterns of language decline in non-fluent primary progressive aphasia. *Aphasiology, 11*(4/5), 297–321.

Thompson, C. K., Ballard, K. J., & Shapiro, L. P. (1998). Role of syntactic complexity in training wh-movement structures in agrammatic aphasia: Optimal order for promoting generalization. *Journal of the International Neuropsychological Society, 4*, 661–674.

Thompson, C. K., & Kearns, K. P. (l981). An experimental analysis of acquisition, generalization and maintenance of naming behavior in a patient with anomia. In R. H. Brookshire (Ed.), *Clinical aphasiology conference proceedings* (pp. 35–45). Minneapolis: BRK.

Thompson, C. K., Shapiro, L. P., Ballard, K. J., Jacobs, B. J., Schneider, S. L., & Tait, M. (1997). Training and generalized production of wh and NP movement structures in agrammatic aphasia. *Journal of Speech and Hearing Research, 40*, 228–244.

Thompson, C. K., Shapiro, L. P., Kiran, S., & Sobecks, J. (2003). The role of syntactic complexity in treatment of sentence deficits in agrammatic aphasia: The complexity account of treatment efficacy (CATE). *Journal of Speech, Language, and Hearing Research, 46*, 587–595.

Thompson, C. K., Shapiro, L. P., Tait, M. E., Jacobs, B., & Schneider, S. S. (1996). Training wh- question production in agrammatic aphasia: Analysis of argument and adjunct movement. *Brain and Language, 52*, 175–228.

Thompson, C. K., & Weintraub, S. (2004). *The Northwestern Naming Battery*. Manuscript in preparation.

Thulborn, K. R., Carpenter, P. A., & Just, M. A. (1999). Plasticity of language-related brain function during recovery from stroke. *Stroke, 30*, 749–754.

Turner, R. S., Kenyon, L. C., et al. (1996). Clinical, neuroimaging, and pathologic features of progressive nonfluent aphasia. *Annals of Neurology, 39*(2), 166–173.

Tyrrell, P. J., Warrington, E. K., et al. (1990). Heterogeneity in progressive aphasia due to focal cortical atrophy. A clinical and PET study. *Brain, 113*(Pt. 5), 1321–1336.

Wambaugh, J. L., & Thompson, C. K. (1989). Training and generalization of agrammatic aphasic adults: Wh- interrogative productions. *Journal of Speech and Hearing Disorders, 54*, 509–525.

Weintraub, S., Rubin, N. P., et al. (1990). Primary progressive aphasia: Longitudinal course, neuropsychological profile, and language features. *Archives of Neurology, 47*(12), 1329–1335.

Westbury, C., & Bub, D. (1997). Primary progressive aphasia: A review of 112 cases. *Brain Language, 60*(3), 381–406.

World Health Organization. (1980). *International classification of impairments, activities, and handicaps*. Geneva: World Health Organization.

World Health Organization. (1997). *ICIDH-2 International classification of impairments, activities, and participation*. Available at www.ch/programmes/mnh/mnh/ems/icidh/icidh.htm

External Aids

MICHELLE S. BOURGEOIS

When memory deficits interfere with everyday functioning, the recall of familiar words, and the recognition of everyday objects, external memory aids are useful compensatory and supportive strategies for persons with dementia and their caregivers. In contrast to internal memory aids that require effortful cognitive processing, external aids that exist in the physical environment are considered memory prostheses. Their sensory characteristics and structural features may be so strongly associated with past experiences that simply encountering them triggers memories and behaviors relevant to everyday functioning. The challenge for caregivers and professionals is to discover which external cues are important to the individual and then engineer the environment to provide these cues in meaningful contexts. The purpose of this chapter is to review the literature on successful use of external aids with persons with dementia and to suggest future research to further our knowledge of this intervention approach.

WHAT ARE EXTERNAL MEMORY AIDS?

Cognitive rehabilitation therapists have described an extensive array of compensatory external aids as prosthetic devices (i.e., a device that substitutes for a memory function, such as alarm clock, watch, sign, calendar, cards) and cognitive orthotics (i.e., a device that performs a memory function, such as computer software, spell checkers, automated telephone; Harrell, Parente, Bellingrath, & Lisicia, 1992). Others categorize external memory aids as environmental (i.e., part of the person's environment, such as labeled storage units and signs) and portable (i.e., can be moved to another location, such as notebooks and electronic organizers; Kapur, 1995). I (Bourgeois, 2002) organized memory aids within a theoretical model of memory functioning that accounts for the sensory registration of information, the encoding and storage of information, and the retrieval of information, all of which are vulnerable in dementia (Baddeley, 1995). External aids can compensate for sensory, encoding, and retrieval deficits that underlie a variety of behavioral expressions of these memory failures, such as failure to recognize familiar persons, repeated questions, and word retrieval problems.

EXTERNAL MEMORY AIDS FOR MEMORY ENCODING DEFICITS

The hallmark memory symptom in dementia is short-term memory, or encoding, deficits. Caregivers report frequent repetitive questions or demands and having to provide repeated reminders of what to do, where to go, and what they were saying. Typically, desired information is conveyed verbally, is recognized and acknowledged as the answer to a question or a reassuring statement of fact, but is not processed and stored for later retrieval. The information has to be presented repeatedly, often because the amount of information to be processed or encoded exceeds the processing capacity. Complex auditory information may require even more time to process and comprehend. If urged to respond before having processed the instruction completely, the person with memory impairments may provide a negative response reflecting frustration, anger, and lack of comprehension. Reducing the amount of verbal information presented at a time, altering caregivers' expectations for quick responses, and training caregivers to use facilitative methods to encode the desired information are strategies that should improve these interactions. Compensatory memory strategies can facilitate the transfer of new information from working to long-term memory or circumvent the encoding process by providing access to the desired information in such a way that it becomes part of the environment and does not need to be stored for later retrieval.

The primary way to address an encoding deficit is to provide a structured and consistent procedure for ensuring that the information to be remembered is encoded. Rehabilitation therapists have a long history of training persons with memory impairments due to brain injuries to use written strategies, such as memory notebooks, diaries, note taking, appointment calendars, and planners (Harrell et al., 1992; Sohlberg & Mateer, 2001). If important information that is presented verbally is written down immediately, the odds of being able to remember that information (because the person can read it) are increased. This commonsense approach is a typical strategy reported by young and older respondents without diagnosed memory impairments (Harris, 1980). It is only when the frequency of note taking becomes extreme, to the point that family members find handfuls of notes on scraps of paper, that memory concerns are voiced. Persons in the early stage of dementia can be aware of their deficits and use this strategy on their own to mask their symptoms. These written notes become external memory aids for important information that needs to be remembered; having a concrete, tangible written note obviates the need to encode and store it internally. Busy professionals, students, and almost anyone faced with a myriad of facts to remember in their daily life, use appointment calendars and planners routinely to circumvent the need to encode and store all of that information. Audio tape recorders, telephone answering machines, voice message devices, and speech compression tape recorders, several of which use a tape loop feature for continuous reminders, are used for a similar purpose: to record information to be remembered later in a form external to the person. Woods (1983) taught a person with severe memory impairment to use a diary (appointment book) to retrieve personal information; Hanley and Lusty (1984) taught another patient to use a diary and a watch to retrieve orientation information that improved her appointment keeping.

Even though these types of memory aids are commonly used by people in their daily lives, and some people instinctively develop a system that meets their individual needs, there are many others who may require some training to design and implement an efficient and effective system. For example, elders with clinically significant memory impairments may need structured training to use a simple calendar reliably. Camp, Foss, O'Hanlon, and Stevens (1996) demonstrated positive outcomes when training persons with dementia to incorporate calendar use into their daily routine via a spaced-retrieval training protocol. Anecdotal reports of overly complex and cumbersome routines (e.g., multiple bell timers to remember several steps in a task or overly detailed computer calendars) that become the focus of one's daily life, to the detriment of other activities, suggest the need for memory strategy classes or counseling sessions for the general public as well as those with diagnosed memory impairments.

When the person with dementia can no longer write down information reliably for him- or herself, caregivers can use external aids in the form of written notes for a variety of encoding-related problem behaviors. I (Bourgeois, 1994) reported decreasing the repetitive questions of a father to his daughter concerning the whereabouts of his wife with a page in his memory book that said, "My wife, Lilian, died of heart disease in 1967." In another study, I and my colleagues taught caregivers to use a variety of written cues (i.e., memory book pages, cue cards, dry erase memo boards) for reducing the repetitive verbalizations of their spouse with dementia (Bourgeois, Burgio, Schulz, Beach, & Palmer, 1997). Repeated requests to leave the house, to answer a question, and to go home were reduced by having the caregivers redirect their spouse to the memory aid by saying, "The answer is in your memory book [memo board/card]," or "Read this [written instruction for alternate activity]." The frequency of repetitive questions was significantly reduced after treatment. Caregivers reported generalizing the use of reminder cards to a variety of situations; one wife kept index cards in the car on which to write the answer to the constant query, "Where are we going?" Others used cards in church and on a bus trip; another caregiver designed a fake letter from the Internal Revenue Service to remind her husband that he had submitted his tax return and that his refund check had been deposited in his bank account.

Practical applications of these external aids in the nursing home with persons with advanced dementia were reported by Bourgeois, Dijkstra, Burgio, and Allen-Burge (2001). Nursing aides were trained to use communication, or reminder, cards with their resident with dementia when they were providing care, such as showering or feeding. Each resident had a collection of personalized cards that addressed problems identified by their nursing aide, such as "Showering makes me feel warm and clean," "My nurse Betty helps me get dressed every day," or "Eating helps me stay strong and healthy." Nursing aides presented the appropriate card to residents, asked them to read it, and then asked them to proceed with the activity. Nursing aides reported increased compliance and cooperation with care activities and decreased negative reactions subsequent to using the cards. An interactive CD-ROM program for training reminder card use by nursing aides in the nursing home has been demonstrated to increase nursing aide knowledge of, and intention to use, the strategy and perceived self-efficacy in managing resident problem behaviors (Irvine, Bourgeois, & Ary, 2003).

When written cues are found to be successful with the person with dementia, and the caregiver has many cards and written notes around the house, it may become important to organize the individual statements or cards into a memory wallet or memory book for more efficient access whenever desired (Bourgeois, 1990, 1992a). At this point, the collection of facts to be remembered serves an external memory storage function for the retrieval of information that may be or should be stored in long-term memory.

EXTERNAL MEMORY AIDS FOR LONG-TERM
MEMORY AND RETRIEVAL DEFICITS

Anomia, or word-finding difficulty—a failure to retrieve words from long-term storage—is typically the earliest language and memory symptom in dementia. Because normally aging adults compensate for word-finding problems by substituting similar words or talking around the missing word, it is often overlooked as one of the early warning signs of the pervasive loss of semantic information in dementia (Craik, Anderson, Kerr, & Li, 1995). The retrieval of other factual, conceptual, and procedural information thought to be stored in long-term memory becomes increasingly impaired as the disease progresses. The difference between the experience of normal forgetting and memory loss associated with dementia is that once the retrieval problem interrupts their train of thought, individuals with memory impairment often digress to another topic and forget the earlier topic. Over the degenerative course of the disease, word-finding and other semantic retrieval problems become more obvious and in need of strategies that provide alternate access routes to the information. External memory aids in print and electronic formats have been developed to access semantic storage via alternate pathways.

The electronics boom has triggered a plethora of devices to store information, to prompt owners to attend to the information with a variety of alarm and messaging features, and to retrieve the relevant or desired information. Electronic calculators, planners (e.g., Daytimers, Dayrunners, Franklin), personal data storage devices (e.g., Rolodex, Texas Instruments, Casio) and watches (e.g., Telememo watch; Naugle, Prevey, Naugle, & Delaney, 1988) are available in infinite combinations of size, price, keyboard style, alarm, and ease of manipulation features (Harrell et al., 1992; Kapur, 1995; Parente & Hermann, 1996). Computerized systems add another level of complexity and multiplicity of features, including the transfer of information from one device to another (e.g., Palm Pilot, the Timex Data Link Watch, and the NeuroPage; Glisky, 1995; Sohlberg & Mateer, 2001). To date, the efficacy literature on these electronic storage devices is limited to persons with memory impairments due to brain injury, encephalitis, epilepsy, multiple sclerosis, and Parkinson's disease, with mixed results (Kapur, 1995). The complexity of training multiple performance steps and the time required to master the routines led to cautious endorsement of these products by the trainers. The cost of training, in addition to the cost of the devices themselves, may prevent the routine use of electronic devices unless the person had been a proficient user premorbidly. Low-cost and low-tech print formats seem to be more feasible alternatives for persons with dementia.

The most commonly used external memory aids for long-term memory storage and retrieval are the memory book and memory wallet (Bourgeois, 1990, 1992a, 1992b). Memory books and wallets present factual information in a written and picture format, activating visual pathways through reading. In one study (Bourgeois, 1990), memory wallets contained 30 pages with one sentence and one picture depicting a single statement of fact on each page. In baseline conversations without a memory wallet, subjects with moderate dementia provided limited and repetitive information when prompted to talk about their family, their life, and their daily schedule. Access to the memory wallet during the treatment condition enabled them to read aloud each sentence and then elaborate about the topic, increasing the number of factual statements significantly and decreasing repetitiveness and ambiguity. Systematic replications of this study with patients more impaired cognitively and with greater sensory deficits revealed the efficacy of this approach as long as the visual-stimulus characteristics of the memory aid matched the patients' deficits (Bourgeois, 1992a). That is, the font size of the type was increased until it was read easily, and the size of the memory aid was prescribed for ease of physical manipulation; some persons required 8 × 11-inch pages and plastic page protectors to improve page turning, whereas others required lightweight, laminated 3 × 5-inch pages in a portable format (i.e., on a book ring and lanyard, necklace, wristband, or belt). Also, the number of pages varied depending on the extent of the content desired to be included in the aid; persons with more severe impairments required fewer pages (i.e., 10–15). McPherson et al. (2001) replicated the effects of these studies with subjects who had severe memory deficits.

External aids for storing important information about the person with dementia for future retrieval have also been developed for safety purposes. Information pendants, medic alert devices, and safe-return bracelets containing personal information (i.e., name, address) and medical information (i.e., diagnosis, allergies) are widely advocated and distributed by the Alzheimer's Association and other supportive organizations (Alzheimer's Association, 2003). To date, there has been no research on the ability of persons with dementia themselves to retrieve relevant information from these external aids.

EXTERNAL MEMORY AIDS TO MODIFY BEHAVIOR AND SUPPORT FUNCTION

External memory aids have successfully modified a variety of problem behaviors, such as wandering, lack of initiation/cooperation, and sundowning, which could be explained as problems with the integration of sensory input, encoding, and retrieval processes. For example, wanderers may not remember what they could be doing (e.g., a favorite pasttime or hobby) or where they are going (e.g., to the kitchen for a drink, to the bathroom). The cues that initially may have suggested a trip to the kitchen for a drink may be supplanted by new cues along the route (e.g., a picture on the piano, the laundry basket on the counter). A portable memory aid consisting of cards with activity suggestions or a single instruction card that states, for example, "I'm going to the kitchen for a drink," could help keep the relevant information in focus until the task was completed. Similarly, a person's apathy or inactivity may be due to the fact that access to long-term memory for familiar favorite activities is impaired and activity materials are not recognizable or too complex. Simple, written activity instructions and labels on the materials could increase recognition and participation. Alternatively, a memory album consisting of pictures of a favorite hobby or interest (e.g., "All about Roses," "My Book of Baseball," "My Trips around the World") could capture the person's attention, enabling him or her to engage with the materials for a significant amount of time.

Agitated behaviors may reflect problems with several memory systems simultaneously. For example, agitation attributed to boredom may reflect an inability to access words (long-term retrieval) to explain the need for a purposeful activity in the presence of an object that is no longer familiar (i.e., a sensory memory deficit; Volicer & Bloom Charette, 1999); a memory book with pages depicting preferred activities with specific objects could help patients communicate their needs. Resistance or lack of cooperation may result from patients not understanding verbal directions and not being able to explain that they do not understand what is expected of them; the communication cards used by nursing aides addressed this problem (Bourgeois et al, 2001). Persons who exhibit sundowning behaviors, such as saying they need to go home, packing a suitcase or shopping bags, or exit seeking, may not remember that they are in their own home because familiar visual cues have lost their salience; I (Bourgeois, 1990) reported a caregiver independently using a page in his wife's memory book to remind her that she was at home ("I have lived at 123 Elm Street for 45 years" + picture of home).

Lack of access to the words to express wants, needs, frustration, boredom, loneliness, and confusion results in many problem behaviors, such as sundowning, restless pacing, or yelling and crying out for help (i.e., disruptive vocalization). The range of challenging behaviors of persons with dementia is thought to be the result of unmet needs (Algase et al., 1996, Beck et al., 1998; Cohen-Mansfield, 2000). These communication problems are often responded to by concerned questioning, but when the person is unable to express a specific need, the need remains unmet, resulting in increased disruptive behavior. External memory aids in the form of memory books with pages depicting desired activities, typical need resolutions, and comforting messages could mediate these deficits. At late stages of dementia, when access to vocabulary is severely limited, it is imperative that disruptive vocalization be interpreted by caregivers as communicative attempts, albeit unsuccessful ones, and strategies be attempted to address clients' needs.

EXTERNAL AIDS FOR SENSORY MEMORY AND REGISTRATION DEFICITS

When the person with dementia has trouble recognizing familiar objects or persons . . . when he or she loses his or her way inside his or her own home . . . when a shadow in a darkened room creates the delusion of a stranger . . . or when the waste basket is mistaken for the toilet, he or she may be experiencing a failure of sensory input to be registered, recognized, and understood. The salience of visual features may degrade over time, causing familiar objects to look strange or new. Auditory information can become distorted or inaudible due to age-related sensory-neural hearing deficits. In the latter stages of dementia, persons may attempt to gain sensory information from objects they pick up and fondle or from patting a tabletop. Failure to recognize the familiar can create confusion, frustration, or apathy. Rehabilitative strategies—particularly external aids that address the sensory features of stimuli by enhancing them, making them more salient, visible, heard, and felt in order to activate the visual, auditory, and tactile pathways that access their semantic counterparts—should be helpful.

External memory aids can enhance sensory or environmental features and signal or cue behavior by triggering associations between auditory, visual, or tactile features and past experiences of the person with memory impairment (Garrett & Yorkston, 1997; Sohlberg & Mateer, 2001). Auditory signals such as doorbells, car door alarms, ringing telephone, kitchen/oven timers, and whistling tea kettles, may have been experienced for so many years that recognition of the meaning of these signals is automatic, unconscious, and resistant to memory decay. Caregivers have reported using door alarms that emit loud, noxious sounds to prompt the person with dementia to recognize a dangerous situation and to reduce exit-seeking behaviors. Auditory cueing systems exist along a continuum of sound-enhancing technology, from personal hearing aids, to assistive listening devices for the television and telephone, and signaling/alerting systems such as bells, ringers, and vibrating devices (Weinstein, 1991). Voice mail and telephone reminding systems, in addition to pill dispensers with timed alarms, have successfully increased medication adherence and appointment attendance (Azrin & Powell, 1969; Leirer, Morrow, Pariante, & Doksum, 1988; Leirer, Morrow, Tanke, & Pariante, 1991). Two caveats concerning external aids in the form of auditory cues should be noted. First, if the cue is nonspecific (i.e., a kitchen timer or alarm clock), it may remind the person that *something*, but not *what*, needs to be remembered, causing frustration or confusion (Woods, 1996). Secondly, the compromised hearing status of many elderly persons can adversely impact cognitive performance based on auditory or verbal cues; and persons with dementia are at increased risk for disorientation, confusion, and impaired comprehension when information has not been processed completely due to reduced hearing (Weinstein, 1991). These individuals may be cued more effectively using their visual and tactile modalities or cue combinations.

Visual external aids such as written signs for labeling the contents of drawers and closets, name tags, grocery lists, activity schedules, wall calendars, orientation and message boards, cue cards and Post-it notes, medication organizers, maps and floor plans take advantage of the unconscious, automatic, and relatively preserved processes involved in reading comprehension (Bourgeois, 2001). Other visual cues such as clocks, single-button dialing telephones, traffic signs, and photographs trigger long-term memories for iconic symbols that are recognized with little effort. When stimuli are altered to enhance their visibility, associated stored memories can be triggered. For example, enlarging the print, using bright or neon colors, highlighting, creating high-contrast situations, or using personal objects can increase a person's attention to the importance of the cue. Visual cueing in its simplest form may well be the use of a routine place and location for specific objects; hanging the car keys by the door to the garage, keeping a note pad for messages by the telephone, and placing bills to be paid in a specific letter tray on the desk are strategies used by many individuals who report using memory strategies routinely (Harris, 1980). Organizational strategies similarly address the visual salience of objects in specific locations; for example, silverware trays, desk supply organizers, and closet organizers for ties and belts facilitate finding and recognizing desired objects.

Caregivers are often advised to place a particular activity or materials along the pacing route of an individual to cue him or her to engage in an alternate activity (e.g., a laundry basket with towels to be folded). Bourgeois et al. (1997) taught caregivers to place important written messages and activity suggestions on an erasable memo board magnetically attached to the refrigerator for persons whose pacing route included the kitchen. A variety of disruptive behaviors were decreased and desired behaviors increased with this simple visual strategy. When the cue is visual and in the environment, the opportunity for it to be noticed and recognized by the individual is enhanced without overt prompting to look at it or to use it. Smith (1988) used cue cards to reduce disruptive behaviors of persons with dementia. Park and Kidder (1996) reviewed the literature on external aids for medication adherence, including 1-day and 7-day (with and without times—morning, noon, dinner, evening) medication organizers. The most effective aids for elderly users were those with the most compartments (7 days with time; 28 places; Rehder, McCoy, Blackwell, Whitehead, & Robinson, 1980) and those used in combination with a visual organizational chart (Park, Morrell, Frieske, & Kincaid, 1992). Other researchers have found that external visual aids in the form of a tear-off calendar (MacDonald, MacDonald, & Phoenix, 1977) and a check-off chart (Gabriel, Gagnon, & Bryan, 1977) increased adherence by elderly users. Hussian and Brown (1987) placed a two-dimensional grid pattern on the floor in front of an exit and thereby reduced the hazardous ambulation of nursing home patients. Similarly, Namazi, Rosner, and Calkins (1989) found that visual concealment in the form of a cloth panel was successful at preventing exit through an emergency door. Leseth and Meader (1995) used a vase of bright red flowers to cue a person to her assigned table in the dining room. Nursing home residents were cued effectively to find their own rooms and prevent unwanted access to other resident rooms using personal photographs and large-print name plates (Nolan, Mathews, & Harrison, 2001). Visual cues have become a popular marketing strategy for residential facilities; color schemes, street signs, personalized front doors and mailboxes, and mail baskets or flower boxes are designed to enhance recognition memory for the familiar in the context of a new environment (Zeisel, Hyde, & Shi, 1999). Researchers have found, however, that simply placing visual cues in the path of the person with dementia may not ensure that he or she sees it, recognizes it, and responds to it, as desired. Some concerted effort to point out, identify, and rehearse the cue with the person may be necessary to keep it salient. The use of signs, signposts, and labels on drawers and cupboards was found to be enhanced when staff members were involved in practicing the environmental cues with patients (Gilleard, Mitchell, & Riordan, 1981; Hanley, 1981; Josephsson et al. 1993; Lam & Woods, 1986).

Tactile cues in the form of objects and textures have also been found useful for triggering associated memories, particularly with the most impaired individuals. Hopper, Bayles, and Tomoeda (1998) found that tangible stimuli in the form of dolls and stuffed animals improved the meaningfulness and relevance of conversations of persons with dementia. External aids in the form of dolls have also been used to prompt positive alternative behaviors in persons who exhibited troublesome behaviors (Ehrenfeld, 2003; Godfrey, 1994). Similarly, Buettner (1999) demonstrated decreased patient agitation and improved family visiting with a variety of handmade, therapeutically based sensory-motor recreational items (e.g., activity apron, electronic busy box, "look inside purse," "squeezies") were given to nursing home residents with dementia.

External memory aids that combine sensory features may have increased salience. The keyless car door opener that beeps and causes the headlights of the car to flash when the doors are locked and unlocked remotely is one of the latest external memory aids—in effect, a car finding device for those who lose their cars in large parking lots. Medication organizers may have alarms to signal when to look for the appropriate medication for that time period. The NeuroPage device is an auditory pager that signals the user to look at the message screen for the next written appointment prompt (Hersh & Treadgold, 1994).

Although most caregiver guidebooks recommend the use of these commonsense strategies that are based on positive anecdotal reports (i.e., Hoffman & Platt, 1991; Mace & Rabins, 1981), more experimental research is needed to document the effectiveness of visual external aids, especially with persons who have dementia or memory impairments. Empirical investigations have suggested that enhanced stimuli alone cannot produce desired changes in patient functioning, training, or routine, and that repetitive exposure is required (Cohen & Weisman, 1991; Zeisel et al., 1999).

TRAINING CONSIDERATIONS

Many of the external memory aids described above may require training to ensure their routine use and to retain their recognition, organizational, and memory-supporting value.

The range of aids—from computers, electronic organizers, and personal data storage devices to written planning systems, organizers, and memory notebooks with divided sections for daily, weekly, and monthly events, telephone directory, and notes—may require a significant amount of time to learn how to use and to incorporate into daily life. Even simple environmental aids, such as signs and labels, may need periodic time investments so that the person can practice identifying, reading, and discussing them to maintain their salience and intended function. A deterrent to the use and training of many memory aids, however, is the belief that persons with dementia and encoding memory deficits are unable to acquire new information and demonstrate new learning. This belief, however, has been challenged by Camp (1999) and others with evidence that persons with dementia can learn new information using spaced retrieval (described extensively in Camp, Chapter 12, this volume).

Spaced retrieval involves recalling information over increasingly longer periods of time and has been used to teach persons with dementia (1) to remember the names of common objects (Abrahams & Camp, 1993), (2) to remember to perform a future action (Camp, Foss, Stevens, & O'Hanlon, 1996), (3) face–name and object–location associations (Camp & Stevens, 1990), (4) to use a strategy (e.g., "Look at the calendar"; Camp, Foss, O'Hanlon, & Stevens, 1996), and (5) to use external memory aids (Bourgeois et al., 2003). In a spaced-retrieval training session, the therapist prompts the person with dementia to produce the target response by saying, "How do you remember where your room is?" The person with dementia responds, "I look at my reminder card." The therapist replies, "That's correct, and I want you to remember that because I will be asking you again in a few minutes." After a specified time interval, the therapist repeats the prompt, "How do you remember where your room is?" Each correct response results in doubling the time interval time before the next prompt. Incorrect responses elicit the modeling and repetition of the correct response. This procedure results in rapid and durable acquisition of the target response (Bourgeois et al., 2003; Camp, Foss, O'Hanlon, & Stevens, 1996).

Factors to consider before selecting an external memory aid and a potential training regimen include the individual's level of literacy, prior experience with reminding systems, degree and severity of cognitive impairment, level of awareness regarding the memory problems, and motivation to compensate for them. As described in Attix (Chapter 10, this volume), intervention targets and training techniques vary depending on stage and severity of the cognitive deficits. Persons with a mild cognitive impairment may begin to reactivate formerly useful reminding systems independently (e.g., the retired businessman who starts to use a planner again, or the retired college professor who keeps a small notebook to record people's names and words he has stumbled over recently). Persons with mild memory impairment usually request memory rehabilitation efforts and participate in the development and evaluation of their own functional systems. As memory deficits worsen, successful memory-enhancing systems require premorbid familiarity, salient multisensory features, or specific training protocols (e.g., spaced retrieval). When introducing a novel cueing system, such as an enlarged plate switch with a picture of a nurse taped to it as an alternative call button, training the person with dementia "to touch the picture when you need a nurse" would be necessary (Garrett & Yorkston, 1997). Many examples of successful training in the use of external memory aids have been reported in the literature, including the use of a palmtop computer to get to scheduled appointments and take medication (Kim, Burke, Dowds, & George, 1999), and a portable paging and text screen system, the NeuroPage (Hersh & Treadgold, 1994). Enwefa (1999) trained 10 persons with dementia to use communication wallets and the Alpha Talker, an augmentative communication device with preprogrammed phrases, and measured more conversational content with the electronic device. Lekeu, Wojtasik, Van der Linden, and Salmon (2002) used cue cards and spaced retrieval to teach two persons with dementia to use a mobile phone; although both eventually learned to use their phones correctly, one person required much more training than the other.

Not all efforts at training the use of electronic memory aids have been successful, however. Kapur (1995) detailed efforts to train patients with a range of memory disorders to use electronic organizers; two of five subjects failed to learn and two others only reduced their memory lapses by 50%. The only successful user was a bank clerk who learned to use a Tandy organizer in two training sessions; she then used it daily in performing the duties of her job. The educational level of the participants, degree of impairment, motivation to use the devices, and degree of appropriateness of the training techniques were thought to contribute to the difficulties encountered by the unsuccessful participants. Sohlberg and Mateer (2001) have suggested the use of training protocols that incorporate a variety of effective instruction techniques, including functional task selection, task analysis, errorless instruction, prompting, cueing, feedback, and reinforcement. In addition, the role of the caregiver in facilitating the use of external aids cannot be overlooked. Many of the reports of successful aid use have involved family and nursing aides who ensured that the aids were available and prompted their use at appropriate times (Bourgeois et al., 1997, 2001). Much of the literature on training external aid use has been with persons who have sustained memory loss due to head injury or other etiologies; more research is needed to find efficacious ways to enable persons with memory loss due to the degenerative process of dementia to use external aids effectively.

Although additional research is still needed, this emerging literature is encouraging in the diversity of evidence that is accumulating, debunking the myths that persons with cognitive deficits could not learn new information or maintain treatment effects over the long term. It should be clear from this review that the maintenance of functional memory skills is possible when individuals are provided with the appropriate system of external cues and training procedure for their condition.

REFERENCES

Abrahams, J. P., & Camp, C. J. (1993). Maintenance and generalization of object naming training in anomia associated with degenerative dementia. *Clinical Gerontologist, 12,* 57–72.

Algase, D. L., Beck, C., Kolanowski, A., Whall, A., Berent, S., Richards, K., et al. (1996). Need-driven dementia-compromised behavior: An alternative view of disruptive behavior. *American Journal of Alzheimer's Disease, 11,* 10–19.

Alzheimer's Association. (2003). *Safe return.* Retrieved August 18, 2003, www.alz.org/ResourceCenter/Programs/SafeReturn.htm

Azrin, N., & Powell, J. (1969). Behavioral engineering: The use of response priming to improve prescribed self-medication. *Journal of Applied Behavior Analysis, 2,* 39–42.

Baddeley, A. (1995). The psychology of memory. In A. D. Baddeley, B. A. Wilson, & F. N. Watts (Eds.), *Handbook of memory disorders* (pp. 3–26). New York: Wiley.

Beck, C., Frank, L., Chumbler, N. R., O'Sullivan, P., Vogelpohl, T. S., Rasin, J., et al. (1998). Correlates of disruptive behavior in severely cognitively impaired nursing home residents. *Gerontologist, 38,* 189–198.

Bourgeois, M. (1990). Enhancing conversation skills in Alzheimer's disease using a prosthetic memory aid. *Journal of Applied Behavior Analysis, 23,* 29–42.

Bourgeois, M. (1992a). Evaluating memory wallets in conversations with patients with dementia. *Journal of Speech and Hearing Research*, 35, 1344–1357.

Bourgeois, M. (1992b). *Enhancing the Conversations of Memory-Impaired Persons: A Memory Aid Workbook*. Gaylord, MI: Northern Speech Services.

Bourgeois, M. (1994). Teaching caregivers to use memory aids with patients with dementia. In M. Bourgeois (Ed.), Caregiving in Alzheimer's disease: II. Caregiving interventions. *Seminars in Speech and Language*, 15(4), 291–305.

Bourgeois, M. (2001). Is reading preserved in dementia? *ASHA Leader*, 6(9), 5.

Bourgeois, M. (2002). Where is my wife and when am I going home? The challenge of communicating with persons with dementia. *Alzheimer Care Quarterly*, 3, 132–144.

Bourgeois, M., Burgio, L., Schulz, R., Beach, S., & Palmer, B. (1997). Modifying repetitive verbalization of community dwelling patients with AD. *Gerontologist*, 37, 30–39.

Bourgeois, M., Camp, C., Rose, M., White, B., Malone, M., Carr, J., et al. (2003). A comparison of training strategies to enhance use of external aids by persons with dementia. *Journal of Communication Disorders*, 36, 361–378.

Bourgeois, M., Dijkstra, K., Burgio, L., & Allen-Burge, R. (2001). Memory aids as an AAC strategy for nursing home residents with dementia. *Augmentative and Alternative Communication*, 17, 196–210.

Buettner, L. (1999). Simple pleasures: A multilevel sensorimotor intervention for nursing home residents with dementia. *American Journal of Alzheimer's Disease*, 14, 41–52.

Camp, C. (1999). Memory interventions for normal and pathological older adults. In R. Schulz, G. Maddox, & M. P. Lawton (Eds.), *Annual review of gerontology and geriatrics: Focus on intervention research with older adults* (pp. 155–189). New York: Springer.

Camp, C. J., Foss, J. W., O'Hanlon, A. M., & Stevens, A. B. (1996). Memory interventions for persons with dementia. *Applied Cognitive Psychology*, 10, 193–210.

Camp, C. J., Foss, J. W., Stevens, A. B., & O'Hanlon, A. M. (1996). Improving prospective memory task performance in persons with Alzheimer's disease. In M. A. Brandimonte, G. Einstein, & M. McDaniel (Eds.), *Prospective memory: Theory and applications* (pp. 351–367). Hillsdale, NJ: Erlbaum.

Camp, C. J., & Stevens, A. B. (1990). Spaced-retrieval: A memory intervention for dementia of the Alzheimer's type (DAT). *Clinical Gerontologist*, 10, 658–661.

Cohen, U., & Weisman, G. (1991). *Holding on to home: Planning environments for the elderly and the confused*. Owings Mills, MD: National Health Publishing.

Cohen-Mansfield, J. (2000). Theoretical frameworks for behavioral problems in dementia. *Alzheimer's Care Quarterly*, 1, 8–21.

Craik, F., Anderson, N., Kerr, S., & Li, K. (1995). Memory changes in normal ageing. In A. D. Baddeley, B. A. Wilson, & F. N. Watts (Eds.), *Handbook of memory disorders* (pp. 211–242). Chichester, UK: Wiley.

Ehrenfeld, M. (2003). Using therapeutic dolls with psychogeriatric patients. In C. E. Schaefer (Ed.), *Play therapy with adults* (pp. 291–297). New York: Wiley.

Enwefa, R. L. (1999). An investigative study of the efficacy of an external aid (conversation wallet) and augmentative communication (alpha talker device) on the communicative functions of middle stage Alzheimer's disease populations. *Dissertation Abstracts International*, 59(11-B), 5801.

Gabriel, M., Gagnon, J. P., & Bryan, C. K. (1977). Improved patient compliance through use of a daily drug reminder chart. *American Journal of Public Health*, 67, 968–969.

Garrett, K., & Yorkston, K. (1997). Assistive communication technology for elders with cognitive and language disabilities. In R. Lubinski & D. J. Higginbotham (Eds.), *Communication technologies for the elderly* (pp. 203–234). San Diego, CA: Singular Press.

Gilleard, C., Mitchell, R. G., & Riordan, J. (1981). Ward orientation training with psychogeriatric patients. *Journal of Advanced Nursing*, 6, 95–98.

Glisky, E. L. (1995). Computers in memory rehabilitation. In A. D. Baddeley, B. A. Wilson, & F. N. Watts (Eds.), *Handbook of memory disorders* (pp. 557–575). New York: Wiley.

Godfrey, S. (1994). Doll therapy. *Australian Journal on Ageing, 13*, 46.

Hanley, I. G. (1981). The use of signposts and active training to modify ward disorientation in elderly patients. *Journal of Behavior Therapy and Experimental Psychiatry, 12*, 241–247.

Hanley, I. G., & Lusty, K. (1984). Memory aids in reality orientation: A single-case study. *Behavior Research Therapy, 22*, 709–712.

Harrell, M., Parente, F., Bellingrath, E. G., & Lisicia (1992). *Cognitive rehabilitation of memory: A practical guide.* Gaithersburg, MD: Aspen.

Harris, J. E. (1980). Memory aids people use: Two interview studies. *Memory and Cognition, 8*, 31–38.

Hersch, N., & Treadgold, L. (1994). NeuroPage: The rehabilitation of memory dysfunction by prosthetic memory and cueing. *Neuropsychological Rehabilitation, 4*, 187–197.

Hoffman, S. B., & Platt, C. A. (1991). *Comforting the confused: Strategies for managing dementia.* New York: Springer.

Hopper, T., Bayles, K., & Tomoeda, C. (1998). Using toys to stimulate communicative function in individuals with Alzheimer's disease. *Journal of Medical Speech–Language Pathology, 6*, 73–80.

Hussian, R. A., & Brown, D.C. (1987). Use of two-dimensional grid patterns to limit hazardous ambulation in demented patients. *Journals of Gerontology, 42*, 558–560.

Irvine, A. B., Bourgeois, M., & Ary, D. V. (2003). An interactive multi-media program to train professional caregivers. *Journal of Applied Gerontology, 22*, 269–288.

Josephsson, S., Backman, L., Borell, L., Bernspang, B., Nygard, L., & Ronnberg, L. (1993). Supporting everyday activities in dementia: An intervention study. *International Journal of Geriatric Psychiatry, 8*, 395–400.

Kapur, N. (1995). Memory aids in the rehabilitation of memory disordered patients. In A. D. Baddeley, B. A. Wilson, & F. N. Watts (Eds.), *Handbook of memory disorders* (pp. 534–556). Chichester, UK: Wiley.

Kim, H. J., Burke, D. T., Dowds, M. D., & George, J. (1999). Utility of a microcomputer as an external memory aid for a memory impaired head injury patient during in-patient rehabilitation. *Brain Injury, 13*, 147–150.

Lam, D. H., & Woods, R. T. (1986). Ward orientation training in dementia: A single-case study. *International Journal of Geriatric Psychiatry, 1*, 145–147.

Leirer, V. O., Morrow, D. G., Pariante, G. M., & Doksum, T. (1988). Increasing influenza vaccination adherence through voice mail. *Journal of the American Geriatric Society, 37*, 1147–1150.

Leirer, V. O., Morrow, D. G., Tanke, E. D., & Pariante, G. M. (1991). Elders' nonadherence: Its assessment and medication reminding by voice mail. *Gerontologist, 31*, 514–520.

Lekeu, F., Wojtasik, V., Van der Linden, M., & Salmon, E. (2002). Training early Alzheimer patients to use a mobile phone. *Acta Neurologica Belgica, 102*, 114–121.

Leseth, L., & Meader, L. (1995). Utilizing an AAC system to maximize receptive and expressive communication skills of a person with Alzheimer's disease. *ASHA AAC Special Interest Division Newsletter, 4*, 7–9.

MacDonald, E. T., MacDonald, J. B., & Phoenix, M. (1977). Improving drug compliance after hospital discharge. *British Medical Journal, 2*, 618–621.

Mace, N. L., & Rabins, P. V. (1981). *The 36-hour day.* Baltimore, MD: Johns Hopkins University Press.

McPherson, A., Furniss, F. G., Sdogati, C., Cesaroni, F., Tartaglini, B., & Lindesay, J. (2001). Effects of individualized memory aids on the conversation of persons with severe dementia. *Aging and Mental Health, 5*, 289–294.

Namazi, K., Rosner, T., & Calkins, M. (1989). Visual barriers to prevent ambulatory Alzheimer's patients from exiting through an emergency door. *Gerontologist, 29*, 699–702.

Naugle, R., Prevey, M., Naugle, C., & Delaney, R. (1988). New digital watch as a compensatory device for memory dysfunction. *Cognitive Rehabilitation, 6*, 22–23.

Nolan, B., Mathews, M., & Harrison, M. (2001). Using external memory aids to increase room finding by older adults with dementia. *American Journal of Alzheimer's Disease, 16*, 251–154.

Parente, R., & Hermann, D. (1996). *Retraining cognition: techniques and applications*. Gaithersburg, MD: Aspen.

Park, D. C., & Kidder, D. P (1996). Prospective memory and medication adherence. In M. Brandimonte, G. Einstein, & M. McDaniel (Eds.), *Prospective memory: Theory and applications* (pp. 369–390). Hillsdale, NJ: Erlbaum.

Park, D. C., Morrell, R. W., Frieske, D., & Kincaid, D. (1992). Medication adherence behaviors in older adults: Effects of external cognitive supports. *Psychology and Aging, 7*, 252–256.

Rehder, T. L., McCoy, L. K., Blackwell, B., Whitehead, W., & Robinson, A. (1980). Improving medication compliance by counseling and special prescription container. *American Journal of Hospital Pharmacy, 37*, 379–384.

Smith, W. L. (1988, May). *Behavioral interventions in gerontology: Management of behavior problems in individuals with Alzheimer's disease living in the community*. Paper presented at the Association for Behavior Analysis Convention, Philadelphia.

Sohlberg, M. M., & Mateer, C. A. (2001). *Cognitive rehabilitation: An integrative neuropsychological approach*. New York: Guilford Press.

Weinstein, B. E. (1991). Auditory testing and rehabilitation of the hearing impaired. In R. Lubinski (Ed.), *Dementia and communication* (pp. 223–237). Philadelphia: B. C. Decker.

Woods, R. T. (1983). Specificity of learning in reality orientation sessions: A single-case study. *Behaviour Research and Therapy, 21*, 173–175.

Woods, R. T. (1996). Psychological "therapies" in dementia. In R. T. Woods (Ed.), *Handbook of the clinical psychology of ageing* (pp. 575–600). New York: Wiley.

Volicer, L., & Bloom-Charette, L. (1999). Assessment of quality of life in advanced dementia. In L. Volicer & L. Bloom-Charette (Eds.), *Enhancing the quality of life in advanced dementia* (pp. 3–20). Philadelphia: Taylor & Francis.

Zeisel, J., Hyde, J., & Shi, L. (1999). Environmental design as a treatment for Alzheimer's disease. In L. Volicer & L. Bloom-Charette (Eds.), *Enhancing the quality of life in advanced dementia* (pp. 206–222). Philadelphia: Taylor & Francis.

Section B

Psychotherapeutic Interventions

In Section B of Part II we primarily focus on psychotherapeutic interventions that target emotional distress or behavioral problems. Although these symptoms remain our primary targets, we also recognize that their amelioration has other tangible impact beyond symptom relief. We thus encourage consideration of important secondary outcomes that follow from the successful treatment of depression and problem behaviors: namely, improved quality of life, reduction of family and caregiver stress, and potentially reduced health care utilization, given the well-established link between depression and health care status.

In the chapters that follow as well as those in the preceding section, it again becomes clear that different methodologies or treatment modalities can be used to address similar problems. The reader is thus referred to the general intervention model in Chapter 10 for consideration of the variables that assist in the selection of intervention targets and techniques.

Chapter 16 leads off with discussion of nonpharmacological behavioral approaches to reduce depression. This contribution is by authors whose work historically sets strong examples of rigorously designed intervention outcomes research, which the field urgently needs. It also nicely demonstrates our belief that *inactivity breeds depression*.

Chapter 17 focuses on modifying problematic or maladaptive behavior rather than emotional distress. This work is included in this section rather than the cognitive training section because the methodology involves application of behavioral principles and techniques to achieve improved functional outcomes. This is in contrast to the functional skills training described earlier in the book (Chapter 11), which directly trains the specific skill using a combination of cognitive techniques and practice of functional skills. This chapter is an essential component of this text, given that so much of intervention draws upon behavioral techniques and principles.

Chapter 18 outlines the literature and provides details from experience in conducting psychotherapeutic group therapy with geriatric patients who have neuropsychological deficits. The chapter explores important conceptual issues involving the application of these approaches with cognitively impaired groups and discusses the patient and caregiver perspectives of treatment.

Finally, realizing that this type of intervention work occurs within the context of other types of approaches, Chapter 19 concludes the text with a review of pharmacologi-

347

cal treatments in memory-impaired patients. The chapter discusses the impact of pharmacotherapy on symptom expression and progression in Alzheimer's disease and related dementias. Considered in this chapter is the design of clinical trials for treatment of dementia as well as for primary prevention of disorders in normal older groups who do not express the disease or who are experiencing mild symptoms suggestive of prodromal disease, so-called "secondary prevention." The chapter provides a broad overview of the medications currently on the market or in clinical trial and also considers approaches that show future promise for either delaying symptom onset or slowing rates of progression so as to maintain optimal function for extended periods of time. We include this chapter to consider the larger treatment context within which intervention work proceeds.

Behavioral Treatment of Affective Disorders and Associated Symptoms

REBECCA G. LOGSDON
SUSAN M. MCCURRY
LINDA TERI

Although memory loss and other cognitive changes are the defining indices of dementia, disruptive or distressing behaviors are often cited as the most difficult aspect of care, leading to greater functional impairment in the person with dementia and increased burden in the caregiver (Burns, 1996; Cummings & Kaufer, 1996; Fitz & Teri, 1994; Teri, 1992). Affective disturbances such as depression, anxiety, and sleep difficulties may particularly interfere with care and decrease quality of life of both the affected individual and his or her family (Teri et al., 1992; Vitaliano, Young, & Russo, 1991; Wagner, Logsdon, Pearson, & Teri, 1997). Thus it is essential that mental health providers are aware of the most effective ways to assess and treat these problems. Failure to do so may compound the disability of patients and their caregivers. Furthermore, when behavioral and mood disturbances are severe or cause safety concerns, the use of behavioral or social support interventions may delay the need for institutionalization (Carlson, Fleming, Smith, & Evans, 1995; Mittelman et al., 1993; Mittelman, Ferris, Shulman, Steinberg, & Levin, 1996; Steele, Rovner, Chase, & Folstein, 1990).

This chapter provides a review of affective problems seen in cognitively impaired older adults, focusing on depression, anxiety, and sleep difficulties, and describes a framework for an empirically validated behavioral approach to care. We focus on the behavioral treatment of community-residing individuals with Alzheimer's disease (AD) or related dementia. Practitioners interested in pharmacological treatment approaches are referred elsewhere (Sano, Chapter 19, this volume; Raskind & Peskind, 2001; Teri, Logsdon, & Schindler, 1999; Weiner, Schneider, Gray, & Stern, 1996), as are those who are working in residential care settings (Allen-Burge, Stevens, & Burgio, 1999; Camp, Cohen-Mansfield, & Capezuti, 2002; Snowden, Sato, & Roy-Byrne, 2003; Sutor, 2002).

COMMON AFFECTIVE DISTURBANCES IN DEMENTIA

The constellation of behavioral disturbances that includes depression, anxiety, and sleep difficulties affects up to 80% of individuals with dementia during the progression of the disease, and comorbidity is the rule, rather than the exception (Lyketsos et al., 2001; Teri et al., 1999).

Depressive symptoms in clinical and population-based studies have been reported to occur in 30–70% of individuals diagnosed with dementia (Lyketsos et al., 2002; Lyketsos et al., 2001; Teri, Baer, & Reifler, 1991; Weiner, Edland, & Luszczynska, 1994). Unhappiness, withdrawal, inactivity, fatigue, expressions of guilt and worthlessness, tearfulness, and loss of interest are all symptoms of depression and contribute to excess disability, compounding the distress of both the person with dementia and the caregiver (Brodaty & Luscombe, 1998; Fitz & Teri, 1994; Teri et al., 1992).

Studies of community-residing individuals with dementia, using a variety of well-established scales, have found that as many as 71% of subjects had anxiety symptoms, including irritability, agitation, day/night disturbance, and motor restlessness (Eustace et al., 2002; Lyketsos et al., 2002; Mega, Cummings, Fiorello, et al., 1996; Reisberg et al., 1987). The rates of anxiety symptoms among both hospitalized and community-dwelling patients with AD are higher than in healthy elderly peers (Mega et al., 1996; Orrell & Bebbington, 1996).

Comorbidity of depression and anxiety is common in older adults, with 30–60% of older adults who are diagnosed with clinically significant anxiety or depression meeting DSM-IV (American Psychiatric Association, 1994) criteria for both disorders (Schneider, 1996). This relationship also holds for individuals with dementia (Teri, Ferretti, et al., 1999). Anxiety in dementia is associated with increased behavioral disturbances, and comorbid anxiety and depression are associated with greater functional impairment (Ferretti, McCurry, Logsdon, Gibbons, & Teri, 2001; Teri, Ferritti, et al., 1999).

Sleep and nighttime behavioral disturbances are also common among persons with dementia and are associated with both depression and anxiety. Among outpatients with dementia, prevalence rates of 11–51% for sleep disturbances have been reported (Carpenter, Strauss, & Patterson, 1995; Eustace et al., 2002; Ferretti et al., 2001; Lyketsos et al., 2002; Zubenko et al., 2003). The co-occurrence of sleep complaints in nondemented adults who have depressive or anxiety disorders is well known (Foley, Monjan, Izmirlian, Hays, & Blazer, 1999; Ohayon, Cauclet, & Lemoine, 1998), and there is evidence that these conditions also impact the sleep quality of affected demented individuals (McCurry, Gibbons, Logsdon, & Teri, 2003a; Zubenko et al., 2003).

ASSESSMENT OF AFFECT: IDENTIFYING PROBLEMS

The most common method for assessing affective disturbance in cognitively impaired older adults is a detailed clinical interview with the patient and an informant familiar with the patient's day-to-day functioning, such as a family member or caregiver. It is essential to interview an informant because patients who have memory loss often have difficulty accurately describing the frequency and severity of their own symptoms. It is usually helpful to interview the patient and informant together initially to obtain an overview of the patient's history and to observe the interaction between the two of them. Whenever possible, it is also advisable to interview them individually, to give each an opportunity to discuss problems or concerns privately. Often family members are hesitant to bring up topics that may be "sensitive" in front of the affected person, and the person with dementia may have important information to provide privately about his or her concerns or relationship with the caregiver. In the interview, the patient and informant are generally asked about the occurrence, frequency, and severity of typical problems, including depression, tearfulness, sleep disturbance, loss of interest in activities, verbal expressions of hopelessness, sighing, complaining, etc. To assure that the full spectrum of problems is assessed in an efficient and thorough manner, a standardized inquiry list is recommended as a valuable tool. By asking about the presence or absence of a variety of potential problems, the clinician can focus on the ones that are of greatest concern. This type of assessment provides an objective method for evaluating outcomes of any interventions that are attempted.

A variety of mood and behavior assessment measures with good psychometric properties have been developed. Table 16.1 shows a representative sampling of instruments that has been used to measure affective disturbances in clinical controlled trials with dementia subjects. Some measures are paper-and-pencil informant report; others require

TABLE 16.1. Common Affective Assessment Instruments for Dementia

	Informant report questionnaire	Interviewer administered	Reliability/validity data	Used in clinical controlled trials
Cornell Scale for Depression in Dementia (CSDD; Alexopoulos et al., 1988)		×	Mack & Patterson, 1994; Perrault et al., 2000	Lyketsos, Lindell Veiel, Baker, & Steele, 1999; Teri et al., 1997
Dementia Mood Assessment Scale (DMAS; Sunderland, Hill, Lawlor, & Molchan, 1988)	×		Onega & Abraham, 1997; Perrault et al., 2000	Lawlor, Aisen, Green, Fine, & Schmeidler, 1997
Geriatric Depression Scale (GDS; Yesavage et al., 1983)	×		Logsdon & Teri, 1995	Teri et al., 1997
Hamilton Depression Rating Scale (HDRS; Hamilton, 1960)		×	Logsdon & Teri, 1995	Teri et al., 1997; Teri, McCurry, et al., 1998
Neuropsychiatric Inventory (NPI; Cummings et al., 1994)		×	Perrault et al., 2000	Olin & Schneider, 2001; Teri et al., 2002
Revised Memory and Behavior Problem Checklist (RMBPC; Teri et al., 1992)	×		Weiner et al., 2000	Teri et al., 1997; Teri, Logsdon, et al., 1998
Epworth Sleepiness Scale (ESS; Johns, 1991)	×		Johns, 1991; Johns, 2000; Osman, Osborne, Hill, & Lee, 1999	Lind et al., 2003; Massie & Hart, 2003
Time-Based Behavioral Disturbance Questionnaire (Bliwise, Yesavage, & Tinklengerg, 1992)	×		Friedman et al., 1997	

structured interviews with trained clinicians or direct behavioral observation. Some (e.g., the Cornell Scale for Depression in Dementia; Alexopoulos, Abrams, Young, & Shamoian, 1988) provide information on the severity of symptoms; others (e.g., the Revised Memory and Behavior Problems Checklist [RMBPC]; Teri et al., 1992) rate behaviors on the frequency of their occurrence and provide information on caregiver distress about specific behaviors when they do occur. For some measures (e.g., the Neuropsychiatric Inventory; Cummings et al., 1994), subscale information is computed from a combination of frequency and severity ratings for individual behavioral symptoms. A number of self-report instruments also have been shown to be valid when completed by surrogate informants such as dementia caregivers (Logsdon & Teri, 1995).

As can be seen from Table 16.1, no single instrument has been adopted for universal use with patients who have dementia. In selecting an appropriate strategy for behavioral assessment, clinicians and researchers should consider the length of the measure, its reported sensitivity to change, and specific behaviors of concern for their clinical population. Providers caring for populations that include non-English-speaking individuals from multicultural backgrounds or persons with limited education or reading skills particularly need to evaluate the validity of a given instrument for their patients. A number of excellent comprehensive reviews of behavioral screening instruments used in dementia care and research is available for those who require additional information (Katz, 1998; Kluger & Ferris, 1991; Perrault, Oremus, Demers, Vida, & Wolfson, 2000; Sky & Grossberg, 1994; Snowden et al., 2003; Teri & Logsdon, 1995; Weiner et al., 1996).

Once specific problems are identified, a thorough assessment of possible causes is essential. Common causes of affective disturbance in dementia include medical illness or medication side effects, loss of pleasant activities due to cognitive and functional decline, environmental changes, or interpersonal conflicts. For example, anxiety or restlessness may be triggered by an acute medical condition, such as a urinary tract infection, or by a change in medication. Restlessness may also result from changes in brain functioning secondary to the dementing process, or it may be related to environmental triggers, such as lack of appropriate activity, too much noise or stimulation, or conflicts with people with whom the patient comes into contact. Thus assessing affective disorders often involves behavioral observation to obtain a baseline profile and identify the antecedents and consequences of problem behaviors. In turn, this assessment leads directly to the development of behavioral treatment programs.

RATIONALE AND THEORETICAL BASIS FOR BEHAVIORAL TREATMENT OF AFFECTIVE DISTURBANCES IN DEMENTIA

Although antidepressants have been widely used in treating depression in dementia, reports of their effectiveness have been mixed, and many older adults experience side effects or interactions with other medications (Lyketsos & Olin, 2002; Raskind, 1993). Furthermore, as noted, cognitive and environmental factors (e.g., lack of pleasant events) or interpersonal factors (e.g., conflicts with caregivers) are frequently the primary triggers of depressive or anxious behaviors, and lack of activity or poor sleep hygiene practices often lead to sleep disturbances. Caregiver education, support, and training in behavioral strategies for management can be quite effective in alleviating or preventing affective disturbances. Consequently, nonpharmacological treatments are often the most appropriate initial strategy for dealing with these disturbances (Rabins, 1994; Teri, 1986; Teri, Logsdon, & McCurry, 2002).

Behavioral theory postulates a cycle of affective disturbance that is applicable to individuals with dementia. As formulated by Lewinsohn and colleagues with nondemented older adults, decreased positive person–environment interactions and increased aversive interactions trigger depressed or anxious behaviors (Lewinsohn, Antonuccio, Steinmetz, & Teri, 1984; Lewinsohn, Sullivan, & Grosscup, 1980). The depressed person is often withdrawn and apathetic, showing little interest in activities he or she once enjoyed; the less active he or she is, the more depressed he or she becomes; the more depressed, the less active, and so on. Likewise, lack of activity may lead to restlessness or anxiety, which in turn may lead to agitation or other behavioral disturbances that further limit the availability of opportunities to engage with other people or activities. This same cycle can be seen in individuals with dementia and depression (Teri, 1986, 1994). Due to cognitive impairment, these individuals lose the ability to do many of the activities they once enjoyed. They can no longer function as independently as they once did, and they must rely on others to initiate and maintain activities. The fewer pleasant events they experience, the more depressed or anxious they feel; the more depressed or anxious they become, the less they do, and so on. Furthermore, family members or caregivers may perceive the affected individual as increasingly difficult and therefore be less likely to engage in pleasant social interactions with him or her.

Behavioral treatment of affective disturbance in dementia disrupts this cycle by altering the contingencies that initiated and maintain the depressive or anxious behavior (i.e., antecedents and consequences; Teri, 1986; Teri et al., 2002) in two salient ways: (1) by identifying and reinforcing incompatible nondepressive behaviors (i.e., pleasant events; Logsdon & Teri, 1997; Teri & Logsdon, 1991); and (2) by changing the caregiver–care recipient interaction that is the context in which the nonadaptive contingencies are maintained (Logsdon, McCurry, Moore, & Teri, 1997). The frequency and severity of affective disturbances are thus decreased.

Emotional and cognitive symptoms of depression are not ignored under this conceptualization. They are simply viewed as other forms of behavior that respond to behavioral principles and therefore are equally modifiable. This is not to imply that individuals with dementia will "learn" new skills, but rather that their behavior responds to reinforcement, and modifying the contingencies of a given behavior will alter that behavior. Although individuals with dementia have difficulty learning and may not "remember" the reinforcements, they still respond to them.

OVERVIEW OF NONPHARMACOLOGICAL
TREATMENT STRATEGIES IN DEMENTIA CARE

Providing education, support, and advice to help families better understand and cope with dementia has a long clinical history. Practitioners often advise families to adapt the environment and modify their own behaviors in order to provide better care for patients. The amount and popularity of this kind of information have grown exponentially in recent years, as evidenced by the proliferation of books, training materials, informational handouts, videos and websites. For example, *The 36-Hour Day* (Mace & Rabins, 1991), long considered a staple of information to families, is in its second printing with over one-half million copies sold worldwide. The Alzheimer's Association, another popular resource, provides extensive information for health care providers, families, and affected individuals on its website (www.alz.org).

Published reports of behavioral treatment of dementia span two decades. Early case studies demonstrated that caregivers were able to learn specific techniques and successfully reduce problematic behaviors (Aronson, Levin, & Lipkowitz, 1984; Haley, 1983; Pinkston & Linsk, 1984; Zarit, Anthony, & Boutselis, 1987). Later, case-controlled and randomized controlled trials investigated the effectiveness of behavioral treatment in reducing agitation and depression or delaying institutionalization in patients with dementia. Three investigations included behavior training as part of a larger psychoeducational and social support program that examined general behavioral outcomes and delayed patient institutionalization (Carlson et al., 1995; Mittelman et al., 1996; Mohide et al., 1990). One study provided focused behavioral training to reduce patient depression (Teri, Logsdon, Uomoto, & McCurry, 1997), and another compared nonpharmacological to pharmacological approaches to reduce patient agitation (Teri et al., 2000; Teri, Logsdon, et al., 1998). Although certainly not conclusive, results thus far suggest that nonpharmacological interventions can significantly reduce general patient behavioral problems (Mohide et al., 1990; Teri, Logsdon, et al., 1998), decrease patient depression (Teri et al., 1997), delay institutionalization (Mittelman et al., 1996), and increase caregiver satisfaction (Mittelman et al., 1993). (For more detailed reviews of nonpharmacological treatments, see Bourgeois, Schulz, & Burgio, 1996; Teri, Logsdon, et al., 1999.)

GENERAL GUIDELINES FOR BEHAVIORAL INTERVENTION IN DEMENTIA

Since patients with progressive dementia are significantly limited in their ability to learn new material, behavioral treatment focuses on teaching caregivers strategies to use in working with the patient on a daily basis. Caregivers may include family members, unpaid caregivers, and paid caregivers who have a role in the patient's day-to-day care. In planning management strategies it is important to have a good understanding of the resources of both the patient and the caregiver. In particular, the degree of the patient's cognitive impairment impacts his or her ability to perform particular behaviors, and the degree of stress the caregiver is experiencing will impact his or her ability to carry out recommended changes. The past and present relationship between patient and caregiver will also influence the occurrence and treatment of depressive behaviors. Programs must be tailored to the individual in order to be most effective. Flexibility and creativity are needed to find solutions to problems, and because dementia typically progresses over time, it is necessary to repeatedly modify and adapt solutions to the patient's current problems. Finally, it is important to respect the dignity of both the patient and the caregiver when developing behavioral management strategies, and to encourage each of them to participate as much as possible in the treatment.

SPECIFIC INTERVENTIONS FOR AFFECTIVE DISTURBANCES IN DEMENTIA

We have developed systematized behavioral interventions to train caregivers to reduce depression (Teri et al., 1997), agitation (Teri et al., 2000; Teri, Logsdon, et al., 1998) and sleep disturbances (McCurry, Gibbons, Logsdon, Vitiello, & Teri, 2005; McCurry,

Logsdon, Vitiello, & Teri, 1998; McCurry, Reynolds, Ancoli-Israel, Teri, & Vitiello, 2000) in patients with dementia. As described above, affective disturbances are viewed as a series of observable and modifiable behaviors that are initiated and maintained by person–environment interactions. Caregivers are taught to alter these interactions in a way that results in decreased problem behaviors. Treatment is systematic but individualized, focusing on the current observable interactions of direct relevance to the problem under consideration.

A video training program, "Managing and Understanding Behavior Problems in Alzheimer's Disease and Related Disorders" (Teri, 1990), teaches caregivers to use a behavior management approach with individuals with dementia. This series of videotapes uses didactic information along with vignettes of specific problems and solutions to guide caregivers through a systematic process called the "A-B-C's of Behavior Change." In this approach, caregivers learn that "A" is the antecedent or triggering event that precedes the problem behavior, "B" is the behavior of concern, and "C" is the consequence of that behavior. Caregivers are thus introduced to the importance of behavioral observation and are taught problem-solving strategies. This video series has been successfully used with both family members and professional caregivers as an adjunct to one-on-one and group training in behavior therapy.

Once the caregiver understands and can identify the A-B-C's of a problem, a step-by-step problem-solving strategy is implemented. The following six steps can be applied to a variety of problems, including affective disturbances such as social withdrawal, tearfulness, restlessness, aggression, anxiety, and sleep disturbances.

1. Identify the problem. A clear definition of the problem behavior is the first step in changing it. This is the "B" of the A-B-C's. The more clearly a caregiver can define a problem, the more likely he or she will be able to carry out an effective course of action. It is best to begin with one specific problem that occurs frequently and is easily observable.

2. Gather information about the problem. Once the problem is identified and can be observed, gather as much information as possible about it: When does it happen? How often? Where does it happen most? Caregivers may be able to recall the last few weeks and provide some information about the problem, but it is also often helpful to have them keep notes, or a "diary," about the behavior for a few days.

3. Identify what happens before and after the problem. While observing the person with dementia, the caregiver should carefully note what happens immediately before the problem occurs and what happens immediately after the problem begins. These are the "A" (antecedents) and "C" (consequences) of the A-B-C's. Many problems will have more than one antecedent and consequence, and the more the therapist and the caregiver understand how they fit together, the more likely they will be able to intervene successfully.

4. Set realistic goals and make plans. For a plan to work it must be creative but realistic and tailored to the individual patient and caregiver. Involve the patient as much as possible, and work closely with the caregiver to establish the goals. Start with a small, achievable goal and proceed step by step. Be practical and allow plenty of time for change to occur. Do not expect major changes overnight. Work with the caregiver to anticipate problems that may occur and discuss how they may be solved.

5. Acknowledge and reinforce any effort on the part of both the patient and caregiver to make changes. Changing behavior is hard work for everyone involved. It is very

important for caregivers to feel good about their accomplishments, no matter how small. The patient with AD will also benefit from being praised for doing a good job.

6. Repeatedly evaluate and modify plans. It is important that caregivers be consistent yet flexible in carrying out plans. Strategies will change as they discover what does and does not work. Decide how to determine whether the plan is working—by monitoring the amount of time the behavior occurs, the number of instances of the behavior, or whatever makes the most sense.

Depression

Many of the behavioral triggers of depressive behaviors in dementia are associated with inappropriate activities or with too little activity. Identifying activities that the person with dementia finds enjoyable and providing opportunities for him or her to engage in them successfully on a daily basis, may be effective alternatives to medication. This approach appeals to many caregivers because it provides opportunities for positive interactions and social contact and contributes to a more pleasant environment for both the person with dementia and the caregiver. However, identifying pleasant activities that are appropriate to the person's level of functioning can be difficult, particularly for caregivers who are already taxed by routine daily responsibilities. The challenge is also an ongoing process because as dementia progresses, activities must be modified to fit the changing needs and abilities of the individual. Behavior therapy with the caregiver and person with dementia can facilitate this process.

In a controlled clinical investigation of behavioral treatment for depression in patients with AD, Teri et al. (1997) compared two active behavioral interventions, one emphasizing patient pleasant events (BT-PE) and one emphasizing caregiver problem solving (BR-PS), to an equal-duration-typical-care control condition (TC) and a wait-list control (WL). Seventy-two patient–caregiver dyads were randomly assigned to one of the four conditions and assessed pre-, post-, and at 6-month follow-up. A significant overall treatment effect was obtained for patient depression, $F(3,71) = 4.52$, $p < .001$. Post hoc analysis indicated that subjects in the two active treatment conditions (BT-PE and BT-PS) did not differ significantly from one another, but that each active treatment resulted in significant improvement, as compared to the two control conditions.

In this investigation no significant changes were hypothesized for caregivers, because the focus of intervention was the patients. Unexpectedly, an overall treatment effect *was* found for caregiver depression on the Hamilton Depression Rating Scale (HDRS), $F(3,66) = 4.73$, $p < .01$. Post hoc analysis revealed that BT-PE and BT-PS caregivers did not significantly differ from one another, but that caregivers in either of the active conditions improved significantly more than caregivers in the control conditions.

The clinical significance of change in test scores was also examined by evaluating change in depression diagnosis. Twenty-five subjects (60%) in the active treatment conditions showed clinically significant improvement, whereas only six subjects (20%) in the TC or WL conditions showed improvement. Twenty-one subjects in the control conditions (70%) showed no change in diagnosis, and three (10%) worsened. No subject in active treatment worsened, $\chi^2(6, n = 72) = 18.48$, $p < .005$.

Six month follow-up data on subjects in the active treatment conditions (BT-PE and BT-PS) indicated that both patients and caregivers maintained significant improvement over pretest scores (patient HDRS: $F(60,2) = 31.47$, $p < .001$; caregiver HDRS: $F(60,2) = 4.28$, $p < .05$). The clinical significance of these change scores was evaluated by examining depression diagnosis at 6-month follow-up as compared to posttreatment. Twenty-two (69%) subjects maintained their improvement or improved further, whereas 10 (31%) relapsed during the 6-month follow-up period.

Methods to modify antecedents and alter consequences to depressive behaviors include the following:

- Increase and encourage enjoyable activities by identifying activities that the person has enjoyed in the past and modifying them to be appropriate for the patient's current level of functioning. The Pleasant Events Schedule—AD (Logsdon & Teri, 1997; Teri & Logsdon, 1991), a 53-item inventory, was designed to help caregivers identify simple, everyday pleasant activities that might be incorporated into the daily care of patients with dementia. Items include being outside, listening to music, having meals with family or friends, helping around the house, exercising, and going for a ride in the car.

- Use redirection and distraction to help depressed patients stay focused on positive experiences and pleasant memories. Memory books (Bourgeois, 1992) with pictures of happier times, reminiscing of pleasant experiences, or having cheerful conversations can be quite helpful.

- Initiate pleasant social activities that keep the patient alert and involved, such as outings with someone whose company the patient enjoys, particularly if the patient complains of feeling isolated or lonely. If the patient has had to stop driving, arrange transportation to activities the patient enjoys but is no longer able to attend without assistance.

- Eliminate sources of conflict and frustration by helping caregivers recognize and modify activities the patient can no longer perform successfully. By ensuring that patients are not continually challenged and frustrated, sources of conflict and frustration can be alleviated (and sometimes eliminated), fostering a more contented patient.

- If the patient lives with a caregiver, evaluate and discuss the caregiver's own affective state. Depressed patients often have depressed caregivers (Teri & Truax, 1994), and improving caregiver mood is likely to have a positive outcome on the patient's behavioral problems.

Anxiety

Symptoms of anxiety, such as worrying, tension, somatic symptoms, fearfulness, excessive concern about health, anger, irritability, and psychomotor agitation affect between 70 and 90% of patients with dementia at some point during the course of the disease (Devanand et al., 1997; Lyketsos et al., 2002; Mega et al., 1996). As with depression, anxiety may have a variety of causes, including physiological, environmental, and interpersonal triggers. Furthermore, these causes often interact. For example, patients may have decreased tolerance for stimulation, fearfulness caused by environmental changes, or decreased inhibition of inappropriate behaviors due to neurological changes. They may experience anxious or catastrophic reactions in response to environmental triggers such as overstimulation or activities they do not understand (e.g., being bathed by a caregiver they do not know or remember). The key to nonpharmacological intervention for episodes of anxiety is to identify and avoid their triggers, thus reducing their frequency and impact.

Research on behavioral interventions that specifically target anxiety (as distinguished from agitation or other more severe behavioral disturbances) in patients with dementia is virtually nonexistent. In a post hoc analysis of data from the depression treatment study described previously (Teri et al., 1997), anxiety was measured using seven items from the Schedule for Affective Disorders and Schizophrenia (worrying, somatic anxiety, psychic anxiety, excessive concern about health, anger, irritability, and psychomotor agitation). Fifty percent of subjects experienced at least mild levels of anxiety, and 30% experienced moderate levels of these symptoms. Although the depression intervention did not specifically target anxiety, a significant overall treatment effect on reduction of anxiety was found, $F(1,68) = 17.84$, $p < .000$. Factors predictive of improvement on anxiety symptoms included behavioral depression treatment ($AR^2 = .18$), lower level caregiver of burden ($AR^2 = .03$), and lower patient Mini-Mental State Examination (MMSE) score ($AR^2 = .08$). Thus it appears that for many patients with AD, it is important to address both depression and anxiety in evaluating and treating psychological distress; behavioral treatment may successfully reduce symptoms of both.

Specific methods for modifying antecedents and altering consequences to anxious behaviors include the following:

- Identify triggers and intervene early to prevent anxiety and catastrophic reactions.
- Work with caregivers to develop new communication skills; for example, using a reassuring and gentle voice to help calm the patient. Approach an anxious patient slowly, from the front, and tell him or her what you are going to do, to avoid startling him or her.
- Distract the patient with questions about the problem and gradually turn his or her attention to something unrelated and pleasant. Change activities, go to another room, or temporarily leave the situation.
- Use touch judiciously and gently. Sometimes a touch can be reassuring or comforting to an anxious person. Other times, a touch will be unwelcome and may trigger an aggressive response.
- Use nonthreatening postures when dealing with an anxious patient. Stand or sit at eye level, rather than standing over the person.
- Establish a calm, quiet environment with soft lighting and music.
- Avoid arguing or trying to reason with the person to allay anxiety. Arguing almost always causes anxious behaviors to escalate.
- Avoid physical restraint. Restraints can increase the patient's perception of threat and cause anxiety to escalate into agitation or aggression.

Sleep Disturbances

Wandering at night, bedtime agitation, disturbed sleep, and night–day reversal are common problems for persons with dementia (McCurry et al., 1999). Patients with AD are more likely to awaken during the night, nap during the day, and in some cases develop complete day–night sleep pattern reversals (Prinz, Poceta, & McCurry, 2002). Sleep problems in patients with dementia can be caused by physical conditions such as incontinence and chronic pain; they are also highly correlated with anxiety and depression (McCurry, Gibbons, Logsdon, Vitiello, & Teri, 2003b; Vitiello & Borson, 2001). Whatever the cause, sleep disturbances are very stressful for family members (McCurry et al., 1999). Caregivers who are awakened frequently during the night to reassure or assist the patient eventually become exhausted. This exhaustion, and its associated impact on physical and emotional health, is one of the most common reasons caregivers are forced to institutionalize their loved ones (Hope, Keene, Gedling, Fairburn, & Jacoby, 1998; Pollak & Perlick, 1991).

Like depression and anxiety symptoms, sleep disturbances in dementia can have environmental and behavioral activators that lend themselves well to behavior therapy. For example, Alessi and colleagues (Alessi, Yoon, Schnelle, Al-Samarrai, & Cruise, 1999) found that a combination of light physical exercise and other behavioral strategies (e.g., keeping patients out of bed in the late afternoon and evening or providing quiet nighttime incontinence care) produced significant improvements in actigraphic measures of percent of total sleep and duration of sleep episodes in nursing home residents. There is also a growing literature suggesting that timed bright light exposure may be helpful in reducing the sleep disturbances found in institutionalized patients with AD (Ancoli-Israel et al., 2003; Ancoli-Israel, Martin, Kripke, Marler, & Klauber, 2002; McCurry et al., 2000; van Someren, Kessler, Mirmiran, & Swaab, 1997).

Two studies conducted in community settings support the efficacy of teaching family caregivers of patients with dementia to use behavioral interventions for sleep disturbances. In the first, subjective caregiver sleep self-reports were improved with a 4- to 6-week program that provided education about good sleep habits, training in management of patient nighttime disruptive behaviors, and caregiver support (McCurry et al., 1998). More recently, a randomized controlled clinical trial, called NITE-AD (*Nighttime Insomnia Treatment and Education for Alzheimer's Disease*), examined whether caregivers could carry out a behavioral intervention using structured activity and increased daytime light exposure to reestablish normal sleep patterns in community-dwelling persons with dementia (McCurry et al., 2005). Subjects were 36 patients with AD (mean age = 77.7 years; mean AD duration = 5.8 years; 56% male) and their family caregivers, who were randomly assigned into either an active treatment or a contact control condition. Mean patient MMSE score was 11.8. Caregivers (mean age = 63.6 years; 72% female; 58% spouses) reported all patients had at least two sleep problems, occurring three or more times per week (mean = 4.1; range 2–8 problems).

All participants received six 1-hour in-home treatment sessions over a 2-month period, which included written information about standard principles of good sleep hygiene, sleep changes associated with normal aging, and general strategies for improving the sleep of persons with dementia. Caregivers in active treatment were also guided to develop a sleep hygiene program for the patient, with a particular emphasis on establishing a consistent bed and rising time, reducing daytime napping, and walking 30 minutes per day. Active treatment patients were further instructed to sit for an hour a day in front of a light box at an exposure level of 2,500 lux during a 3-hour window before each patient's habitual bedtime.

Longitudinal analyses were conducted at 3 and 6 months. Patients in active treatment were found to have significantly fewer total nighttime awakenings ($p < .05$), fewer awakenings per hour ($p < .05$), and spent less time awake at night ($p < .05$) than control subjects. Forty-four percent of NITE-AD subjects who entered treatment with average nighttime wakefulness greater than 1 hour were awake less than 1 hour at posttest, compared to 14% of controls, representing a treatment effect size of 0.65 for the primary outcome in the proposed study. Patient depression on the RMBPC was also significantly lower ($p = .01$) at 6 months, compared to control subjects. Of the six patients (17%) who were institutionalized during the study period, all were either control subjects ($n = 4$) or treatment subjects who dropped out immediately after baseline testing ($n = 2$) before receiving any active treatment, indicating that behavioral treatment may have a positive impact on caregivers' ability to keep patients at home for longer periods of time. These results support the use of nonpharmacological interventions for sleep problems in community-dwelling patients with AD (McCurry et al., 2005).

Specific suggestions for modifying antecedents and altering consequences associated with sleep disturbances in persons with dementia include the following:

- Strive for consistent bedtime and rising times. Regular sleep time habits and routines help reinforce time cues for individuals with dementia, and may also promote circadian rhythmicity by maximizing cues to the brain's time-keeping system. Although there have been no clinical trials demonstrating the value of consistent sleep habits in patients with dementia, sleep regularity and prevention of sleep disturbances in all older adults are considered important aspects of the treatment (Taylor, Friedman, Sheikh, & Yesavage, 1997).

- Limit daytime napping. In the later stages of disease, many persons with dementia spend a significant proportion of their daytime hours asleep (Ancoli-Israel, Klauber, Gillin, Campbell, & Hofstetter, 1994; Dowling & Wiener, 1997). Reduced daytime napping, particularly when combined with increased physical activity, can increase the likelihood that the patient will have longer, more consolidated nighttime sleep.

- Restrict use of alcohol and caffeinated beverages (including chocolate products). When consumed close to bedtime, these can disrupt sleep and exacerbate the preexisting tendency of patients to awaken more often and spend less time in deep (slow-wave) sleep. However, a light bedtime snack on foods that promote sleep, such as milk, bananas, or cheese, may reduce patient awakenings that are caused by nighttime hunger.

- Avoid excessive evening fluid intake and assure emptying of the bladder before patient retires for the night. For patients with nocturia, scheduled nighttime bathroom trips can be helpful.

- Eliminate or reduce environmental nuisance factors that may interrupt sleep. Reductions in light levels and nighttime noise have been shown to be critical for the alleviation of sleep disturbances for nursing home residents (Alessi & Schnelle, 2000). In community home settings, potential environmental causes of disturbed patient sleep that should also be evaluated include the impact of household pets, live-in adult children or grandchildren, caregiver snoring, and outside traffic noise.

- Be aware that changes in daily routine, such as family get-togethers or holidays, may produce a worsening in nighttime sleep. Try to plan ahead and build in some quiet "catch up" time following any out-of-the-ordinary planned activity.

SUMMARY

In summary, patients with AD and their caregivers are confronted with a variety of affective disturbances that may have a devastating impact on all involved. It is important for clinicians to assess the occurrence and impact of these behaviors, in order to best care for their patients with AD. Measurement tools can augment the clinical interview to help the practitioner obtain a thorough assessment of behavioral problems and provide a means of evaluating the success of interventions. Once they are identified, affective problems are often responsive to a coordinated behavioral treatment plan that teaches caregivers to analyze the antecedents and consequences of behavioral problems and to develop effective strategies for amelioration. The studies described in this chapter represent a behavioral treatment approach used in clinical practice and research with community-residing patients and caregivers. Existing research is promising, and similar interventions have been used in institutional care settings. Further, these interventions offer an alternative to pharmacological interventions and are often just as effective as medications, with fewer side effects. However, we have only just begun to understand and successfully apply behavioral treatment to patients with dementia and their caregivers. Additional controlled clinical research is needed to clarify how to best use these approaches and how to maximize their effectiveness and clinical significance with this population.

ACKNOWLEDGMENT

Preparation of this chapter was supported in part by grants from the National Institutes of Health (Nos. AG10483, AG10845, and MH01644).

REFERENCES

Alessi, C. A., & Schnelle, J. F. (2000). Approach to sleep disorders in nursing home setting. *Sleep Medicine Reviews*, 4(1), 45–56.

Alessi, C. A., Yoon, E. J., Schnelle, J. F., Al-Samarrai, N. R., & Cruise, P. A. (1999). A randomized trial of a combined physical activity and environmental intervention in nursing home residents: Do sleep and agitation improve? *Journal of the American Geriatrics Society*, 47(7), 784–791.

Alexopoulos, G. S., Abrams, R. C., Young, R. C., & Shamoian, C. A. (1988). Cornell Scale for Depression in Dementia. *Biological Psychiatry*, 23, 271–284.

Allen-Burge, R., Stevens, A. B., & Burgio, L. D. (1999). Effective behavioral interventions for decreasing dementia-related challenging behavior in nursing homes. *International Journal of Geriatric Psychiatry*, 14, 213–232.

American Psychiatric Association. (1994). *Diagnostic and statistical manual of mental disorders* (4th ed.). Washington, DC: Author.

Ancoli-Israel, S., Gehrman, P. R., Martin, J. L., Shochat, T., Marler, M., Corey-BLoom, J., et al. (2003). Increased light exposure consolidates sleep and strengthens circadian rhythms in severe Alzheimer's disease patients. *Behavioral Sleep Medicine*, 1, 22–36.

Ancoli-Israel, S., Klauber, M. R., Gillin, J. C., Campbell, S. S., & Hofstetter, C. R. (1994). Sleep in non-institutionalized Alzheimer's disease patients. *Aging, Clinical and Experimental Research*, 6, 451–458.

Ancoli-Israel, S., Martin, J. L., Kripke, D. F., Marler, M., & Klauber, M. R. (2002). Effect of light treatment on sleep and circadian rhythms in demented nursing home patients. *Journal of the American Geriatrics Society*, 50(2), 282–289.

Aronson, M. K., Levin, G., & Lipkowitz, R. (1984). A community based family/patient group program for Alzheimer's disease. *Gerontologist*, 24, 339–342.

Bliwise, D. L., Yesavage, J. A., & Tinklengerg, J. R. (1992). Sundowning and rate of decline in mental function in Alzheimer's disease. *Dementia*, 3, 335–341.

Bourgeois, M. S. (1992). Evaluating memory wallets in conversations with persons with dementia. *Journal of Speech and Hearing Research*, 35, 1344–1357.

Bourgeois, M. S., Schulz, R., & Burgio, L. (1996). Interventions for caregivers of patients with Alzheimer's disease: A review and analysis of content, process, and outcomes. *International Journal of Aging and Human Development*, 43(1), 35–92.

Brodaty, H., & Luscombe, G. (1998). Psychological morbidity in caregivers is associated with depression in patients with dementia. *Alzheimer's Disease and Associated Disorders*, 12(2), 62–70.

Burns, A. (1996). The Institute of Psychiatry Alzheimer's disease cohort 1986–1992: Part I. Clinical observations. *International Journal of Geriatric Psychiatry, 11*, 309–320.

Camp, C. J., Cohen-Mansfield, J., & Capezuti, E. A. (2002). Use of nonpharmacologic interventions among nursing home residents with dementia. *Psychiatric Services, 53*(11), 1397–1401.

Carlson, D. L., Fleming, K. C., Smith, G. E., & Evans, J. M. (1995). Management of dementia-related behavioral disturbances: A nonpharmacological approach. *Mayo Clinic Proceedings, 70*, 1108–1115.

Carpenter, B. D., Strauss, M. E., & Patterson, M. B. (1995). Sleep disturbances in community-dwelling patients with Alzheimer's disease. *Clinical Gerontologist, 16*(2), 35–49.

Cummings, J. L., & Kaufer, D. (1996). Neuropsychiatric aspects of Alzheimer's disease: The cholinergic hypothesis revisited. *Neurology, 47*, 876–883.

Cummings, J. L., Mega, M., Gray, K., Rosenberg-Thompson, S., Carusi, D. A., & Gornbein, J. (1994). The Neuropsychiatric Inventory: Comprehensive assessment of psychopathology in dementia. *Neurology, 44*(12), 2308–2314.

Devanand, D. P., Jacobs, D. M., Tang, M.-X., Del Castillo-Castaneda, C., Sano, M., Marder, K., et al. (1997). The course of psychopathologic features in mild to moderate Alzheimer's disease. *Archives of General Psychiatry, 54*(3), 257–263.

Dowling, G. A., & Wiener, C. L. (1997). Roadblocks encountered in recruiting patients for a study of sleep disruption in Alzheimer's disease. *Image: Journal of Nursing Scholarship, 29*(1), 59–64.

Eustace, A., Coen, R., Walsh, C., Cunningham, C. J., Walsh, J. B., Coakley, D., et al. (2002). A longitudinal evaluation of behavioural and psychological symptoms of probable Alzheimer's disease. *International Journal of Geriatric Psychiatry, 17*, 968–973.

Ferretti, L., McCurry, S. M., Logsdon, R., Gibbons, L., & Teri, L. (2001). Anxiety and Alzheimer's disease. *Journal of Geriatric Psychiatry and Neurology, 14*(1), 52–58.

Fitz, A. G., & Teri, L. (1994). Depression, cognition, and functional ability in patients with Alzheimer's disease. *Journal of the American Geriatrics Society, 42*, 186–191.

Foley, D. J., Monjan, A. A., Izmirlian, G., Hays, J. C., & Blazer, D. G. (1999). Incidence and remission of insomnia among elderly adults in a biracial cohort. *Sleep, 22*(Suppl. 2), S373–S378.

Friedman, L., Kraemer, H. C., Zarcone, V., Sage, S., Wicks, D., Bliwise, D. L., et al. (1997). Disruptive behavior and actigraphic measures in home-dwelling patients with Alzheimer's disease: Preliminary report. *Journal of Geriatric Psychiatry and Neurology, 10*(2), 58–62.

Haley, W. E. (1983). A family-behavioral approach to the treatment of the cognitively impaired elderly. *Gerontologist, 23*(1), 18–20.

Hamilton, M. (1960). A rating scale for depression. *Journal of Neurology and Neurosurgical Psychiatry, 23*, 56–62.

Hope, T., Keene, J., Gedling, K., Fairburn, C. G., & Jacoby, R. (1998). Predictors of institutionalization for people with dementia living at home with a carer. *International Journal of Geriatric Psychiatry, 13*(10), 682–690.

Johns, M. W. (1991). A new method for measuring daytime sleepiness: The Epworth Sleepiness Scale. *Sleep, 14*(6), 540–545.

Johns, M. W. (2000). Sensitivity and specificity of the multiple sleep latency test (MSLT), the maintenance of wakefulness test and the Epworth Sleepiness Scale: Failure of the MSLT as a gold standard. *Journal of Sleep Research, 9*(1), 5–11.

Katz, I. R. (1998). Diagnosis and treatment of depression in patients with Alzheimer's disease and other dementias. *Journal of Clinical Psychiatry, 59*(Suppl. 9), 38–44.

Kluger, A., & Ferris, S. H. (1991). Scales for the assessment of Alzheimer's disease. *Psychiatric Clinics of North America, 14*, 309–326.

Lawlor, B. A., Aisen, P. S., Green, C., Fine, E., & Schmeidler, J. (1997). Selegiline in the treatment of behavioural disturbance in Alzheimer's disease. *International Journal of Geriatric Psychiatry, 12*(3), 319–322.

Lewinsohn, P. M., Antonuccio, D. O., Steinmetz, J., & Teri, L. (1984). *The coping with depression course.* Eugene, OR: Castalia.

Lewinsohn, P. M., Sullivan, J. M., & Grosscup, S. J. (1980). Changing reinforcing events: An approach to the treatment of depression. *Psychotherapy: Theory, Research and Practice, 17*, 322–334.

Lind, B. K., Goodwin, J. L., Hill, J. G., Ali, T., Redline, S., & Quan, S. F. (2003). Recruitment of healthy adults into a study of overnight sleep monitoring in the home: Experience of the Sleep Heart Health Study. *Sleep and Breathing, 7*(1), 13–24.

Logsdon, R., McCurry, S., Moore, A., & Teri, L. (1997). Family and caregiver issues in the treatment of patients with Alzheimer's disease. *Seminars in Clinical Neuropsychiatry, 2*(2), 138–151.

Logsdon, R. G., & Teri, L. (1995). Depression in Alzheimer's disease patients: Caregivers as surrogate reporters. *Journal of the American Geriatrics Society, 43*, 150–155.

Logsdon, R. G., & Teri, L. (1997). The Pleasant Events Schedule—AD: Psychometric properties and relationship to depression and cognition in Alzheimer's disease patients. *Gerontologist, 37*(1), 40–45.

Lyketsos, C. G., Lindell Veiel, L., Baker, A., & Steele, C. (1999). A randomized, controlled trial of bright light therapy for agitated behaviors in dementia patients residing in long-term care. *International Journal of Geriatric Psychiatry, 14*(7), 520–525.

Lyketsos, C. G., Lopez, O., Jones, B., Fitzpatrick, A. L., Breitner, J., & DeKosky, S. (2002). Prevalence of neuropsychiatric symptoms in dementia and mild cognitive impairment. *Journal of the American Medical Association, 288*(12), 1475–1483.

Lyketsos, C. G., & Olin, J. (2002). Depression in Alzheimer's disease: Overview and treatment. *Biological Psychiatry, 52*, 243–252.

Lyketsos, C. G., Sheppard, J. E., Steinberg, M., Tschanz, J. A. T., Norton, M. D., Steffens, D. C., et al. (2001). Neuropsychiatric disturbance in Alzheimer's disease clusters into three groups: The Cache County study. *International Journal of Geriatric Psychiatry, 16*, 1043–1053.

Mace, N. L., & Rabins, P. V. (1991). *The 36-hour day.* Baltimore, MD: Johns Hopkins University Press.

Mack, J. L., & Patterson, M. B. (1994). The evaluation of behavioral disturbances in Alzheimer's disease: The utility of three rating scales. *Journal of Geriatric Psychiatry and Neurology, 7*(2), 99–115.

Massie, C. A., & Hart, R. W. (2003). Clinical outcomes related to interface type in patients with obstructive sleep apnea/hypopnea syndrome who are using continuous positive airway pressure. *Chest, 123*(4), 1112–1118.

McCurry, S. M., Gibbons, L. E., Logsdon, R. G., & Teri, L. (2003a). Anxiety and nighttime behavioral disturbances in Alzheimer's disease. *Journal of Gerontological Nursing, 30*(1), 12–20.

McCurry, S. M., Gibbons, L. E., Logsdon, R. G., Vitiello, M. V., & Teri, L. (2003b). Training caregivers to change the sleep hygiene practices of patients with dementia: The NITE–AD Project. *Journal of the American Geriatrics Society, 10*, 1455–1460.

McCurry, S. M., Gibbons, L. E., Logsdon, R. G., Vitiello, M. V., & Teri, L. (2005). Nighttime Insomnia Treatment and Education for Alzheimer's Disease (NITE–AD): A randomized controlled trial. *Journal of the American Geriatrics Society, 53*, 793–802.

McCurry, S. M., Logsdon, R. G., Teri, L., Gibbons, L. E., Kukull, W. A., Bowen, J. D., McCormick, W. C., & Larson, E. B. (1999). Characteristics of sleep disturbance in community-dwelling Alzheimer's disease patients. *Journal of Geriatric Psychiatry and Neurology, 12*, 53–59.

McCurry, S. M., Logsdon, R. G., Vitiello, M. V., & Teri, L. (1998). Successful behavioral treatment for reported sleep problems in elderly caregivers of dementia patients: A controlled study. *Journals of Gerontology B: Psychological Sciences and Social Sciences, 53B*(2), P122–P129.

McCurry, S. M., Reynolds, C. F., Ancoli-Israel, S., Teri, L., & Vitiello, M. V. (2000). Treatment of sleep disturbance in Alzheimer's disease. *Sleep Medicine Reviews, 4*(6), 603–608.

Mega, M. S., Cummings, J. L., Fiorello, T., & Gornbein, J. (1996). The spectrum of behavioral changes in Alzheimer's disease. *Neurology, 46*, 130–135.

Mittelman, M. S., Ferris, S. H., Shulman, E., Steinberg, G., & Levin, B. (1996). A family intervention to delay nursing home placement of patients with Alzheimer's disease: A randomized controlled trial. *Journal of the American Medical Association, 276*, 1725–1731.

Mittelman, M. S., Ferris, S. H., Steinberg, G., Shulman, E., Mackell, J., Ambinder, A., et al. (1993). An intervention that delays institutionalization of Alzheimer's disease patients: Treatment of spouse-caregivers. *Gerontologist, 33*(6), 730–740.

Mohide, E. A., Pringle, D. M., Streiner, D. L., Gilbert, J. R., Muir, G., & Tew, M. (1990). A randomized trial of family caregiver support in the home management of dementia. *Journal of the American Geriatrics Society, 38*, 446–454.

Ohayon, M. M., Cauclet, M., & Lemoine, P. (1998). Comorbidity of mental and insomnia disorders in the general population. *Comprehensive Psychiatry, 39*(4), 185–197.

Olin, J., & Schneider, L. (2001). *Galantamine for Alzheimer's disease (Cochrane Review)*. Cochrane Database System Review 1:CD001747.

Onega, L. L., & Abraham, I. L. (1997). Factor structure of the Dementia Mood Assessment Scale in a cohort of community-dwelling elderly. *International Psychogeriatrics, 9*(4), 449–457.

Orrell, M., & Bebbington, P. (1996). Psychosocial stress and anxiety in senile dementia. *Journal of Affective Disorders, 39*, 165–173.

Osman, E. Z., Osborne, J., Hill, P. D., & Lee, B. W. (1999). The Epworth Sleepiness Scale: Can it be used for sleep apnoea screening among snorers? *Clinical Otolaryngology, 24*(3), 239–241.

Perrault, A., Oremus, M., Demers, L., Vida, S., & Wolfson, C. (2000). Review of outcome measurement instruments in Alzheimer's disease drug trials: Psychometric properties of behavior and mood scales. *Journal of Geriatric Psychiatry and Neurology, 13*(4), 181–196.

Pinkston, E. M., & Linsk, N. (1984). Behavioral family intervention with the impaired elderly. *Gerontologist, 24*, 576–583.

Pollak, C. P., & Perlick, D. (1991). Sleep problems and institutionalization of the elderly. *Journal of Geriatric Psychiatry and Neurology, 4*, 204–210.

Prinz, P. N., Poceta, J. S., & McCurry, S. (2002). Sleep in the dementing disorders. In T. L. Lee-Chiong, M. J. Sateia, & M. A. Carskadon (Eds.), *Sleep medicine* (pp. 497–507). Philadelphia: Hanley & Belfus.

Rabins, P. V. (1994). Non-cognitive symptoms in Alzheimer's disease. In R. D. Terry, R. Katzman, & K. L. Bick (Eds.), *Alzheimer's disease* (pp. 419–429). New York: Raven Press.

Raskind, M. A. (1993). Geriatric psychopharmacology. *Psychiatric Clinics of North America, 16*(4), 815–827.

Raskind, M. A., & Peskind, E. R. (2001). Alzheimer's disease and related disorders. *Medical Clinics of North America, 85*(3), 803–817.

Reisberg, B., Borenstein, J., Salob , S. P., Ferris, S. H., Franssen, E., & Georgotas, A. (1987). Behavioral symptoms in Alzheimer's disease: Phenomenology and treatment. *Journal of Clinical Psychiatry, 48*(Suppl. 5), 9–15.

Schneider, L. S. (1996). Overview of generalized anxiety disorder in the elderly. *Journal of Clinical Psychiatry, 57*(Suppl. 7), 34–45.

Sky, A. J., & Grossberg, G. T. (1994). The use of psychotropic medication in the management of problem behaviors in the patient with Alzheimer's disease. *Medical Clinics of North America, 78*(4), 811–822.

Snowden, M., Sato, K., & Roy-Byrne, P. (2003). Assessment and treatment of nursing home residents with depression or behavioral symptoms associated with dementia: A review of the literature. *Journal of the American Geriatrics Society, 51*(9), 1305–1317.

Steele, C., Rovner, B., Chase, G. A., & Folstein, M. (1990). Psychiatric symptoms and nursing home placement of patients with Alzheimer's disease. *American Journal of Psychiatry, 147*(8), 1049–1051.

Sunderland, T., Hill, J. L., Lawlor, B. A., & Molchan, S. E. (1988). NIMH Dementia Mood Assessment Scale (DMAS). *Psychopharmacology Bulletin, 24*(4), 747–751.

Sutor, B. (2002). Behavior problems in demented nursing home residents: A multifaceted approach to assessment and management. *Comprehensive Therapy, 28*(4), 183–188.

Taylor, J. O., Friedman, L., Sheikh, J., & Yesavage, J. A. (1997). Assessment and management of "sundowning" phenomena. *Seminars in Clinical Neuropsychiatry, 2*(2), 113–122.

Teri, L. (1986, August). *Treating depression in Alzheimer's disease: Teaching the caregiver behavioral strategies*. Paper presented at the annual meeting of the American Psychological Association, Washington, DC.

Teri, L. (1990). *Managing and understanding behavior problems in Alzheimer's disease and related disorders* [Training program with video tapes and written manual]. Seattle: University of Washington.

Teri, L. (1992). Clinical problems in older adults: Behavioral treatment of depression in patients with dementia. *Clinician's Research Digest, 9*, 1–2.

Teri, L. (1994). Behavioral treatment of depression in patients with dementia. *Alzheimer's Disease and Associated Disorders, 8*, 66–74.

Teri, L., Baer, L., & Reifler, B. (1991). Depression in Alzheimer's patients: Investigation of symptom patterns and frequency. *Clinical Gerontologist, 11*, 47–57.

Teri, L., Ferretti, L. E., Gibbons, L. E., Logsdon, R. G., McCurry, S. M., Kukull, W. A., et al. (1999). Anxiety in Alzheimer's disease: Prevalence and comorbidity. *Journals of Gerontology: Medical Sciences, 54A*(7), M348–M352.

Teri, L., & Logsdon, R. G. (1991). Identifying pleasant activities for Alzheimer's disease patients: The Pleasant Events Schedule—AD. *Gerontologist, 31*, 124–127.

Teri, L., & Logsdon, R. G. (1995). Methodologic issues regarding outcome measures for clinical drug trials of psychiatric complications in dementia. *Journal of Geriatric Psychiatry and Neurology, 8*(Suppl. 1), S8–S17.

Teri, L., Logsdon, R. G., & McCurry, S. M. (2002). Nonpharmacologic treatment of behavioral disturbance in dementia. *Medical Clinics of North America, 86*, 641–656.

Teri, L., Logsdon, R. G., Peskind, E., Raskind, M., Weiner, M. F., Tractenberg, R. E., et al. (2000). Treatment of agitation in Alzheimer's disease: A randomized placebo controlled clinical trial. *Neurology, 55*, 1271–1278.

Teri, L., Logsdon, R. G., & Schindler, R. (1999). Treatment of behavioral and mood disturbances in dementia. *Generations, 23*(3), 50–56.

Teri, L., Logsdon, R. G., Uomoto, J., & McCurry, S. (1997). Behavioral treatment of depression in dementia patients: A controlled clinical trial. *Journals of Gerontology B: Psychological Sciences and Social Sciences, 52B*(4), P159–P166.

Teri, L., Logsdon, R. G., Whall, A. L., Weiner, M. F., Trimmer, C., Peskind, E., et al. (1998). Treatment for agitation in dementia patients: A behavior management approach. *Psychotherapy, 35*(4), 436–443.

Teri, L., McCurry, S. M., Buchner, D., Logsdon, R. G., LaCroix, A., Kukull, W. A., et al. (1998). Exercise and activity level in Alzheimer's disease: A potential treatment focus. *Journal of Rehabilitation Research and Development, 35*(4), 411–419.

Teri, L., & Truax, P. (1994). Assessment of depression in dementia patients: Association of caregiver mood with depression ratings. *Gerontologist, 34*, 231–234.

Teri, L., Truax, P., Logsdon, R. G., Uomoto, J., Zarit, S., & Vitaliano, P. P. (1992). Assessment of behavioral problems in dementia: The Revised Memory and Behavior Problems Checklist. *Psychology and Aging, 7*, 622–631.

van Someren, E. J. W., Kessler, A., Mirmiran, M., & Swaab, D. F. (1997). Indirect bright light improves circadian rest–activity rhythm disturbances in demented patients. *Biological Psychiatry, 41*, 955–963.

Vitaliano, P. P., Young, H. M., & Russo, J. (1991). Burden: A review of measures used among caregivers of individuals with dementia. *Gerontologist, 31*, 67–75.

Vitiello, M. V., & Borson, S. (2001). Sleep disturbances in patients with Alzheimer's disease: Epidemiology, pathophysiology and treatment. *CNS Drugs, 15*(10), 777–796.

Wagner, A. W., Logsdon, R. G., Pearson, J. L., & Teri, L. (1997). Caregiver expressed emotion and depression in Alzheimer's disease. *Aging and Mental Health, 1*(2), 132–139.

Weiner, M. F., Edland, S. D., & Luszczynska, H. X. (1994). Prevalence and incidence of major depression in Alzheimer's disease. *American Journal of Psychiatry, 151*, 1006.

Weiner, M. F., Schneider, L. S., Gray, K. F., & Stern, R. G. (1996). Pharmacologic management and treatment of dementia and secondary symptoms. In M. F. Weiner (Ed.), *The dementias: Diagnosis, management, and research* (2nd ed., pp. 175–210). Washington, DC: American Psychiatric Press.

Weiner, M. F., Tractenberg, R., Teri, L., Logsdon, R., Thomas, R. G., Gamst, A., et al. (2000). Quantifying behavioral disturbance in Alzheimer's disease patients. *Journal of Psychiatric Research*, *34*(2), 163–167.

Yesavage, J. A., Brink, T. L., Rose, T. L., Lum, O., Huang, V., Adey, M. B., et al. (1983). Development and validation of a Geriatric Depression Screening Scale: A preliminary report. *Journal of Psychiatric Research*, *17*, 37–49.

Zarit, S., Anthony, C., & Boutselis, M. (1987). Interventions with care givers of dementia patients: Comparison of two approaches. *Psychology and Aging*, *2*(3), 225–232.

Zubenko, G. S., Zubenko, W. N., McPherson, S., Spoor, E., Marin, D. B., Farlow, M., et al. (2003). A collaborative study of the emergence and clinical features of major depressive syndrome of Alzheimer's disease. *American Journal of Psychiatry*, *160*, 857–866.

17

Behavioral Treatment of Impaired Functioning and Behavioral Symptoms

ANN LOUISE BARRICK

Most individuals with dementia display behaviors that challenge personal and professional caregivers. Dementia causes progressive cognitive changes that make a wide range of behavioral challenges likely. The person may have difficulty carrying out everyday activities such as looking up a phone number and dialing it, grocery shopping, keeping track of his or her schedule, or picking up the mail, as described in Marson, Chapter 7, this volume. The person may also misunderstand what other people say, have difficulty initiating activities or keeping occupied, have problems sleeping, or may even become violent. An estimated 23% of individuals over age 65 living in the community have difficulty performing at least one activity of daily living. It is not always clear whether these deficits are physical, cognitive, environmental, or a combination of these factors (National Center for Health Statistics, n.d.).

The accumulation of deficits often leads to nursing home placement. As many as 88% of residents in nursing homes require assistance (National Center for Health Statistics, n.d.). Although the reported prevalence of physically and verbally aggressive behavior varies considerably, depending on methods, as many as 50–90% of persons with moderate to severe dementia exhibit clinically significant behaviors sometime during their illness (Allen-Burge, Stevens, & Burgio, 1999). Physically and verbally aggressive behaviors occur most frequently during assistance with personal care, because these activities involve touch and invasion of personal space. Such behaviors do not occur in a vacuum; dementia can best be understood as an interaction of medical, psychological, social, and environmental processes. Even though we cannot alter the medical mechanism of dementia, we can change how we interact with the person who has dementia as well as aspects of his or her environment, which may result in a substantial change in the person's level of functioning. In the absence of effective biological treatments, behavioral strategies are often a powerful approach for treating the challenging behaviors that emerge with dementia.

367

This chapter reviews the behavioral symptoms commonly found in persons with dementia and discusses interventions that have been found to be helpful with specific behaviors. Strategies for developing individualized behavioral intervention plans are also described.

TYPES OF BEHAVIORAL SYMPTOMS

Behaviors associated with dementia have been defined in different ways. Early in the disease process we typically find impairments in functional skills such as higher-level activities of daily living. As the disease progresses, behaviors requiring intervention have usually been classified in one of two categories: deficits or excesses.

Behavioral deficits are those behaviors that are absent despite the physical ability to carry out the components of the behavior. An example would be the failure to self-feed in a person who has preserved motor control and moderate dementia. Agitation and aggression are the most common behavioral "excesses" requiring intervention. These disruptive or problem behaviors include pacing, grabbing, hitting, and verbal abuse. Also included in this category are screaming and repetitive requests, which have been called disruptive vocalizations. However, when considering the behavior of a person with dementia within the context of cognitive impairment, it can be argued that the behavior is actually a method of communicating and therefore adaptive. The behaviors are not always disruptive, as in pacing or "wandering." Because these behaviors can teach us about the internal state of the person and the person's needs, they may actually be more accurately described as behavioral symptoms. The most common behavioral symptoms requiring intervention are described in Table 17.1.

IMPACT OF BEHAVIORAL SYMPTOMS

Behavioral symptoms have been found in individuals who live in both community and institutional settings. From the perspective of family caregivers, these challenging behaviors can impact relationships by exacerbating conflicts, increasing anxiety and depression of the caregiver, and often resulting in institutionalization (Aneshensel, Pearlin, & Schuler, 1993; Davis, 1997; Schulz, O'Brien, Bookwala, & Fleissner, 1995). In fact, behavioral symptoms have been found to be among the main reasons for institutionalization (Moak & Fisher, 1990; Petrie, Lawson, & Hollendar, 1982). Nursing facility staff also experience stress when dealing with these behaviors. Aggressive behaviors are the most distressing form of behavioral symptom that occurs during caregiving (Everitt, Fields, Soumerai, & Avorn, 1991). Being subjected repeatedly to such behavior has been linked to declines in physical and mental health status (Miller, 1997), frustration with caregiving (Mentes & Ferraro, 1989), job dissatisfaction and burnout (Colenda & Hamer, 1991), and turnover (Burgio, Butler, & Engel, 1988). However, the reaction of staff members differs with their understanding and interpretation of aggressive behavior within the context of the disease process and the caregivers' experience (Hallberg & Norberg, 1993) and is possible to change (Feldt & Ryden, 1992; Hallberg & Norberg, 1993; Hoeffer, Rader, McKenzie, Lavelle, & Stewart, 1997). For example, Hoeffer et al. (2005) investigated caregiver outcomes as part of a larger study of person-centered interventions to reduce aggression and agitation during bathing. They found that they were able to teach nursing

TABLE 17.1. Common Behavioral Symptoms in Persons with Dementia

Behavior	Examples
Difficulty with personal tasks	Failure to dress or bathe self despite physical and cognitive ability to do so
Urinary incontinence	Urinating outside the bathroom facilities; frequent wetness
Sleep problems	Difficulty falling asleep, getting up during the night, wakes and dresses at night, early morning awakening
Wandering	Attempts to exit; excessive pacing trying to get to a different place
Agitation	General restlessness, excessive fidgeting;, performing repetitive mannerisms or activities; constant unwarranted requests; resists ADLs; repeatedly dresses and undresses; picking behavior
Aggression	Physical aggression: grabbing, kicking, hitting, and dangerous assaulted behaviors Verbal aggression: verbal threats, cursing
Excessive vocalization	Loud screaming, excessive self-talk, frequent loud requests
Suspiciousness, paranoia	Fear of harm, theft, spousal affair; family/staff seen as imposters; misinterpreting actions or words of others; talks to the TV
Inappropriate or impulsive sexual behavior	Touching another person sexually; excessive requests for sexual contact; repetitive obscene gestures, remarks; kisses or attempts to kiss others

Note. ADLs, activities of daily living.

assistants to use a person-centered approach that viewed behaviors as symptoms of unmet needs. This approach decreased the distress experienced by the nursing assistants and increased satisfaction with, and preparedness for, assisting during bathing. Improving the understanding of behavioral symptoms is thus critical to improving the experience of caregivers as well as the care they give recipients.

Behavioral symptoms can also affect the person with dementia. Additionally, these behaviors can affect the staff–resident relationship and result in the reduction of caregiving services (Burgio, 1996) and the avoidance of residents (Meddaugh, 1990). Individuals who display behavioral symptoms tend to deteriorate faster than those without symptoms.

ETIOLOGY OF BEHAVIORAL SYMPTOMS

One of the most important factors in treating behavioral symptoms in persons with dementia is understanding the triggers or causes of the behavior. These include both personal and environmental factors and are described below. A list of some of the common triggers to behavioral symptoms can be found in Table 17.2.

Personal Factors

Neurological Factors

The relationship of cognitive deficits to behavioral symptoms remains somewhat unclear. For example, not surprisingly, Teri, Borson, Kiyak, & Yamagishi (1989) found that confusion, disorientation, and memory loss were the symptoms most strongly associated with level of cognitive functioning. Additionally, persons with more cognitive impairment

TABLE 17.2. Common Triggers of Behavioral Symptoms

Physical	Emotional/ psychological	Interpersonal	Environmental	Cognitive/ neurological
• Response to medication • Pain • Thirst • Hunger • Cold • Acute illness • Infection • Touch • Fatigue • Poor sleep • Poor vision • Hearing loss	• Fear/anxiety • Depression • Loneliness • Boredom • Grief • Frustration • Irritability • Apathy • Suspiciousness	• Lack of attention to personal preferences • Perceived loss of personal control • Changes in caregiver • Confrontation • Rushed approach • Perceived invasion of space • Reinforced dependency	• Overstimulation • Understimulation • Change in routine • Task demands that exceed capacity • Overcrowding • Noise	• Misinterpretation of environmental cues • Unable to understand words • Unable to express needs verbally • Inability to start or stop a task • Short attention span • Failure to recognize caregiver • Lack of insight • Impaired decision making • Poor impulse control

had more difficulties with instrumental activities. However, in this study, no single behavioral symptom such as aggression was related to overall level of cognitive impairment.

Other authors have found that the types of behavioral symptoms vary with the level of cognitive impairment. Wandering has been associated with greater cognitive impairment in language, memory, orientation, and concentration (Algase, 1992). Hoeffer et al. (1997) reported that physical aggression was more common during caregiver activities among persons with moderate to severe levels of dementia. Barrick, Rader, Hoeffer, and Sloane (2002) reported different kinds of behavioral symptoms during bathing at different stages of dementia. For example, a person in the early stages of dementia is more likely to verbally refuse the bath by saying, "I've already had a bath." Persons with moderate dementia may say "Stop!" as they approach the bathroom or hold firmly to the doorjamb and refuse to enter the bathroom. Severely demented persons often moan or cry when they enter the bathroom. Matteson, Linton, and Barnes (1997) prescribed behavioral interventions based on the Piaget model, suggesting that interventions could be linked to disease stage.

Behavioral symptoms have also been associated with different disorders. For example, in Alzheimer's disease (AD), agitation and psychosis have been associated with neurofibrillary tangles in the frontal lobes (Tekin et al., 2001). Persons with frontotemporal dementia (FTD) are often apathetic or disinhibited (Levy et al., 1996). Other symptoms seen in FTD include inappropriate affect with unusual laughter, tactlessness, and lack of concern for others. The neurobehavioral features of vascular dementia are variable; psychomotor retardation and emotional lability are common. These illnesses are detailed in Welsh-Bohmer and Warren (Chapter 3, this volume).

Persons with central nervous system dysfunction frequently misinterpret what others are doing or saying and can respond in a way that is inappropriate to the situation. For example, disinhibition from neurological damage may cause some persons to engage in inappropriate sexual behavior. Misperception may result in such behaviors as a woman following a man she thinks is her husband. The man, not recognizing her or understanding that she is cognitively impaired, may then hit the woman in an effort to keep her away from him. Other behaviors may actually be the result of self-care deficits, as when a person with dementia looks disheveled and is unaware of his or her poor hygiene.

Physical Factors

Several basic physical factors can trigger or worsen behavioral symptoms (Hall, Gerdner, Zwygart-Stauffacher, & Buckwalter, 1995). These include fatigue, pain, infection, acute illness, and sensory and perceptual deficits. Infectious or other processes may cause delirium and a sudden change in behavior. Urinary tract infections can produce pain that may go undetected because the person is unable to express discomfort. Other frequent causes of pain include arthritis, osteoporosis, back problems, constipation, contractures, and dental problems. The anticipation of pain has also been reported as a cause of behavioral symptoms (Cohen-Mansfield et al., 1990b). Other sources of discomfort include sensitivity to cold, sensitive skin and feet, and problems with mobility such as stiffness on movement.

Sensory and perceptual deficits may affect perception of situations or requests. For example, a person may not have a hearing aid turned on during personal care and therefore be unable to understand what the caregiver is telling him or her. He or she may respond aggressively out of fear and a perceived need for self-defense. Perceptual deficits can also make it difficult for a person to do such tasks as sitting down in a bathtub. Visual neglect due to a stroke may contribute to poor food intake and other deficits in self-care.

Emotional/Psychological Factors

Several emotions are related to the occurrence of behavioral symptoms. Frustration with ability to perform daily tasks independently has been reported to cause behavioral symptoms (Cohen-Mansfield, Marx, & Rosenthal, 1990). Swearer, Drachman, O'Donnell, and Mitchell (1988) noted that angry outbursts were significantly related to anxiety. A cognitively impaired person may misjudge the dangerousness of a situation, and this error in judgment may result in anxiety. Given the limited ability of the person to cope with anxiety-provoking situations, he or she may become aggressive.

Other behaviors, particularly those not related to suffering, such as aimless wandering, occur under normal conditions and may be adaptive and provide stimulation. Individual differences that have been associated with wandering behavior include stress and coping patterns and tendencies toward greater socialization needs (Goldsmith, Hoeffer, & Rader, 1995). Although wandering can cause safety and health problems, it also provides both stimulation and exercise and is therefore reinforcing for residents of nursing homes (Cohen-Mansfield et al., 1998). Individuals find different objects, such as doorknobs, to touch and rub as they explore their environment, or they may be following other persons who are walking around, modeling the behavior they see from others.

Interpersonal Factors

Relationships with individuals in the care environment can often trigger dependency or distress. Behavioral deficits are often the result of interpersonal factors. Available evidence suggests that there is a relationship between functional abilities and the need for interpersonal contact in residents in nursing homes (Willis et al., 1998). Everyday tasks such as bathing and dressing involve social interaction with staff. Dependency is reinforced as it increases staff contact (Baltes & Baltes, 1990). Baltes labeled the patterns of overcare displayed by caregivers the dependency–support script (Baltes & Wahl, 1992). Older adults learn that being dependent allows them to gain control, attention from others, and the opportunity to choose where to expend their energies.

Caregivers may also reinforce many dependent behaviors when they underestimate the person's resources and provide more care than is necessary (Baltes & Werner-Wahl, 1987). Caregivers, believing that older adults are in need of help, may feel altruistic providing this assistance. However, this extension of assistance can result in increased social, physical, and psychological dependency (Wilson, Cockburn, & Halligan, 1987). Neumann (as cited in Baltes & Werner-Wahl, 1987) also found that staff in institutions gave immediate help to residents rather than giving them time to perform the task independently, thus reinforcing dependent behavior. There is pressure to complete tasks quickly, such as dressing or bathing, and caregivers often find it faster to provide extensive assistance to the person rather than encouraging independence, thus reinforcing passive–dependent behaviors.

Studies of resistive and aggressive behavior during activities of daily living (ADLs) indicate that caregivers often unknowingly initiate or perpetuate inappropriate responses. Caregiver behaviors that impact the relationship include tone of voice, facial expressions, and gestures that often communicate more than words. Burgener and colleagues (Burgener, Jirove, Murrell, & Barton, 1992) found that rigid and tense caregiver behaviors were significantly associated with agitated behaviors, whereas relaxed and smiling caregiver behaviors during ADL care were significantly associated with calm and attending behaviors of residents. Change of caregiver can also trigger behavioral symptoms (Hall et al., 1995). Other documented causes of behavioral symptoms, particularly aggression toward staff during care include touch or the invasion of personal space (Marx, Werner, & Cohen-Mansfield, 1989; Rossby, Beck, & Heacock, 1992; Ryden, Bossenmaier, & McLachlan, 1991), perceived loss of personal control or choice (Meddaugh, 1990; Winger, Schirm, & Steward, 1987), efforts to attain or share control (Kovach & Meyer-Arnold, 1996), attempts to avoid a stimulus such as a nurse's request (Bridges-Parlet, Knopman, & Thompson, 1994), and lack of attention to personal needs or preferences (Chrisman, Tabar, Whall, & Booth, 1991). Social factors such as poor quality of relationships or a decrease in social contacts have also been predictive of a change in aggression (Cohen-Mansfield & Werner, 1998). Finally, providing less compensation for the person's disabilities—in other words, doing less for the person—has been related to calmer and more functional behaviors (Burgener et al., 1992).

Environmental Factors

The environment can impact behavior; ADL deficits may be related to the surrounding environment. An environment that demands more independence or presents more stimuli than a person with cognitive deficits is capable of managing may result in maladaptive or reduced functioning. For example, too many clothing choices may overwhelm the person, leaving him or her unable to make a decision. Equipment may not match physical needs; for example, the handles on eating utensils may be too small to grasp easily. Shower chairs may be unpadded and cause pain. Other physical environmental factors that contribute to behavioral symptoms include lighting, noise level, temperature of the room, cluttered or crowded space, and unpleasant odors.

Rigid administrative policies and practices impact behavior and the environment of care. Both anecdotal and research findings report that task completion and adherence to a strict care schedule are often a priority. A philosophy of care that does not allow for flexibility in determining when and how care activities such as dressing and bathing are performed may result in residents feeling coerced, triggering aggression or agitation. An emphasis on the completion of personal care tasks, at the expense of the emotional needs of the person, can have a similar result.

THE INTERVENTION PROCESS

Behavioral treatments have been found to be effective for many different behaviors. Nonpharmacological interventions are often used because they avoid the adverse side effects and drug–drug interactions of medications. In addition, medications have limited efficacy in treating these problems. In persons with dementia, it is sometimes possible to use a traditional behavioral approach and intervene directly. Following are helpful types of interventions:

- *Differential reinforcement of other behavior* (DRO). Reinforce the nonoccurrence of a prespecified problem behavior by scheduling reinforcement on a fixed interval of time and omitting the next scheduled reinforcer if the problem behavior occurs during the interval.
- *Extinction of positively reinforced behavior.* Identify a reinforcer that maintains a problem behavior and remove it.
- *Stimulus control.* Reinforce a behavior only in the presence of an antecedent event or stimulus that facilitates the behavior, and provide no reinforcement in the absence of that stimulus. This approach is helpful when a behavior exists but in the wrong situations, or occurs too frequently or not frequently enough.
- *Shaping.* Reinforce successive approximations to desired behavior, until the desired behavior occurs.
- *Prompting.* Provide extra verbal or physical cues to elicit the behavior. Prompts for appropriate behavior may include gesturing or pointing, verbalizations, manual guidance, and praise for desired behavior. Once the behavior occurs consistently with prompting, the caregiver needs to fade out prompts until the behavior occurs without prompts.

For example, independence in ADL care (e.g., dressing, bathing) may be increased by giving prompts for each step of the process (prompting). Providing a reinforcer, such as giving praise or something to eat, when the person performs each step of the process can be used to shape behavior. For example, a person fearful of bathing in the tub can be given candy as a reinforcer for each successive step toward the goal of bathing in the tub. Or if a person has too many somatic complaints, it may be helpful to establish a plan allowing the person to make these complaints only to the nurse (stimulus control).

More often when working with someone who has dementia, impairments in memory, communication, and reasoning limit the effectiveness of behavioral interventions that require learning new information, language comprehension, or the formation of insights. It is then necessary to focus on preventing maladaptive behavior by changing the environment or how other people respond to the person to optimize the person's functioning. Moreover, behaviors may look alike (e.g., hitting by two different persons) but have very different etiologies and respond to very different interventions. The main objective is to identify treatable or modifiable aspects of the particular situation for the individual and develop a plan that promotes specific, individualized goals.

Behavioral interventions focus on the interaction between the person and the environment. The process includes three steps: (1) assessment to identify the behavior and factors related to its occurrence; (2) development and implementation of the plan; and (3) monitoring and revising the plan, as needed. Treatment recommendations are designed to change antecedent conditions and/or provide different consequences for different responses in order to compensate for losses while preserving remaining abilities. Monitoring is essential to track the success of the plan and guide the revision process.

Assessment

Understanding the Person

Knowing as much as possible about the person will help determine why the behavior might be occurring as well as develop individualized strategies to change it. The most common personal causes of distress and behavioral symptoms are related to physical and emotional needs and problems related to cognitive deficits. Identification of factors such as physical health, personality, psychosocial well-being and mood, personal history, and neurocognitive deficits is essential to understanding the behavior and developing a plan that will be effective. The assessment described in Marson and Hebert (Chapter 7, this volume) provides much of the information about personal factors that may be associated with behavioral symptoms.

Describing the Behavior

The assessment begins with identifying the behavior. Many scales have been developed that focus on the identification of target behaviors and the frequency and intensity of these behaviors in older adults. These scales are useful for obtaining baseline levels of behavior and for monitoring the effects of interventions. Instruments vary in length, time frames, domains covered, and ease of administration. The final choice of instrument depends on the purpose of the assessment. Those with adequate interrater reliability and demonstrated usefulness in the assessment of behavioral symptoms are listed in Table 17.3.

As with all geriatric cases, it is helpful to consult with those who know the person best. Sources of information include the family; friends; other caregivers; other staff such as housekeepers, social workers, activity coordinators; and the medical record. If the person is only mildly impaired, he or she can provide useful input as well. Ratings can be subjective, with some informants underreporting and others overreporting, depending on their level of stress and their beliefs about the consequences of the assessment. However, if accuracy can be stressed, they can provide useful data to measure the occurrence of behaviors and the effect of interventions.

TABLE 17.3. Sample of Behavior Rating Scales for Older Adults

Scale name	Primary reference	Rater source	Population rated	Behaviors measured
Behavioral Pathology in Alzheimer's Disease Scale (BEHAVE-AD)	Reisberg et al. (1987)	Clinician (interview with patient and caregiver)	Patients with AD	Paranoid and delusional ideation, hallucinations, activity disturbance, aggressiveness, diurnal disturbance, and anxieties/phobias exhibited 2 weeks prior to interview and global rating of distress to caregiver
Caretaker Obstreperous Behavior Rating Assessment Scale (COBRA)	Drachman et al. (1992)	Caregiver (questionnaire)	Outpatients, nursing home residents, with dementia	Frequency and severity of aggressive/assaultive behavior, disordered ideas/personality, mechanical/motor and vegetative behaviors (including hyper/hyposexuality)
Cohen-Mansfield Agitation Inventory (CMAI)	Cohen-Mansfield et al. (1989)	Nursing staff	Nursing home residents	Frequency of physical aggression toward self or others; physically or verbally disruptive, but not aggressive, behavior; socially inappropriate behaviors
Cornell Scale for Depression in Dementia (CSDD)	Alexopoulos et al. (1988)	Clinician (interview with caregiver) or caregiver questionnaire	Older adults with dementia	A broad spectrum of depressive signs and symptoms observed during the prior week: mood-related signs, behavior disturbance, physical signs, cyclic disturbance, and ideational disturbance
Dementia Behavior Disturbance Scale (DBD)	Baumgarten et al. (1990)	Clinician (interview with caregiver) or caregiver questionnaire	Community-residing older adults	Frequency of a broad range of behaviors
Disruptive Behavior Rating Scale (DBRS)	Mungas et al. (1989)	Nursing staff	Nursing home residents	Severity of verbally and physically aggressive behaviors, agitation, and wandering; Ratings made weekly
Pittsburgh Agitation Scale	Burgio et al. (1994)	Direct observation by clinical staff	Older adults with dementia	Aberrant vocalizations, motor agitation, aggressiveness, and resisting care
Pleasant Events Schedule—AD (PES-AD)	Teri & Logsdon (1991)	Caregiver (questionnaire)	Outpatients with AD	Helps identify and monitor participation in pleasurable activities
Ryden Aggression Scale (RAS)	Ryden (1988)	Caregiver (questionnaire)	Community-residing older adults	Frequency of physical, verbal, and sexual aggression

Looking for Causes

Behavioral symptoms can be caused by antecedent factors that trigger the behavior; they can also be the result of consequences that maintain the behavior through positive or negative reinforcement. Rarely is there only one cause to a behavior. Identification of the causes of the symptoms can be particularly challenging when an individual has a degenerative condition such as AD, because similar behaviors may have different etiologies over the course of the disease. Given the significant variation in cognitive abilities and health of older adults, the identification of the causes of behavioral symptoms is best considered within an interactional model that includes personal, interpersonal, and environmental factors. The Behavior Observation Record (BOR) or the Behavior Tracking Log (BTL) (see Figures 17.1 and 17.2) can be used when assessing these factors. Observations related to the ABC's of behavior as well as the duration of specific behaviors are documented on the BOR. The behavior, its antecedents, any interventions tried, and the person's response to interventions are recorded over the course of a 24-hour period on the BTL. Using these kinds of tools can give the clinician a baseline measure of the percentage of time in which the behavior is occurring as well as clues to the causes of the behavior. Other data-gathering tools can also be designed. The important point is to select a method that will provide reasonably accurate data on the factors described below.

Personal Factors. Assessing and treating physical symptoms first may eliminate the behavior and avoid the need for more in-depth assessment. For example, does the person have a urinary track infection or is he or she dehydrated? If pain is suspected, it would be helpful to complete a thorough pain assessment. If the person is able to communicate, use a verbally administered questionnaire such as the McGill Pain Questionnaire (Melzack, 1975). If the person is severely impaired, it is usually necessary to rely on direct observation methods, such as the Discomfort Scale—Dementia of the Alzheimer's Type (Hurley, Volcier, Hanrahan, Houde, & Volcier, 1992). In addition, the direct caregiver can complete a pain flow sheet with all possible behavioral manifestations of the pain experience.

It is important to consider medications and any changes in them. Older adults are at increased risk for iatrogenic effects associated with drug toxicity, drug interactions, and drug withdrawal. (Gerdner & Buckwalter, 1994). One medication may negate or alter the effects of another and result in behavioral symptoms. Neuroleptics, benzodiazepines, and nonprescription medication with anticholinergic properties have been found to contribute to agitation in older adults (Fisher, Swingen, & Harsin, 2001). Psychiatric review of medications can often be quite instrumental in identifying the causes of behavioral symptoms.

There is a great deal of variance in how people with dementia communicate their psychological needs. Watch for signals that suggest that the person is generally fearful or afraid of specific objects or events. Look for such clues as wide open eyes, open or tense mouth, or eyebrows in a straight line. The need for control may be expressed through demands, threats, or refusals to cooperate. Depression may be expressed through restlessness, irritability, numerous complaints, and lack of interest in doing things or being with people. Always keep in mind the personal history and preferences of the individual. For example, a resident of a facility who refused to attend activities went happily when given the role of "judge" of a teddy bear contest. She was used to being "in charge," and the role fit her perception of herself. A person who has always bathed in the evening may refuse a bath offered in the morning but accept it in the evening, just before bedtime.

Patient: _____ Date: _____

Behavior(s) being monitored: _____

Location: _____

Date	Time	ANTECEDENT What was going on before the behavior?	BEHAVIOR Describe what the person did.	Duration of the incident (minutes)	CONSEQUENCE What happened after, or as a result of, the behavior? What did peers or staff say or do?

FIGURE 17.1. Behavior observation record.

Interpersonal Factors. Relationships with individuals in the care environment can often trigger distress. Watch to see if caregivers respond promptly with apologies or change of technique to complaints of pain or cold. Are caregivers calm or moving too fast, frowning, or talking to someone else in the room? Does the person get caregiver attention only when this behavior occurs? Does the level of assistance fit the needs of the person? Do the behaviors occur only when specific caregivers are present? Are interactions culturally appropriate?

Environmental Factors. Assess all aspects of the environment in order to understand causes of behavioral symptoms. Check to see if there is enough nonglare lighting for the older person to be able to see, that room temperature and the equipment are comfortable, and that the area is not noisy or cluttered. Do the demands of the environment exceed the person's ability to cope? Does the behavior result in the termination of the task and removal of an aversive stimuli? Assess the effect on the behavior of the daily schedule, caregiver support and education, and the availability of adaptive equipment and supplies.

Name/Date: _____

BEHAVIOR:	1 = calm	2 = yelling	3 = cursing	4 = physically aggressive	5 = other— describe	
INTERVENTION:	1 = 1:1	2 = music	3 = offered snack	4 = ignored	5 = distracted with activity	6 = other— describe
RESULTS:	1 = made it worse	2 = didn't help	3 = helped			

Time	Behavior	If not calm, what happened (trigger) before he/she became upset?	Interventions tried	Results	Initials
6:00 A.M.– 7:00 A.M.					
7:00 A.M.– 8:00 A.M.					
8:00 A.M.– 9:00 A.M.					
9:00 A.M.– 10:00 A.M.					
10:00 A.M.– 11:00 A.M.					
11:00 A.M.– 12:00 noon					
12:00 noon– 1:00 P.M.					
1:00 P.M.– 2:00 P.M.					
2:00 P.M.– 3:00 P.M.					
3:00 P.M.– 4:00 P.M.					
4:00 P.M.– 5:00 P.M.					
5:00 P.M.– 6:00 P.M.					
6:00 P.M.– 7:00 P.M.					
7:00 P.M.– 8:00 P.M.					
8:00 P.M.– 9:00 P.M.					
9:00 P.M.– 10:00 P.M.					
10:00 P.M.– 11:00 P.M.					
11:00 P.M.– 12:00 A.M.					
12:00 A.M.– 1:00 A.M.					
1:00 A.M.– 2:00 A.M.					
2:00 A.M.– 3:00 A.M.					
3:00 A.M.– 4:00 A.M.					
4:00 A.M.– 5:00 A.M.					
5:00 A.M.– 6:00 A.M.					

FIGURE 17.2. Behavior tracking log.

INTERVENTION PLANNING AND IMPLEMENTATION

Behavior can have many causes and respond to different interventions depending on whether the cause is personal, interpersonal, environmental, or a combination of these factors. When developing a plan, utilize available data to specify goals and interventions, monitor the results, and revise the plan as needed.

Behavioral Interventions in the Literature

Research is available on methods of addressing functional behavioral deficits such as incontinence, sleep disturbances, wandering, physical and verbal aggression, excessive vocalizations, and inappropriate sexual behavior. Much of this research has limitations due to small samples and the implementation of interventions by research staff rather than regular staff. However, there are many promising interventions. Overall, the studies that show the most promise incorporate comprehensive environmental interventions with careful assessment of the individual.

Behavioral Deficits

Independence in self-care skills such as bathing, eating, dressing, and toileting are important for older adults living in the community as well as those in nursing facilities. Various types of behavioral approaches have been used to increase these self-help behaviors. Operant techniques such as verbal prompting, combined with stimulus control, immediate reinforcement, and time out for inappropriate behavior, have resulted in an increase in self-feeding (Baltes & Zerbe, 1976). Hussian and Davis (1985) were able to increase appropriate eating behavior by reinforcing these behaviors with favorite foods or drinks.

A series of studies conducted by Cornelia Beck and her associates over several years has demonstrated that behavioral interventions can increase the functional ability of persons with cognitive impairment. Seven out of eight cognitively impaired persons living at home required less assistance with dressing after caregivers were taught behavioral strategies such as stimulus control, reinforcement, and verbal prompts to increase independence of participants (Beck, 1988). Similar results were found in long-term care studies (Beck, Heacock, Rapp, & Mercer, 1993).

Hussian and Davis (1985) suggested the use of stimulus control to increase dressing and grooming competence in persons with severe memory loss. These activities were performed in a consistent manner, at the same time each day, in the same area, with the same materials. Performing these tasks in the presence of a specific antecedent stimulus (i.e., the same area, the same materials) increased the likelihood that the behavior would occur.

Urinary Incontinence

Prompted voiding, a procedure that uses verbal prompts and positive reinforcement, has been successful in improving bladder control. However, studies are very limited. Adkins and Mathews (1997) taught in-home caregivers to use prompted voiding to reduce the incontinence of two cognitively impaired older adults. Hussian (1981) successfully used stimulus control, feedback, and positive reinforcement contingent on appropriate voiding to reduce urinary incontinence in 12 residents of a long-term care facility. Residents were toileted 15 minutes after awakening, every hour unless no voiding occurred in 4 hours, then every half hour, then every 15 minutes after an accident. Residents were praised for dryness and told if they had not voided or if they were wet. Although successful with some persons, such a prompted voiding system is difficult to maintain and requires a specialized program with careful monitoring and supervisory feedback to staff when done in facilities.

Sleep Disturbance

Environmental interventions have also been effective in increasing sleep. For example, Alessi et al. (1999) increased daytime activities and introduced a nighttime program to decrease disruptive noises; this approach resulted in a 10% increase in nighttime sleep and a 32% decrease in time in bed during the day. White noise has been effective in some cases in decreasing nocturnal wandering and increasing sleep (Young, Muir-Nash, & Ninos, 1988).

Physically Aggressive Behaviors

Techniques such as differential reinforcement of incompatible behavior (DRI) and stimulation have been effective in reducing aggression. Rosenberger and MacLean (1983) were able to reduce the aggressive behavior of a 79-year-old stroke patient who was partially paralyzed by using DRI. Prior to the intervention, this person received caregiver attention primarily when she was aggressive toward others; this pattern seemed to be maintaining the behavior. The plan involved staff members greeting and praising her for appropriate behaviors. Aggressive behaviors were followed by brief periods of time out. In 3 weeks the woman was no longer aggressive. Fisher (1995) found that aggressive behavior was an effort to escape from an aversive situation or event. Reducing the anxiety-provoking characteristics of the demand tasks was accomplished by the use of a stimulus to distract the person from the aversive situation. For example, during caregiving activities persons with dementia were presented with a stimulus that interested them, such as a live animal, a magazine, or a stuffed toy. This added stimulus altered the situation, refocused attention, and reduced aggression.

Behavioral techniques designed to fit individual resident needs have also been successful in the reduction of physical aggression (Burgio & Bourgeois, 1992; Burgio & Stevens, 1999; Sloane et al., 2004). For example, in a controlled trial of two bathing interventions in 15 nursing homes, Sloane et al. (2004) found a 29% reduction in the rate of physical aggression during showering of persons with dementia. Personal, interpersonal, and environmental factors were examined to determine antecedents and consequences of aggressive and agitated behaviors. This information was used to develop a person-centered care plan that focused on patient comfort and preferences. The caregiver sought to individualize the experience of the bath to change the bathing environment and meet the physical and emotional needs of the person by using the wide variety of techniques that modified the setting events or antecedent stimuli. These included such simple changes as covering the person with towels to maintain warmth, distracting attention (e.g., providing food), using bathing products recommended by family and staff, using no-rinse soap, offering choices, and modifying the shower spray to soften its impact. Similar results were found in a small sample intervention study with 10 intermediate care residents by Hoeffer et al. (1997). In both studies the larger interpersonal and environmental systems in which physically aggressive behaviors occurred were considered when developing the intervention.

Wandering

Environmental interventions have been useful in curbing wandering behavior. The use of a stimulus control, such as a picture of a toilet on the bathroom door, as well as contingent staff attention for nonwandering have shown some success in reducing wandering (Hussian, 1981; Hussian & Davis, 1985). Cohen-Mansfield and Werner (1998) enhanced the nursing home environment with visual, auditory, and olfactory stimuli that simulated the home and natural outdoor environment. Results indicated that residents spent more time in enhanced environments than regular nursing home space. There were also trends toward less trespassing, exit seeking, and agitated behavior as well as an increase in pleasure when the residents were at the nature scene in comparison with the regular nursing home unit. Rather than try to reduce wandering, Burgio, Cotter, and Stevens (1996) provided residents of a nursing facility with a secure place to walk.

Another intervention to decrease wandering is increasing staff–resident interactions. Goldsmith et al. (1995) reported that an increase in the amount of staff time spent interacting with residents reduced wandering behavior. Similarly, Okawa et al. (1991) found a 30% reduction in wandering of persons with dementia with increasing social interaction with nursing staff.

Finally, Heard and Watson (as cited in Cohen-Mansfield, 2001) used differential reinforcement and extinction to reduce wandering. Tangible reinforcers (e.g., food) and attention were given when subjects were not wandering

Excessive Vocalizations

Excessive vocalizations are often the result of overstimulation, understimulation, or affective or physiological pain. When excessive vocalizations were thought to result from a lack of, or excess, environmental stimulation, Burgio et al. (1994) tried adding auditory and tactile stimulation, but none of their interventions was reliably associated with decrease in the vocalizations. However, the researchers noted that some subjects responded to each of the interventions, suggesting that an individualized approach is necessary. An unexpected finding of this study revealed that residents under the hairdryer had a very low rate of vocalizations, suggesting that white noise might be effective in reducing vocalizations. Burgio, Scilley, Harding, Hsu, and Yancy (1996) piloted the use of white noise by using gentle ocean and mountain stream audio tapes, played through headphones, to decrease the frequency of vocalizations among residents displaying significant baseline rates of vocalizations. Although this was a very small study, there was a 23% decrease in vocalizations when listening to the audiotapes.

Buchanan and Fisher (2002) reported a decrease in excessive vocalizations by two elderly persons with dementia who were residing in a nursing home. These researchers used noncontingent reinforcement (NCR), a procedure that involves presenting a stimulus with a known reinforcing value on a specific schedule regardless of what the person is doing. A functional analysis was performed to determine stimuli that were reinforcing. Music and attention were provided continuously to one subject, and attention alone on a fixed schedule (every 160 seconds) to the other subject. The intervention resulted in a decrease in vocalizations for both subjects. Unfortunately, only modest reductions were achieved for the second subject, despite a significant amount of attention. Behavioral techniques can thus be effective. However, as this study highlights, the positive effects gained need to be considered within the context of the labor required to accomplish the results. In situations where the behavior is very disruptive, it is often worth the added effort and improves the quality of life of all involved.

Woods and Ashley (1995) reported a significant reduction of vocalizations through the use of simulated presence therapy (SPT). A "significant other's" presence is simulated in the person's environment via an audiotape that plays half of a normal spontaneous conversation and recounts cherished memories. Nursing staff turned on the audiotape when an individual's vocalizations were most likely to occur. Audiotape use is intended to increase social interaction. Other studies have not found significant results using SPT. However, treatment fidelity data indicated very low use of the audiotapes, which may have contributed to the lack of significant results. Video respite (VR), a technique involving simple, engaging videotapes made professionally or informally by family members, has been used as a distraction for older adults with vocalizations. Lund, Hill, Caserta, and Wright (1995) reported a decrease in vocalizations and agitation with the use both a 53-minute music tape made by a professional music therapist inviting the listener to sing along, and a 33-minute "friendly visitor" tape that asked questions about familiar things such as parents, childhood, animals, and holidays. Although these studies have limitations, the interventions show promise and are being investigated in newer, better controlled studies.

Sexually Inappropriate Behavior

Although relatively infrequent, when this behavior does occur, it is particularly troublesome to family members and observers. Few studies of behavioral techniques to manage this behavior have been conducted. Stimulus control has been effective with brain-injured clients (Zencius, Wesolowshki, Burke, & Hough, 1990) and may be helpful in persons with dementia.

Goal Setting

Behavioral interventions are designed to change factors in the environment in order to eliminate, decrease, increase, or change countable and observable behaviors. Identify specific, measurable changes in the behavior that indicate that the intervention has been successful in meeting the goal. These can described in terms of an increase in positive behaviors, such as engagement in conversation when approached by a caregiver for a person who has been withdrawn. They may also be stated as a decrease in the number of negative behaviors, such as the number of times a person hits or yells in a specified time frame.

Developing the Plan

Information gathered during the assessment phase should be used to develop hypotheses about the factors related to the behavior. For example, a person's polite refusal to take a bath may be ignored by the caregiver. This failure to comply with the person's wishes may lead to resistance or aggression when the caregiver attempts to proceed with the unwanted bath. Interventions are designed using hypotheses regarding the etiology of the behavior as well as knowledge of the person's skills, deficits, and preferences. For instance, if it appears that the person's behavior is the result of specific cognitive deficits, a method for utilizing the person's cognitive strengths to compensate for these deficits should be devised. If the person's distress is caused by pain, treatment of physical illnesses and medication adjustments may be needed. Other interventions for pain include altering the response of caregivers or suggesting the purchase of different equipment and supplies. As stated in Attix (Chapter 10, this volume), interventions must be developed with input from those involved and be both practical and realistic. Discuss the pros and cons of each potential intervention with the caregiver to judge which is most likely to be effective.

Monitoring and Revising the Plan

Once interventions have been implemented, monitor the results closely. Data on the success of the interventions can be gathered on the same instruments used for assessment, or a special record sheet can be developed and completed by the caregiver. Other useful tools for monitoring progress and assess changes in antecedents and consequences of the behavior are the BTL and the BOR (see Figures 17.1 and 17.2).

If the plan is successful and the behavior improves, continue with the plan. If the targeted behavior gets worse or does not improve, then look for other possible causes and interventions. Change the plan as new hypotheses emerge. For example, a Spanish-speaking, cognitively impaired patient at a local hospital refused to wear his identification bracelet. Because this bracelet was essential for identification of his medications and other treatments, the team referred the patient for a behavior plan. On initial assessment, we learned from an interpreter that the reason for the refusal was that the patient's name was misspelled. A new bracelet was made, but the patient still would not wear it. When talking with nursing staff, we learned that the patient liked jewelry. A metal identification bracelet was considered, but we decided to try a watch with the patient's name and hospital number on the band first, because it would be something that was familiar to the patient. The patient was delighted with his new watch and has been wearing it without problem for over 2 months.

The intervention planning and implementation process is highlighted in a case study described in Table 17.4. As with many cases, working with the person involved a trial-and-error process, and the initial plan needed revision. However, the result was an individualized bathing care plan that kept Mrs. P comfortable and warm. She no longer cried in the shower, and her complaints of pain and cold were greatly reduced.

GENERAL GUIDELINES AND TIPS FOR SPECIFIC BEHAVIORAL SYMPTOMS

Simple interventions can often be surprisingly effective in reducing behavioral symptoms. Although similar behaviors may have different etiologies and meanings for different individuals, there are some general strategies that are helpful when working who display persons with behavioral symptoms. These include the following:

- *Assess and treat physical factors first.* Changes in medication, sudden illness, nutritional deficiency, and sensory/perceptual changes can all impact the person's behavior. Check these before initiating behavioral treatment.

TABLE 17.4. Case Study of Implementation and Planning

Describe the behavior

Mrs. P did not want to shower and refused to be showered at least 50% of the time. She had an odor, her hair looked dirty, and her son asked that she be showered more frequently. When transferred to the shower chair, she looked anxious and shouted. While being showered, she cried and complained of pain and being cold almost constantly. She also asked staff to hurry up. Sometimes she mixed up words, saying, for example, that the water was too hot when she really meant too cold.

Describe personal factors

Mrs. P was 93 years old and very proud of having been a school teacher. She had one son, who visited regularly. She had been very active in her church and had also enjoyed reading, cooking, and baking. She made women's clothes, liked fashion, and was careful about her appearance. She had entered a nursing home 2 years prior, after fracturing her hip. Her affect was usually bright and she enjoyed activities and visiting with friends and family. Her diagnoses included arthritis, peripheral neuropathy (from diabetes), limited vision and hearing, and AD. The diabetes was controlled by diet. She had an order for acetaminophen four times a day, as necessary, for pain, but she rarely received it. She was nonambulatory and incontinent of both urine and stool. She could feed herself but required assistance. Neuropsychological testing was not done because the diagnosis was clear. She had severe deficits in memory and executive functioning. She could understand one-step instructions but sometimes had difficulty expressing her needs verbally. She lacked insight into her deficits but was cooperative with care, with the exception of showering.

Describe environmental factors

The bathing chair in the bathroom was a standard one, made of plastic pipe with a hard seat, and the room temperature was cool. There were no wall decorations and the room had an institutional look.

Develop a hypothesis regarding the antecedents/triggers to the behavior

After this initial assessment, it was felt that her major sources of distress came from her needs for comfort, warmth, and security. She had many possible sources of pain—arthritis, her previous hip fracture, and peripheral neuropathy. The initial plan, therefore, focused on personal and environmental triggers and interventions to reduce pain and increase warmth.

Plan

It was recommended that acetaminophen be given routinely early in the morning, so that it would be effective by shower time. The shower chair was cushioned with a padded seat, and the room was warmed by turning on the heat lamp before bringing her in. She was kept covered with towels while showering; the caregiver lifted the towels to wash small areas and then rinsed them with a hand-held nozzle. In addition, church music was played softly in an effort to distract and relax her, though it was difficult to know how much she understood because of her hearing loss and the fact that the music echoed in the bathroom.

Assessment and modification of plan

Mrs. P's complaints decreased, but she continued to cry for at least 50% of the shower. Additional pain medication (a narcotic) was tried prior to the shower, but her pain complaints, mostly related to being moved, did not change, and the medication only made her drowsy. Looking again at the physical environment, the water spray of the hand-held nozzle seemed to trigger her cries and increase her discomfort and her leg pain. In response to this observation she was washed with baby-soft washcloths, using a no-rinse soap solution in a basin; the caregiver kept her covered and warm the entire time, lifting the towels to wash each area.

At the same time, different distraction interventions were tried when she appeared anxious. The nursing assistant sang hymns with her; "The Old Rugged Cross" was a favorite. Mrs. P was given small plastic figurines to hold and comment on, and the nursing assistant talked with her about her son or her work in the church. This plan worked especially well just before a difficult procedure, such as washing her buttocks. Before the nursing assistant touched an area that might be painful or experienced as intrusive, she also told Mrs. P that she was going to touch her and assured her that she would be careful. If Mrs. P complained, the nursing assistant apologized and adjusted her approach to address Mrs. P's need, such as covering an area or readjusting her in the shower chair. Her feet were soaked in a basin of comforting warm water while other parts of her body were being washed, and she found this soothing.

We consulted a physical therapist to learn techniques to make transfers less painful. A sliding board transfer was recommended. This method decreased Mrs. P's complaints slightly. Because it seemed that fear and anxiety were also playing a role, we asked her to count with the nursing assistant before being transferred; this yielded fewer complaints of pain and fear.

Finally, recalling that she had been careful about her appearance in the past, we gave her a mirror to hold. As Mrs. P held the mirror, the nursing assistant commented on how nice she would look after the bath. The nursing assistant also shared simple jokes with her and sometimes could get her to laugh.

Because Mrs. P disliked having her hair washed, an appointment was made for her at the beauty parlor. Since this was an activity she enjoyed prior to the onset of dementia, she tolerated the process and expressed few complaints.

Results

This was a trial-and-error process. The result was an individualized bathing care plan that worked for Mrs. P. Measurable improvements included the following behaviors:

- She showered willingly.
- She no longer cried.
- Complaints of pain decreased from 10 per bath to fewer than 5 per bath.
- Complaints of being cold decreased from 15 per bath to fewer than 3.
- She showed interest in the conversation with the nursing assistant and in the objects presented to her as a means of distraction.
- She thanked the nursing assistant for her help.

Note. Adapted from Barrick, Rader, Hoeffer, and Sloane (2002). Copyright 2002 by Springer Publishing Company. Adapted by permission.

- *Keep it simple.* Simple, well-established routines can help persons with dementia remain calm and perform to the best of their abilities.
- *Reduce environmental stress.* Environments can be confusing to persons with dementia. Reduce unnecessary noise and extra people and remove misleading stimuli.
- *Be flexible.* Modify the approach to meet the person's need. Modification may involve adapting the method, the physical environment, and/or the procedure. For example, a bed bath rather than a shower may be indicated if a person is anxious, afraid, or in pain due to the equipment or the procedure of showering.
- *Focus more on the person than the task.* The process and relationship are more important than the task; meeting the individual preferences of the person requires observing his or her feelings and reactions and adapting the approach to fit his or her needs.
- *Respond to the person's feelings rather than the facts of the situation.* The person may misperceive the situation; empathize and reassure rather than trying to explain.

In difficult cases, to get the best results, tailor interventions to the specific needs of the person and symptom. Suggested strategies for potential causes of specific behaviors are listed in Table 17.5. These strategies are based primarily on clinical experience and are not exhaustive.

TABLE 17.5. Suggested Strategies for Management of Behavior Problems in Patients with Dementia

Behavior	Potential causes or antecedents	Management strategies
Difficulty with personal care tasks	• Task too difficult or overwhelming • Caregiver impatience, rushing • Cannot remember task • Pain involved with movement • Cannot understand or follow caregiver instructions • Fear of task; cannot understand need for task or instructions • Inertia, apraxia; difficulty initiating and completing a task	• Divide task into small, successive steps. • Be patient, allow ample time, or try again later. • Demonstrate action or task; allow person to perform parts of the task that can still be accomplished. • Treat underlying condition; consider pain medication or physiotherapy; modify or assist the movement needed. • Repeat request simply; state instructions one step at a time. • Reassure, comfort, distract from task with music or conversation; ask patient to help perform the task. • Set up task sequence by arranging materials (such as clothing) in the order to be used; help begin the task.
Incontinence	• Infection, prostate problem, chronic illness, medication side effect, stress or urge incontinence • Difficulty in finding bathroom • Lack of privacy • Difficulty undressing • Difficulty in seeing toilet • Impaired mobility • Dependence created by socialized reinforcement • Cannot express need • Task overwhelming	• Evaluate medically. • Place signs/picture on door; ensure adequate lighting. • Provide for privacy. • Simplify clothing; use elastic waistbands. • Use contrasting colors on toilet and floor. • Evaluate medically, treat associated pain (include physiotherapy); provide a commode; reduce diuretics when possible. • Provide increased attention for continence rather than incontinence; allow independence whenever possible, even if time consuming. • Schedule toileting (such as every 2 hours while awake); reduce diuretics and bedtime liquids when possible. • Simplify; establish step-by-step routine.
Sleep disturbance	• Illness, pain, medication effect (e.g., causing daytime sleep or nocturnal awakening) • Depression • Less need for sleep • Too hot, too cold • Disorientation from darkness • Caffeine or alcohol effect • Hunger • Urge to void • Normal age- and disease-related fragmentation of sleep (like that of an infant or toddler) • Daytime sleeping • Fear of darkness; restless	• Evaluate medically. • Prescribe antidepressant (consider bedtime sedative such as trazodone). • Schedule later bedtime; allow activities or tasks safely done at night; plan more daytime exercise. • Adjust temperature. • Use night-lights. • Reduce or eliminate alcohol; limit caffeine after noon. • Provide nighttime snack. • Ensure clear, well-lit pathway to bathroom. • Accept; plan for safety. • Eliminate or limit naps; provide activity and exercise instead; for naps, use recliner rather than bed. • Provide soft music, massage, night-light.

Wandering	• Stress—noise, clutter, crowding • Lost; looking for someone or something familiar • Restless, bored—no stimuli • Medication side effect • Lifelong pattern of being active or usual coping style • Needing to use the toilet • Environmental stimuli—exit signs, people leaving	• Reduce excessive stimulation. • Provide familiar objects, signs, pictures; offer to help find objects or place; reassure. • Provide meaningful activity. • Monitor, reduce, or discontinue medication. • Respond to underlying mood or motivation; provide safe area to move about (e.g., secured circular path). • Institute toileting schedule (such as every 2 hours); place signs or pictures on bathroom door. • Remove or camouflage environmental stimuli; provide identification or alarm bracelets.
Agitation (also "sundowning," catastrophic reactions)	• Discomfort, pain • Physical illness (such as urinary tract infection) • Fatigue • Overstimulation—noise, overhead paging, people, radio, television, activities • Mirroring of caregiver's affect • Overextending capabilities (resulting in failure); caregiver expectations too high • Patient is being "quizzed" (multiple questions that exceed abilities) • Medication side effect • Patient is thwarted from desired activity (e.g., attempting to escape) • Lowered stress threshold • Unfamiliar people or environment; change in schedule or routine • Restless	• Assess and manage sources of pain, constipation, infection, or full bladder; check clothing for comfort. • Evaluate medically; eliminate caffeine and alcohol. • Schedule adequate rest; monitor activity. • Reduce noise, stress; remove from situation; use television sparingly; limit crowding (e.g., dining hallways just before meals). • Control affect; model calmness with low tone and slow rate; use support system and groups for outlet. • Do not put person in failure-oriented situations or tasks; understand losses and reduce expectations accordingly. • Avoid persistent testing of memory; pose one question at a time; eliminate questions that require abstract thought, insight, or reasoning. • Assess, monitor, and reduce medication if possible; monitor health concerns • Redirect energy to similar activity; ask patient to help with meaningful activity; have diversionary tactics for outbursts; choose battles—assess whether behavior is merely irritating, rather than compromising patient safety or obstructing care. • Simplify tasks, create calm; lower expectations and demands; avoid arguments and reprimands. • Be consistent; avoid changes, surprises; introduce any change gradually. • Plan calming music, massage, or meaningful activities; assign tasks that provide exercise.

(continued)

TABLE 17.5. (*continued*)

Behavior	Potential causes or antecedents	Management strategies
Aggression (physical, verbal)	• Discomfort, pain • Doesn't understand what's happening • Fatigue • Fear • Physical illness • Feeling lack of sense of control • Hunger • Cannot inhibit behavior	• Assess and manage source of pain; provide ample support on transfers; adapt equipment; stop what you are doing; apologize; warn; distract. • Explain each step; match communication to abilities; slow down; distract. • Come back later. • Provide physical and verbal support; reassure; distract (e.g., engage in singing, give something of interest to hold, take to quiet environment). • Evaluate medically. • Honor preferences; give choices; be flexible and stay calm; have the person help; ask permission; tell the person firmly that the behavior is unacceptable, such as "Stop hitting" or "That hurts." • Give something to eat or drink. • Identify mildly agitated behaviors and take action before behavior escalates.
Suspiciousness, paranoia	• Forgot where objects were placed • Misinterpreting actions or words • Misinterpreting who people are; suspicious of their intentions • Change in environment or routine • Misinterpreting environment • Physical illness • Social isolation • Someone is actually taking something from patient	Offer to help find; have more that one of same object available; have a list where objects should be placed; learn favorite hiding places. • Do not argue or try to reason; do not take personally; distract. • Introduce self and role routinely; draw on old memory, connections; do not argue. • Reassure, familiarize, set routine. • Assess vision, hearing; modify environment, as needed; explain misinterpretation simply; distract. • Evaluate medically. • Encourage and provide familiar social opportunities. • Verify the situation.
Inappropriate or impulsive sexual behavior	• Dementia-related decreased judgment and social awareness • Misinterpreting caregiver's interaction • Uncomfortable—too warm, clothing too tight; need to void, genital irritation • Need for attention, affection, intimacy • Self-stimulating, reacting to what feels good	Do not overreact or confront; respond calmly and firmly; distract and redirect. • Do not give mixed sexual message (e.g., double entendres and innuendos, even in jest); avoid nonverbal messages; distract while performing personal care, bathing. • Check room temperature; assist with comfortable weather-appropriate clothing; ensure that elimination needs are met; examine for groin rash, perineal skin problems, stool impaction. • Increase or meet basic need for touch and warmth; model appropriate touch; offer soothing objects (such as stuffed animals); provide hand or back massage. • Offer privacy; remove from inappropriate place.

Note. Adapted from Carlson, Fleming, Smith, and Evans (1995). Copyright 1995 by the Mayo Clinic. Adapted by permission.

PHARMACOLOGICAL TREATMENTS

When a person is not responding well to behavioral treatment alone, a psychiatric referral for consideration of medication may be necessary and beneficial. Individuals vary greatly in their response to medication, and several factors must be considered. These include stability of medical problems, past response to medications, family history of response to medications, and tolerance for side effects. Expert consensus guidelines have been developed to assist in the selection of first- and second-line treatments (Alexopoulus, Abrams, Young, & Shamoian, 1998). For example, in the guidelines conventional high-potency antipsychotics such as Haldol in small doses have been recommended for psychosis and severe aggression. For mild, long-term aggression, selective serotonin reuptake inhibitors (SSRIs), trazodone, and busiprone may be beneficial. Depakote has been helpful in the treatment of aggression, anger, and hypersexual behavior. Trazodone, although technically an antidepressant, is commonly prescribed for insomnia. Benzodiazepines can be used but are recommended for only short periods.

SUMMARY

Dementia is often accompanied by noncognitive symptoms such as combativeness, agitation, and functional behavioral deficits. These symptoms have a significant impact on the lives of those with the disease and their caregivers. The causes of these symptoms are often an interaction between the person, individuals in the care environment, and physical environmental factors. Behavioral interventions can be very effective in managing these symptoms and improving the quality of day-to-day life. Several researchers have reported promising results in the prevention of functional behavioral deficits, incontinence, and sleep disorders as well as the reduction of agitation, aggression, and other behavioral "excesses."

Implementation of behavioral interventions requires assessment of the person, the behavior, and the possible causes or triggers of the behavior; identification of specific, measurable goals; development and implementation of an individualized plan; and revision of the plan, as needed. Methods for assessment, intervention, and evaluation are described as well as a number of interventions that have been successful in clinical practice and research studies. A case study is included that illustrates this process.

Behavioral interventions, although efficacious, can be labor intensive. The realities of clinical practice often mean that time is limited and data are incomplete. Caregivers may need to be trained in such areas as gathering data and assessing causes. They may also have to learn to make consistent, supportive responses when behaviors occur. Available equipment may have to be adapted when resources are limited. However, there are a variety of ways to deal with a problem, and interventions can be adapted to fit the needs of the situation.

Often simple, safe, and practical behavioral interventions can result in significant improvement in symptoms. Sometimes something as simple as attending to a person's needs by using towels to keep him or her warm during a bath or distracting a person with candy or conversation during a painful care task can reduce agitation by as much as 50%. At other times a combination of behavioral and pharmacological treatments, such as pain medication or neuroleptics, is necessary. The improved care experience can have a very favorable effect on both the person with dementia and his or her caregivers. It is a "win–win" situation!

REFERENCES

Adkins, V. K., & Matthews, R. M. (1997). Prompted voiding to reduce incontinence in community dwelling older adults. *Journal of Applied Behavioral Analysis, 30*(1), 153–156.

Alessi, C. A., Yoon, E. J., Schnelle, J. F., Al-Samarrai, N. R., & Cruise, P. A. (1999). A randomized trial of a combined physical activity and environmental intervention in nursing home residents: Do sleep and agitation improve? *Journal of the American Geriatrics Society, 47*(7), 784–791.

Alexopoulos, G. S., Abrams, R. C., Young, R. C., & Shamoian, C. A. (1988). Cornell Scale for Depression in Dementia. *Biological Psychiatry, 23*, 271–284.

Algase, D. L. (1992). Cognitive discriminants of wandering among nursing home residents. *Nursing Research, 41*(2), 78–81.

Allen-Burge, R., Stevens, A. R., & Burgio, L. D. (1999). Effective behavioral interventions for decreasing dementia-related challenging behavior in nursing homes. *International Journal of Geriatric Psychiatry, 14*, 213–232.

Aneshensel, L., Pearlin, L., & Schuler, R. (1993). Stress, role captivity and the cessation of caregiving. *Journal of Health and Social Behavior, 34*, 54–70.

Baltes, M. M., & Werner-Wahl, H. W. (1987). Dependence in Aging. In L. Carstensen & B. Edelstein (Eds.), *Handbook of Clinical Gerontology* (pp. 204–221). New York: Pergamon Press.

Baltes, M. M., & Wahl, H. W. (1992). The dependency support script in institutions: Generalization to community settings. *Psychology and Aging, 7*, 409–418.

Baltes, M. M., & Zerbe, M. (1976). Independence training in the nursing home resident. *Gerontologist, 16*, 428–432.

Baltes, P. B., & Baltes, M. M. (1990). Psychological perspectives on successful aging: The model of selective optimization with compensation. In P. B. Baltes & M. M. Baltes (Eds.), *Successful aging: Perspectives from the behavioral sciences (pp. 1–34). New York: Cambridge University Press.

Barrick, A. L., Rader, J., Hoeffer, B., & Sloane, P. D. (2002). *Bathing without a battle: Personal care of individuals with dementia.* New York: Springer.

Baumgarten, M., Becker, R., & Gauthier, S. (1990). Validity and reliability of the Dementia Behavior Disturbance Scale. *Journal of the American Geriatrics Society, 38*, 221–226.

Beck, C. (1988). Measurement of dressing performance in persons with dementia. *American Journal of Alzheimer's Care and Related Disorders and Research, 3*(3), 21–25.

Beck, C. K., Heacock, P., Rapp, C. G., & Mercer, S. O. (1993). Assisting cognitively impaired elders with activities of daily living. *American Journal of Alzheimer's Care and Related Disorders and Research, 8*(6), 11–20.

Bridges-Parlet, S., Knopman, D., & Thompson, T. (1994). A descriptive study of physically aggressive behavior in dementia by direct observation. *Journal of the American Geriatrics Society, 42*, 192–197.

Buchanan, J. A., & Fisher, J. E. (2002). Functional assessment and noncontingent reinforcement in the treatment of disruptive vocalization in elderly dementia patients. *Journal of Applied Behavior Analysis, 35*(1), 99–103.

Burgener, S. C., Jirove, M., Murrell, L., & Barton, D. (1992). Caregiver and environmental variables related to difficult behaviors in institutionalized, demented elderly persons. *Journal of Gerontology, 47*(4), 242–249.

Burgio, L. D. (1996). Direct observation of behavioral disturbances of dementia and their environmental context. *International Journal of Psychogeriatrics, 8*(3), 343–349.

Burgio, L. D., & Bourgeois, M. (1992). Treating severe behavioral disorders in geriatric residential settings. *Behavioral Residential Treatment, 7*(2), 145–168.

Burgio, L. D., Butler, F., & Engel, B. T. (1988). Nurses' attitudes towards geriatric behavior problems in long-term care settings. *Clinical Gerontologist, 7*(3/4), 23–34.

Burgio, L. D., Cotter, E. M., & Stevens, A. B. (1996). Treatment in residential settings. In M. Hersen & V. Van Hasselt (Eds.), *Psychological treatment of older adults: An introductory textbook* (127–145). New York: Plenum Press.

Burgio, L. D., Scilley, K., Hardin, J. M., Hsu, C., & Yancy, J. (1996). Environmental "white noise": An intervention for verbally agitated nursing home residents. *Journals of Gerontology: Psychological Sciences, 51B*, P364–P373.

Burgio, L. D., Scilley, K., Hardin, J. M., Janosky, J., Bonino, P., Cadman, S., et al. (1994). Studying disruptive vocalization and contextual factors in the nursing home using computer-assisted real-time observation. *Journal of Gerontological and Psychological Sciences, 49*, 230–239.

Burgio, L. D., & Stevens, A. B. (1999). Behavioral interventions and motivational systems in the nursing home. *Annual Review of Gerontology and Geriatrics, 18*, 284–320.

Carlson, D. L., Fleming, K. C., Smith, G. E., & Evans, J. M. (1995). Management of dementia-related behavioral disturbances: A nonpharmacologic approach. *Mayo Clinic Proceedings, 70*, 1108–1115.

Chrisman, M., Tabar, D., Whall, A. L., & Booth, D. E. (1991). Agitated behavior in the cognitively impaired elderly. *Journal of Gerontological Nursing, 17*(12), 9–13.

Cohen-Mansfield, J., Marx, M. S., & Rosenthal, A. S. (1989). A description of agitation in a nursing home. *Journals of Gerontology, 44*, M77–M84.

Cohen-Mansfield, J., Marx, M. S., & Rosenthal, A. S. (1990). Dementia and agitation in nursing home residents: How are they related? *Psychology and Aging, 5*, 3–8.

Cohen-Mansfield, J., & Werner, P. (1998). The effects of an enhanced environment on nursing home residents who pace. *Gerontologists, 38*, 199–208.

Cohen-Mansfield, J. C. (2001). Nonpharmacologic interventions for inappropriate behaviors in dementia. *American Journal of Psychiatry, 9*(4), 361–381.

Colenda, C. C., & Hamer, R. M. (1991). Antecedents and intervention for aggressive behavior of patients: A geropsychiatric state hospital. *Hospital and Community Psychiatry, 42*, 287–292.

Davis, L. (1997). Family conflicts around dementia home care. *Families, Systems, and Health, 15*, 85–98.

Drachman, D. A., Swearer J. A., O'Donnel, B. F., Mitchell A. L., & Malloon, A. (1992). The Caretaker Obstreperous-Behavior Rating Assessment (COBRA) scale. *Journal of the American Geriatrics Society, 40*, 463–470.

Everitt, D. E., Fields, D. R., Soumerai, S. S., & Avorn, J. (1991). Resident behavior and staff distress in the nursing home. *Journal of the American Geriatrics Society, 39*, 792–798.

Feldt, K., & Ryden, M. (1992). Aggressive behaviors: Educating nursing assistants. *Journal of Gerontological Nursing, 18*(5), 3–12.

Fisher, J. E. (1995, August). *Agitation and adaptation: Functional characteristics of the behavior of dementia patients.* Paper presented at the annual convention of the American Psychological Association, New York.

Fisher, J. E. (1997). Contextual factors in the assessment and management of aggression in dementia patients. *Cognitive and Behavioral Practice, 4*(1), 171–190.

Fisher, J. E., Swingen, D. N., & Harsin, C. M. (2001). Agitated and aggressive behavior. In A. S. Bellack & M. Hersen (Eds.), *Comprehensive Clinical Psychology: Vol 7. Clinical Geropsychology* (pp. 413–432). New York: Elsevier Science.

Gerdner, L. A., & Buckwalter, K. C. (1994). A nursing challenge: Assessment and management of agitation in Alzheimer's patients. *Journal of Gerontological Nursing, 20*, 11–12.

Goldsmith, S. M., Hoetter, B., & Rader, J. (1995). Problematic wandering behavior in the cognitively impaired elderly: A single-subject case study. *Journal of Psychosocial Nursing Mental Health Services, 33*(2) 6–12.

Hall, G. R., Gerdner, L., Zwygart-Stauffacher, M., & Buckwalter, K. C. (1995). Principles of nonpharmacological management: Caring for people with Alzheimer's disease using a conceptual model. *Psychiatric Annals, 25*(7), 432–440.

Hallberg, I. R., & Norberg, A. (1993). Strain among nurses and their emotional reactions during one year of systematic clinical supervision combined with the implementation of individualized care in dementia care: Comparison between an experimental ward and a control ward. *Journal of Advanced Nursing, 18,* 1860–1875.

Hoeffer, B., Rader, J., McKenzie, D., Lavelle, M., & Stewart, B. (1997). Reducing aggressive behavior during bathing cognitively impaired nursing home residents. *Journal of Gerontological Nursing, 23*(5), 16–23.

Hoeffer, B., Talerico, K. A., Rasin, J., Mitchell, C. M., Stewart, B., McKenzie, D., et al. (2005). *The effects on caregiver outcomes of a person-centered approach with shower and towel bath methods for reducing agitated and aggressive behaviors of cognitively impaired nursing home residents during bathing.* Manuscript in preparation.

Hurley, A. C., Volcier, J., Hanrahan, P. A., Houde, S., & Volcier, L (1992). Assessment of discomfort in advanced Alzheimer patients. *Research in Nursing and Health, 15*(5), 369–377.

Hussian, R. A. (1981). *Geriatric psychology: A behavioral perspective.* New York: Van Nostrand Reinhold.

Hussian, R. A., & Davis, R. L. (1985). *Responsive care: Behavioral interventions with elderly persons.* Champaign, IL: Research Press.

Kovach, C. R., & Meyer-Arnold, E. A. (1996). Coping with conflicting agenda: The bathing experience of cognitively impaired older adults. *Scholarly Inquiry for Nursing Practice: An International Journal, 10*(1), 23–42.

Levy, M. L., Miller, B. L., Cummings, J. L., Fairbanks, L. A., & Craig, A. (1996). Alzheimer disease and frontotemporal dementias: Behavioral distinctions. *Archives of Neurology, 53,* 687–690.

Lund, D. A., Hill, R. D., Caserta, M. S., & Wright, S. D. (1995). Video respite: An innovative resource for family, professional caregivers, and persons with dementia. *Gerontologist, 35,* 683–687.

Marx, M. S., Werner, P., & Cohen-Mansfield, J. (1989). Agitation and touch in the nursing home. *Psychological Reports, 64*(3, Pt. 2), 1019–1026.

Matteson, M. A., Linton, A. D., & Barnes, S. J. (1997). Management of problematic behavioral symptoms associated with dementia: A cognitive developmental approach. *Aging and Clinical and Experimental Research, 9,* 342–355.

Meddaugh, D. I. (1990). Reactance: Understanding aggressive behavior in long-term care. *Journal of Psychosocial Nursing, 28*(4), 28–33.

Melzack, R. (1975). The McGill Pain Questionnaire: Major properties and scoring methods. *Pain, 1,* 277–299.

Mentes, J. C., & Ferraro, J. (1989). Calming aggressive reactions: A preventive program. *Journal of Gerontological Nursing, 15*(2), 22–27.

Miller, M. F. (1997). Physically aggressive behavior during hygienic care. *Journal of Gerontological Nursing, 23*(5), 24–39.

Moak, G. S., & Fisher, W. H. (1990). Alzheimer's disease and related disorders in state mental hospitals: Data from a nationwide survey. *Gerontologist, 30*(6), 798–802.

Mungas, D., Weiler, P., Franzi, C., & Henry, R. (1989). Assessment of disruptive behavior associated with dementia: The Disruptive Behavior Rating Scales. *Journal of Geriatric Psychiatry and Neurology, 2,* 196–202.

National Center for Health Statistics. (n.d.). *Data warehouse on trends in health and aging.* Retrieved January 22, 2004, from www.cdc.gov/nchs/agingact.htm.

Okawa, M., Mishima, K., Hishikawa, Y., Hozumi, S., Hori, H., & Takahashi, K. (1991). Circadian rhythm disorders in sleep–waking and body temperature in elderly patients with dementia and their treatment. *Sleep, 14,* 478–485.

Petrie, W., Lawson, E., & Hollendar, M. (1982). Violence in geriatric patients. *Journal of the American Medical Association, 248,* 443–444.

Reisberg, B., Borenstein, J., Salob, S. P., Ferris, S. H., Franssen, E., & Georgotas, A. (1987). Behavioral symptoms in Alzheimer's disease: Phenomenology and treatment. *Journal of Clinical Psychiatry, 48*(Suppl. 5), 9–15.

Rosenberger, Z., & MacLean, J. (1983). Behavioral assessment and treatment of "organic" behaviors in an institutionalized geriatric patient. *International Journal of Behavioral Geriatrics, 1*, 33–46.

Ryden, M. B. (1988). Aggressive behavior in persons with dementia who live in the community. *Alzheimer's Disease and Associated Disorders, 2*, 342–355.

Ryden, M. B., Bossenmaier, M., & McLachlan, C. (1991). Aggressive behavior in cognitively impaired nursing home residents. *Research in Nursing and Health, 14*(2), 87–95.

Schulz, R., O'Brien, A. T., Bookwala, J., & Fleissner, K. (1995). Psychiatric and physical morbidity effects of dementia caregiving: Prevalence, correlates, and causes. *Gerontologists, 35*, 771–791.

Sloane, P. D., Hoeffer, B., Mitchell, C. M., McKensie, D. A., Barrick, A. L., Rader, J., et al. (2004). Effect of person-centered showering and the towel bath on bathing-associated aggression, agitation and discomfort in nursing home residents with dementia: A randomized, controlled trial. *Journal of the American Geriatrics Society, 52*, 1795–1804.

Swearer, J. M., Drachman, D. A., O'Donnell, B. F., & Mitchell, A. L. (1988). Troublesome and disruptive behaviors in dementia: Relationships to diagnosis and disease severity. *Journal of the American Geriatrics Society, 36*, 784–790.

Tekin, S., Mega, M. S., Masterman, D. M., Chow, T., Garakain, J., Vinter, H. V., et al. (2001). Orbitofrontal and anterior cingulated cortex: Neurofibrillary tangle burden is associated with agitation in Alzheimer's disease. *Annals of Neurology, 49*, 355–361.

Teri, L., Borson, S., Kiyak, A., & Yamagishi, M. (1989). Behavioral disturbance, cognitive dysfunction, and functional skill: Prevalence and relationship in Alzheimer's disease. *Journal of the American Geriatrics Society, 37*, 109–116.

Teri, L., & Logsdon, R. G. (1991). Identifying pleasant activities for Alzheimer's disease patients: The Pleasant Events Schedule—AD. *Gerontologist, 31*, 124–127.

Willis, S. L., Allen-Burge, R., Dolan, M., Bertrand, R., Yesavage, J., & Taylor, J. (1998). Everyday problem solving among individuals with Alzheimer's disease. *Gerontologist, 38*, 569–577.

Wilson, B. A., Cockburn, J., & Halligan, P. (1987). *Behavioral Inattention Test.* Bury St. Edmunds, UK: Thames Valley Test Company.

Winger, J., Schirm, V., & Steward, D. (1987). Aggressive behavior in long-term care. *Journal of Psychosocial Nursing, 25*(4), 28–33.

Woods, P., & Ashley, J. (1995). Simulated presence therapy: Using selected memories to manage problem behaviors in Alzheimer's disease patients. *Geriatric Nursing, 16*, 9–14.

Young, S. H., Muir-Nash, J., & Ninos, M. (1988) Managing nocturnal wandering behavior. *Journal of Gerontological Nursing, 14*, 6–12.

Zencius, A., Wesolowshki, M. D., Burke, W. H., & Hough, S. (1990). Managing hypersexual disorders in brain-injured clients. *Brain Injury, 4*(2), 175–181.

18

Group Psychotherapy Approaches for Dementia

GUY G. POTTER
DEBORAH K. ATTIX
CORY K. CHEN

As has been well expressed in other chapters of this book, cognitive impairment in older adults has multiple etiologies that produce a range of neuropsychological and behavioral manifestations. Because of this range, treatment of cognitive impairment in older adults, particularly with regard to dementia, requires multimodal intervention strategies that are informed by a solid scientific understanding of the etiology and symptomatology of this condition. Although there have been significant advances in identifying the neuropsychological and behavioral sequelae of geriatric cognitive disorders, less is known about intrapersonal factors and how these contribute to treatment outcome. What is known is that these individuals experience depression, social isolation, grief, family discord, and other forms of psychological distress that can exacerbate cognitive and functional disability when left untreated (Koltai & Branch, 1999). Behavior problems resulting from psychological distress are associated with decreased caregiver well-being (Ballard, Lowery, Powell, O'Brien, & James, 2000) and increased likelihood of institutionalization (Balesteri, Grossberg, & Grossberg, 2000). Fortunately, psychological distress is a modifiable factor that can often be improved through psychotherapy—which makes this mode of intervention an important part of a comprehensive strategy for managing dementia.

Psychotherapeutic treatments for geriatric cognitive disorders include individual, group, and caregiver-based interventions. Interventions for patients with Alzheimer's disease (AD) predominate over those for other cognitive disorders, owing to its prevalence and the care demands associated with its typical course of progressive debilitation. Although interventions for dementia and other geriatric cognitive disorders have long been practiced, empirical studies of treatment outcomes have been slower to emerge. In the current care climate, however, the increasing number of individuals diagnosed at early stages of cognitive impairment, in conjunction with demand for clinically efficacious treatments, has highlighted the need for psychotherapeutic interventions that have empirical support. Reviews of the psychotherapeutic treatments for dementia do identify interventions that appear efficacious, but conclude that, on the whole, there is still limited empirical support to guide treatment planning for the diverse treatment needs of individuals and families living with dementia (Kasl-Godley & Gatz, 2000; Scott & Clare, 2003).

This chapter focuses on the conceptualization of group-based approaches to treating the psychological and behavioral symptoms of geriatric cognitive impairment, principally represented by AD and related dementias. According to Cheston (1998), group-based interventions for dementia have traditionally been more prevalent than individually oriented interventions, and Scott and Clare (2003) note that group therapies were important in establishing the usefulness of therapy for people with dementia. We discuss the merits of group psychotherapy for addressing emotional and behavioral issues in people with dementia, as well as modifications that may be necessary for conducting group work with a cognitively impaired population. We discuss how factors such as treatment targets, neuropsychological function, and diagnosis contribute to the conceptualization of group interventions for individuals with cognitive impairment, and we also review the extant literature on group psychotherapies for this population. The chapter is written from the perspective that the implementation of empirically guided psychotherapies for dementia groups is still a work in progress. We approach these issues with the belief that clinical practice with the best available evidence will move the field toward greater use of evidence-based treatment in general. Finally, we offer examples from our own clinical experience in conducting group psychotherapy with cognitively impaired individuals to illustrate vital caregiver and patient perspectives regarding the role and significance of this type of intervention, as well as some of the challenges of applying empirical principles to clinical practice.

GROUP PSYCHOTHERAPY

There are many characteristics of group psychotherapy that make it a desirable treatment option for individuals living with cognitive impairment. One characteristic is that group therapy offers a sense of belonging to individuals who may be feel isolated by their impairments (LaBarge & Trtanj, 1995). Isolation often arises from social withdrawal, such as when an individual avoids interacting with others out of sensitivity to his or her cognitive decline. Loss of mobility and independence, such as might occur when an individual stops driving, can also limit social interaction and increase feelings of isolation. Therapy groups offer a positive response to social isolation because they provide a context for meaningful interactions and a supportive forum for sharing the problems of cognitive impairment with others who have similar experiences. Such social stimulation is associated with positive cognitive and emotional responses in normally aging people (Fillit et al., 2002) as well as those with dementia (Koh et al., 1994), which suggests that social interaction alone can be therapeutic. Whereas certain group interventions do rely primarily on social interaction as the therapeutic catalyst, nearly all group formats provide this benefit to some extent.

Another therapeutic characteristic of group psychotherapy is the beneficial effects of social learning. The benefits of social learning in group therapy occur via: (1) interpersonal exchange, (2) behavioral modeling, and (3) information sharing. Saiger (2001), for instance, described the therapy group as a social microcosm in which the positive and negative effects of an individual's interpersonal behavior can be identified and discussed in a supportive context. The dynamics of interpersonal exchange and the feedback received from these interactions are essential aspects of social learning. The therapy group can also function as a learning environment in which individuals can observe and model the coping strategies of successful peers (Solomon & Szwabo, 1992). Finally, an important aspect of social learning that is a primary component of many therapy groups is sharing knowledge of resources that are available outside of the group setting per se (Yale, 1999). As with the social interaction benefits of group therapy, social learning benefits are present to some extent across most groups, though some approaches make this a more explicit focus of the intervention than do others (Barton, Levene, Kladakis, & Buttersworth, 2002; Bednar, Weet, Evensen, Lanier, & Melnick, 1974; Diamond, 1974).

One characteristic of group interventions that is more pragmatic than therapeutic is that group treatment is often more cost-effective than individual therapy. Although the rates of group therapy vary depending on the therapist and type of intervention, the average group therapy session is approximately half the cost of an individual session (American Group Psychotherapy Association, 2004). Additionally, across a wide variety of populations, group interventions have been found to produce treatment outcomes comparable to individual interventions (DeRubeis & Crits-Christoph, 1998; Dugas et al., 2003; Marques & Formigoni, 2001; Yalom, 1995). The lower cost of group therapy combined with equal and sometimes better outcomes relative to individual interventions can mean higher cost-effectiveness across a variety of intervention approaches and patient populations (Bastien, Morin, Ouellet, Blais, & Bouchard, 2004; McFarlane et al., 1995; Shapiro, Sank, Shaffer, & Donovan, 1982). The lower cost associated with group treatment can be important to individuals with financial limitations, especially when extensive diagnostic workups often precede the treatment-planning stage. Group therapy is used effectively in inpatient settings, where time and budget constraints preclude extensive one-to-one treatment. It is important to note, however, that group therapy should not serve as a substitute treatment for those individuals whose treatment needs clearly require a one-to-one relationship.

CONCEPTUALIZING GROUP INTERVENTIONS

Yalom (1995) advises clinicians to develop group intervention plans that are informed by a clear understanding of the relevant clinical issues, with attention to specific treatment goals and the methods most appropriate for achieving them. As detailed by Attix's intervention model (Chapter 10, this volume), the efficacy of a particular intervention is facilitated by proper matching of a patient's characteristics to his or her treatment. In the case of group therapy, several factors play a role in determining the suitability of an individual for a particular intervention approach: (1) potential to engage in treatment, (2) treatment targets, (3) neuropsychological profile, (4) diagnosis, (5) symptom severity, and (6) therapeutic context.

Potential to Engage in Treatment

Group therapy is not appropriate for every individual living with cognitive impairment (Cheston, Jones, & Gilliard, 2003). Many individuals find the experience of sharing their emotions within a group to be threatening and thus can be resistant to engaging in the key therapeutic experiences of a group. In addition, the lack of engagement on the part of one individual may hinder the treatment progress of the group as a whole. Some individuals may engage emotionally but still not acknowledge their disorder. The capacity to acknowledge the presence of cognitive difficulties is not necessarily a prerequisite for joining a therapy group, but progress on many treatment targets is likely to remain limited if the individual does not eventually accept his or her condition. Challenges also exist when the lack of acknowledgment is one of the actual features of the condition, as is the case with anosognosia (Koltai, Welsh-Bohmer, & Schmechel, 2001).

An individual's motivation to actively participate in group psychotherapy is essential to treatment success. One source of poor motivation stems from the fact that behaviors that are viewed as problematic by caregivers may not necessarily be distressing to the patient (Lyman, 1989). Thus, resistance is not uncommon for individuals who attend therapy based on the wishes of others. Resistance that results in poor group participation can be detrimental to the progress of other group members and should be promptly addressed by the therapist; however, this problem can be minimized through careful assessment and intervention planning. Different issues arise when motivational problems reflect a stable feature of an individual's condition, such as the amotivational tendencies and apathy that occur in many dementias. Individuals with acquired deficits in motivation or insight are typically better suited for more behaviorally oriented groups and/or those in which the therapist is a directive presence (Teri & Gallagher-Thompson, 1991).

Treatment Targets

The selection of an appropriate group intervention depends in large measure on treatment targets. It is important to recognize in this context that although a condition such as AD is not currently reversible, it is possible to treat associated behaviors and feelings that create additional distress, burden, or disability. Zarit and colleagues (Zarit, Femia, Watson, Rice-Oeschger, & Kakos, 2004) have identified several global targets for individuals with dementia and their caregivers, including:

- Facilitating communication between patient and caretaker.
- Addressing relationship issues with other friends and family members.
- Developing coping strategies for memory loss.
- Finding ways for the patient to feel useful.
- Dealing with grief and loss.
- Acquiring disease- and treatment-related knowledge.

Indeed, we find these targets to be accurate. In addition, we have found the following goals to be important to treatment success:

- Forging relationships/friendships (for patients as well as caregivers).
- Providing a sanctuary from fear and criticism—an environment of acceptance and support.
- Learning behaviorally appropriate methods of interacting with and supporting others.
- Generating appropriate ideas to maintain and enhance behavioral activity.

Although there is growing appreciation of the needs and experiences of individuals diagnosed with cognitive impairment (Woods, 2001), treatment targets have been historically defined by the perspective of the caregiver. One survey of caregivers of individuals with AD found that over 70% of those with early-stage symptoms manifest behavioral disturbance during the course of their illness (Harrell et al., 1995). Most often, the problem behaviors relate to anxiety and mood disturbance, not to more intractable symptoms such as delusions and hallucinations. Teri and colleagues (Teri et al., 1992) found that whereas memory-related behaviors such as repetitive question asking were reported by caregivers as most frequent in occurrence, depression was rated as most distressing. Similar to the findings of Harrell and colleagues (1995), behaviors such as delusions and hallucinations were found to be infrequent prior to the latter stages of dementia. Although the problems with depression and anxiety that cause most distress for caregivers in the early stages of dementia can be addressed in the context of numerous group-based approaches, hallucinations and delusions are often more idiosyncratic in their presentation (Teri et al., 1992) and would be better targeted by an individually oriented intervention and possibly pharmacological management.

From a patient-oriented perspective, the range of individual responses to dementia is varied and personal. For instance, catastrophic reactions have been reported to occur in approximately 16% of individuals in response to their diagnosis (Tiberti et al., 1998). In contrast, other individuals minimize or deny their deficits. These responses have been interpreted as a protective reaction to a frightening threat to one's sense of self (Clare, 2003). Several authors have recognized depressive symptomatology as the most prevalent emotional response among individuals with dementia, frequently associated with grief about lost cognitive and functional abilities (Cheston & Bender, 1999; Solomon, 1982). In this context, depression may be accompanied by anxiety regarding the consequences of the cognitive and functional losses, as well as by feelings of anger and frustration. Other common experiences reported by individuals with dementia include (1) fear of being out of control or perceived as out of control, (2) feeling lost, (3) losing a sense of meaning, and (4) concerns about being a burden on family members (Kitwood, 1997).

Many studies of the coping process of individuals with dementia identify a progression of stages similar to that of other individuals confronted with the anticipated and actual losses of serious illnesses: denial, anger, guilt, sadness, and eventually adaptation (Cohen, Kennedy, & Eisdorfer, 1984; Kubler-Ross, 1969). Similarly, Clare (2003) outlines five types of reactions to changes caused by dementia: (1) registering, (2) reacting, (3) explaining, (4) experiencing, and (5) adjusting. She describes the interaction among these responses as an individual attempts to balance fighting his or her illness against accepting it. This model does not posit a stage-like progression of responses, but rather emphasizes the importance of understanding the implications of each of these responses for the individual. These models of coping provide an effective framework for group therapy, where the principles of modeling, sharing, social feedback, and validation can facilitate therapeutic change.

We have found that the intervention process often yields a transformation in the patient's perception of self and role identities. As noted in Attix (Chapter 10, this volume), our definition of intervention involves a restructuring of the individual's responsibilities, expectations, and sense of self, largely to yield a transformation in role identity that is adaptive in the behavioral context of the illness. Although this transformation may be a direct target of treatment in certain cases, it often occurs as a secondary result of moving through grief stages and adopting alternative behaviors and activities in line with new realities of living with cognitive impairment. We have found it instructive and beneficial in treatment planning to periodically consider a patient's standing in this regard, because it is a useful marker of intervention progress.

Neuropsychological Profile

Assessing an individual's level of general neurocognitive functioning is an essential consideration in formulating a treatment plan for group therapy, but the presence of even moderate deficits should not necessarily preclude an individual from benefiting from some form of group psychotherapy. Because mild cognitive impairment often takes months to years to progress, there is a substantial amount of time during which individuals can productively engage in a cognitively demanding task such as psychotherapy (Jutagir, 1993). In addition, individuals with mild cognitive impairment can be expected to comprehend treatment goals, engage in therapeutic discourse, and complete assignments between sessions in a manner similar to noncognitively impaired peers (Teri & Gallagher-Thompson, 1991). Impairments in areas such as memory, executive function, or language are often specific targets for intervention, but they are also treatment modifiers because these deficits can alter an individual's retention, conceptualization, or communication in therapy (see Kasl-Godley & Gatz, 2000, for additional discussion of how cognitive impairment may influence specific therapeutic approaches for dementia). Whereas there are numerous modifications that can be made to compensate for deficits in memory and other cognitive processes that accompany early cognitive decline, the progression to moderate decline produces deficits in domains such as attention, self-monitoring, and language, which make it difficult to implement approaches that rely on insight or extensive therapeutic dialogue. This progression of cognitive impairment may narrow the range of appropriate interventions to supportive and behavioral strategies. The restriction of strategies for intervention is typically concomitant with a parallel evolution of treatment needs.

Memory

In addition to considering an individual's general level of cognitive functioning in treatment planning, patterns of impaired and preserved abilities also dictate the choice of group intervention. Because memory loss is a defining characteristic of most dementing disorders, many interventions are specific to memory skills training (see chapters in Part II, Section A: Cognitive Training and Compensatory Techniques). Although compensating for mild memory loss with note taking and audiotaping can help some individuals improve carryover from session to session, our experience with the former has been that group members often find note taking to be an additional cognitive burden that detracts from their ability to focus on therapy in the present moment. Individuals with more profound memory loss can of course be expected to demonstrate decreased retention of complex themes, but in our experience they can retain general themes if they are repeated within a session or over the course of several sessions. In fact, we have been surprised at the degree of retention and integration of therapeutic themes, as is evidenced by current group members when they orient new members to therapy. Finally and importantly, specific memory problems can be used therapeutically. For instance, it is not uncommon for individuals to experience difficulty remembering the names of other group members. Such events provide an opportunity for the therapist to normalize episodes of forgetfulness, and in certain groups they may present an entrance point for discussing and practicing mnemonic strategies.

Executive Functions

Decline in executive functions can present challenges in psychotherapy due to problems with abstraction and insight, but additional challenges exist in group psychotherapy due to the potentially overstimulating and distracting nature of group dialogue. Because individuals with deficits in executive functions may have difficulty with the cognitive demands of tracking a dialogue among multiple participants (Alberoni et al., 1992), therapists must be attentive to managing the group dialogue by using core therapeutic techniques such as reframing. In relation to this point, Morris (1994) suggests that keeping group membership small is a useful accommodation to executive and other neurocognitive deficits. Executive deficits that involve impulsivity, which can be seen in conditions such as frontotemporal dementia, may further affect group dynamics. Impulsive or disinhibited comments can be disruptive and/or inadvertently offensive, but a therapist can often address these in context, using therapeutic techniques such as modeling or reinforcement to teach appropriate alternative responses. Severe deficits in executive functions, however, may prove too disruptive for group therapy and require one-to-one treatment.

Language

In contrast to memory, moderate to severe language deficits such as those associated with stroke or primary progressive aphasia indicate a poor prognosis for most group therapies, but some specialized groups do exist (see Johnson, Chapter 14, this volume, for a more detailed review of interventions for language deficits). Mild word-finding problems are common across many cognitive disorders, and these often can be addressed through the therapist's ability to facilitate communication during sessions. In one clinical experience, however, we had an individual who could not participate productively in group therapy because of declining insight and language abilities, but who ultimately found a social and experiential outlet through art therapy. This non-language-based activity proved to be a soothing counterpoint to the individual's verbal struggles and had a notable impact on quality of life through his enjoyment of producing art and interacting with others.

Diagnosis

As mentioned previously, most group interventions for geriatric cognitive disorders are targeted to patients with AD, so one important treatment planning issue is whether individuals with different dementia diagnoses can be combined in the same treatment group. Unfortunately, there is limited research on psychotherapeutic intervention with diagnoses other than AD from which evidence-based conclusions can be drawn. Diagnostic research, however, informs us that many dementing conditions are similar to each other in that multiple cognitive and functional domains are affected, along with relatively consistent intrapersonal reactions of depression, anxiety, and adjustment issues. We have also experienced this similarity in our clinical practice, where we have had success integrating individuals with different diagnoses but similar cognitive and behavioral profiles (e.g., primary executive and memory deficits accompanied by depression). The key elements appear to be that all members can engage in personal reflection, share their reflections with the group, and validate the reflections of others.

When individuals lack the cognitive capacity to reflect, share, and validate emotional experiences, the progress and benefits associated with group treatment are likely to be compromised. For instance, during one phase of group treatment in our practice, a new participant with deficits in insight and verbal expressive abilities initially found it socially stimulating to attend therapy sessions, but his inability to respond meaningfully to other group members limited the treatment progress of both the individual and the group as a whole. Although some current group members were able to discern that this individual's upbeat denials of deficit were related to his particular disease presentation and direct their questions to him accordingly, other members found it difficult to relate to an individual who did not appear to be experiencing the same processes of frustration, confrontation, and adaptation that were central group themes. As this example illustrates, the prospects for successfully integrating individuals with different diagnoses become more challenging when neuropsychological profiles differ substantially across group members, or when specific behavioral deficits such as anosognosia are prominent. Groups interventions designed specifically for conditions such as stroke (Welterman et al., 2000) or Parkinson's disease (Charlton & Barrow, 2002) reflect increasing recognition of the benefits of selecting group members who have similar experiences and display similar symptom presentations. Although promising, additional research on the efficacy of these treatments is needed.

Symptom Severity

Assuming that homogeneity in specific diagnoses of group members is less important than ensuring that group members share comparable cognitive ability and treatment needs, it is important to consider the impact of differing levels of dementia severity on the dynamics and productivity of a treatment group. Goldwasser and colleagues (Goldwasser, Auerbach, & Harkins, 1987) comment from experience with outcome research that treatment difficulties can arise when mildly impaired but functional individuals share a group with individuals whose behavioral and functional deficits are more profound. For instance, less impaired group members may resent being placed with more impaired individuals and find their greater confusion and disruptiveness to be a distraction; however, Goldwasser and colleagues also noted that positive therapeutic changes occurred among group members, despite these difficulties. Divergence in the severity of cognitive impairment among group members should be anticipated in groups with stable membership that are conducted on an ongoing basis. LaBarge and Trtanj (1995), for instance, reported the experience of having specific group members demonstrate cognitive decline over the course of several group sessions, and noted that other group members were able to respond with appropriate emotional support. As the divergence in severity grows, however, the focus and composition of group membership may need to be reconsidered.

Therapeutic Context

The therapeutic context in which group psychotherapy occurs often plays a significant role in the selection of treatment goals and intervention strategy. Much of early empirical research on group psychotherapy for persons with dementia was conducted in inpatient settings. Because greater cognitive and behavioral symptoms increase the probability of institutionalization, these settings tend to have a more cognitively impaired population than community settings. Depending on the resources of an inpatient facility, there may not be enough individuals who can participate in a cognitively demanding, insight-oriented therapy. Inpatient groups may by necessity have a greater range of dementia severity and intermingling of treatment goals and diagnoses, which can make intervention planning more challenging. On the other hand, individuals in an inpatient setting can often meet longer and more frequently than is feasible on an outpatient basis, and some treatment goals can be reinforced by staff members outside of the therapy session. Availability of consistent reinforcement becomes particularly important in the latter stages of dementing illnesses, when behavioral and environmental modifications tend to be the predominant method of intervention.

Outpatient therapy groups provide a different set of benefits and challenges. One advantage is that individuals may be more specifically matched to groups based on their deficits and treatment needs. In an active therapy practice, individuals may be able to make transitions between groups as their level of function and treatment targets change. There are also challenges to conducting outpatient groups, many of which are practical in nature. One of these is that as individuals progress in a dementing illness, they may become more reliant on a caregiver for scheduling and transportation. Often, the continuity of a group depends in part on the therapist's ability to establish rapport with caregivers. In our practice we encourage caregivers, typically spouses, to meet at the end of therapy sessions for a brief summary of therapeutic issues and to address subsequent scheduling. This approach is consistent with research highlighting the benefits of including caregivers in treatment planning (Teri, Logsdon, Wagner, & Uomoto, 1994). Caregivers often remain in our clinic for all or part of the patient's session, and it is not uncommon for a secondary "support group" to emerge from their dialogue with each other. We have found that facilitating the development of these informal relationships among spouses enhances the overall commitment to the patients' therapy.

THERAPIST ADJUSTMENTS FOR GROUP THERAPY

The previous sections illustrate that conducting psychotherapy among individuals with cognitive impairment requires an awareness of the common neurocognitive deficits and an ability to make appropriate modifications for them. Although this awareness is also required in conducting individual therapy, it becomes more salient in the group setting because of the multiple and competing stimuli that are inherent in group interactions; hence the adjustments highlighted in the previous discussion of group conceptualization are summarized here in brief. In terms of cognitive modifications, therapists should be mindful to speak in concrete and specific terms. Deficits in memory, attention, and receptive language capabilities require simplified explanations of psychological constructs that may need to be repeated throughout a session in order to bolster retention. Therapists should also be prepared to "direct traffic" by verbally guiding individuals back to the prevailing discussion of the group and assisting participants with expressive difficulties by interpreting and reframing their comments for the benefit of other group members. Therapists should look for opportunities to validate adaptive behaviors that can be modeled by other group members. Behavioral modifications such as handouts, diagrams, and even audio- or videotaping may be appropriate in certain situations to complement or reinforce the verbal content of the therapy session.

There are also several practical issues to consider when planning a therapy group for patients with cognitive compromise. Whereas some authors have suggested that briefer sessions may be more effective for patients in individual therapy as their cognitive impairment progresses (Hausman, 1992; Solomon & Szwabo, 1992), we and others (LaBarge & Trtanj, 1995) have found 60- to 90-minute sessions to be appropriate for groups involving mildly impaired participants with capacity for verbal engagement. Consistency in time, day, and place of session meetings can provide important structure for individuals. Our group sessions are typically held in the morning, which is the time of day when most older adults are at their peak cognitive efficiency (May, Hasher, & Stoltzfus, 1993). The quality of the room environment—good lighting, proper ventilation, and quiet surroundings—can help minimize cognitive distractions and the effects of vision and hearing deficits. It is also important to allow adequate space for individuals with mobility problems.

EMPIRICAL REVIEW OF GROUP THERAPY APPROACHES

The preceding discussion focused on conceptualization and application of group therapy principles to individuals with dementia and other geriatric cognitive disorders. This section focuses on the outcomes of several approaches to group psychotherapy with patients having cognitive compromise. As mentioned previously, there are presently limited data on approaches that would meet a codified definition of treatment efficacy (Chambless et al., 1998; Gatz et al., 1998), much less Camp's (2001) definition of treatment effectiveness, which requires positive effects across diagnostic groups and real-world treatment contexts. Extant studies are limited by unclear distinctions between levels of dementia severity, lack of controlled designs, and inconsistent use of quantifiable outcome measures. Scott and Clare (2003) raise important questions about which outcomes best capture the effects of group intervention and how to properly operationalize these outcomes. In addition, they note that individuals differ in their response to the same group experience, and that this difference requires a particular flexibility in clinical practice to balance individual and group needs. Thus, whereas some empirical standards for treatment outcome research will be challenging to attain in the reality of clinical care, we nevertheless believe that an empirically informed approach to conceptualizing and treating dementia should be practiced, even when the idealized environment of a controlled trial cannot be achieved. We also recognize that qualitative observations of therapeutic process can be valuable sources of information when they are systematically obtained. As a result, we do not limit the following reviews to quantitative outcomes alone, and we leave it to the reader to draw an informed opinion from these appraisals.

Behavioral and Cognitive-Behavioral Groups

Although distinctions can be made between purely cognitive and purely behavioral treatment approaches, in practice these interventions draw upon a mix of cognitive and behavioral elements. On the cognitive end of the spectrum, interventions focus on changing maladaptive patterns of thinking that contribute to depression, anxiety, and undesirable behaviors. Behavioral interventions focus on learning and reinforcement principles to increase positive experiences and decrease negative ones. Common treatment targets include management of depression, anxiety, and agitation. Although behavioral approaches to treating targets such as depression in patients with dementia have among the strongest empirical support (e.g., Teri, Logsdon, Uomoto, & McCurry, 1997; Teri & McCurry, 2000), these findings are largely based on interventions with individuals and patient–caregiver dyads.

Among the studies that focus on group interventions, Abraham et al. (Abraham, Neundorfer, & Currie, 1992) divided 76 depressed individuals with mild to moderate cognitive impairment into three treatment groups: (1) cognitive-behavioral therapy (CBT), (2) visual imagery, and (3) a psychoeducational discussion group. They found no change in measures of depression, hopelessness, or life satisfaction across the three conditions over the course of the treatment; however, individuals in both CBT and imagery groups demonstrated an increase in cognitive performance on a brief mental status measure. The negative findings for the noncognitive treatment targets are in contrast to positive findings with healthy older adults (Teri & McCurry, 2000), and with those from one small study of demented individuals (Kipling, Bailey, & Charlesworth, 1999). The lack of noncognitive treatment effects in the Abraham et al. study may have been due to the inclusion of the physically frail along with both mildly and moderately impaired group members, the latter of which could have been a poor neuropsychological fit for the intervention. This explanation would be consistent with Kasl-Godley and Gatz's (2000) argument that mildly impaired individuals can be successful with interventions based on cognitive and learning principles, whereas individuals with moderate or greater impairment may respond best to more simplified principles of reinforcement.

Psychodynamic Psychotherapy

Like other therapeutic approaches, the goal of psychodynamic psychotherapy is to ameliorate psychological distress. As described by Hausman (1992), the therapeutic techniques to achieve treatment goals include (1) establishing a validating relationship, (2) providing an outlet for emotional catharsis, (3) promoting self-esteem and self-efficacy, (4) promoting adaptive over maladaptive defense and coping mechanisms, (5) and promoting self-insight. Whereas these goals are achieved in individual therapy through the dynamic of the relationship between therapist and patient, the dynamic in group therapy is additionally influenced by relationships among group members and between the group and the therapist. In this way, group psychodynamic therapy is similar to other approaches that use the dynamic of the group to achieve therapeutic effects, but a psychodynamic orientation specifically includes the therapist's interpretations of the emotional content of a group's conversations (Solomon & Szwabo, 1992). With regard to an individual's appropriateness for a psychodynamic group, Hausman argues that entry into therapy at the earliest indication of a dementing illness offers the best prognosis for effective engagement in treatment. Solomon and Szwabo, however, argue that psychodynamic treatment becomes increasingly difficult beyond the stage of mild impairment.

Evidence for the efficacy of psychodynamic therapy groups with cognitively impaired patients comes largely from qualitative analysis of therapist notes and observation of sessions. For instance, Akerlund and Norberg (1986) described improvement in their treatment group after changing from a reality orientation (RO) model to a psychodynamic model. Based on retrospective clinical observations and review of session videotapes, the authors identified a pattern of more active participation and more cognitively sophisticated processing, compared to behavior during the RO period of treatment. From a methodological perspective, criticisms include a lack of psychometrically sound outcome measures, nonblinded raters, and a small sample ($n = 9$), but the authors' impressions are consistent with expectations of a psychodynamic treatment model. An older but larger study (Birkett & Boltuch, 1973) included random assignment of patients to psychodynamic group therapy versus another treatment (remotivation therapy). After weekly 1-hour sessions over a 12-week period, raters blinded to treatment condition found improvement for both groups but no difference between groups.

Support Groups

The basic premise of most support groups is that sharing common experiences is therapeutic. Yale (1995), who has written extensively about grief work in AD, stated that treatment targets for support groups often include working through grief issues, decreasing social isolation, and encouraging group members to adopt a positive identity regarding their diagnosis. Support groups have long been available to family members of individuals with dementia, but there has been a more recent increase in the availability of support groups for the patients themselves, as well as for groups that include both patients and caregivers (Snyder, Quayhagen, Shepard, & Bower, 1995). Support groups can vary widely in format, from nondirective process groups driven by patients' current concerns, to structured, topic-driven groups directed by the therapist. Because a key element of support groups is the shared coping experience, they are not necessarily organized around a specific psychological model. According to Yale (1995), individuals with moderate to severe dementia would be less likely to benefit from support groups.

Drawing conclusions from the empirical literature on support groups is challenging because of the diversity of support group formats. Further, most outcome measures are based on clinical observations and the self-report of participants. In one of the more comprehensive studies of support groups, Yale (1995) reported a treatment–control study of 15 individuals with early AD. The treatment condition involved eight weekly sessions lasting 90 minutes, with caregivers included in the final session. The control condition was care as usual. The authors assessed cognitive and social functioning, but did not find significant group differences for posttreatment or follow-up intervals. Process notes from the therapists were qualitatively assessed and indicated that the members of the treatment group were more likely to discuss illness-related issues, and that they provided an overall positive report of their experience. Other studies (e.g., LaBarge & Trtanj, 1995) from small samples offer similar findings of positive experiences by participant report and observations of increased discussion of illness-related issues, but no clear change for specific treatment targets such as depression or anxiety. Studies of groups including both patients and caregivers are similar in methodology and outcome (Snyder et al., 1995). Studies of conjoint support group approaches (e.g., McAfee, Ruh, Bell, & Martichuski, 1989) report positive evaluations from both patients and caregivers, but they do not address the issue of whether the conjoint approach improves communication between the patient and the caregiver—often a key treatment goal.

Reminiscence Groups

Whereas the act of reminiscence was at one time considered a negative sign among demented individuals (Watt & Wong, 1991), reminiscence therapy is actually supported by a number of empirical studies. The goal of reminiscence therapy is to help demented patients recall past events and experiences as a means to improve social interaction and promote a general sense of well-being. Although these groups do not typically emphasize treatment of specific psychological issues or behaviors, they have been found to be associated with increases in meaningful discourse among individuals with mild to moderate impairment (Moss, Polignano, White, Minichello, & Sunderland, 2002). Reminiscence groups may tap some of the residual cognitive abilities of individuals who have the most common forms of dementia, later into the disease course than other types of intervention (Rentz, 1995).

Regarding empirical studies of reminiscence therapy, Goldwasser and colleagues (Goldwasser et al., 1987) compared a reminiscence group to a nonspecific support group and a no-treatment group ($n = 27$) and found an improvement in depression among reminiscence treatment group members compared to those in the other two groups. They did not, however, find a significant treatment effect after a 5-week follow-up period. Interestingly, the authors describe a technique that incorporates behavioral training elements: guiding patients to generate internal retrieval cues. Baines and colleagues (Baines, Saxby, & Ehlert, 1987) compared a reminiscence therapy group to an RO group and a no-treatment group in a nursing home setting ($n = 15$). They used a crossover design in which each group received the intervention for a half-hour each day over a 4-week period, with a 4-week no-treatment period between the intervention periods. Patients in the reminiscence group demonstrated maintenance of cognitive function after treatment and 4-week follow-up, but no changes on behavioral or life satisfaction measures. On the whole, reminiscence groups may have positive effects on depression as well as other nonspecific effects on the overall function of individuals with moderate levels of dementia.

Reality Orientation Therapy

Like reminiscence therapy, RO therapy is used with individuals who have greater levels of cognitive impairment (Donahue, 1984; Taulbee, 1984). The goal of RO is to reorient patients by means of continual stimulation and repetitive orientation to their environment. Typically, daily group sessions are held that contain a didactic component designed to help orient and engage group members (Holden & Woods, 1988). A number of studies have reported positive changes associated with RO, including improvements in orientation, memory of personal facts and appointments, and general cognitive functioning (Hanley, 1981; Hanley & Lusty, 1984). Two studies have shown that RO may slow the decline in global cognitive status over time, as measured by change in Mini-Mental State Examination (MMSE) scores (Baldelli et al., 1993; Zanetti et al., 1995), but there were no effects for improving affective status or activities of daily living (see also Bates, Boote, & Beverley, 2004). Although there is empirical support for RO therapy, some authors report that certain patients may become emotionally upset during treatment and that an alternative approach may be more appropriate (Zanetti et al., 1995). Validation therapy, which is based on empathic listening, has been proposed for patients with greater levels of cognitive impairment who do not respond well to RO (Dietch, Hewett, & Jones, 1989; Zanetti et al., 1995); however, few well-designed studies have examined its effectiveness.

ECLECTIC PSYCHOTHERAPIES

In the reality of current clinical practice, an eclectic approach to group therapy may be more common than one that strictly follows a single treatment methodology. Koltai and

Branch (1999), for instance, argue that combining elements from different therapeutic approaches enhances the potential for clinical gain. Eclectic intervention strategies, when systematically designed and implemented, offer flexibility in responding to the specific needs of the individuals in the group. Given the nature of progressive neurodegeneration and the shifting needs and challenges faced by many individuals and families as they attempt to cope with the changing nature of symptoms and impairments, intervention approaches that have access to a wide variety of tools allow the person with dementia to remain central in defining the intervention. Dhooper and colleagues (Dhooper, Green, Huff, & Austin-Murphy, 1993) reported the outcome of an eclectic treatment approach that combined elements of reminiscence, emotional processing, and problem-solving skills in 16 elderly nursing home residents experiencing mild to moderate depression. They reported significant changes in depression following the intervention when compared to a no-treatment control group. Despite these positive findings, the lack of an active treatment control condition limits the support that these findings provide for their assertion that an eclectic treatment approach is more broadly effective than other treatment modalities. Our experience with one eclectic approach (Koltai et al., 2001) combined empirically guided intervention strategies and clinical approaches involving multiple cognitive, compensatory, and coping strategies. These results revealed significant improvement in perceived memory functioning among individuals with dementia who had intact insight. Other combined cognitive coping approaches are reviewed in Clare (Chapter 13, this volume).

Cheston and colleagues (2003) recently described a psychotherapeutic intervention for individuals with dementia called the Dementia Voice Group Psychotherapy Project. The project involved a 10-week therapy group that was conducted at several different sites. Groups consisted of individuals with AD and other dementias who were characterized as mildly impaired and who all had MMSE scores greater than 18. Participants in these groups were asked to reflect on the emotional significance of their experience of memory loss, with a focus on "here-and-now" issues, such as the impact of memory difficulties on their interpersonal relationships. Data were reported for 19 individuals who participated in preintervention testing, the full course of therapy, and a 10-week follow-up assessment. Although the study lacked a control group, the authors found that group members had decreased levels of depressive symptomatology from baseline, both for the duration of therapy and follow-up assessment. Marginally significant treatment effects for anxiety were reported as well.

GROUP PERSPECTIVES FROM CLINICAL PRACTICE

Our psychotherapeutic intervention group has been meeting for approximately 3 years. The group was initiated when three patients were referred to one of us (DKA) for intervention to address depression, anger, and memory compensatory strategy training. The three were all considerably distressed, having experienced recent declines and diagnoses. All had similar cognitive profiles at the time (primary executive dysfunction, memory deficits, and word-finding difficulties), as well as similar losses of role function (sudden unanticipated retirement, cessation of driving privileges) and accompanying emotional responses (primarily depression, with some anger and anxiety). One individual was in his early 50s, another in his mid-50s, and the third in his early 60s. Over the course of the group to date, three others have joined and participated from 2 to 12 months, but the original three members have remained the consistent core of the group.

The group has met every 2–3 weeks over the past 3 years. The themes and goals of treatment have evolved over time to accommodate the cognitive and functional changes of the group members. It is best described as utilizing a combination of behavioral and grief models of psychotherapy. We often integrated the two approaches; for instance, emphasizing participation in pleasant and rewarding activities as a behavioral response to negative feelings about functional loss or perceptions of decreased usefulness. Like Teri and colleagues (1997), we found promoting or maintaining rewarding activity to be a particularly valuable component of the treatment.

Consistent with the perspective of this chapter, we have attempted to conduct our treatment in accordance with empirical knowledge about the symptoms and expressions of cognitive impairment, and to integrate therapeutic models that have been honed by research; however, quantifying treatment progress in small groups such as ours has been challenging. In part, this is because a small group does not necessarily have a normative experience on a specific outcome measure. For instance, although the Geriatric Depression Scale was useful in assessing baseline distress and subsequent improvement among most group members, one member who entered therapy with a "motivated denial" about his deficits actually reported increased depression as treatment progressed. In this case, the increase in negative affect was a reflection of the patient's evolving acceptance of his dementia and its implications, which reflects treatment success in terms of insight and adaptation. Because of similar experiences, we have found that our empirical outcome measures are a useful adjunct to treatment when they are interpreted in the context of feedback from patients, spouses, and often the referring physicians. To this purpose, and also to highlight the personal and experiential nature of group treatment, we present perspectives of group members and spouses on the process of therapy

The quotes in the following section are from our group members (directly or with assistance) and their spouses, which we have obtained from taped conversations and written responses. These couples have previously shared their experiences with a large audience at a regional AD conference. They continue to remember this experience well and fondly, and have been eager for other outlets to express themselves. Although their ability to articulate their message has changed over time, the message itself has remained consistent with themes discussed previously in this chapter.

Regarding Loss and Adaptation

"We know there are things we cannot do that we wish we could do, and it is not an easy process to let these go. There are a lot of things we can do, though, and we need you to see this."

"By being in group—it helps each other. Others can get by with better help. Others can feel better once they knock the wall down, by being mad and mean and crying . . . you've done that and you can put it back together."

"There is no point of focusing on the negative and the losses. Yes, they are there, but where do we get thinking only about these? We have to focus on who we are and what we can do."

On the Interpersonal Experience of Therapy

"The friendships we have forged are extremely powerful emotionally."

"We offer each other ideas. We offer each other acceptance. We will confront each other when that is needed, in instances of unsafe or unhealthy behavior. We do not give up on each other."

"This group has been *very* important to me because I don't have to worry about making mistakes. . . . It's okay not to remember and not to be able to get the words out. . . . It has been the most helpful thing for me, other than my wife. . . . I think this type of group would help anyone with our problems, and I hope there will be more groups like this everywhere."

"We are here. Our memories and words might not always be, but we are."

The following quotes about group therapy are from the spouses' perspectives.

On the Significance of Group Therapy to Healthy Adjustment

"He knows that no matter how overwhelming things seem for him sometimes, he can go to group and talk about it and be heard and understood. There is no criticism in group, but there is encouragement and support. The group's themes of accepting yourself the way you are and realizing that you can't do the things you used to do but you are still the person you always were have been very helpful to him. . . . "

"[My husband] was very depressed, negative, angry, and lethargic. . . . Group has been very beneficial in processing the fear and anger and moving [him] on to the acceptance stage. . . . The consistent support over the years has provided an understanding that they are not alone in their challenges . . . they have shed their tears, expressed their frustrations, and faced their fears together. . . . The group sessions have enabled him to process the stages of grief and loss of himself. . . . I cannot begin to tell you how important [group] is to the well-being of the patient. . . . Without group, we probably would have isolated ourselves and wallowed in our rollercoaster of emotions."

On the Meaning of Group to the Spouses

"For me, as a spouse, group has meant the opportunity for wives to have regular 'meetings of the minds,' 'sharings of the heart,' and 'barings of the soul'—in essence—to form a unique sisterhood of support for one another. I can share with [the other spouses] things about daily struggles, discoveries, resources, and dark nights that I share with no one else."

On What Patients and Spouses Want Care Providers to Know

"Group support has not been wasted on the 'forgetful.' Even though communication and remembering are very difficult, the messages are still inside the heart and soul.

These guys have tremendous value and can still make a contribution. Friends, family members, and caregivers must recognize and respect the individual as a wonderful value and a gift to life. Although the challenges are great, there is much still to be learned if we just spend time and listen."

The preceding perspectives from group members and their spouses express important aspects of the group therapeutic process that we as scientist-practitioners often find challenging to capture empirically. Treatment providers need to balance both idiographic (individually oriented) and nomothetic (normatively based) methods of conceptualizing and evaluating outcomes. They are not mutually exclusive, but complementary, and methods such as case studies and treatment outcome research can contribute to the advancement of group therapy for dementia and other geriatric cognitive disorders. Regardless of the approach, it is important to integrate clinical techniques with empirical knowledge of brain–behavior relationships to promote optimal growth for patients and to consistently assess progress with attention to cognition, function, affect, and quality of life as they pertain to the individual and those within the care environment.

REFERENCES

Abraham, I. L., Neundorfer, M. M., & Currie, L. J. (1992). Effects of group interventions on cognition and depression in nursing home residents. *Nursing Research*, *41*, 196–202.

Akerlund, B. M., & Norberg, A. (1986). Group psychotherapy with demented patients. *Geriatric Nursing*, *7*, 83–84.

Alberoni, M., Baddeley, A. D., Della Sala, S., Logie, R. H., & Spinnler, H. (1992). Keeping track of a conversation: Impairments in Alzheimer's disease. *International Journal of Geriatric Psychiatry*, *7*, 639–646.

American Group Psychotherapy Association. (2004). *About group psychotherapy*. Available at www.groupsinc.org/group/consummerguide2000.html

Baines, S., Saxby, P., & Ehlert, T. K. (1987). Reality orientation and reminiscence therapy: A controlled cross-over study of elderly confused people. *British Journal of Psychiatry*, *151*, 222–231.

Baldelli, M. V., Pirani, A., Motta, M., Abati, E., Mariani, E., & Manxi, V. (1993). Effects of reality orientation therapy on elderly patients in the community. *Archives of Gerontology and Geriatrics*, *17*, 211–218.

Balesteri, L., Grossberg, A., & Grossberg, G. T. (2000). Behavioral and psychological symptoms of dementia as a risk factor for nursing home placement. *International Psychogeriatrics*, *12*, 59–62.

Ballard, C., Lowery, K., Powell, I., O'Brien, J., & James, I. (2000). Impact of behavioral and psychological symptoms of dementia on caregivers. *International Psychogeriatrics*, *12*, 93–105.

Barton, J., Levene, J., Kladakis, B., & Butterworth, C. (2002). Stroke: A group learning approach. *Nursing Times*, *98*, 34–35.

Bastien, C. H., Morin, C. M., Ouellet, M. C., Blais, F. C., & Bouchard, S. (2004). Cognitive-behavioral therapy for insomnia: Comparison of individual therapy, group therapy, and telephone consultation. *Journal of Consulting and Clinical Psychology*, *72*, 653–659.

Bates, J., Boote, J., & Beverley, C. (2004). Psychosocial interventions for people with a milder dementing illness: A systematic review. *Journal of Advanced Nursing*, *45*, 644–658.

Bednar, R. L., Weet, C., Evensen, P., Lanier, D., & Melnick, J. (1974). Empirical guidelines for group therapy: Pretraining, cohesion, and modeling. *Journal of Applied Behavioral Science*, *10*, 149–165.

Birkett, D. P., & Boltuch, B. (1973). Remotivation therapy. *Journal of the American Geriatrics Society*, *21*, 368–371.

Camp, C. J. (2001). From efficacy to effectiveness to diffusion: Making the transitions in dementia intervention research. *Neuropsychological Rehabilitation*, 11, 495–517.

Chambless, D. L., Baker, M. J., Baucom, D. H., Beutler, L. E., Calhoun, K. S., Crits-Christoph, P., et al. (1998). Update on empirically validated therapies, II. *Clinical Psychologist*, 51, 3–16.

Charlton, G. S., & Barrow, C. J. (2002). Coping and self-help group membership in Parkinson's disease: An exploratory qualitative study. *Health and Social Care in the Community*, 10, 472–478.

Cheston, R. (1998). Psychotherapeutic work with people with dementia: A review of the literature. *British Journal of Medical Psychology*, 71, 211–231.

Cheston, R., & Bender, M. (1999). Brains, minds and selves: Changing conceptions of the losses involved in dementia. *British Journal of Medical Psychology*, 72, 203–216.

Cheston, R., Jones, K., & Gilliard, J. (2003). Group psychotherapy for people with dementia. *Aging and Mental Health*, 7, 452–461.

Clare, L. (2003). Managing threats to self: Awareness in early stage Alzheimer's disease. *Social Science and Medicine*, 57, 1017–1029.

Cohen, D., Kennedy, G., & Eisdorfer, C. (1984). Phases of change in the patient with Alzheimer's dementia: A conceptual dimension for defining health care management. *Journal of the American Geriatrics Society*, 32, 11–15.

DeRubeis, R. J., & Crits-Christoph, P. (1998). Empirically supported individual and group psychological treatments for adult mental disorders. *Journal of Consulting and Clinical Psychology*, 66, 37–52.

Dhooper, S. S., Green, S. M., Huff, M. B., & Austin-Murphy, J. (1993). Efficacy of a group approach to reducing depression in nursing home elderly residents. *Journal of Gerontological Social Work*, 20, 87–100.

Diamond, M. J. (1974). From Skinner to Satori? Towards a social learning analysis of encounter group behavior change. *Journal of Applied Behavioral Science*, 10, 133–148.

Dietch, J. T., Hewett, L. J., & Jones, S. (1989). Adverse effects of reality orientation. *Journal of the American Geriatrics Society*, 37, 974–976.

Donahue, E. M. (1984). Reality orientation: A review of the literature. In I. Burnside (Ed.), *Working with the elderly: group process and techniques* (pp. 165–176). Monterey, CA: Wadworth Health Sciences.

Dugas, M. J., Ladouceur, R., Leger, E., Freeston, M. H., Langlois, F., Provencher, M. D., et al. (2003). Group cognitive-behavioral therapy for generalized anxiety disorder: Treatment outcome and long term follow-up. *Journal of Consulting and Clinical Psychology*, 71, 821–825.

Fillit, H. M., Butler, R. N., O'Connell, A. W., Albert, M. S., Birren, J. E., Cotman, C. W., et al. (2002). Achieving and maintaining cognitive vitality with aging. *Mayo Clinic Proceedings*, 77, 681–696.

Gatz, M., Fiske, A., Fox, L. S., Kaskie, B., Kasl-Godley, J., McCallum, T., et al. (1998). Empirically-validated psychological treatments for older adults. *Journal of Mental Health and Aging*, 4, 9–46.

Goldwasser, A. N., Auerbach, S. M., & Harkins, S. W. (1987). Cognitive, affective, and behavioral effects of reminiscence group therapy on demented elderly. *International Journal of Aging and Human Development*, 25, 209–232.

Hanley, I. (1981). The use of signposts and active training to modify ward disorientation in elderly patients. *Journal of Behavior Therapy and Experimental Psychiatry*, 12, 241–247.

Hanley, I., & Lusty, K. (1984). Memory aids in reality orientation: A single case study. *Behavior Research and Therapy*, 22, 709–712.

Harrell, L. E., Marson, D., Duke, L., Foster, J., Burgard, S., Anderson, B., et al. (1995). Behavioral changes in early Alzheimer's disease. In K. Iqbal, J. A. Mortimer, B. Winblad, & H. M. Wisniewski (Eds.), *Research advances in Alzheimer's disease and related disorders* (pp. 219–224). New York: Wiley.

Hausman, C. P. (1992). Dynamic psychotherapy with elderly demented patients. In G. M. M. Jones, & B. M. L. Miesen (Eds.), *Care-giving in dementia: Research and applications* (pp. 181–198). New York: Tavistock/Routledge.

Holden, U. P., & Woods, R. T. (1988). *Reality orientation: Psychological approaches to the confused elderly* (2nd ed.). Edinburgh: Churchill Livingstone.

Jutagir, R. (1993). Geropsychology and neuropsychological testing: Role in evaluation and treatment of patients with dementia. *Mount Sinai Journal of Medicine, 60,* 528–531.

Kasl-Godley, J., & Gatz, M. (2000). Psychosocial interventions for individuals with dementia: An integration of theory, therapy, and a clinical understanding of dementia. *Clinical Psychology Review, 20,* 755–782.

Kipling, T., Bailey, M., & Charlesworth, G. (1999). The feasibility of a cognitive behavioural therapy group for men with mild/moderate cognitive impairment. *Behavioural and Cognitive Psychotherapy, 27,* 189–193.

Kitwood, T. (1997). *Dementia reconsidered: The person comes first.* Buckingham, UK: Open University Press.

Koh, K., Ray, R., Lee, J., Nair, A., Ho, T., & Ang, P. (1994). Dementia in elderly patients: Can the 3R mental stimulation programme improve mental status? *Age and Ageing, 23,* 195–199.

Koltai, D. C., & Branch, L. G. (1999). Cognitive and affective interventions to maximize abilities and adjustment in dementia. In R. Cacabelos, C. Fernandez, & E. Giacobini (Eds.), *Annals of psychiatry: Basic and clinical neurosciences* (pp. 241–255). Barcelona: Prous Science.

Koltai, D. C., Welsh-Bohmer, K. A., & Schmechel, D. E. (2001). Influence of anosognosia on treatment outcome among dementia patients. *Neuropsychological Rehabilitation, 11,* 455–475.

Kubler-Ross, E. (1969). *On death and dying.* London: Collier-Macmillan.

LaBarge, E., & Trtanj, F. (1995). A support group for people in the early stages of dementia of the Alzheimer's type. *Journal of Applied Gerontology, 14,* 289–301.

Lyman, K. A. (1989). Bringing the social back in: A critique of the biomedicalization of dementia. *Gerontologist, 29,* 597–605.

Marques, A. C., & Formigoni, M. L. (2001). Comparison of individual and group cognitive behavioral therapy for alcohol and/or drug-dependent patients. *Addiction, 96,* 835–846.

May, C. P., Hasher, L., & Stoltzfus, E. R. (1993). Optimal time of day and the magnitude of age differences in memory. *Psychological Science, 4,* 326–330.

McAfee, M. E., Ruh, P. A., Bell, P. A., & Martichuski, D. K. (1989). Including persons with early stage Alzheimer's disease in support groups and strategy planning. *American Journal of Alzheimer's Care and Research, 4,* 18–22.

McFarlane, W. R., Lukens, E., Link, B., Dushay, R., Deakins, S. A., Newmark, M., et al. (1995). Multiple-family group and psychoeduation in the treatment of schizophrenia. *Archives of General Psychiatry, 52,* 679–687.

Morris, R. G. (1994). Working memory in Alzheimer-type dementia. *Neuropsychology, 8,* 544–554.

Moss, S. E., Polignano, E., White, C. L., Minichiello, M. D., & Sunderland, T. (2002). Reminiscence group activities and discourse interaction in Alzheimer's disease. *Journal of Gerontological Nursing, 28,* 36–44.

Rentz, C. A. (1995). Reminiscence: A supportive intervention for the person with Alzheimer's disease. *Journal of Psychosocial Nursing and Mental Health Services, 33,* 15–20.

Saiger, G. M. (2001). Group psychotherapy with older adults. *Psychiatry, 64,* 132–145.

Scott, J., & Clare, L. (2003). Do people with dementia benefit from psychological interventions offered on a group basis? *Clinical Psychology and Psychotherapy, 10,* 186–196.

Shapiro, J., Sank, L. I., Shaffer, C. S., & Donovan, D. C. (1982). Cost effectiveness of individual vs. group cognitive behavior therapy for problems of depression and anxiety in an HMO population. *Journal of Clinical Psychology, 28,* 674–677.

Snyder, L., Quayhagen, M. P., Shepherd, S., & Bower, D. (1995). Supportive seminar groups: An intervention for early stage dementia patients. *Gerontologist, 35,* 691–695.

Solomon, K. (1982). The subjective experience of the Alzheimer's patient. *Geriatric Consultant, 1,* 22–24.

Solomon, K., & Szwabo, P. (1992). Psychotherapy for patients with dementia. In J. E. Morley, R. M.

Coe, R. Strong, & G. T. Grossberg (Eds.), *Memory function and aging-related disorders* (pp. 295–319). New York: Springer.

Taulbee, L. R. (1984). Reality orientation and clinical practice. In I. Burnside (Ed.), *Working with the elderly: Group process and techniques* (pp. 177–186). Monterey, CA: Wadworth Health Sciences.

Teri, L., & Gallagher-Thompson, D. G. (1991). Cognitive-behavioral interventions for treatment of depression in Alzheimer's patients. *Gerontologist, 31,* 413–416.

Teri, L., Logsdon, R. G., Uomoto, J., & McCurry, S. M. (1997). Behavioral treatment of depression in dementia patients: A controlled clinical trial. *Journals of Gerontology: Psychological Sciences, 82B,* P159–P166.

Teri, L., Logsdon, R. G., Wagner, A., & Uomoto, J. (1994). The caregiver role in behavioral treatment of depression in dementia patients. In E. Light, B. Lebowtiz, & G. Niederehe (Eds.), Stress effects on family caregivers of Alzheimer's patients (pp. 185–204). New York: Springer.

Teri, L., & McCurry, S. M. (2000). Psychosocial therapies with older adults. In C. E. Coffey & J. L. Cummings (Eds.), *Textbook of geriatric neuropsychiatry* (2nd ed., pp. 861–890). Washington, DC: American Psychiatric Press.

Teri, L., Traux, P., Logsdon, R., Uomoto, J., Zarit, S., & Vitaliano, P. (1992). Assessment of behavioral problems in dementia: The Revised Memory and Behavioral Problems Checklist. *Psychology and Aging, 7,* 622–631.

Tiberti, C., Sabe, L., Kuzis, G., Cuerva, A. G., Leiguarda, R., & Starkstein, S. E. (1998). Prevalence and correlates of the catastrophic reaction in Alzheimer's disease. *Neurology, 50,* 546–548.

Watt, L. M., & Wong, P. T. P. (1991). A taxonomy of reminiscence and therapeutic implications. *Journal of Gerontological Social Work, 16,* 37–57.

Welterman, B. M., Homann, J., Rogalewski, A., Brach, S., Voss, S., & Ringelstein, E. B. (2000). Stroke knowledge among stroke support group members. *Stroke, 31,* 1230–1233.

Woods, R. T. (2001). Discovering the person with Alzheimer's disease: cognitive, emotional and behavioural aspects. *Aging and Mental Health, 5,* S7–S16.

Yale, R. (1995). *Developing support groups for individuals with early-stage Alzheimer's disease.* Baltimore, MD: Health Professional Press.

Yale, R. (1999). Support groups and other services for individuals with early-stage Alzheimer's disease. *Generations, 23,* 57–61.

Yalom, I. D. (1995). *The theory and practice of group psychotherapy* (4th ed.). New York: Basic Books.

Zanetti, O., Frisoni, G. B., De Leo, D., Buono, M. D., Bianchetti, A., & Trabucchi, M. (1995). Reality orientation therapy in Alzheimer's disease: Useful or not? A controlled study. *Alzheimer's Disease and Associated Disorders, 9,* 132–128.

Zarit, S. H., Femia, E. E., Watson, J., Rice-Oeschger, L., & Kakos, B. (2004). Memory Club: A group intervention for people with early-stage dementia and their partners. *Gerontologist, 44,* 262–269.

19

Pharmacological and Other Treatment Strategies for Alzheimer's Disease

Kathleen Hayden
Mary Sano

The treatment of Alzheimer's disease (AD) has a modern-day history that begins in the early 1990s and continues to expand today, with clinical research initiatives addressing preventive strategies and treatments for other forms of dementia and memory loss. To this end, it is now generally recognized that AD is a protracted process in which the neuropathological events occur years, and perhaps decades, before diagnosis. As such, there are three distinct stages along the pathological cascade at which point interventions may be implemented: (1) a "preclinical" asymptomatic phase; (2) a "prodromal" or early symptom state; and (3) the fully expressed disease stage. It cannot be assumed that treatments for AD are equally effective at all stages of the disease; in fact, there is evidence that some pharmacological interventions are potentially useful in primary and secondary AD prevention but essentially ineffective at the later stages of the illness in affecting disease progression (e.g., Zandi, Anthony, et al., 2002). The situation is not unique to AD. Analogous scenarios exist for many progressive medical illnesses, for which the aggressiveness of the indicated therapy depends on the stage of the underlying disease state.

This chapter focuses on the pharmacological treatment of AD and similar disorders. First, we provide a review of the drug development and approval process for AD compounds and discuss the currently available treatment options for patients affected by the disease. We then address the notion of extending current treatment to new indications, which includes disease prevention options and suggested therapeutic mechanisms for slowing progression. This section summarizes some of the new and novel approaches that are aimed at the fundamental neuropathological mechanisms of the disease and hold potential promise of treating the disease even when it is fairly advanced. We conclude the chapter with a discussion of topical areas in which clinical trials can provide important answers. Our intention in this chapter is to provide practicing neuropsychologists with information regarding the treatment options for currently affected dementia patients and an overview of ongoing research directions in developing effective treatment options for the future.

TREATING LATE-LIFE COGNITIVE DISORDERS

Medical treatment of the last two decades includes pharmacological interventions for patients with AD. Although still in its infancy, five drugs are approved for use in the United States, and there is robust interest in development of better agents that may modify disease progression and prevent disease onset. Researchers have experienced monumental steps forward as well as disappointing results, and enthusiasm remains high—which is not surprising given the estimates of growth in prevalence and incidence of this disease (Brookmeyer, Gray, et al., 1998). Perhaps in part due to the availability of treatment for cognitive symptoms, there is growing interest in identifying treatment of other forms of memory loss and dementia associated with diseases of aging. These include vascular disease, neurodegenerative diseases, prodromes to disease such as mild cognitive impairment (MCI), and other forms of age-related cognitive decline. The success in identifying treatments for AD has been aided by regulatory guidelines for drug approval. A review of this process may outline the efforts needed to make similar progress for drug approval for other indications.

THE REGULATORY APPROVAL PROCESS

In the United States, the Food and Drug Administration (FDA) approves new drugs for marketing based on a New Drug Application (NDA) that provides evidence of (1) efficacy for the specified indication and (2) safety in the population for which it is to be used. Based on draft guidelines from 1990, the FDA requires that the efficacy of drugs for this indication be demonstrated in at least two separate randomized, double-blind, placebo-controlled trials that are each of at least 3–6 months' duration. A further requirement is that efficacy should be determined by demonstrating benefit in two prespecified primary outcome measures, one of which should assess cognitive function and the other should be either a clinician's overall impression of benefit (including cognition, function or behavior) or a measure of activities of daily living (ADLs). The guidelines recommend that superiority of treatment over placebo be demonstrated for each of the two prestated outcomes by statistical significance at the $p < .05$ level (Mani, 2004).

Currently there are four drugs approved for the treatment of mild to moderate dementia of the AD type; all are of the same class of cholinesterase inhibition. Memantine, an (NMDA) receptor antagonist (mechanism of action explained on p. 432), has been approved for the treatment of moderate to severe dementia. It is unclear how useful the indication by disease stage will be in clinical practice. The specific labeling for these treatments includes statements that there is no evidence that the drug in question alters the course of the underlying dementia.

At present there are no guidelines for the approval process for other dementias such as vascular and mixed dementias. One limitation is inadequate knowledge about appropriate outcome measures. Approaches to trial design in these diseases consist of using assessments developed for patients with mild to moderate AD, which may not be the most appropriate for capturing benefit in other conditions.

Interest in the prevention of AD has grown, and the identification of mildly symptomatic individuals typically labeled with MCI has provided a model for trials of secondary prevention of AD. Methodological reports from such studies describe these individuals and have estimated the likelihood of their progression to AD. Results from clinical trials in patients with MCI are becoming available and may provide information to determine the best approach to treatment. By and large, the agents under study have been those used to treat AD or which theoretically could treat AD.

TOOLS FOR ASSESSING DEMENTIA IN CLINICAL TRIALS

The FDA requires a demonstration of improvement in cognition and either clinical global change or improvement in ADLs. As awareness of the breadth of symptomatology and social and economic impact has grown, clinical trials for AD have come to include measures of behavioral disturbance, quality of life, and cost effectiveness. In addition, several efforts have been made to specify the nature of cognitive benefit. Table 19.1 summarizes instruments that have been used to assess efficacy in these domains in clinical trials for AD.

Numerous tests are available to evaluate each of these domains. The cognitive subscale of the Alzheimer's Disease Assessment Scale—Cognitive subscale, or ADAS-Cog, is the most widely used scale to evaluate cognition. This scale evaluates spoken language ability, comprehension, recall of test instructions, word finding, following commands, naming objects, constructional praxis, ideational praxis, orientation, word recall, and word recognition. The Mini-Mental State Examination (MMSE) is frequently used by clinicians in practice as a screening device in research studies and as a secondary outcome measure of cognition in clinical trials. The Severe Impairment Battery (SIB) has been used to demonstrate efficacy in patients with low MMSE scores and consists of praxis items as well as simple memory items. Like the ADAS-Cog, it has been used to support an NDA application for a currently approved drug. The Syndrome Kurtz Test (SKT) has also been used in clinical trials to evaluate cognitive change, although it is not commonly used in the United States. All of these tests are administered to the patient and therefore are direct assessments of cognitive function.

An estimate of a clinician's impression of change is generally measured via the Clinical Global Impression of Change (CGI) or the Clinician's Interview-Based Impression of Change plus Caregiver Input (CIBIC-Plus). These tests are standardized ratings given by a clinician after interviewing the patient, and caregiver input is considered as well. Other tests of global function include the Clinical Dementia Rating Scale (CDR), which uses a semistructured interview to independently assess patient and informant. The Global Deterioration Scale (GDS) is a staging instrument that is completed after a clinical examination.

The most commonly used measure of functional ability is the Alzheimer's Disease Cooperative Study—Activities of Daily Living (ADCS-ADL). This scale was empirically derived and has specific versions for disease stage. It has been useful in many trials in demonstrating efficacy in the functional domain. Other measures include the Interview for Deterioration in Daily Living Activities in Dementia (IDDD), the Functional Activities Questionnaire (FAQ), and the Disability Assessment for Dementia scale (DAD). These tests are administered to an informant or caregiver. Finally, the Physical Self Maintenance Scale (PSMS), which can be self-rated, is typically rated by an observer in AD trials.

Behavioral symptoms are an important clinical aspect of dementia, and outcome

TABLE 19.1. Instruments and outcome measures commonly used in clinical trials for Alzheimer's disease

Domain	Test	Reference	Score	Outcome measures	Comments
Cognition[a]	ADAS-Cog (Alzheimer's Disease Assessment Scale—Cognitive subscale)	Mohs et al. (1997); Rosen et al. (1984)	• Range: 0–70 • Higher scores indicate increased severity	Severity of symptoms	• "Gold standard" cognitive outcome measure for AD • Administered to patient
	MMSE (Mini-Mental State Examination)	Folstein et al. (1975)	• Range: 0–30 • Low scores indicate increased severity	Onset, stability, and severity of cognitive symptoms	• Secondary outcome measure; used for screening • Administered to patient
	SIB (Severe Impairment Battery)	Schmitt et al. (1997)	• Range: 0–100 • Higher scores reflect higher cognitive ability	Cognitive function in severe dementia	• Primary outcome measure for severe impairment • Administered to patient
	SKT (Syndrom Kurtz Test)	Erzigkeit (1989); Lehfeld & Erzigkeit (1997)	• Range: 0–27 • Lower scores show improvement	Memory and attention	• Primary outcome measure • Administered to patient Timed test
Clinical global change[a]	CGI (Clinical Global Impression of Change)	Schneider et al. (1997)	• Range: 1–7 • Higher scores indicate increased severity	Cognitive, behavioral, social, and daily functioning	• Alzheimer's Disease Cooperative Study (ADCS) version • Standardized rating given by clinician; patient and informant interviewed
	CIBIC-Plus (Clinician's Interview-Based Impression of Change Plus Caregiver Input)	Knopman et al. (1994)	• Range: 1–7 • Higher scores indicate increased severity	Four major areas of function: general, cognitive, behavioral, and ADLs	• Semistructured review • Rating of patient given by clinician with informant input
	CDR-SB (Clinical Dementia Rating—Sum of Boxes)	Berg (1988)	• Range: 0–18 • Higher scores indicate increased severity	Presence and severity of dementia	• Structured interview • Evaluates six categories of function: memory, orientation, judgment and problem solving, community affairs, personal care • Administered to patient and informant
	GDS (Global Deterioration Scale)	Reisberg et al. (1982)	• Range: 1–7 • Higher scores indicate increased severity	Rates seven stages of dementia	• **Informant not required** • Structured interview not required

(continued)

TABLE 19.1. (*continued*)

Domain	Test	Reference	Score	Outcome measures	Comments
Functional	IDDD (Interview for Deterioration in Daily Living Activities in Dementia)	Teunisse & Derix (1991)	• Range: 1–7 • Higher scores indicate increased severity	Severity of functional impairment; ability to perform activities of daily living (ADLs and IADLs)	• Structured interview • Administered to informant
	ADCS-ADL (Alzheimer's Disease Cooperative Study—Activities of Daily Living)	Galasko et al. (1997)	• Range: 0–78 • Higher scores indicate higher function	Assesses level of independence	• Administered to informant • Inventory of items varies according to severity of dementia being assessed
	FAQ (Functional Activities Questionnaire)	Pfeffer et al. (1982)	• Range: 1–7 • Higher scores indicate increased severity	Evaluates performance on ten complex activities of daily living	• Administered to informant
	DAD (Disability Assessment for Dementia Scale)	Gelinas et al. (1999)	• Range: 0–100 • Higher scores indicate improvement	Assesses basic and instrumental ADLs, leisure activities, initiation, planning, organization, and effective performance	• Administered to informant
	PSMS (Physical Self Maintenance Scale)	Lawton & Brody (1969)	• Range: 6–30 • Lower scores indicate better self-maintenance	Assesses ability to feed, toilet, dress, groom, walk, and bathe	• Observer version and self-rated versions available
Behavioral	BEHAVE-AD (Behavioral Pathology in Alzheimer's Disease Scale)	Reisberg et al. (1987)	• Range: 0–75 plus global rating • Higher scores indicate more severe problems	Assesses behavioral symptoms	• Able to distinguish cognitive symptomatology from pharmacologically remediable behavioral symptoms • Administered to informant

	NPI (Neuropsychiatric Inventory)	Cummings et al. (1994)	• Range: 0–120 • Higher scores indicate increased severity	Assesses delusions, hallucinations, agitation/ aggression, depression, anxiety, elation, apathy, disinhibition, irritability, aberrant motor behavior, sleep, and appetite	• Behavioral change usually within a defined period of time • Administered to informant
	CMAI (Cohen-Mansfield Agitation Inventory)	Cohen-Mansfield (1986)	• Range: 1–7 • Higher scores indicate increased severity	Rating of agitated behaviors	
Quality of life	ADRQL (Alzheimer Disease-Related Quality of Life)	Rabins et al. (1999)	• Range: 0–100 • Higher scores indicate better QoL	Evaluates behaviors associated with five domains	• Administered to primary caregiver
	QOL-AD (Quality of Life—Alzheimer's Disease scale)	Logsdon et al. (2002)	• Range: 13–52 • Higher scores indicate greater quality of life	Assesses domains of behavioral competence, psychological status, physical function, and interpersonal environment	• Administered to patient
	DQOL (Dementia Quality of Life instrument)	Brod et al. (1999)	• 29 items scored on 5-point Likert scale	Five subscales assess 10 domains of quality of life	• Administered to patients with MMSE scores >12
	CBS (Cornell–Brown Scale for Quality of Life in dementia)	Ready et al. (2002)	• Range: −38–+38 • Negative scores represent poor QoL ratings	Rating based on positive/ negative affect, physical complaints, and satisfaction	• Semistructured interview • Administered to patient and informant
Caregiver measures	BGP—Care Dependency subscale (Behavioral Rating Scale for Geriatric Patients, Care Dependency subscale)	van der Kam et al. (1971)	• Range: 0–70 • Higher scores indicate increased severity	Assesses cognitive and functional characteristics associated with need for care	• Reflects cognitive and functional characteristics associated with increased need for care
	SCB (Screen for Caregiver Burden)	Vitaliano et al. (1991)	• Range: 0–25 for objective burden; 0–75 for subjective burden • Higher scores indicate greater burden	Rapidly identifies distressing caregiver experiences	• Administered to caregiver

[a] FDA requires evidence of benefit in these domains.

measures in clinical trials frequently include assessment of this domain. The Neuropsychiatric Inventory (NPI), currently the most commonly used instrument, is a structured interview administered to a caregiver or knowledgeable proxy informant that addresses 12 domains of behavior, including agitation, irritability, anxiety, dysphoria, hallucinations, delusions, apathy, euphoria, disinhibition, aberrant motor behavior, nighttime disturbances, and abnormalities in appetite or eating habits. The score is a composite of frequency and severity ratings of each item. Caregiver distress is rated for each item, although it is not typically included in the overall score. The Behavioral Pathology in Alzheimer's Disease Scale (BEHAVE-AD) is a 25-item scale that uses input from the caregiver and direct observation to assess the behavioral symptoms of delusional ideation, hallucinations, activity disturbances, aggressiveness, sleep disturbance, affective symptoms, and anxiety. The Cohen-Mansfield Agitation Inventory (CMAI) is a caregiver questionnaire that provides an overall measure of agitation and behavioral problems.

Recently, several scales have been developed to evaluate the quality of life (QOL) of patients with dementia. These scales are being incorporated in clinical trials. Tests include Alzheimer Disease-Related Quality of Life (ADRQL), Quality of Life—Alzheimer's Disease scale (QOL-AD), Dementia Quality of Life instrument (DQoL), and the Cornell–Brown Scale for Quality of Life in dementia (CBS). Finally, changes in the level of caregiver burden can be evaluated with the Behavioral Rating Scale for Geriatric Patients (BGP)—Care Dependency subscale and the Screen for Caregiver Burden (SCB).

TREATMENT FOR AD WITH APPROVED AGENTS

Cholinergic Stimulation

Observed deficits in cholinergic neurotransmission in AD led to the development of the first symptomatic treatments for the disease. These treatments are designed to inhibit the breakdown of acetylcholine in the synaptic cleft, thus enhancing cholinergic neurotransmission. To date, there are four FDA-approved cholinergic agents available in the United States.

Tacrine

In September 1993 tacrine became the first agent approved by the FDA in the cholinesterase inhibitor class. Tacrine requires multiple daily dosing (four times per day) from initial doses of 10 mg, four times per day, to a maximum total of 160 mg/day. Titration should be done at 4-week intervals, with slow titration of dose into the effective range (i.e., 16 weeks) in order to minimize cholinergic side effects. Tacrine has 5–30% absolute bioavailability after absorption and is diminished with food, requiring administration on an empty stomach. Tacrine has limited tolerability of about 65% at the highest dose and requires monitoring of liver enzymes (Knapp, Knopman, et al., 1994). Contraindications include hepatic impairment, cardiac arrhythmias or cardiac disease, chronic obstructive pulmonary disease, gastrointestinal (GI) bleeding, hepatic disease, hypotension, jaundice, and Parkinson's disease, among others. Interactions with antimuscarinic agents, other cholinesterase inhibitors, estrogens, general or local anesthetics, neuromuscular blockers, nonsteroidal anti-inflammatory drugs, parasympathomimetics, phenothiazines, sedating H$_1$ blockers, tricyclic antidepressants, and others are noted. Side effects associated with tacrine include nausea, diarrhea, vomiting, exacerbation of hypotension or syncope, weight loss, elevation of liver enzymes, seizures, vagotonic effects, bronchoconstriction, and exaggerated muscle relaxation. Due to the profile of side effects, the need to monitor liver enzymes with routine blood tests, and compliance problems associated with multiple daily dosing, tacrine is generally no longer prescribed. Newer cholinergics require less frequent daily dosing and do not require monitoring of liver enzymes.

Donepezil

The second agent to be approved by the FDA (November 1996), donepezil, is a reversible inhibitor of the enzyme acetyl cholinesterase, and is used for symptomatic management of mild to moderate AD. Donepezil is administered once daily and does not require monitoring of liver enzymes. Maximum dosage is 10 mg/day, although there is no clinical evidence of greater effect at 10 mg/day than 5 mg/day. Titration from 5 mg to 10 mg can occur after an interval of 4–6 weeks. Donepezil is well absorbed with 100% bioavailability and no food limitations to absorption. The most common adverse events are nausea, diarrhea and vomiting, insomnia, muscle cramps, and anorexia, with more study withdrawals from those on 10 mg than 5 mg. Side effect rates were reduced at the 10-mg dose when the titration interval between 5 and 10 mg was increased from 1 to 6 weeks. Sleep disturbance may occur, perhaps because recommended dosing instructions suggest evening administration; modification of the time of administration may minimize this effect (Geldmacher, 1997).

A number of randomized clinical trials has been conducted to evaluate the efficacy of donepezil for patients with AD. A recent meta-analysis of 16 trials examined donepezil use in 4,365 patients with mild, moderate, or severe AD (Birks & Harvey, 2003). The trials varied in length from 12 to 52 weeks. Outcomes studied included cognitive function and global clinical state, the two outcomes required by the FDA for approval. Statistically significant improvements in cognition were shown for both 5- and 10-mg/day treatment. Clinical global measures also showed improvement, and some studies reported benefit in ADLs and behavior, mostly with the 10-mg/day treatment.

There are few long-term randomized controlled trials, but efficacy has been demonstrated in a 1-year study (Winblad, Engedal, et al., 2001). More recently, the AD2000 Collaborative Group studied long-term donepezil treatment in 565-community residing patients and reported findings of better cognition and functionality compared to a placebo over a 2-year period, though there were no differences in behavioral and psychological symptoms, time to nursing home placement, caregiver psychopathology, formal care costs, unpaid caregiver time, adverse events, or deaths (Courtney, Farrell, et al., 2004).

Rivastigmine

The next agent to appear on the market was rivastigmine (approved April 2000), also a reversible acetylcholinesterase inhibitor. Rivastigmine inhibits both acetyl- and butyl-cholinesterase; however, there is little information on the relationship of the latter to the clinical impact of the drug. The maximum dose administered is 12 mg/day. The drug is completely absorbed, and absolute bioavailablity is 36%. Food helps to enhance the bioavailability and increases tolerability of the medication. Patients take 1.5 mg twice daily with food and may increase to 3 mg after 2 weeks. Usual maintenance dosages are between 3 and 6 mg twice a day. If medication is discontinued at any point for more than a few days, it is recommended that the treatment be reinitiated at the lowest dose and titrated as described above. Side effects include dizziness and GI disorders such as nausea, vomiting, and diarrhea. Drug interactions may occur with antimuscarinics, other cholinesterase inhibitors, general and local anesthetics, and other drugs.

A Cochrane Review of eight trials of rivastigmine use in mild to moderate AD showed benefits in cognition, global measures, and ADLs with 6–12 mg/day over an interval of 26 weeks (Birks, Grimley Evans, et al., 2004). Although higher doses showed greater benefits, patients on higher doses experienced more side effects. The authors suggest that smaller doses administered more frequently may ameliorate this problem. Patients who took lower doses (4 mg/day) showed statistically significant improvements in cognition.

Galantamine

The most recent cholinesterase inhibitor to receive approval from the FDA for treatment of mild to moderate AD is galantamine (February 2001). This drug is a specific, reversible, competitive acetylcholinesterase inhibitor and an allosteric modulator at nicotinic cholinergic receptor sites. Originally isolated from various plants, including daffodil bulbs, galantamine is now synthesized (Olin & Schneider, 2004). The maximum dose administered is 24 mg/day. Galantamine is completely absorbed, and the bioavailability approaches 90%. The initial dose is 4 mg twice a day taken with food. After 4 weeks the dose can be increased to 8 mg two times per day and increased in 4-mg increments to the maximum of 24 mg/day.

A systematic review of seven trials, varying in length from 12 weeks to 6 months, showed improvements in cognition, global ratings, ADLs, and behavior. Doses above 8 mg/day showed statistically significant results; however, no dose–response effect was found among higher doses. The most common adverse effects, similar to other cholinesterase inhibitors, were nausea, vomiting, diarrhea, anorexia, and weight loss. Dosage increases were associated with GI symptoms and discontinuation. Galantamine was best tolerated when there was a slow titration (4 weeks) to a dose of 16 mg/day (Olin & Schneider, 2004). Administration with food, the use of antiemetic medication, and ensuring adequate fluid intake may reduce the impact of GI disturbance.

Considerations for Cholinesterase Inhibitor Use in AD

In the treatment of mild to moderate AD, cholinesterase inhibitors are efficacious in slowing cognitive decline and may be effective for up to 2 years. Side effects tend to be relatively benign and can be mitigated by slow titration to optimal dosages. Practical issues of drug administration, such as the availability of a caregiver to administer and/or supervise treatment and manage side effects, and the frequency of dosing may be important in the selection of an agent. Patients should be monitored for side effects. Improvement or stabilization may not be apparent for several months after the initiation of treatment.

No guidelines currently exist for the selection of one drug over another, and few studies have been conducted to compare treatments. Recently, a study by Jones et al. (Jones & Soininen, 2004) compared donepezil and galantamine in a head-to-head open-label trial. Donepezil showed greater effects on cognition, ADLs, and tolerability than galantamine. Although the galantamine group was older and had a greater number of females—both potential reasons for poor tolerability—the authors reported that no treatment-by-gender interactions were found. Generally, the experience of the family members as well as patients will play a key role in weighing benefits of any treatment. Although data support benefits in areas that should have an important impact on quality of life and economic value, no such results have been observed.

Glutamate and the NMDA Receptor

Memantine, the newest drug on the market for treatment of AD symptoms, is different from cholinesterase inhibitors in two respects: mechanism of action and specific indication. First, memantine is a noncompetitive N-methyl-D-aspartate (NMDA) receptor antagonist. The action of this drug is to protect cells from excitotoxicity by blocking the uptake of glutamate at the NMDA receptor site. Second, the drug has been approved for use in moderate to severe AD. (It should be noted that the cognitive assessment used in clinical trials of patients at this stage of the disease is the SIB rather than the ADAS-Cog). The half-life of memantine is 60–80 hours with the peak concentration reached in 3–7 hours. The recommended starting dose is 5 mg once a day with an increment of 5 mg/day at weekly intervals until the maximum dose of 20 mg/day is achieved. It is recommended that twice-daily dosing be observed with the first dose escalation.

Three trials, including 973 patients with moderate to severe AD and lasting 12–28 weeks, have been published. In one, memantine alone demonstrated benefits in cognition over placebo (Reisberg, Doody, et al., 2003). In another randomized trial, the combined use of memantine plus donepezil demonstrated benefits over donepezil alone, in terms of effects on cognition, a clinical global measure, and behavior (Tariot, Farlow, et al., 2004). Although a third study did not use a cognitive measure (Winblad & Poritis, 1999), all three studies assessed clinical global benefits. Two of the three studies demonstrated a statistically significant benefit of memantine over placebo using an intention-to-treat (ITT) analysis. Additionally, all three studies demonstrated efficacy in analyses of completers. Memantine was well tolerated in clinical trials. An increase in confusion (7.9 vs. 2%) was reported in one study (Tariot, Farlow, et al., 2004) but no consistent pattern of side effects has emerged. Clinical exposure to this agent is minimal compared to cholinesterase inhibitors, and it may be too early to know the complete side effect profile.

Early reports of the use of memantine in mild to moderate AD in combination with a cholinesterase inhibitor failed to demonstrate efficacy, though the details of the study are not available at this writing. A study examining the effect of memantine in this patient population in the absence of other treatments yields small but significant effects on cognition and clinical global measures (Pomara, Peskind, et al., 2004). Additional studies are needed to provide support for the use of this agent in patients at milder stages of the disease.

Table 19.2 summarizes the data on FDA-approved therapeutic agents for treatment of AD.

TREATMENT OF OTHER DEMENTIA AND COGNITIVE DEFICITS

Vascular Dementia

The development of treatments for AD was advanced by uniform diagnostic criteria (American Psychiatric Association, 1987; McKhann, Drachman, et al., 1984). In the absence of biomarkers, these clinical criteria play a key role in identifying a homogeneous population in which to demonstrate reliable treatment effects. Such criteria are less well established for other conditions, though there is a growing awareness of the need and many attempts to develop consensus around diagnoses.

TABLE 19.2. FDA-Approved Therapeutic Agents

Agent[a]	Action	Indication	Dosing	Most frequent adverse events	Beneficial effects: mean difference in change score for treated vs. nontreated	
					Cognitive	Global impression of change
Tacrine (Cognex)	Cholinesterase inhibitor (inhibits acetyl- and butylcholinesterase)	Mild to moderate DAT	160 mg/day	Nausea Diarrhea Vomiting Syncope	ADAS-Cog 2.07 for average doses of 39–135 mg/day	CIBIC-Plus 0.58 for average doses of 39–135 mg/day
Donepezil (Aricept)	Reversible selective acetylcholinesterase inhibitor	Mild to moderate DAT	5–10 mg/day at night	Nausea Diarrhea Vomiting	ADAS-Cog 2.7–3.1 for doses of 5 to 10 mg/day	CIBIC-Plus 0.35–0.39 for doses of 5–10 mg/day
Rivastigmine (Exelon)	Pseudo-irreversible noncompetitive acetylcholinesterase inhibitor	Mild to moderate DAT	6–12 mg/day with food	Nausea Vomiting Dizziness Diarrhea	ADAS-Cog 0.2–4.9 for doses of 1–12 mg/day	CIBIC-Plus 0.14–0.41 for doses of 1–12 mg/day
Galantamine (Reminyl)	Specific, reversible, competitive acetylcholinesterase inhibitor	Mild to moderate DAT	16–24 mg/day with food	Nausea Vomiting Diarrhea	ADAS-Cog 1.7–4.1 for doses of 8–32 mg/day	CIBIC-Plus 0.15–0.47 for doses of 8–32 mg/day
Memantine (Namenda)	Uncompetitive NMDA-receptor antagonist	Moderate to severe DAT	20 mg/day	Dizziness Headache Confusion Constipation	SIB 3.3–5.7 for doses of 5–20 mg/day	ADCS-ADL 1.6–3.4 for doses of 5–20 mg/day

Note. ADAS-Cog, Alzheimer's Disease Assessment Scale, Cognitive subscale; ADCS-ADL, Alzheimer's Disease Cooperative Study—Activities of Daily Living inventory, used here to assess day-to-day function; CIBIC-Plus, Clinician's Interview-Based Impression of Change Plus Caregiver Input; DAT, dementia of the Alzheimer's type; SIB, Severe Impairment Battery, used to assess cognitive performance. Data sources: for tacrine, Qizilbash et al. (1998); for donepezil, rivastigmine, galantamine, and memantine, FDA package labeling.

[a] Trade name in parentheses.

One such condition of interest for treatment is vascular dementia (VaD), driven in part by the advances made in the diagnosis and treatment of AD. Clinically it can be very difficult to make the distinction between AD and VaD, as noted in previous sections of this text. Briefly, the two entities frequently coexist, and it is not obvious to what degree each contributes to the dementia symptomatology. Also, it is less clear what role memory impairment plays in VaD. There may be similarities in the pattern of cognitive deterioration in AD and VaD, and these have led to comparable clinical trial designs. Clinical, pilot, and open longitudinal studies (Li, Meyer, et al., 2002; Mendez, Younesi, et al., 1999; Meyer, Chowdhury, et al., 2002) showed the potential for the use of cholinesterase inhibitors in VaD. Several studies have examined agents in patients with AD and some degree of vascular disease as well as in individuals described as having probable or possible vascular disease (see Table 19.3). Perhaps the largest database exists for donepezil, with published clinical trials including over 1,200 individuals with possible or probable VaD or cognitive decline (Birks & Harvey, 2003).

To date, two large randomized, double-blind, placebo-controlled trials for the use of donepezil in VaD have been completed (Black, Roman, et al., 2003; Wilkinson, Doody, et al., 2003). These two studies recruited 1,219 patients diagnosed with probable or possible vascular cognitive impairment, based on the National Institute of Neurological Disorders and Stroke–Association Internationale pour la Recherche et l'Enseignement en Neurosciences (NINDS–AIREN; Roman, Tatemichi, et al., 1993) criteria, for a 24-week trial. Results demonstrated significant improvement from baseline in ADAS-Cog scores for a 5-mg/day treatment group compared to placebo ($p = .003$). Of those VaD patients receiving 5-mg/day treatment, 41% showed improvement in global function on the CIBIC-Plus after 24 weeks compared to placebo, whereas 38% showed no change and 21% worsened (Goldsmith & Scott, 2003). Wilkinson et al. (2003) reported even greater drug–placebo differences in dementia severity with a 10-mg/day treatment. A Cochrane meta-analysis evaluated these two studies looking at both completers and ITT analysis (Malouf & Birks, 2004). Significant improvement was shown for both analyses on the ADAS-Cog and the MMSE. When ITT analyses were applied, only the 10-mg/day group showed benefit. Both studies reported acceptable tolerability for the drug. Clinical global improvement in the ITT analysis was observed in one study (Wilkinson et al., 2003) but not in others, although significance was observed at 5 mg but not at 10 mg in an observed cases analysis.

There have been no randomized trials of rivastigmine for the treatment of VaD. A reanalysis of a trial of patients with AD (Kumar, Anand, et al., 2000) suggested that benefit may still be apparent when a mild amount of vascular risk factor, as measured by the modified Rosen–Hachinski Scale (Rosen, Terry, et al., 1980), is present. A 22-month open study of rivastigmine conducted by Moretti et al (Moretti, Torre, et al., 2002) evaluated treatment of VaD with rivastigmine at 3–6 mg/day. All subjects met NINDS–AIREN criteria for probable VaD and subcortical VaD as determined by computed tomography (CT) scan. In this small study ($n = 16$), patients on rivastigmine showed improvement over baseline on the Ten-Point Clock Test (Tuokko, Hadjistavropoulos, et al., 1992), the Neuropsychiatric Inventory (NPI), and the Clinical Dementia Rating (CDR). However, in open trial designs it is difficult to rule out practice and attention effects. The results support the need to conduct rigorous studies to determine efficacy with this agent in a VaD population.

Erkinjuntti, Kurz, et al. (2002) conducted a multicenter, placebo-controlled, double-blind trial for the use of galantamine in patients with dementia and vascular disease. Centers in 10 countries participated in this study, which had a 4-week run-in period followed by 6-week titration at 4 mg/day for the first week to 24 mg/day in the sixth week and continued for 6 months. The ITT analysis demonstrated significant benefit on the ADAS-Cog ($p < .0001$) and on the CIBIC-Plus ($p = .001$) in those receiving galantamine compared to those receiving placebo. In a post hoc analysis, subjects were subdivided into those with possible AD and vascular disease ($n = 239$) and those with probable VaD (NINDS–AIREN criteria; $n = 188$). In this secondary analysis the VaD group showed improvement from baseline, which did not reach significance on the ADAS-Cog (2.4 points, $p = .06$), whereas the possible AD plus vascular disease group showed significant benefit in cognition. The opposite was true for measures of global function. On the CIBIC-Plus, the VaD group showed no improvement at 6 months over placebo ($p = .23$), and the possible AD plus vascular disease group showed significant benefit ($p = .019$). In an open-label extension of this trial, Erkinjuntti et al. (Erkinjuntti, Kurz, et al., 2003) showed sustained benefits in cognition, functional ability, and behavior after 12 months for both the VaD and AD groups, as measured by the ADAS-Cog, the Disability Assessment for Dementia scale (DAD), and the NPI.

TABLE 19.3. Clinical Trials for Vascular Dementia Treatments

Author (year)	Primary diagnoses	No. of subjects	Analytic approach	Study design	Duration	Dropout rate (%)	Daily dose	Treatment	Primary outcome measures	Secondary outcome measures
Kumar et al. (2000)	DAT with vascular	699	OC	Randomized, double-blind, placebo-controlled	26 weeks	22	12 mg/day 4 mg/day	Rivastigmine	ADAS-Cog, CIBIC-Plus, PDS	MMSE, GDS
Pantoni et al. (2000)	Subcortical VaD	259	LOCF	Randomized, double-blind, placebo-controlled	6 months	8	30 mg/day	Nimodipine	GBS, ADL, IADL, RDRS, CDR	ZVT-G, FOM, digit span, MMSE
Erkinjuntti et al. (2002)	VaD and mixed dementua	592	ITT	Randomized, double-blind, placebo-controlled	6 months	22.8	24 mg/day	Galantamine	ADAS-Cog, CIBIC-Plus	
Moretti et al. (2002)	Subcortical VaD	16	OC	Open label	22 months	0	6 mg/day	Rivastigmine	MMSE, TPC, WFs, WFp	ADL, IADL, CDR, NPI, RSS
Wilcock et al. (2002)	Probable VaD	579	ITT	Randomized, double-blind, placebo-controlled, parallel group	28 weeks	20	20 mg/day	Memantine	ADAS-Cog, CGI-C	MMSE, NOSGER, GBS

(continued)

TABLE 19.3. (*continued*)

Author (year)	Primary diagnoses	No. of subjects	Analytic approach	Study design	Duration	Dropout rate (%)	Daily dose	Treatment	Primary outcome measures	Secondary outcome measures
Black et al. (2003)	VaD	603	ITT	Randomized, double-blind, placebo-controlled. parallel group	24 weeks	20.3	10 mg/day 5 mg/day	Donepezil	ADAS-Cog, CIBIC-Plus	MMSE, CDR-SB, ADFACS
Erkinjuntti et al. (2003)	VaD and mixed dementia	459	ITT	Open label	6 months	18.5	24 mg/day	Galantamine	ADAS-cog, DAD, NPI	
Wilkinson et al. (2003)	VaD	616	ITT	Randomized, double-blind, placebo-controlled parallel group	24 weeks	20.3	10 mg/day 5 mg/day	Donepezil	ADAS-Cog, CIBIC-Plus	MMSE, CDR-SB, ADFACS

Note. DAT, dementia of the Alzheimer's type; ITT, intent-to-treat; LOCF, last observation carried forward; OC, observed cases; VaD, vascular dementia; outcome measures: ADAS-Cog, Alzheimer's Disease Assessment Scale—Cognitive subscale (Mohs et al., 1997; Rosen et al., 1984); ADFACS, Alzheimer's Disease Functional Assessment and Change Scale (Mohs et al., 2001); ADL, Activities of Daily Living for Dementia (Katz et al., 1963); CDR, Clinical Dementia Rating (Hughes et al., 1982); CDR-SB, Clinical Dementia Rating—Sum of Boxes (Berg, 1988); CGI-C, Clinical Global Impression of Change (Guy, 1976); CIBIC-Plus, Clinician's Interview-Based Impression of Change Plus Caregiver Input (Knopman et al., 1994); DAD, Disability Assessment for Dementia scale (Gelinas et al., 1999); FOM, Fuld Object–Memory Evaluation (Fuld, 1978; LaRue, 1989); GBS, Gottfries–Bråne–Steen scale (Gottfries et al., 1982); GDS, Global Deterioration Scale (Reisberg et al., 1982); IADL, Instrumental Activities of Daily Living (Lawton & Brody, 1969); MMSE, Mini-Mental State Examination (Folstein et al., 1975); NOSGER, Nurses' Observation Scale for Geriatric Patients (Spiegel et al., 1991); NPI, Neuropsychiatric Inventory (Cummings et al., 1994); PDS, Progressive Deterioration Scale (DeJong et al., 1989); RDRS, Rapid Disability Rating Scale (Linn, 1967); RSS, Relative Stress Scale (Greene et al., 1982); TPC, Ten-Point Clock Test (Manos, 1997); WFp, Word Fluency—Phonological (Wechsler, 1981); WFs, Word Fluency—Semantic (Wechsler, 1981); ZVT-G, Zahlen–Verbindungs Test—Geriatric (Oswald & Roth, 1978).

Memantine has also been examined in trials of patients with VaD. Currently, several ongoing clinical trials are attempting to determine the efficacy of memantine use in mild to moderate (MMM) VaD. Initial results reported in a Cochrane Review (Areosa & Sherriff, 2003) showed findings from two studies: MMM300 (Orgogozo, Rigaud, et al., 2002) and MMM500 (Wilcock, Mobius, et al., 2002). A significant change from baseline in cognition was reported with 20 mg/day ($p < .0001$); however, there were no significant differences for ADLs assessed with the Nurses' Observation Scale for Geriatric Patients (NOSGER) scale (Spiegel, Bruner, et al., 1991), the Gottfries–Brane–Steen (GBS) scale (Gottfries, Brane, et al., 1982), or clinical impression of change with the CIBIC-Plus. The authors correctly note that the cognitive tests used for AD may not be sensitive to the pattern of cognitive deterioration in VaD. They propose that measures of executive function would be more appropriate for the evaluation of VaD. More trials with clearly defined patient groups are suggested.

Although stabilization and treatment of cardiovascular conditions have been shown to slow cognitive decline in VaD (Forette, Seux, et al., 1998; Meyer, Judd, et al., 1986), other agents have been studied. Aside from cholinergic treatments, aspirin has often been prescribed to VaD patients, although there is little empirical evidence for its efficacy in treating cognitive symptoms in VaD (Rands, Orrel, et al., 2004). One retrospective case study reported that regular low-dose aspirin may be beneficial (Devine & Rands, 2003). Others have noted that depending on the underlying cause of the VaD, treatment with aspirin may increase the risk of cerebral hemorrhage (Rands et al., 2004; Sachdev, Brodaty, et al., 1999). Nimodipine, a calcium channel blocker that crosses the blood–brain barrier, is another agent that has been studied for treatment of VaD. Lopez-Arrieta and Birks' (2004) Cochrane review of nimodipine identified nine clinical trials conducted on patients with cerebrovascular dementia. At doses of 90 mg/day, they concluded that nimodipine can be an option for treatment and offers some improvement in overall global impression on the CGI, and cognitive function using the Sandoz Clinical Assessment— Geriatric (SCAG) scale (Shader, Harmatz, et al., 1974, 1976). There was no improvement in ADLs or disease status. Pantoni, Rossi, et al. (2000) studied the effects of nimodipine specifically in cases of subcortical VaD in a post hoc analysis of data from the Scandinavian Multi-Infarct Dementia Trial. They concluded that individuals with subcortical VaD benefited, showing significant differences on several neuropsychological tests, whereas those with multi-infarct dementia did not benefit.

Other agents have been studied in the past, including vinpocetine and hydergine, but these older studies did not offer differentiation of dementia subtypes or have enough power to determine effects (Schneider & Olin, 1994; Szatmari & Whitehouse, 2003). Propentofylline has been studied as a treatment for both AD and VaD. Although results from several trials appeared promising (Kittner, Rossner, et al., 1997; Mielke, Moller, et al., 1998; Rother, Erkinjuntti, et al., 1998), a systematic review by Frampton, Harvey, et al (2003) showed that there was limited evidence of benefit.

Lewy Body Dementia and Parkinson's Disease Dementia

Work with other dementias, beyond AD and VaD, has been more obscure. Lewy body dementia (LBD) is now recognized as a common type of progressive dementia (McKeith, Mintzer, et al., 2004), and patients with Parkinson's disease (PD) often have cognitive symptoms, with dementia occurring in approximately 20–30% of PD cases (Parkinson's disease dementia [PD-D]; Aarsland, Andersen, et al., 2001; Mayeux, Denaro, et al.,

1992). Both LBD and PD-D are synucleinopathies and are likely part of the same disease spectrum (McKeith & Burn, 2000). They share characteristic motor impairments and features, including hallucinations and delusions (see Welsh-Bohmer & Warren, Chapter 3, this volume, for more detail). The cognitive profiles of the two diseases are similar (Aarsland, Litvan, et al., 2003). Treatment is often focused on reduction of behavioral and psychotic symptoms and motor disturbances in addition to treatment of cognitive symptoms. Although LBD may have a presentation of cognitive deficits similar to that of AD, treatment of LBD is difficult because antipsychotics worsen the extrapyramidal features and in 50% of cases can trigger severe neuroleptic sensitivity reactions, with an increased risk of mortality (McKeith, Del Ser, et al., 2000). Treatment with anti-Parkinsonian medication to improve motor symptoms may increase confusion and hallucinations (McKeith 2000). Because the treatment of one symptom can exacerbate another, patients and caregivers should decide which problem is the most distressing before deciding upon a treatment (Burn & McKeith, 2003). Currently, criteria in clinical trials for treatment of LBD are similar to those of AD, requiring improvement in cognition and a clinical global measure of improvement.

There are few randomized clinical trials in the literature for the treatment of cognitive problems in LBD and PD-D (see Table 19.4). One study (McKeith, Del Ser, et al., 2000) involved a 20-week randomized, double-blind, placebo-controlled trial of 120 male and female patients with probable LBD. Patients were randomized to rivastigmine or placebo for 20 weeks followed by a 3-week rest period. Doses were titrated to 6 mg twice a day over an 8-week period. More of the patients on rivastigmine had adverse cholinergic effects. Using ITT analysis, differences between the treatment and placebo groups were not significant; however, differences on the NPI-4 showed a significant percentage of patients with a $\geq 30\%$ improvement from baseline to week 20. Effects were reversed after the 3-week rest period. Clinically relevant improvements included decreases in apathy, anxiety, delusions, and hallucinations. No change was seen on the Unified Parkinson Disease Rating Scale (UPDRS; Fahn, Elton, et al., 1987). In another open-label study (Minett, Thomas, et al., 2003), patients with LBD and PD-D were treated with 10 mg/day donepezil for 20 weeks followed by a 6-week withdrawal period. The aim of the trial was to compare the responses of LBD and PD-D and to determine the effects of donepezil withdrawal. Although the trial was small, significant improvements were shown on the MMSE at week 20 for both LBD and PD-D groups compared to baseline scores (LBD mean difference = 4.1, $p = .007$; PD-D mean difference 3.8, $p = .002$). There were no statistically significant changes from baseline on the NPI, although clinically significant changes were seen in most of the LBD patients and about a third of the PD-D patients.

There has been at least one double-blind, placebo-controlled trial of donepezil for cognitive impairment in Parkinson's disease (Aarsland, Laake, et al., 2002). Fourteen patients with mild to severe Parkinson's disease and evidence of memory impairment (MMSE scores 16–26) participated in the trial. Significant improvement on the MMSE ($p = .013$) and the CIBIC-Plus ($p = .034$) were shown in the treatment groups compared to placebo. The crossover design showed no carryover effects from treatment. Leroi, Brandt, et al. (2004) conducted a small randomized, double-blind, placebo-controlled study of donepezil in PD-D. Sixteen PD patients with clinical diagnoses of dementia or cognitive impairment were randomized to placebo or treatment with 10 mg donepezil per day, titrated over 6 weeks and continued for a total of 18 weeks. There were no significant differences between groups on psychiatric measures or in cognition measured with the MMSE and DRS total scores. A significant improvement with treatment over placebo

TABLE 19.4. Clinical Trials for Lewy Body Dementia and Parkinson's Disease Dementia

Author (year)	Primary diagnoses	No. of subjects	Analytic approach	Study design	Duration	Dropout rate (%)	Daily dose (mg/day)	Treatment	Primary outcome measures	Secondary outcome measures
McKeith, Del Ser, et al. (2000)	LBD	120	ITT, LOCF, OC	Randomized, double-blind, placebo-controlled, multicenter	23 weeks	23	12	Rivastigmine	NPI-4, computerized tests of attention, working memory, and episodic memory	NPI-10, MMSE
Aarsland et al. (2002)	PD	12	LOCF	Randomized, double-blind, placebo-controlled, crossover study	2 periods, 10 weeks each	14	10	Donepezil	MMSE, CIBIC-Plus, UPDRS—Motor subscale	NPI
Leroi et al. (2004)	PD and cognitive impairment	16	LOCF	Randomized, double-blind, placebo-controlled	18 weeks	25	10	Donepezil	NART, MMSE, DRS, BTA, DRS Attention subscore, TMT-A/B, DRS Initiation–Perseveration subscore, DRS Conceptualization subscore, Verbal Fluency, HVLT, DRS Memory subscale, VMI	NPI, CSDD, UPDRS Motor subscale, Hoehn and Yahr Stage, UPDRS, ADL & Complications of Therapy subscale
Minett et al. (2003)	LBD, PD-D	19	OC	Open label	12 months	21	10	Donepezil	MMSE, NPI, UPDRS	

Note. LBD, dementia with Lewy bodies; PD, Parkinson's disease; PD-D, Parkinson's disease with dementia; ITT, intent-to-treat; LOCF, last observation carried forward; OC, observed cases; outcome measures: BTA, Brief Test of Attention (Schretlen, Bobholtz, et al., 1996; Schretlen, Brandt, et al., 1996); CIBIC-Plus, Clinician's Interview-Based Impression of Change Plus Caregiver Input (Knopman et al., 1994); CSDD, Cornell Scale for Depression in Dementia (Alexopoulos et al., 1988); DRS, Dementia Rating Scale (Mattis, 1976; Mattis, 1989); Hoehn and Yahr Stage (Hoehn & Yahr, 1967); HVLT, Hopkins Verbal Learning Test (Brandt, 1991); MMSE, Mini-Mental State Examination (Folstein et al., 1975); NART, National Adult Reading Test (Nelson, 1982); NPI, Neuropsychiatric Inventory (Cummings et al., 1994); NPI-4, Neuropsychiatric Inventory 4-item subscore: delusions, hallucinations, apathy, and depression; NPI-10, Neuropsychiatric Inventory total of items 1–10; TMT-A, Trail Making Test—Part A (Lezak, 1995); TMT-B, Trail Making Test—Part B (Lezak, 1995); UPDRS, Unified Parkinson Disease Rating Scale (Fahn et al., 1987); Verbal Fluency (Barr & Brandt, 1996); VMI, Visual–Motor Integration (Beery, 1989).

was found in the Dementia Rating Scale (DRS) Memory subscore ($p < .05$). There was also a trend toward improvements in processing speed and attention. The authors noted a high dropout rate in both groups and suggested this may be due to the frailty of these older patients. Four of seven randomized to donepezil dropped out for adverse side effects and one for relapse of a preexisting mood disorder. There were no significant changes in UPDRS Motor or ADL subscales. Taken together, these studies show encouraging results for the use of cholinergics in the treatment of cognitive impairments in LBD and PDD. Future work in this area should consider appropriate outcomes, side effects of cholinergic treatment, and the effect of dropouts on study results.

Frontotemporal Dementia

Another form of dementia, frontotemporal dementia (FTD), is estimated to be present in up to 20% of patients appearing in memory clinics (Snowden, Neary, et al., 2002) and can be mistaken for AD (see Welsh-Bohmer & Warren, Chapter 3, this volume). Because the first symptoms of FTD are often behavior changes, treatment of the disorder is initiated for behavioral problems. However, it has been argued that the action of cholinesterase inhibitors would likely benefit FTD patients if the benefit were mediated via the nucleus basalis of Meynert (nbM), where cholinergic activity is decreased in both AD and FTD (Perry & Miller, 2001).

Large-scale trials of standard treatments in FTD are difficult to conduct, due in part to traditionally low rates of case ascertainment in clinical settings. The recent development of diagnostic criteria has led to the appearance of case reports of patients with standardized diagnoses (McKhann, Albert, et al., 2001). One such report of nine FTD patients suggested that cholinesterase inhibitors had a beneficial effect on cognitive testing and single-photon emission computed tomography (SPECT) imaging in approximately half of the patients (Lampl, Sadeh, et al., 2004). The need to conduct well-controlled multicenter trials is apparent and likely to occur in the near future, now that diagnostic criteria have been established.

Mild Cognitive Impairment

Another recently recognized entity is MCI (see Smith & Rush, Chapter 2, this volume). This condition is initially characterized by the presence of significant memory impairment with other aspects of cognition and function remaining relatively intact (Petersen, Smith, et al., 1999). MCI is different from age-associated memory impairment (AAMI) in that the former characterizes impairment in comparison to others of a comparable age, whereas the latter defines impairment with age when compared to a young normative sample. Several studies have demonstrated that individuals with MCI are at increased risk for a diagnosis of dementia, and some studies have suggested that about 25–45% of the MCI population will have a diagnosis of AD within in 3 years. Clinical trials have recruited individuals with this condition to determine if specific agents could delay the time to dementia onset. These trials constitute a form of secondary prevention of dementia, with MCI defining the early, symptomatic stage of disease.

The baseline characteristics of one multicenter clinical trial population of subjects with MCI have been described (Grundman, Petersen, et al., 2004), and several large clinical trials of MCI have been reported in abstract form (Gold, Francke, et al., 2004; Petersen, Grundman, et al., 2004; Visser, Thal, et al., 2003). The first to be reported (Visser et al.,

2003) examined the selective cyclooxygenase-2 (COX-2) inhibitor, rofecoxib, and found no effect in conversion to dementia, with mildly increased risk of dementia in those on drug. A significant difference in conversion to AD, was found with more conversion in the treatment group (6.4% vs. 4.5%; hazard ratio [HR] = 1.46; confidence interval [CI]: 1.09–1.94; p = .11). Secondary outcomes of cognition and function showed no treatment effect.

A large multicenter trial, by the AD2000 Collaborative Group (Petersen, Thomas, et al., 2005) sponsored by the National Institute on Aging (NIA) examined the cholinesterase inhibitor donepezil and vitamin E and found a reduction of conversion to AD in the first 18 months of treatment with donepezil. In addition, a benefit on cognitive measures was noted, lasting about the same time. However, the initial trial proposed to assess outcomes at 3 years, and there was no treatment effect in these a priori analyses. Also, the study was unable to detect any effect with vitamin E. Similar findings have been reported with other cholinesterase inhibitors. The largest effect is seen in those with poorest performance at baseline, and the duration of efficacy parallels that seen in the AD2000 trial. Taken together these results suggest that these studies capture a very early stage of dementia and not necessarily a prodromal phase.

DEVELOPING NEW APPROACHES TO AD TREATMENT

Attacking Amyloid

The hallmark of AD pathology is the amyloid plaque found in the brain. The development and build up of amyloid plaques are generally considered the primary underlying mechanism and etiology of the disease. Interventions that reduce amyloid plaque burden by altering amyloid metabolism or by maximizing clearance are potential mechanisms, although they remain theoretical. Plaque formation may be determined by the metabolism of an amyloid precursor protein (APP). Non-amyloidogenic, soluble APP (sAPP) is created when APP is cleaved by the β-secretase enzyme. Cleavage of APP by amyloid-β cleaving enzyme and then by γ-secretase leads to the formation of two species of amyloid-β(Aβ): $A\beta_{1-40}$ and $A\beta_{1-42}$, the latter of which is prone to self-aggregation, leading to plaque formation. Although environmental factors may influence the ratio of $A\beta_{1-40}$ to $A\beta_{1-42}$, therapeutic development has focused on affecting these pathways via enzyme modulators. Although selective enzyme inhibitors have been proposed, to date, clinical trials with such molecules have not gone forward because the targeted enzymes are ubiquitous and involved in other necessary processes, and inhibition of these processes could lead to mechanism-based toxicity.

Protein phosphorylation regulates APP cleavage by stimulating the α-secretase pathway, leading to the relatively nontoxic sAPP. Stimulation of protein kinase-C through steroid hormones such as 17-β-estradiol or DHEA have been shown to stimulate this pathway *in vitro*, but attempts to examine these approaches in clinical trials have not been fruitful, suggesting either that the model is not viable or the specific agents are not sufficiently selectively effective.

Active vaccination strategies in animal models have examined vaccination with Aβ and demonstrated that antibodies can be generated and can achieve clearance of plaque with some behavioral benefit. Human trials have not demonstrated very clear evidence of selective clearance, however. The only trial of the vaccine examined, to date, has shown reduced amyloid levels in some subjects as well as reduced brain volume, making it difficult to interpret these results (Fox & Schott, 2004).

Lowering Homocysteine

Recent studies have suggested that there may be an overlap in risks for cardiac disease and risks for AD, even when VaD is excluded. One potential risk factor is elevated homocysteine. This amino acid is involved in methionine and cysteine metabolism, and it plays a role in methylation reactions. The role of homocysteine as risk factor for atherosclerosis, cardiovascular disease (Bostom, Silbershatz, et al., 1999; Bots, Launer, et al., 1997) and stroke has been well established. Several studies have demonstrated that hyperhomocysteinemia is associated with AD in the absence of folate or vitamin B_{12} deficiency (Quadri, Fragiacomo, et al., 2004; Seshadri, Beiser, et al., 2002). When age-based norms for plasma homocysteine are divided into tertiles, the risk of AD in subjects in the highest tertile of homocysteine levels is more than four times higher than those in the lowest (McCaddon, Davies, et al., 1998; Seshadri et al., 2002). However, recent prospective epidemiological studies have not been able to find this association (Luchsinger, Tang, et al., 2004). Other evidence for a role for homocysteine in AD comes from data indicating that elevated plasma homocysteine occurs in neuropathologically confirmed cases of AD, in the absence of any vascular neuropathology (Clarke, Smith, et al., 1998). Also, among AD cases, higher levels of homocysteine are associated with more rapid radiological disease progression.

Folate, as well as vitamins B_{12} and B_6, are cofactors in metabolic reactions involving homocysteine and are very effective in lowering homocysteine levels (Homocysteine Lowering Trialists' Collaboration, 1998). In addition, folate improves nitric oxide availability in the brain. It also plays a number of other roles, such as acting as a coenzyme in the synthesis of serotonin and catecholamine neurotransmitters and of S-adenosylmethionine, and these have been reported to have antidepressant properties. Thus the use of folate may offer benefits through several mechanisms. It is therefore reasonable to postulate that lowering homocysteine with these vitamins would provide cognitive benefit or protection from cognitive decline. It has been demonstrated that supplementation with folate, vitamin B_{12}, and vitamin B_6 can lower homocysteine levels in patients with AD, even in those with already normal levels (Aisen, Egelko, et al., 2003), although the ability to affect cognition has not yet been demonstrated.

Several clinical trials have assessed folate effects on cognition in a range of populations. Four randomized trials were identified in a recent review (Malouf, Grimley, Evans, et al., 2003); one enrolled healthy women only (Bryan, Calvaresi, et al., 2002), and three others recruited people with mild to moderate cognitive impairment or dementia (Clarke et al., 1998; Fioravanti, Ferrario, et al., 1997; Sommer, Hoff, et al., 1998). Although folic acid plus vitamin B_{12} was effective in reducing serum homocysteine concentrations, a meta-analysis of these studies found no benefit from folic acid with or without vitamin B_{12} in comparison with placebo on any measures of cognition or mood for healthy, cognitively impaired, or demented people. Folic acid was well tolerated, and no adverse effects were reported. Several limitations of these studies include brief exposure periods, lack of standardized diagnosis, and lack of surety about appropriate outcome measures.

Effective lowering of homocysteine levels can be achieved with folate and vitamins B_{12} and B_6, even when levels are in the relatively normal range and in the presence of fortified grain (Aisen, Egelko et al., 2003). On this basis, and given its relative safety, it is reasonable to hypothesize that vitamin supplementation may lower the risks of cognitive decline and dementia in older adults. Because ongoing trials of high doses of supplementation continue to prove safe in aging populations, intervention with these supplements is worthy of study as a treatment strategy for primary prevention of cognitive loss and dementia in aging.

Lowering Lipids

There is compelling evidence from laboratory research in animal models and cell-culture systems, observational epidemiological studies, and small clinical trials that lowering cholesterol may reduce the pathology of AD. In support of the link between cholesterol and AD are *in vitro* studies demonstrating that cholesterol levels modulate the enzymatic processing of APP and, consequently, $A\beta$ production. Dietary manipulation to increase cholesterol in rabbits, rats, and transgenic mice demonstrated that high cholesterol yields increased secretion of amyloidagenic $A\beta_{1-40}$ and $A\beta_{1-42}$, as well as increasing size and number of amyloid plaques. Lipid lowering agents can reduce these findings both in cell cultures and in animals.

Epidemiological data have suggested that use of some lipid-lowering drugs is associated with a reduced risk of AD. Observational studies using existing clinical practice registries have reported an inverse association between statin use and risk of AD. Wolozin, Kellman, et al. (2000) reported cross-sectional examination of computerized medical records from 3 hospitals and demonstrated that the prevalence of diagnosed AD in patients taking lovastatin or pravastatin was 60–73% lower than the entire patient population during the period from 1996–1998. Jick, Zornberg, et al. (2000) examined the General Practice Research Database in the United Kingdom and reported reduced risk of AD with statin use. In this study the 284 cases were patients who developed a first-time diagnosis of dementia or AD between 1992 and 1998. Rockwood, Kirkland, et al. (2002) reported a reduced risk of AD among those using statins and other lipid-lowering agents (odds ratio [OR] = 0.26; 95% CI: 0.08–0.88). These authors noted no effect of statins among those over 80, though very few in that age group were taking statins. It is not clear that lowering cholesterol can help patients with AD, and retrospective studies have not supported that connection. However, well-controlled clinical trials could answer this question directly.

Despite these epidemiological findings, two recent large-scale trials conducted "add-on" studies to assess cognition. The Heart Protection Study (HPS, 2002) also examined the effect of simvastatin, a cholesterol-lowering agent, on the large cohort with the Telephone Interview for Cognitive Status (TICS). There were no difference in the percentages of participants classified as cognitively impaired (23.7% simvastatin-allocated vs. 24.2% placebo-allocated) or having incident dementia during follow-up (0.3% vs. 0.3%). In a trial of pravastatin in over 5,000 individuals ages 70–82, cognitive testing administered before and after treatment found no effect on measures of learning, memory, attention, speed of processing, mental status, or ADLs (Shepherd, Blauw, et al., 2002). Although these studies used large samples, the studies may have been too brief to observe the transition from normal cognition to dementia, resulting in insufficient power to observe an effect in this intact population.

The relative safety of these drugs has led to their use in trials to slow disease progression in AD. A single-site study of atorvastatin in patients with mild to moderate AD suggested a beneficial effect in cognitive and clinical global outcome measures (Sparks, Connor, et al., 2002). At this writing there are two ongoing multicenter trials of statins that will examine the rate of change on cognition and clinical global benefit over an 18-month period in patients with mild to moderate disease. Changes in cognition in dementia are rapid enough that trials of this duration should have sufficient power to detect effects.

PRIMARY PREVENTION OF AD

Although the exact cause of AD and some other dementias is not known, researchers can still investigate the efficacy of preventive agents that may have been identified in cohort studies. These agents include estrogens, antioxidants, anti-inflammatory drugs, and omega-3 fatty acids. We review the status of each agent as of December 2004 in the text that follows. The final analyses of these studies are projected into 2005 or beyond, and hence definitive information regarding safety and efficacy is forthcoming.

Estrogen

The surprising results of the Women's Health Initiative (WHI) illustrate the need to conduct randomized clinical trials to obtain accurate information about efficacy. Although efforts to examine the role of estrogen in many laboratory models and observational studies of dementia led to the expectation of benefit, such effects have not been realized in clinical trials. Estrogen receptors are colocalized with neurotrophin receptors in the basal forebrain, center of AD pathology. Estrogen has been associated with enhancing cholinergic neurons and promoting survival of hippocampal neurons exposed to excitotoxins, oxidative stress, or amyloid-β (Aβ). This hormone may also reduce the generation of Aβ_{1-40} and Aβ_{1-42} fragments. Animal studies demonstrate increased levels of Aβ_{1-40} and Aβ_{1-42} following ovariectomy, suggesting that menopause may accelerate Aβ formation in a period in which accumulation would be incipient. Observational studies supported the notion that estrogen use by women during the postmenopausal period may substantially reduce their risk of developing clinically diagnosed AD (e.g., LeBlanc, Janowsky, et al., 2001; Yaffe, Gawaya, et al., 1998; Zandi, Carlson, et al., 2002).

However, randomized clinical trials (RCTs) tell a very consistent story that contradicts these results. In women with AD, negative results have been reported repeatedly from studies of conjugated equine estrogens (CEE) for periods ranging from 3 months to 1 year and included 42, 50, and 120 subjects, respectively (Henderson, Paganini-Hill, et al., 2000; Mulnard, Cotman, et al., 2000; Wang, Liao, et al., 2000).

Most disappointing has been the results in prevention trials. Results of the Women's Health Initiative Memory Study (WHIMS), an add-on to the WHI, suggest that treatment with combined estrogen and progesterone (hormone replacement therapy or HRT) increases the risk of dementia and has a deleterious effect on mental status test scores (Rapp, Espeland, et al., 2003; Shumaker, Legault, et al., 2003). In the cohort of 4,532 women over the age of 65, followed for 4 years, the incidence of dementia with HRT was increased two-fold (relative risk [RR] = 2.0; CI: 1.2–3.5) compared to placebo (Shumaker et al., 2003). Although both the HRT and placebo groups demonstrated improved scores over time, the HRT group had smaller increases (annual point change: 0.15 vs. 0.21; $p = .03$) in mental status testing over time (Rapp et al., 2003). Results from the estrogen only arm of this study are equally disappointing, and although smaller sample sizes provided less power to see a statistical effect, the trend toward increased dementia, MCI, and declining performance on mental status examinations was apparent (Espeland, Rapp, et al., 2004; Shumaker, Legault, et al., 2004). Given that these agents apparently increase risk of vascular disease, it is possible that the dementia result is mediated through vascular mechanisms. This distinction may be important if positive and negative effects of the molecule are mediated through separate receptors. This possibility might permit the identification of a molecule with selective receptor modulation that could offer specific benefit without the associated vascular risk.

Antioxidants

The role of oxidative stress as a pathological mechanism in aging and dementia is supported by several lines of evidence. Biological studies demonstrate that the accumulation of free radicals is associated with damage to lipids, cell membranes, and proteins, including DNA and RNA. These oxidative byproducts induce the production of APP, already noted as the hallmark of AD pathology. The accumulation of Aβ fragments may reduce compensatory antioxidant ability resulting in further increases in Aβ deposition, synapse loss, DNA damage, neuronal dysfunction, and cell death. Free radical scavengers sequester free radicals, thereby rendering them impotent, minimizing oxidative reactions, and minimizing cellular damage (for a review of these potential mechanisms, see Butterfield, Griffin, et al., 2002).

Compelling support for the link between oxidative stress and Aβ comes from a recent study which crossed mice that had a knockout of one allele of a critical antioxidant enzyme (manganese superoxide dismutase: MnSOD) with a mouse that overexpressed a doubly mutated human β-amyloid precursor protein (i.e., Tg19959). Previous work established the MnSOD to cause elevated oxidative stress; the mice of the resulting cross demonstrated increases in both amyloid plaque burden and amyloid levels (Li, Calingasan, et al., 2004).

Evidence for a benefit of antioxidant agents comes from observational studies. Two prospective studies examined the association of dietary antioxidants and incident AD and provided evidence of reduced risk of AD (Engelhart, Geerlings, et al., 2002; Morris, Evans, et al., 2002). Daily intake of antioxidants, including vitamin E, vitamin C, beta-carotene, and flavenoids, was assessed with food-frequency questionnaires. In one study of over 800 subjects, followed for a mean of nearly 4 years, the group in the highest quintile of vitamin E intake had a relative risk of AD of 0.36 (95% CI: 0.11–1.17) compared to the group in the lowest quintile (Morris et al., 2002). Other antioxidants had no effect. In another study of more than 5,000 individuals followed for a mean of 6 years, a reduced risk of AD was reported with vitamin E and vitamin C intake (RR = 0.82; 95% CI: 0.66–1.00). Both reports failed to demonstrate a benefit to the use of antioxidant supplements, even though they increased the intake levels by 50% or more (Sano, 2002).

Data from the multi-ethnic cohort of the Washington Heights–Inwood Columbia Aging Project, in New York City, examined both dietary intake and supplemental use of antioxidant vitamins. Elderly subjects ($n = 980$) were followed for a mean of 4 years and nutrient data was gathered with a standardized food-frequency questionnaire, which also gathered data on supplement intake. This report found neither evidence of risk reduction nor a trend toward reduction with vitamins E, C, or carotenoids in any combination (Luchsinger, Tang, et al., 2003). Recently, a study from the well-described cohort of the Cache County Study of Memory, Health and Aging in Utah examined the effect of supplement intake on both prevalent and incident dementia. This report described a reduction in both prevalence and incidence with the combination of vitamins C and E, but not with either alone. A trend toward lower incidence of AD was associated with vitamin E in combination with a multivitamin possibly containing C, but not with a multivitamin alone (Zandi, Anthony, et al., 2004).

Typically, we move from observational studies to clinical trials to test hypotheses about potential treatments. A range of agents has been tried in clinical trials for the treatment of AD. As described below, early trials provided promising evidence of benefit with antioxidant therapies, but longer and larger trials have been disappointing.

Vitamin E

One study reported a benefit to AD with vitamin E, which was associated with a delay in clinical milestones compared to a placebo group among moderately impaired patients with AD, though no benefit was observed on standardized cognitive tests (Sano, Ernesto, et al., 1997). In the same study selegiline, a selective inhibitor of monoamine oxidase-B, was also effective, but the combination of drugs had no additional benefit. Physicians commonly recommend vitamin E as treatment for AD. Although no data are available for the combination, it is often given along with cholinesterase inhibitors, probably based on its perceived safety.

Two trials have reported the outcome of cognitive add-ons to other studies. One is the antioxidant arm of the HPS (1999). This large trial of over 20,000 enrollees, ages 40–80 years, selected subjects who were at risk for cardiovascular disease. The study used a 2×2 factorial design in which one agent was simvastatin and the other was an antioxidant combination of vitamin E (600 mg), vitamin C (250 mg), and beta-carotene (20 mg). Although no initial cognitive assessment was conducted, at the final visit the modified TICS (TICS-m) (Brandt, Spencer, et al., 1988; Welsh, Breitner, et al., 1993) was administered. Using an established cutoff score to identify cognitive impairment (22 of 39), no significant difference was found between the treatment groups in the percentages of the cognitively impaired (23.4% vitamin group vs. 24.4% placebo group). There was also no difference in the mean TICS-m score, and similar numbers of participants in each treatment group were reported to have developed dementia (0.3%) or other psychiatric disorders (0.6%). This rate of incident cases appears quite low, given the age range of the subject population, suggesting that this methodology may have been inadequately sensitive to cognitive change. Interestingly, these supplemental doses are far above the range in which dietary antioxidants were reported to have an effect.

The DATATOP study was a trial of over 800 subjects, newly diagnosed with Parkinson's disease, who were treated with selegiline or vitamin E (2000 international units [IU]) in a 2×2 factorial design. Cognitive assessments consisted of a battery of tests, including memory tests. No significant difference was noted among the groups (Kieburtz, McDermott, et al., 1994). Whether these results from this specialized population can be generalized is difficult to know, because the study population was relatively young and all had early/mild Parkinson's disease. Nevertheless, in this cognitively fragile cohort, high-dose vitamin E was unable to modify cognition.

An ongoing study known as PREADVISE, an "add-on" study, is examining the preventive effect of various antioxidants on prostate cancer (Kryscio, Mendiondo, et al., 2004). The parent study recruits men ages 60 years and over, who are randomly assigned to receive 200 micrograms of selenium and 400 IU of vitamin E per day, and are then monitored for prostate cancer. Participants randomized to assess antioxidant effects on prostate cancer may enroll in this cognitive add-on study, which will assess cognition and dementia with a brief screen followed by a more comprehensive workup. The relatively young age of the cohort may make it difficult to observe a cognitive change, and follow-up may be confounded by results or new findings with bearing on prostate treatment. Nevertheless, this study offers an opportunity to observe cognition in this unique cohort.

A recent meta-analysis of vitamin E trials suggests that high doses (400 IU) may be associated with increased risk of mortality, whereas lower doses might provide reduced risk of mortality (Miller, Pastor-Barriuso, et al., 2004). The mortality effect was not observed in persons with neurodegenerative disease, although these studies were included in the meta-analysis. The highest risk appears in studies that include individuals with cardiovascular risk factors, which increase with age and therefore may overlap with dementia risk. This observation will add additional caution to future research of vitamin E as a preventive measure for dementia.

Ginkgo Biloba

Ginkgo biloba is a plant extract containing flavenoids, which act as free radical scavengers that may protect cells from excessive lipid peroxidation and neuronal membrane breakdown (Scholtyssek, Damerau, et al., 1997). Laboratory studies indicate that Ginkgo biloba may maintain neuronal function in the hippocampus, with evidence of neurotrophic effects in mossy fibers and maintenance of age-related adrenergic and serotonergic receptor loss (Barkats, Venault, et al., 1995). Clinical trials of this drug (Table 19.5) in cognitively impaired populations have yielded mixed results, with reports of benefit in some but not all outcomes (van Dongen, van Rossum, et al., 2000).

A meta-analysis by Oken et al. (Oken, Storzbach, et al., 1998) found small but significant improvements in cognition in patients with AD who received 3–6 months of treatment with 120–240 mg of Ginkgo biloba extract (mean effect size = 0.41, 95% CI = 0.22–0.61). Evidence of improvement in other outcomes was inconclusive. These trials suggest that antioxidants, which appear to be well tolerated, may have a role in the treatment of AD, though sufficient evidence is not yet available (Oken et al., 1998).

A recent Cochrane Review of Ginkgo biloba for cognitive impairment and dementia expanded on the Oken analysis, identifying 33 studies (Birks & Grimley Evans, 2004). Of these studies, ranging from 3 to 52 weeks in duration, most were 12 weeks long and used comparable standard ginkgo biloba extracts. The review identified benefits on the CGI scale at 24 weeks (OR 2.16, 95% CI = 1.11–4.20, p = .02) and in cognition (standardized mean difference = –0.17, 95% CI = –0.3 to –0.02, p = .03). Measures of ADLs and mood and emotional function also showed benefits. The reviewers noted, however, that there was variation in the methodology of the studies, and evaluation of diagnostic categories was difficult because many trials did not distinguish between them. Few studies used the more rigorous ITT analysis, and thus conclusions were based on completers and may be biased. Because of mixed results in more recent trials and a low profile of side effects, additional large trials with modern methodology, diagnostic categories, and ITT analyses were recommended.

Currently, the Ginkgo Evaluation of Memory (GEM) study, a primary prevention trial sponsored by the National Center for Complementary and Alternative Medicine and the National Institute on Aging, is underway. The GEM study is a large multicenter trial including approximately 3,000 participants in four states, ages 75 years or older, who have been randomized to receive either Ginkgo biloba (240 mg/day) or placebo for 5 years. The primary outcome measure is dementia with a specified analysis for the diagnosis of AD; secondary outcome measures include a cognitive battery and tests of other domains typically used in clinical trials for AD.

In general, although antioxidant treatments appear to be safe, results from supplement trials in the area of cognition have been disappointing. There appear to be many methodological challenges to previously reported trials, so hopefully future studies will utilize more definitive trial designs.

TABLE 19.5. Clinical Trials for Ginkgo Biloba

Author (year)	Primary diagnoses	No. of subjects	Analytic approach	Study design	Duration	Dropout rate (%)	Daily dose	Treatment	Primary outcome measures	Secondary outcome measures
Hofferberth (1994)	AD	40			12 weeks	5	240 mg/day	Egb 761	SKT	SCAG, EEG
Le Bars et al. (1997)	AD, MID	309	ITT	Randomized, double-blind, placebo-controlled, fixed dose, parallel group, multicenter trial	52 weeks	20	120 mg/day	EGb 761	ADAS-Cog	CGI, GERRI
Kanowski et al. (1996)	DAT, MID	216	PP	Randomized, double-blind, placebo-controlled, multicenter	24 weeks	30	240 mg/day	EGb 761	SKT	CGI
Wesnes et al. (1987)	AD	54		Randomized, double-blind, placebo-controlled	12 weeks	7	120 mg/day	Tanakan (Ginkgo)	10-item battery; BVRT, digit symbol, word recall, reaction time	QOL
Rai et al. (1991)	AD	27		Double-blind placebo-controlled, parallel group	24 weeks	9	120 mg/day	Tanakan (Ginkgo)	MMSE, KDCT, KOLT, digit recall, classification task	EEG
Van Dongen et al. (2003)	AD, VaD, AAMI	123	ITT	Randomized, double-blind, placebo-controlled, parallel group, multicenter trial	24 weeks	8	240–160 mg/day	Egb 761	SKT, CGI-2	NAI-NAA

(continued)

TABLE 19.5. (continued)

Author (year)	Primary diagnoses	No. of subjects	Analytic approach	Study design	Duration	Dropout rate (%)	Daily dose	Treatment	Primary outcome measures	Secondary outcome measures
Kanowski & Hoerr (2003)	DAT, MID	205	ITT	Randomized, double-blind, placebo-controlled, fixed dose, parallel group	24 weeks	8	240 mg/day	Egb 761	Estiamted ADAS-Cog scores from SKT, CGI-2	
Solomon et al. (2002)	Healthy 60+	219	ITT	Randomized, double-blind, placebo-controlled	6 weeks	12	40 mg three times per day	Ginkgo OTC formula	CVLT, WAIS-R, WMS-R	

Note. AAMI, age-associated memory impairment; AD, Alzheimer's disease; DAT, dementia of the Alzheimer type; EEG, electroencephalograph; ITT, intent to treat; MID, multi-infarct dementia; PP, per protocol; VaD, vascular dementia; outcome measures: ADAS-Cog, Alzheimer's Disease Assessment Scale—Cognitive subscale (Mohs et al., 1997; Rosen et al., 1984); BVRT, Benton Visual Retention Test (Benton, 1963); CGI-C, Clinical Global Impression of Change (Guy, 1976); CGI-2, Clinical Global Impression of Change, item 2; CVLT, California Verbal Learning Test (Delis et al., 1987); GERRI, Geriatric Evaluation by Relatives Rating Instrument (Schwartz, 1983); KDCT, Kendrick Digit Copying Test (Kendrick et al., 1979); KOLT, Kendrick Object Learning Test (Kendrick et al., 1979); NAI-NAA, Nuremberg Gerontopsychological Rating Scale for Activities of Daily Living, Nurnberger Alters Inventar (Oswald & Fleischmann, 1995); QOL-AD, Quality of Life—Alzheimer's Disease (Logsdon et al., 2002); SCAG, Sandoz Clinical Assessment—Geriatric Scale (Shader et al., 1974; Shader et al., 1976); SKT, Syndrom Kurz Test (Overall & Schaltenbrand, 1992); WAIS-R, Wechsler Adult Intelligence Scale—Revised (Wechsler, 1981); WMS-R, Wechsler Memory Scale—Revised (Wechs er, 1987).

Anti-Inflammatory Agents

The use of anti-inflammatory agents as a preventive measure for AD is supported by several lines of evidence. Inflammatory processes play a role in the development of AD as evidenced by the wide range of proteins that appear in proximity to Aβ plaques in the brain. These proteins include β1–antichymotripsin, ICAM-1, and β2-macroglobuline and are presumed to be produced in the brain. Additionally, messenger ribonucleic acid (mRNA) for complement factors and complement proteins are found in neurons but not glial cells, supporting evidence of an inflammatory response to neural injury. Animal studies have shown that inflammation-related proteins are associated with higher amyloid load (Nilsson, Bales, et al., 2001), and that inhibition of complement factors lowers amyloid burden (Bales, Verina, et al., 1997). Autopsy studies have shown correlations between microglial cells and plaque deposits in the cerebral cortex of brains with AD but not with Aβ or tau markers of disease progression. Thus it is possible that inflammation is an early response to the disease process (Eikelenboom, van Gool, et al., 2004).

Several epidemiological studies support the association between inflammation and AD, based on the finding of lower prevalence and incidence of AD among users of nonsteroidal anti-inflammatory drugs (NSAID; Etminan, Gill, et al., 2003; in t' Veld, Ruitenberg, et al., 2001; Zandi, Anthony, et al., 2002). A meta-analysis of epidemiological studies (Szekely, Thorne, et al., 2004) reported a combined OR of 0.51 (95% [CI] 0.40–0.66) from cross-sectional evaluations in seven studies and a total of 12,979 subjects. Three studies, totaling 11,902 subjects, prospectively examined NSAID use for a duration of ≥ 2 years, and the authors reported a combined relative risk (RR) of AD of 0.42 (95% CI 0.26–0.66). These reports indicate that the strength of the association is in studies with exposure 1–2 years prior to the onset of disease, implying that NSAID protection can only be observed in the intact brain and is not likely to be apparent as a treatment effect.

Thus far, clinical trials of anti-inflammatory drugs in AD (Table 19.6) have been disappointing, although many were designed as treatment studies rather than as prevention trials. Glucocorticoids have not been proven to be beneficial in treating AD in clinical trials. A multicenter randomized clinical trial of prednisone showed no benefit, and significant side effects were observed (Aisen, Davis, et al., 2000). An early NSAID trial demonstrated borderline benefit in the presence of significant side effects with indomethacin (Rogers, Kirby, et al., 1993). A more recent study found no benefit for the NSAID diclofenac in combination with misoprostol and reported nearly a 50% withdrawal rate (Scharf, Mander, et al., 1999). Similarly, a multicenter trial of naproxen showed no benefit in patients with AD (Aisen, Schafer, et al., 2003). Although selective COX-2 inhibitors have reasonable CNS penetrability, two well-designed, year-long, multicenter trials of these agents have not demonstrated efficacy in the treatment of AD (Aisen, Schafer, et al., 2003; Reines, Block, et al., 2004).

It is possible that the effect observed with NSAIDs in epidemiological studies is not due to anti-inflammatory properties but rather to a reduction of Aβ formation. Recently, Weggen, Eriksen, et al. (2001) reported that ibuprofen and indomethacen reduced the amyloidagenic Aβ$_{42}$ formation in cell cultures. Naproxen and COX-2 inhibitors did not have the same effect (Weggen et al., 2001). The authors postulate that this effect may come from subtle mediation of secretase activity. Taken together, the present state of knowledge provides no data to support the use of anti-inflammatory agents for the treatment of AD, and the known side effect profile suggests that the risks may be consider-

TABLE 19.6. Clinical Trials for Anti-Inflammatory Agents

Author (year)	Primary diagnoses	No. of subjects	Analytic approach	Study design	Duration	Dropout rate (%)	Daily dose	Treatment	Primary outcome measures	Secondary outcome measures
Aisen et al. (2000)	Probable AD	138	ITT	Randomized, double-blind, placebo-controlled, two-group parallel, multicenter trial	1 year	22	20–10 mg/day	Prednisone	ADAS-Cog	CDR-SB, BDRS, HAM-D, BPRS
Rogers et al. (1993)	Mild to moderate AD	44	OC	Randomized, double-blind, placebo-controlled trial	6 months	36	100–150 mg/day	Indomethican	MMSE, ADAS-Cog, BNT, TK	
Scharf et al. (1999)	AD	41	ITT	Randomized, double-blind, placebo-controlled trial	25 weeks	34	50 mg diclofenac, 200 mg (D/M) misoprostol	Diclofenac & misoprostol	ADAS-Cog, GDS, CGI	MMSE, IADL, PSMS
Aisen, Schafer, et al. (2003)	Mild to moderate AD	351	ITT	Randomized, double-blind, placebo-controlled, parallel group trial	1 year	24	220 mg 2x/day	Naproxen	ADAS-Cog	CDR-SB, NPI, QOL-AD
Aisen, Schafer, et al. (2003)	Mild to moderate AD	351	ITT	Randomized, double-blind, placebo-controlled, parallel group trial	1 year	24	25 mg/day	Rofecoxib	ADAS-Cog	CDR-SB, NPI, QOL-AD

(continued)

TABLE 19.6. *(continued)*

Author (year)	Primary diagnoses	No. of subjects	Analytic approach	Study design	Duration	Dropout rate (%)	Daily dose	Treatment	Primary outcome measures	Secondary outcome measures
Reines et al. (2004)	Possible or probable AD	692	ITT	Randomized, double-blind, placebo-controlled, parallel group trial	1 year	25	25 mg/day	Rofecoxib	ADAS-Cog, CIBIC-Plus	MMSE, CDR, ADCS-ADL

Note. AD, Alzheimer's disease; ITT, intent-to-treat; OC, observed cases; outcome measures: ADAS-Cog, Alzheimer's Disease Assessment Scale—Cognitive subscale (Mohs et al., 1997; Rosen et al., 1984); ADCS-ADL, Alzheimer's Disease Cooperative Study—Activities of Daily Living (Galasko et al., 1997); BDRS, Blessed Dementia Rating Scale (Blessed et al., 1968); BNT, Boston Naming Test (Kaplan et al., 1976); BPRS, Brief Psychiatric Rating Scale (Overall & Graham, 1962); CDR, Clinical Dementia Rating (Hughes et al., 1982); CDR-SB, Clinical Dementia Rating—Sum of Boxes (Berg, 1988); CGI-C, Clinical Global Impression of Change (Guy, 1976); GDS, Global Deterioration Scale (Reisberg et al., 1982); CIBIC-Plus, Clinician's Interview-Based Impression of Change Plus Caregiver Input (Knopman et al., 1994); HAM-D, Hamilton Depression Rating Scale (Hamilton, 1960); IADL, Instrumental Activities of Daily Living (Lawton & Brody, 1969); MMSE, Mini-Mental State Examination (Folstein et al., 1975); NPI, Neuropsychiatric Inventory (Cummings et al., 1994); PSMS, Physical Self Maintenance Scale (Lawton & Brody, 1969); QOL-AD, Quality of Life—Alzheimer's Disease (Logsdon et al., 2002); TK, Token Test (De Renzi & Vignolo, 1962; Spreen & Benton, 1969).

able, particularly in an elderly population. Interest in these agents for the prevention of AD has led to several secondary and primary prevention trials.

Demonstrating primary prevention with anti-inflammatory agents has also proved challenging. A primary prevention trial, the Alzheimer Disease Anti-Inflammatory Prevention Trial (ADAPT), is a multicenter trial that suspended treatment in December 2004. The ADAPT study is based on observational data (Martin, Meinert, et al., 2002) and explores reduction of incident dementia and mitigation of cognitive decline as the primary outcome measures. The study enrolled 2,625 individuals, ages 70 years and older, with a family history of AD in a first-degree relative and examined two anti-inflammatory agents, the conventional NSAID, naproxen sodium (220 mg twice a day), and the selective COX-2 inhibitor celecoxib (200 mg twice a day) and planned to follow subjects for 7 years. The trial was stopped early due to a finding of increased risk of heart attack in subjects taking celecoxib in an unrelated cancer study. In an analysis of adverse events, the investigators of the ADAPT trial did not find increased risk in those randomized to Celecoxib; however, they did find an increased risk of heart attacks and strokes in the subjects taking naproxen compared to those on placebo. Another primary prevention trial for aspirin, the ASPREE trial (Aspirin in Reducing Events in the Elderly), has begun to follow 15,000 study participants, ages 70 years and older, for 5 years (Nelson, Reid, et al., 2003).

Other Nutritional Supplements

Several approaches to cognitive enhancement have been suggested in the nutritional literature, although few randomized controlled trials are available to assess their efficacy. The following is a sample of potential leads. Though far from comprehensive, it illustrates how leads might be identified and demonstrates the need to conduct well-controlled clinical trials in order to confirm these signals.

Omega-3 fatty acids, the long-chain polyunsaturated fatty acids found in plant and marine sources, have been studied for their beneficial value in a number of contexts. They have been shown to reduce hypertension, coronary artery disease, reduce risk of cardiac arrest, and decrease triglyceride levels (Freeman, 2000). Additionally, they have been shown to have neuroprotective effects in lab studies (Calon, Lim, et al., 2004; Kimura, Saito, et al., 2002).

Docosahexaenoic acid (DHA) is the n-3 polyunsaturated fatty acid that is a component of membrane phospholipids in the brain. An epidemiological study of 815 participants in the Chicago Health and Aging Project showed that subjects who consumed one or more fish meals per week had a 60% reduced risk of AD (Morris, Evans, et al., 2003). Persons with the highest intake of total n-3 polyunsaturated fatty acids had an inverse association with AD compared to those in the group that consumed the lowest (RR = 0.4, 95% CI = 0.1–0.9). In an evaluation of DHA specifically, the reduced risk was similar (RR = 0.3, 95% CI = 0.1–0.9). Thus far, there has been one small treatment trial of omega-3 fatty acids for dementia. In this trial, a total of 20 patients with mild to moderate dementia were randomized to receive 0.72 g of DHA daily for 1 year. Significant differences between groups were shown on the Hasegawa Dementia scale at 3 and 6 months but not at 12 months ($p < .05$). Patients taking DHA also showed significant improvement on the MMSE at 6 months but not 12 months ($p < .05$). Currently, a clinical trial for fish oil and alpha lipoic acid use to treat AD is recruiting patients. This randomized, placebo-controlled, phase I and II trial anticipates an enrollment of 39 patients and will continue for 1 year.

The polyphenol resveratrol (3,5,4'-trihydroxy-*trans*-stilbene) is a sirtuin-activating compound; this compound stimulates the catalytic activity of yeast and human sirtuins and prolong lifespan of yeast (Cohen, Miller, et al., 2004; Howitz, Bitterman, et al., 2003; Wood, Rogina, et al., 2004). It is derived from plants and is found in highest levels in red wine and the skin of red grapes (*Vitis vinifera*). This compound may be responsible for the "French paradox"—epidemiological data demonstrating an inverse correlation between red wine consumption and incidences of cardiovascular disease and of dementia. A small randomized clinical trial using a combination of agents, among which resveriatrol was the most prominent, was reported in abstract form, demonstrating benefit in comparison to a placebo control (Blass & Gordon, 2004).

Taken together, these types of agents offer the possibility for treatment of cognitive loss with potentially safe substances. However, there are many challenges to demonstrating efficacy with these drugs. First, the specific active agent is difficult to identify and is based on many suppositions. Second, there is little known about what dose would reasonably affect cognitive behavior and what the side effect profile of that specific dose might be. Finally, the commercial availability of an apparently safe agent can make it difficult to generate enthusiasm for clinical trials among patient communities, who may opt for using what appears to be a benign treatment.

SUMMARY AND CONCLUSIONS

It is currently recognized that approved and effective treatments exist for AD. It is also recognized that current options are not entirely satisfactory, in that the benefits are small and brief in this degenerative condition. Further the need to maximize cognitive function throughout the lifespan is acknowledged by both young and old. In a society with growing technological demands, even minimal loss of cognitive capacity can create significant functional disability. These forces, along with the aging of the global population, raises awareness and motivates efforts to find interventions to reverse and prevent cognitive loss and dementia. To move these efforts forward will require greater knowledge of the pathophysiology of dementia across the entire disease spectrum as well as early cognitive losses occurring with normal brain aging. The methodology to conduct reliable clinical trials is well established, and clinicians and scientists must work to ensure public understanding and commitment to participating in the clinical trials needed to provide the convincing evidence of efficacy. Only through this partnership will the public health issue be addressed.

REFERENCES

Aarsland, D., Andersen, K., et al. (2001). Risk of dementia in Parkinson's disease: A community-based, prospective study. *Neurology*, 56(6), 730–736.

Aarsland, D., Laake, K., et al. (2002). Donepezil for cognitive impairment in Parkinson's disease: A randomised controlled study. *Journal of Neurology, Neurosurgery, and Psychiatry*, 72(6), 708–712.

Aarsland, D., Litvan, I., et al. (2003). Performance on the Dementia Rating Scale in Parkinson's disease with dementia and dementia with Lewy bodies: Comparison with progressive supranuclear palsy and Alzheimer's disease. *Journal of Neurology, Neurosurgery and Psychiatry*, 74(9), 1215–1220.

Aisen, P. S., Davis, K. L., et al. (2000). A randomized controlled trial of prednisone in Alzheimer's disease. Alzheimer's Disease Cooperative Study. *Neurology, 54*(3), 588–593.

Aisen, P. S., Egelko, S., et al. (2003). A pilot study of vitamins to lower plasma homocysteine levels in Alzheimer disease. *American Journal of Geriatric Psychiatry, 11*(2), 246–249.

Aisen, P. S., Schafer, K. A., et al. (2003). Effects of rofecoxib or naproxen vs. placebo on Alzheimer disease progression: A randomized controlled trial. *Journal of the American Medical Association, 289*(21), 2819–2826.

Alexopoulos, G. S., Abrams, R. C., et al. (1988). Cornell Scale for Depression in Dementia. *Biological Psychiatry, 23*(3), 271–284.

American Psychiatric Association. (1987). *Diagnostic and statistical manual of mental disorders* (3rd ed., rev.). Washington, DC: Author.

Areosa, S. A., & Sherriff, F. (2004). Memantine for dementia. *Cochrane Database of Systematic Reviews* (3): CD003154.

Bales, K. R., Verina, T., et al. (1997). Lack of apolipoprotein E dramatically reduces amyloid beta-peptide deposition. *Nature Genetics, 17*(3), 263–264.

Barkats, M., Venault, P., et al. (1995). Effect of long-term treatment with EGb 761 on age-dependent structural changes in the hippocampi of three inbred mouse strains. *Life Sciences, 56*(4), 213–222.

Barr, A., & Brandt, J. (1996). Word-list generation deficits in dementia. *Journal of Clinical and Experimental Neuropsychology, 18*(6), 810–822.

Beery, K. E. (1989). *Developmental test of visual–motor integration: Administration, scoring and teaching manual.* Cleveland, OH: Modern Curriculum Press.

Benton, A. L. (1963). *The Revised Visual Retention Test: Clinical and experimental applications.* New York: Psychological Corporation.

Berg, L. (1988). Clinical Dementia Rating (CDR). *Psychopharmacology Bulletin, 24*(4), 637–639.

Birks, J., & Grimley Evans, J. (2004). Ginkgo biloba for cognitive impairment and dementia. *Cochrane Database of Systematic Reviews* (3): CD003120.

Birks, J., Grimley Evans, J., et al. (2004). Rivastigmine for Alzheimer's disease. *Cochrane Database of Systematic Reviews* (3): CD001191.

Birks, J. S., & Harvey, R. (2004). Donepezil for dementia due to Alzheimer's disease. *Cochrane Database of Systematic Reviews* (3): CD001190.

Black, S., Roman, G. C., et al. (2003). Efficacy and tolerability of donepezil in vascular dementia: Positive results of a 24-week, multicenter, international, randomized, placebo-controlled clinical trial. *Stroke, 34*(10), 2323–2330.

Blass, J. P., & Gordon, D. (2004). An adjunct treatment for Alzheimer Disease. *Neurobiology of Aging, 25*(S2), 84.

Blessed, G., Tomlinson, B. E., et al. (1968). The association between quantitative measures of dementia and of senile change in the cerebral grey matter of elderly subjects. *British Journal of Psychiatry, 114*(512), 797–811.

Bostom, A. G., Silbershatz, H., et al. (1999). Nonfasting plasma total homocysteine levels and all-cause and cardiovascular disease mortality in elderly Framingham men and women. *Archives of Internal Medicine, 159*(10), 1077–1080.

Bots, M. L., Launer, L. J., et al. (1997). Homocysteine, atherosclerosis and prevalent cardiovascular disease in the elderly: The Rotterdam Study. *Journal of Internal Medicine, 242*(4), 339–347.

Brandt, J. (1991). The Hopkins Verbal Learning Test: Development of a new memory test with six equivalent forms. *Clinical Neurophysiology, 5,* 125–142.

Brandt, J., Spencer, M., et al. (1988). The Telephone Interview for Cognitive Status. *Neuropsychiatry, Neuropsychology, and Behavioral Neurology, 1,* 111–117.

Brod, M., Stewart, A. L., et al. (1999). Conceptualization and measurement of quality of life in dementia: The Dementia Quality of Life instrument (DQoL). *Gerontologist, 39*(1), 25–35.

Brookmeyer, R., Gray, S., et al. (1998). Projections of Alzheimer's disease in the United States and the public health impact of delaying disease onset. *American Journal of Public Health*, 88(9), 1337–1342.

Bryan, J., Calvaresi, E., et al. (2002). Short term folate vitamin B$_{12}$ or vitamin B$_6$ supplementation slightly affects memory performance but not mood in women of various ages. *Journal of Nutrition*, 132(6), 1345–1356.

Burn, D. J., & McKeith, I. G. (2003). Current treatment of dementia with Lewy bodies and dementia associated with Parkinson's disease. *Movement Disorders*, 18(Suppl. 6), S72–S79.

Butterfield, D. A., Griffin, S., et al. (2002). Amyloid beta-peptide and amyloid pathology are central to the oxidative stress and inflammatory cascades under which Alzheimer's disease brain exists. *Journal of Alzheimer's Disease*, 4(3), 193–201.

Calon, F., Lim, G. P., et al. (2004). Docosahexaenoic acid protects from dendritic pathology in an Alzheimer's disease mouse model. *Neuron*, 43(5), 633–645.

Clarke, R., Smith, A. D., et al. (1998). Folate, vitamin B$_{12}$, and serum total homocysteine levels in confirmed Alzheimer disease. *Archives of Neurology*, 55(11), 1449–1455.

Cohen, H. Y., Miller, C., et al. (2004). Calorie restriction promotes mammalian cell survival by inducing the SIRT1 deacetylase. *Science*, 305(5682), 390–392.

Cohen-Mansfield, J. (1986). Agitated behaviors in the elderly: II. Preliminary results in the cognitively deteriorated. *Journal of the American Geriatric Society*, 34(10), 722–727.

Courtney, C., Farrell, D., et al. (2004). Long-term donepezil treatment in 565 patients with Alzheimer's disease (AD2000): Randomised double-blind trial. *Lancet*, 363(9427), 2105–2115.

Cummings, J. L., Mega, M., et al. (1994). The Neuropsychiatric Inventory: Comprehensive assessment of psychopathology in dementia. *Neurology*, 44(12), 2308–2314.

DeJong, R., Osterlund, O., et al. (1989). Measurement of quality of life changes in patients with Alzheimer's disease. *Clinical Therapeutics*, 11, 545–554.

Delis, D. C., Kramer, J., et al. (1987). *California Verbal Learning Test (CVLT) Manual*. San Antonio, TX: Psychological Corporation.

De Renzi, E., & Vignolo, L. A. (1962). The token test: A sensitive test to detect receptive disturbances in aphasics. *Brain*, 85, 665–678.

Devine, M. E., & Rands, G. (2003). Does aspirin affect outcome in vascular dementia? A retrospective case-notes analysis. *International Journal of Geriatric Psychiatry*, 18(5), 425–431.

Eikelenboom, P., & van Gool, W. A. (2004). Neuroinflammatory perspectives on the two faces of Alzheimer's disease. *Journal of Neural Transmission*, 111(3), 281–294.

Engelhart, M. J., Geerlings, M. I., et al. (2002). Dietary intake of antioxidants and risk of Alzheimer disease. *Journal of the American Medical Association*, 287(24), 3223–3229.

Erkinjuntti, T., Kurz, A., et al. (2002). Efficacy of galantamine in probable vascular dementia and Alzheimer's disease combined with cerebrovascular disease: A randomised trial. *Lancet*, 359(9314), 1283–1290.

Erkinjuntti, T., Kurz, A., et al. (2003). An open-label extension trial of galantamine in patients with probable vascular dementia and mixed dementia. *Clinical Therapeutics*, 25(6), 1765–1782.

Erzigkeit, H. (1989). The SKT: A short cognitive performance test as an instrument for the assessment of clinical efficacy of cognitive enhancers. In W. Bergener & B. Reisberg (Eds.), *Diagnosis and treatment of senile dementia* (pp. 164–174). Heidelberg: Springer-Verlag.

Espeland, M. A., Rapp, S. R., et al. (2004). Conjugated equine estrogens and global cognitive function in postmenopausal women: Women's Health Initiative Memory Study. *Journal of the American Medical Association*, 291(24), 2959–2968.

Etminan, M., Gill, S., et al. (2003). Effect of non-steroidal anti-inflammatory drugs on risk of Alzheimer's disease: Systematic review and meta-analysis of observational studies. *British Medical Journal*, 327(7407), 128.

Fahn, S., Flton, R. L., et al. (1987). Unified Parkinson's Disease Rating Scale. In S. Fahn & C. D. Marsden (Eds.), *Recent developments in Parkinson's Disease* (Vol. 2, pp. 153–163). Florham Park, NJ: Macmillan.

Fioravanti, M., Ferrario, E., et al. (1997). Low folate levels in the cognitive decline of elderly patients and efficacy of folate as a treatment for improving memory deficits. *Archives of Gerontology and Geriatrics, 26*(1), 1–13.

Folstein, M. F., Folstein, S. E., et al. (1975). "Mini-Mental state": A practical method for grading the cognitive state of patients for the clinician. *Journal of Psychiatric Research, 12*(3), 189–198.

Forette, F., Seux, M. L., et al. (1998). Prevention of dementia in randomised double-blind placebo-controlled Systolic Hypertension in Europe (Syst-Eur) trial. *Lancet, 352*(9137), 1347–1351.

Fox, N. C., & Schott, J. M. (2004). Imaging cerebral atrophy: Normal ageing to Alzheimer's disease. *Lancet, 363*(9406), 392–394.

Frampton, M., Harvey, R. J., et al. (2003). Propentofylline for dementia. *Cochrane Database of Systematic Reviews* (2): CD002853.

Freeman, M. P. (2000). Omega-3 fatty acids in psychiatry: A review. *Annals of Clinical Psychiatry, 12*(3), 159–165.

Fuld, P. A. (1978). Psychological testing in the differential diagnosis of the dementias. In R. Katzman & R. D. Terry (Eds.), *Alzheimer's disease: Senile dementia and related disorders. Vol. 7. Aging* (pp. 185–193). New York: Raven Press.

Galasko, D., Bennett, D., et al. (1997). An inventory to assess activities of daily living for clinical trials in Alzheimer's disease: The Alzheimer's Disease Cooperative Study. *Alzheimer Disease and Associated Disorders, 11*(Suppl. 2), S33–S39.

Geldmacher, D. S. (1997). Donepezil (Aricept) therapy for Alzheimer's disease. *Comprehensive Therapy, 23*(7), 492–493.

Gelinas, I., Gauthier, L., et al. (1999). Development of a functional measure for persons with Alzheimer's disease: The disability assessment for dementia. *American Journal of Occupational Therapy, 53*(5), 471–481.

Gold, M., Francke, S., et al. (2004). Impact of ApoE genotyping on the efficacy of galantamine for the treatment of mild cognitive impairment. *Neurobiology of Aging, 25*(S2), 521.

Goldsmith, D. R., & Scott, L. J. (2003). Donepezil: In vascular dementia. *Drugs and Aging, 20*(15), 1127–1136.

Gottfries, C. G., Brane, G., et al. (1982). A new rating scale for dementia syndromes. *Gerontology, 28*(Suppl. 2), 20–31.

Greene, J. G., Smith, R., Gardner, M., & Timburg, G. C. (1982). Measuring behavioral disturbance of elderly demented in patients in the community and its effects on relatives: A factor analytic study. *Age and Ageing, 11*, 121–126.

Grundman, M., Petersen, R. C., et al. (2004). Mild cognitive impairment can be distinguished from Alzheimer disease and normal aging for clinical trials. *Archives of Neurology, 61*(1), 59–66.

Guy, W. (Ed.). (1976). *ECDEU Assessment Manual for Psychopharmacology* (Rev. ed.). Rockville, MD: U.S. Department of Health and Human Service, Alcohol Drug Abuse and Mental Health Administration, NIMH Psychopharmacology Research Branch.

Hamilton, M. (1960). A rating scale for depression. *Journal of Neurology, Neurosurgery, and Psychiatry, 23*, 56–62.

Henderson, V. W., Paganini-Hill, A., et al. (2000). Estrogen for Alzheimer's disease in women: Randomized, double-blind, placebo-controlled trial. *Neurology, 54*(2), 295–301.

Hoehn, M. M., & Yahr, M. D. (1967). Parkinsonism: Onset, progression and mortality. *Neurology, 17*(5), 427–442.

Hofferberth, B. (1994). The efficacy of EGb 761 in patients with senile dementia of the Alzheimer type: A double-blind, placebo-controlled study on different levels of investigation. *Human Psychopharmacology, 9*, 215–222.

Homocysteine Lowering Trialists' Collaboration. (1998). Lowering blood homocysteine with folic acid based supplements: Meta-analysis of randomised trials. *British Medical Journal, 316*(7135), 894–898.

Howitz, K. T., Bitterman, K. J., et al. (2003). Small molecule activators of sirtuins extend *Saccharomyces cerevisiae* lifespan. *Nature, 425*(6954), 191–196.

Hughes, C. P., Berg, L., et al. (1982). A new clinical scale for the staging of dementia. *British Journal of Psychiatry, 140*, 566–572.

in t' Veld, B. A., Ruitenberg, A., et al. (2001). Nonsteroidal antiinflammatory drugs and the risk of Alzheimer's disease. *New England Journal of Medicine, 345*(21), 1515–1521.

Jick, H., Zornberg, G. L., et al. (2000). Statins and the risk of dementia. *Lancet, 356*(9242), 1627–1631.

Jones, R. W., Soininen, H., et al. (2004). A multinational, randomised, 12-week study comparing the effects of donepezil and galantamine in patients with mild to moderate Alzheimer's disease. *International Journal of Geriatric Psychiatry, 19*(1), 58–67.

Kanowski, S., Herrmann, W. M., et al. (1996). Proof of efficacy of the ginkgo biloba special extract EGb 761 in outpatients suffering from mild to moderate primary degenerative dementia of the Alzheimer type or multi-infarct dementia. *Pharmacopsychiatry, 29*(2), 47–56.

Kanowski, S., & Hoerr, R. (2003). Ginkgo biloba extract EGb 761 in dementia: intent-to-treat analyses of a 24-week, multi-center, double-blind, placebo-controlled, randomized trial. *Pharmacopsychiatry, 36*(6), 297–303.

Kaplan, E., Goodglass, H., et al. (1976). *The Boston Naming Test*. Boston: Veterans Administration.

Katz S., Ford A. B., et al. (1963). Studies of illness in the aged: The Index of ADL—A standardized measure of biological and psychosocial function. *Journal of the American Medical Association, 185*, 914–919.

Kendrick, D. C., Gibson, A. J., et al. (1979). The Revised Kendrick Battery: Clinical studies. *British Journal of Social and Clinical Psychology, 18*(3), 329–340.

Kieburtz, K., McDermott, M., et al. (1994). The effect of deprenyl and tocopherol on cognitive performance in early untreated Parkinson's disease: Parkinson Study Group. *Neurology, 44*(9), 1756–1759.

Kimura, S., Saito, H., et al. (2002). Docosahexaenoic acid attenuated hypertension and vascular dementia in stroke-prone spontaneously hypertensive rats. *Neurotoxicology and Teratology, 24*(5), 683–693.

Kittner, B., Rossner, M., et al. (1997). Clinical trials in dementia with propentofylline. *Annals of the New York Academy of Sciences, 826*, 307–316.

Knapp, M. J., Knopman, D. S., et al. (1994). A 30-week randomized controlled trial of high-dose tacrine in patients with Alzheimer's disease: The Tacrine Study Group. *Journal of the American Medical Association, 271*(13), 985–991.

Knopman, D. S., Knapp, M. J., et al. (1994). The Clinician Interview-Based Impression (CIBI): A clinician's global change rating scale in Alzheimer's disease. *Neurology, 44*(12), 2315–2321.

Kryscio, R. J., Mendiondo, M. S., et al. (2004). Designing a large prevention trial: Statistical issues. *Statistics in Medicine, 23*(2), 285–296.

Kumar, V., Anand, R., et al. (2000). An efficacy and safety analysis of Exelon in Alzheimer's disease patients with concurrent vascular risk factors. *European Journal of Neurology, 7*(2), 159–169.

Lampl, Y., Sadeh, M., et al. (2004). Efficacy of acetylcholinesterase inhibitors in frontotemporal dementia. *Annals of Pharmacotherapy, 38*(11), 1967–1968.

LaRue, A. (1989). Patterns of performance on the Fuld Object-Memory Evaluation in elderly inpatients with depression or dementia. *Journal of Clinical and Experimental Neuropsychology, 11*, 409–422.

Lawton, M. P., & Brody, E. M. (1969). Assessment of older people: Self-maintaining and instrumental activities of daily living. *Gerontologist, 9*(3), 179–186.

Le Bars, P. L., Katz, M. M., et al. (1997). A placebo-controlled, double-blind, randomized trial of an extract of Ginkgo biloba for dementia: North American EGb Study Group. *Journal of the American Medical Association, 278*(16), 1327–1332.

LeBlanc, E. S., Janowsky, J., et al. (2001). Hormone replacement therapy and cognition: Systematic review and meta-analysis. *Journal of the American Medical Association, 285*(11), 1489–1499.

Lehfeld, H., & Erzigkeit, H. (1997). The SKT: A short cognitive performance test for assessing deficits of memory and attention. *International Psychogeriatrics, 9*(Suppl. 1), 115–121.

Leroi, I., Brandt, J., et al. (2004). Randomized placebo-controlled trial of donepezil in cognitive impairment in Parkinson's disease. *International Journal of Geriatric Psychiatry, 19*(1), 1–8.

Lezak, M. D. (1995). *Neuropsychological assessment.* New York: Oxford University Press.

Li, F., Calingasan, N. Y., et al. (2004). Increased plaque burden in brains of APP mutant MnSOD heterozygous knockout mice. *Journal of Neurochemistry, 89*(5), 1308–1312.

Li, Y., Meyer, J. S., et al. (2002). Feasibility of vascular dementia treatment with cholinesterase inhibitors. *International Journal of Geriatric Psychiatry, 17*(2), 194–196.

Linn, M. W. (1967). A rapid disability rating scale. *Journal of the American Geriatrics Society, 15*(2), 211–214.

Logsdon, R. G., Gibbons, L. E., et al. (2002). Assessing quality of life in older adults with cognitive impairment. *Psychosomatic Medicine, 64*(3), 510–519.

Lopez-Arrieta, J. L. A., & Birks, J. (2004). Nimodipine for primary degenerative, mixed and vascular dementia. *Cochrane Database of Systematic Reviews* (3): CD000147.

Luchsinger, J. A., Tang, M. X., et al. (2003). Antioxidant vitamin intake and risk of Alzheimer disease. *Archives of Neurology, 60*(2), 203–208.

Luchsinger, J. A., Tang, M. X., et al. (2004). Plasma homocysteine levels and risk of Alzheimer disease. *Neurology, 62*(11), 1972–1976.

Malouf, R., & Birks, J. (2004). Donepezil for vascular cognitive impairment. *Cochrane Database of Systematic Reviews* (1): CD004395.

Malouf, R., Grimley Evans, J., et al. (2004). Folic acid with or without vitamin B12 for cognition and dementia. *Cochrane Database of Systematic Reviews* (4): CD004514.

Mani, R. B. (2004). The evaluation of disease modifying therapies in Alzheimer's disease: A regulatory viewpoint. *Statistical Medicine, 23*(2), 305–314.

Manos, P. J. (1997). The utility of the ten-point clock test as a screen for cognitive impairment in general hospital patients. *General Hospital Psychiatry, 19*(6), 439–444.

Martin, B. K., Meinert, C. L., et al. (2002). Double placebo design in a prevention trial for Alzheimer's disease. *Controlled Clinical Trials, 23*(1), 93–99.

Mattis, S. (1976). Mental status examination for organic mental syndrome in the elderly patient. In L. Bellak & T. Karasu (Eds.), *Geriatric psychiatry: A handbook for psychiatrists and primary care physicians* (pp. 77–101). New York: Grune & Stratton.

Mattis, S. (1989). *Dementia Rating Scale.* Odessa, FL: Psychological Assessment Resources.

Mayeux, R., Denaro, J., et al. (1992). A population-based investigation of Parkinson's disease with and without dementia: Relationship to age and gender. *Archives of Neurology, 49*(5), 492–497.

McCaddon, A., Davies, G., et al. (1998). Total serum homocysteine in senile dementia of Alzheimer type. *International Journal of Geriatric Psychiatry, 13*(4), 235–239.

McKeith, I., & Burn, D. J. (2000). Spectrum of Parkinson's disease, Parkinson's dementia, and Lewy body dementia. In S. T. DeKosky (Ed.), *Neurologic clinics: Dementia* (Vol. 18, pp. 865–883). Philadelphia: WB Saunders.

McKeith, I., Del Ser, T., et al. (2000). Efficacy of rivastigmine in dementia with Lewy bodies: A randomised, double-blind, placebo-controlled international study. *Lancet, 356*(9247), 2031–2036.

McKeith, I., Mintzer, J., et al. (2004). Dementia with Lewy bodies. *Lancet Neurology, 3*(1), 19–28.

McKhann, G. M., Albert, M. S., et al. (2001). Clinical and pathological diagnosis of frontotemporal dementia: Report of the Work Group on Frontotemporal Dementia and Pick's Disease. *Archives of Neurology, 58*(11), 1803–1809.

McKhann, G. M., Drachman, D., et al. (1984). Clinical diagnosis of Alzheimer's disease: Report of the NINCDS–ADRDA Work Group under the auspices of Department of Health and Human Services task force on Alzheimer's disease. *Neurology, 34*(7), 939–944.

Mendez, M. F., Younesi, F. L., et al. (1999). Use of donepezil for vascular dementia: Preliminary clinical experience. *Journal of Neuropsychiatry and Clinical Neuroscience, 11*(2), 268–270.

Meyer, J. S., Chowdhury, M. H., et al. (2002). Donepezil treatment of vascular dementia. *Annals of the New York Academy of Sciences, 977,* 482–486.

Meyer, J. S., Judd, B. W., et al. (1986). Improved cognition after control of risk factors for multi-infarct dementia. *Journal of the American Medical Association, 256*(16), 2203–2209.

Mielke, R., Moller, H. J., et al. (1998). Propentofylline in the treatment of vascular dementia and Alzheimer-type dementia: Overview of phase I and phase II clinical trials. *Alzheimer Disease and Associated Disorders, 12*(Suppl. 2), S29–S35.

Miller, E. R., III, Pastor-Barriuso, R., et al. (2005). Meta-analysis: High-dosage vitamin E supplementation may increase all-cause mortality. *Annals of Internal Medicine, 142*(1), 37–46.

Minett, T. S., Thomas, A., et al. (2003). What happens when donepezil is suddenly withdrawn? An open label trial in dementia with Lewy bodies and Parkinson's disease with dementia. *International Journal of Geriatric Psychiatry, 18*(11), 988–993.

Mohs, R. C., Doody, R. S., et al. (2001). A 1-year, placebo-controlled preservation of function survival study of donepezil in AD patients. *Neurology, 57*(3), 481–488.

Mohs, R. C., Knopman, D., et al. (1997). Development of cognitive instruments for use in clinical trials of antidementia drugs: Additions to the Alzheimer's Disease Assessment Scale that broaden its scope. The Alzheimer's Disease Cooperative Study. *Alzheimer Disease and Associated Disorders, 11*(Suppl. 2), S13–S21.

Moretti, R., Torre, P., et al. (2002). Rivastigmine in subcortical vascular dementia: An open 22-month study. *Journal of Neurological Sciences, 203–204,* 141–146.

Morris, M. C., Evans, D. A., et al. (2002). Dietary intake of antioxidant nutrients and the risk of incident Alzheimer disease in a biracial community study. *Journal of the American Medical Association, 287*(24), 3230–3237.

Morris, M. C., Evans, D. A., et al. (2003). Consumption of fish and n-3 fatty acids and risk of incident Alzheimer disease. *Archives of Neurology, 60*(7), 940–946.

MRC/BHF Heart Protection Study of cholesterol-lowering therapy and of antioxidant vitamin supplementation in a wide range of patients at increased risk of coronary heart disease death: Early safety and efficacy experience. (1999). *European Heart Journal, 20*(10), 725–741.

MRC/BHF Heart Protection Study of cholesterol lowering with simvastatin in 20,536 high-risk individuals: A randomised placebo-controlled trial. (2002). *Lancet, 360*(9326), 7–22.

Mulnard, R. A., Cotman, C. W., et al. (2000). Estrogen replacement therapy for treatment of mild to moderate Alzheimer disease: A randomized controlled trial. Alzheimer's Disease Cooperative Study. *Journal of the American Medical Association, 283*(8), 1007–1015.

Nelson, H. E. (1982). *National Adult Reading Test (NART): Test manual.* Windsor, UK: NFER-Nelson.

Nelson, M., Reid, C., et al. (2003). Rationale for a trial of low-dose aspirin for the primary prevention of major adverse cardiovascular events and vascular dementia in the elderly: Aspirin in Reducing Events in the Elderly (ASPREE). *Drugs and Aging, 20*(12), 897–903.

Nilsson, L. N., Bales, K. R., et al. (2001). Alpha-1-antichymotrypsin promotes beta-sheet amyloid plaque deposition in a transgenic mouse model of Alzheimer's disease. *Journal of Neuroscience, 21*(5), 1444–1451.

Oken, B. S., Storzbach, D. M., et al. (1998). The efficacy of Ginkgo biloba on cognitive function in Alzheimer disease. *Archives of Neurology, 55*(11), 1409–1415.

Olin, J., & Schneider, L. S. (2004). Galantamine for dementia due to Alzheimer's disease. *Cochrane Database of Systematic Reviews* (3): CD001747.

Orgogozo, J.-M., Rigaud, A.-S., et al. (2002). Efficacy and safety of memantine in patients with mild to moderate vascular dementia: A randomized, placebo-controlled trial (MMM 300). *Stroke, 33*(7), 1834–1839.

Oswald, W. D., & Fleischmann, U. M. (1995). *Nurnberger-Alters-Inventar (NAI)—Testmanual und Textband* [Nurnberger Age Inventory (NA) test manual and text volume]. Göttingen: Hogrefe.

Oswald, W. D., & Roth, E. (1978). Der Zahlen-Verbindungs-Test (ZVT) [The numbers–connections test]. *Verlag für Psychologie,* 1–58.

Overall, J. E., & Gorham, D. R. (1962). The Brief Psychiatric Rating Scale. *Psychological Reports, 10,* 799–812.

Overall, J. E., & Schaltenbrand, R. (1992). The SKT neuropsychological test battery. *Journal of Geriatric Psychiatry and Neurology, 5*(4), 220–227.

Pantoni, L., Rossi, R., et al. (2000). Efficacy and safety of nimodipine in subcortical vascular dementia: A subgroup analysis of the Scandinavian Multi-Infarct Dementia Trial. *Journal of Neurological Sciences, 175*(2), 124–134.

Perry, R. J., & Miller, B. L. (2001). Behavior and treatment in frontotemporal dementia. *Neurology, 56*(11 Suppl. 4), S46–S51.

Petersen, R. C., Grundman, M., et al. (2004). Donepezil and vitamin E as treatments for mild cognitive impairment. *Neurobiology of Aging, 25*(S2), 20.

Petersen, R. C., Smith, G. E., et al. (1999). Mild cognitive impairment: Clinical characterization and outcome. *Archives of Neurology, 56*(3), 303–308.

Petersen, R. C., Thomas, R. G., et al. (2005). Vitamin E and Donepezil for the treatment of mild cognitive impairment. *New England Journal of Medicine, 352*(23), 2439–2441.

Pfeffer, R. I., Kurosaki, T. T., et al. (1982). Measurement of functional activities in older adults in the community. *Journal of Gerontology, 37*(3), 323–329.

Pomara, N., Peskind, E. R., et al. (2004). Memantine monotherapy is effective and safe for the treatment of mild to moderate Alzheimer disease: A randomized controlled trial. *Neurobiology of Aging, 25*(S2), 19.

Qizilbash, N., Whitehead, A., et al. (1998). Cholinesterase inhibition for Alzheimer disease: A meta-analysis of the tacrine trials. Dementia Trialists' Collaboration. *Journal of the American Medical Association, 280*(20), 1777–1782.

Quadri, P., Fragiacomo, C., et al. (2004). Homocysteine, folate, and vitamin B-12 in mild cognitive impairment, Alzheimer disease, and vascular dementia. *American Journal of Clinical Nutrition, 80*(1), 114–122.

Rabins, P. V., Kasper, J. D., et al. (1999). Concepts and methods in the development of the ADQRL: An instrument for assessing health-related quality of life in persons with Alzheimer disease. *Journal of Mental Health and Aging, 5*, 33–48.

Rai, G. S., Shovlin, C., et al. (1991). A double-blind, placebo controlled study of Ginkgo biloba extract ("tanakan") in elderly outpatients with mild to moderate memory impairment. *Current Medical Research and Opinion, 12*(6), 350–355.

Rands, G., Orrel, M., et al. (2004). Aspirin for vascular dementia. *Cochrane Database of Systematic Reviews* (3): CD001296.

Rapp, S. R., Espeland, M. A., et al. (2003). Effect of estrogen plus progestin on global cognitive function in postmenopausal women: The Women's Health Initiative Memory Study—a randomized controlled trial. *Journal of the American Medical Association, 289*(20), 2663–2672.

Ready, R. E., Ott, B. R., et al. (2002). The Cornell–Brown Scale for Quality of Life in dementia. *Alzheimer Disease and Associated Disorders, 16*(2), 109–115.

Reines, S. A., Block, G. A., et al. (2004). Rofecoxib: No effect on Alzheimer's disease in a 1-year, randomized, blinded, controlled study. *Neurology, 62*(1), 66–71.

Reisberg, B., Borenstein, J., et al. (1987). Behavioral symptoms in Alzheimer's disease: Phenomenology and treatment. *Journal of Clinical Psychiatry, 48*(Suppl.), 9–15.

Reisberg, B., Doody, R., et al. (2003). Memantine in moderate-to-severe Alzheimer's disease. *New England Journal of Medicine, 348*(14), 1333–1341.

Reisberg, B., Ferris, S. H., et al. (1982). The Global Deterioration Scale for assessment of primary degenerative dementia. *American Journal of Psychiatry, 139*(9), 1136–1139.

Rockwood, K., Kirkland, S., et al. (2002). Use of lipid-lowering agents, indication bias, and the risk of dementia in community-dwelling elderly people. *Archives of Neurology, 59*(2), 223–227.

Rogers, J., Kirby, L. C., et al. (1993). Clinical trial of indomethacin in Alzheimer's disease. *Neurology, 43*(8), 1609–1611.

Roman, G. C., Tatemichi, T. K., et al. (1993). Vascular dementia: Diagnostic criteria for research studies. Report of the NINDS–AIREN International Workshop. *Neurology, 43*(2), 250–260.

Rosen, W. G., Mohs, R. C., et al. (1984). A new rating scale for Alzheimer's disease. *American Journal of Psychiatry*, *141*(11), 1356–1364.

Rosen, W. G., Terry, R. D., et al. (1980). Pathological verification of ischemic score in differentiation of dementias. *Annals of Neurology*, *7*(5), 486–488.

Rother, M., Erkinjuntti, T., et al. (1998). Propentofylline in the treatment of Alzheimer's disease and vascular dementia: A review of phase III trials. *Dementia and Geriatric Cognitive Disorders*, *9*(Suppl. 1), 36–43.

Sachdev, P. S., Brodaty, H., et al. (1999). Vascular dementia: Diagnosis, management and possible prevention. *Medical Journal of Australia*, *170*(2), 81–85.

Sano, M. (2002). Do dietary antioxidants prevent Alzheimer's disease? *Lancet Neurology*, *1*(6), 342.

Sano, M., Ernesto, C., et al. (1997). A controlled trial of selegiline, alpha-tocopherol, or both as treatment for Alzheimer's disease. The Alzheimer's Disease Cooperative Study. *New England Journal of Medicine*, *336*(17), 1216–1222.

Scharf, S., Mander, A., et al. (1999). A double-blind, placebo-controlled trial of diclofenac/misoprostol in Alzheimer's disease. *Neurology*, *53*(1), 197–201.

Schmitt, F. A., Ashford, W., et al. (1997). The severe impairment battery: Concurrent validity and the assessment of longitudinal change in Alzheimer's disease. The Alzheimer's Disease Cooperative Study. *Alzheimer Disease and Associated Disorders*, *11*(Suppl. 2), S51–S56.

Schneider, L. S., & Olin, J. T. (1994). Overview of clinical trials of hydergine in dementia. *Archives of Neurology*, *51*(8), 787–798.

Schneider, L. S., Olin, J. T., et al. (1997). Validity and reliability of the Alzheimer's Disease Cooperative Study—Clinical Global Impression of Change. The Alzheimer's Disease Cooperative Study. *Alzheimer Disease and Associated Disorders*, *11*(Suppl. 2), S22–S32.

Scholtyssek, H., Damerau, W., et al. (1997). Antioxidative activity of ginkgolides against superoxide in an aprotic environment. *Chemico-Biological Interactions*, *106*(3), 183–190.

Schretlen, D., Bobholz, J. H., et al. (1996). Development and psychometric properties of the Brief Test of Attention. *Clinical Neuropsychologist*, *10*, 80–89.

Schretlen, D., Brandt, J., et al. (1996). Validation of the Brief Test of Attention in patients with Huntington's disease and amnesia. *Clinical Neuropsychologist*, *10*, 90–95.

Schwartz, G. E. (1983). Development and validation of the geriatric evaluation by relatives rating instrument (GERRI). *Psychological Reports*, *53*(2), 479–488.

Seshadri, S., Beiser, A., et al. (2002). Plasma homocysteine as a risk factor for dementia and Alzheimer's disease. *New England Journal of Medicine*, *346*(7), 476–483.

Shader, R. I., Harmatz, J. S., et al. (1974). A new scale for clinical assessment in geriatric populations: Sandoz Clinical Assessment—Geriatric (SCAG). *Journal of the American Geriatrics Society*, *22*(3), 107–113.

Shader, R. I., Harmatz, J. S., et al. (1976). Sandoz Clinical Assessment—geriatric (SCAG). In w. Guy (Ed.), *ECDEU assessment manual for psychopharmacology* (pp. 568–571). Rockville, MD: National Institutes of Health, Psychopharmacology Research Branch.

Shepherd, J., Blauw, G. J., et al. (2002). Pravastatin in elderly individuals at risk of vascular disease (PROSPER): A randomised controlled trial. *Lancet*, *360*(9346), 1623–1630.

Shumaker, S. A., Legault, C., et al. (2004). Conjugated equine estrogens and incidence of probable dementia and mild cognitive impairment in postmenopausal women: Women's Health Initiative Memory Study. *Journal of the American Medical Association*, *291*(24), 2947–2958.

Shumaker, S. A., Legault, C., et al. (2003). Estrogen plus progestin and the incidence of dementia and mild cognitive impairment in postmenopausal women: The Women's Health Initiative Memory Study: A randomized controlled trial. *Journal of the American Medical Association*, *289*(20), 2651–2662.

Snowden, J. S., Neary, D., et al. (2002). Frontotemporal dementia. *British Journal of Psychiatry*, *180*, 140–143.

Solomon, P. R., Adams, F., et al. (2002). Ginkgo for memory enhancement: A randomized controlled trial. *Journal of the American Medical Association*, *288*(7), 835–840.

Sommer, B. R., Hoff, A. L., et al. (1998, March). *Folic acid supplementation in dementia: A preliminary report*. Proceedings of the 11th annual meeting of the American Association for Geriatric Psychiatry, San Diego.

Sparks, D. L., Connor, D. J., et al. (2002). HMG-CoA reductase inhibitors (statins) in the treatment of Alzheimer's disease and why it would be ill-advised to use one that crosses the blood–brain barrier. *Journal of Nutrition, Health and Aging*, 6(5), 324–331.

Spiegel, R., Brunner, C., et al. (1991). A new behavioral assessment scale for geriatric out- and in-patients: the NOSGER (Nurses' Observation Scale for Geriatric Patients). *Journal of the American Geriatrics Society*, 39(4), 339–347.

Spreen, O., & Benton, A. (1969). *Neurosensory center comprehensive examination for aphasia*. University of Victoria, Department of Psychology, Neuropsychology Laboratory, Victoria, BC.

Szatmari, S. Z., & Whitehouse, P. J. (2003). Vinpocetine for cognitive impairment and dementia. *Cochrane Database of Systematic Reviews* (1): CD003119.

Szekely, C. A., Thorne, J. E., et al. (2004). Nonsteroidal anti-inflammatory drugs for the prevention of Alzheimer's disease: a systematic review. *Neuroepidemiology*, 23(4), 159–169.

Tariot, P. N., Farlow, M. R., et al. (2004). Memantine treatment in patients with moderate to severe Alzheimer disease already receiving donepezil: A randomized controlled trial. *Journal of the American Medical Association*, 291(3), 317–324.

Teunisse, S., & Derix, M. M. (1991). [Measurement of activities of daily living in patients with dementia living at home: Development of a questionnaire]. *Tijdschrift voor Gerontologie en Geriatrie*, 22(2), 53–59.

Tuokko, H., Hadjistavropoulos, T., et al. (1992). The Clock Test: A sensitive measure to differentiate normal elderly from those with Alzheimer disease. *Journal of the American Geriatrics Society*, 40(6), 579–584.

van der Kam, P., Mol, F., et al. (1971). *Beoordelingschaal voor oudere patienten (BOP)*. Deventer, The Netherlands: Van Loghum Slaterus.

van Dongen, M. C., van Rossum, E., et al. (2000). The efficacy of ginkgo for elderly people with dementia and age-associated memory impairment: New results of a randomized clinical trial. *Journal of the American Geriatrics Society*, 48(10), 1183–1194.

van Dongen, M. C.,, van Rossum, E., et al. (2003). Ginkgo for elderly people with dementia and age-associated memory impairment: A randomized clinical trial. *Journal of Clinical Epidemiology*, 56(4), 367–376.

Visser, H., Thal, L., et al. (2003, December). *A randomized double-blind placebo controlled of Rofecoxib in patients with mild cognitive impairment*. Paper presented at the 42nd annual meeting of the American College of Neuropsychopharmacology, San Juan, Puerto Rico.

Vitaliano, P. P., Russo, J., et al. (1991). The screen for caregiver burden. *Gerontologist*, 31(1), 76–83.

Wang, P. N., Liao, S. Q., et al. (2000). Effects of estrogen on cognition, mood, and cerebral blood flow in AD: A controlled study. *Neurology*, 54(11), 2061–2066.

Wechsler, D. A. (1981). *Wechsler Adult Intelligence Scale—R—Manual*. New York: Psychological Corporation.

Wechsler, D. A. (1987). *The Wechsler Memory Scale—Revised*. New York: Psychological Corporation.

Weggen, S., Eriksen, J. L., et al. (2001). A subset of NSAIDs lower amyloidogenic Abeta42 independently of cyclooxygenase activity. *Nature*, 414(6860), 212–216.

Welsh, K., Breitner, J. C. S., et al. (1993). Detection of dementia in the elderly using telephone screening of cognitive status. *Neuropsychiatry, Neuropsychology, and Behavioral Neurology*, 6, 103–110.

Wesnes, K., Simmons, D., et al. (1987). A double blind placebo controlled trial of tanakan in the treatment of idiopathic cognitive impairment in the elderly. *Human Psychopharmacology*, 2, 159–169.

Wilcock, G., Mobius, H. J., et al. (2002). A double-blind, placebo-controlled multicentre study of memantine in mild to moderate vascular dementia (MMM500). *International Clinical Psychopharmacology*, 17(6), 297–305.

Wilkinson, D., Doody, R., et al. (2003). Donepezil in vascular dementia: A randomized, placebo-controlled study. *Neurology, 61*(4), 479–486.

Winblad, B., Engedal, K., et al. (2001). A 1-year, randomized, placebo-controlled study of donepezil in patients with mild to moderate AD. *Neurology, 57*(3), 489–495.

Winblad, B., & Poritis, N. (1999). Memantine in severe dementia: Results of the 9M-Best Study (benefit and efficacy in severely demented patients during treatment with memantine). *International Journal of Geriatric Psychiatry, 14*(2), 135–146.

Wolozin, B., Kellman, W., et al. (2000). Decreased prevalence of Alzheimer disease associated with 3-hydroxy-3-methyglutaryl coenzyme A reductase inhibitors. *Archives of Neurology, 57*(10), 1439–1443.

Wood, J. G., Rogina, B., et al. (2004). Sirtuin activators mimic caloric restriction and delay ageing in metazoans. *Nature, 430*(7000), 686–689.

Yaffe, K., Sawaya, G., et al. (1998). Estrogen therapy in postmenopausal women: Effects on cognitive function and dementia. *Journal of the American Medical Association, 279*(9), 688–695.

Zandi, P. P., Breitner, J. C., & Anthony, J. C. (2002). Is pharmacological prevention of Alzheimer's a realistic goal? *Expert Opinion on Pharmacotherapy, 3*(4), 365–380.

Zandi, P. P., Anthony, J. C., et al. (2002). Reduced incidence of AD with NSAID but not H2 receptor antagonists: the Cache County Study. *Neurology, 59*(6), 880–886.

Zandi, P. P., Anthony, J. C., et al. (2004). Reduced risk of Alzheimer disease in users of antioxidant vitamin supplements: The Cache County Study. *Archives of Neurology, 61*(1), 82–88.

Zandi, P. P., Carlson, M. C., et al. (2002). Hormone replacement therapy and incidence of Alzheimer disease in older women: The Cache County Study. *Journal of the American Medical Association, 288*(17), 2123–2129.

Index